THE PRACTICE OF

Perioperative Transesophageal Echocardiography

ESSENTIAL CASES

EDITORS

ALBERT C. PERRINO, JR., MD
Professor
Department of Anesthesiology
Yale University School of Medicine
Attending Anesthesiologist
VA Connecticut Healthcare System
New Haven, Connecticut

SCOTT T. REEVES, MD, MBA, FACC, FASE
The John E. Mahaffey, MD Professor and Chairman
Anesthesia & Perioperative Medicine
Medical University of South Carolina
Charleston, South Carolina

KATHRYN GLAS, MD, FASE, MBA
Associate Professor
Department of Anesthesiology
Emory University School of Medicine
Atlanta, Georgia

Wolters Kluwer Health | Lippincott Williams & Wilkins

Acquisitions Editor: Brian Brown
Product Manager: Nicole Dernoski
Vendor Manager: Alicia Jackson
Senior Manufacturing Manager: Ben Rivera
Marketing Manager: Angela Panetta
Cover and Interior Design: Teresa Mallon
Compositor: MPS Limited, A Macmillan Company

Wolters Kluwer Health
Two Commerce Square
2001 Market Street
Philadelphia, PA 19103

Printed in China

9 8 7 6 5 4 3 2 1

Library of Congress Cataloging-in-Publication Data

The practice of perioperative transesophageal echocardiography : essential cases/editors, Albert C. Perrino Jr., Scott T. Reeves, Kathryn Glas.

p. ; cm.

Contains focused references to the companion sections in A practical approach to transesophageal echocardiography and other sentinel publications.

Includes bibliographical references and index.

Summary: "The Practice of Perioperative Transesophageal Echocardiography provides over 100 teaching cases ranging from the most common to the most challenging. Each case is succinctly presented in an easy-to-read question-answer, self-test format comprised of three printed pages of text and echo images. Echocardiography technique, interpretation, and case management are emphasized by internationally recognized experts in the field. The cases are organized to cover the gamut of clinical challenges faced by perioperative echocardiographers, including disorders of the aorta, left ventricle, and right ventricle, valvular heart disease, congenital heart lesions, catheter and device placement, and unsuspected masses and thrombi. Case challenges related to technical issues such as image optimization and artifacts are also addressed. The versatility of TEE is represented by 2-D, 3-D, color flow and spectral Doppler, tissue Doppler imaging, and quantitative assessments of volumes, pressures, and the severity of valvular pathologies. A companion website contains the fully searchable text plus echocardiographic video clips for each case presented in the book"—Provided by publisher.

ISBN 978-1-60547-716-9 (pbk. : alk. paper) 1. Transesophageal echocardiography—Case studies. 2. Transesophageal echocardiography—Problems, exercises. I. Perrino, Albert C. II. Reeves, Scott T. III. Glas, Kathryn. IV. Practical approach to transesophageal echocardiography.

[DNLM: 1. Echocardiography, Transesophageal—methods—Case Reports. 2. Echocardiography, Transesophageal—methods—Problems and Exercises. 3. Heart Diseases—ultrasonography—Case Reports. 4. Heart Diseases—ultrasonography—Problems and Exercises. 5. Perioperative Care—Case Reports. 6. Perioperative Care—Problems and Exercises. WG 18.2]

RC683.5.T83P75 2011

616.1'207543—dc22

2010025905

DISCLAIMER

Care has been taken to confirm the accuracy of the information present and to describe generally accepted practices. However, the authors, editors, and publisher are not responsible for errors or omissions or for any consequences from application of the information in this book and make no warranty, expressed or implied, with respect to the currency, completeness, or accuracy of the contents of the publication. Application of this information in a particular situation remains the professional responsibility of the practitioner; the clinical treatments described and recommended may not be considered absolute and universal recommendations.

The authors, editors, and publisher have exerted every effort to ensure that drug selection and dosage set forth in this text are in accordance with the current recommendations and practice at the time of publication. However, in view of ongoing research, changes in government regulations, and the constant flow of information relating to drug therapy and drug reactions, the reader is urged to check the package insert for each drug for any change in indications and dosage and for added warnings and precautions. This is particularly important when the recommended agent is a new or infrequently employed drug.

Some drugs and medical devices presented in this publication have Food and Drug Administration (FDA) clearance for limited use in restricted research settings. It is the responsibility of the health care provider to ascertain the FDA status of each drug or device planned for use in their clinical practice.

To purchase additional copies of this book, call our customer service department at (800) 638-3030 or fax orders to (301) 223-2320. International customers should call (301) 223-2300.

Visit Lippincott Williams & Wilkins on the Internet: http://www.lww.com. Lippincott Williams & Wilkins customer service representatives are available from 8:30 am to 6:00 pm, EST.

CONTENTS

DEDICATION

My parents, who inspired four children.
My wife Anita and our three girls, Mary, Isabella, and Juliana, who have been my great support.
My colleagues, for making a career a joy.
ACP

My Savior, Jesus Christ, who gives me perseverance to run the race before me (Hebrews 12:1-2)
My wife, Cathy, who has been my best friend and supporter for over twenty years.
My children, Catherine, Carolyn, and Townsend, who give me great joy.
My faculty, residents and students, who always keep me on my toes.
My patients, who inspire me to do my best daily!
STR

My parents for teaching me I could do whatever I put my mind to.
My brothers and sisters, and their spouses, who provide constant love and support.
My colleagues, past and present, for helping me learn something new every day,
and my friends who remind me to make a difference.
KEG

ACKNOWLEDGMENTS

Growing from conception to completion, this casebook mirrored many of the experiences of parenting. Wise from the rearing of our first book, *A Practical Approach to Transesophageal Echocardiography*, Scott Reeves and I recognized this ambitious casebook project would benefit from more extended parenting than the two of us alone could offer. Thankfully, Kathryn Glas was just young enough and foolish enough (at the time) to be persuaded to join us in editing the book. Claude Toussignant, Douglas Shook, Livia Marica, Nikolaos Skubas, Roman Sniecinski, Stephane Lambert, and William Whitley, each of them we highly regarded for their particular expertise, were eager to see the casebook concept we presented to them published and to serve as its associate editors. The seeds of the book, the over 100 essential cases selected for publication, came from contributors representing perioperative echocardiography services spanning North America. Such a cooperative effort attests to the success of the professional organizations Society for Cardiovascular Anesthesiologists, American Society of Echocardiography, and American Society of Anesthesiologists to foster educational development in echocardiography. In particular, the efforts of Martin London and his liaison editors of Anesthesia & Analgesia's *Echo Rounds* are recognized for their leading efforts in case-based echocardiography education. Lastly, the entire Philadelphia-based team at Lippincott Williams & Wilkins and especially Nicole Dernoski, our product manager, are thanked for delivering the new book to the public.

ASSOCIATE EDITORS

A. Stephane Lambert, MD, FRCPC
Assistant Professor, Department of Anesthesia, University of Ottawa, Attending Anesthesiologist, Division of Cardiac Anesthesia, University of Ottawa Heart Institute, Ottawa, Ontario, Canada

Livia Sofia Marica, MD
Assistant Professor, Department of Anesthesia and Perioperative Medicine, Medical University of South Carolina, Charleston, South Carolina

Douglas C. Shook, MD
Clinical Instructor, Department of Anesthesiology, Brigham's and Women's Hospital, Harvard Medical School, Boston, Massachusetts

Nikolaos J. Skubas, MD, FASE
Associate Professor, Department of Anesthesiology, Weill Cornell Medical College, Director, Division of Cardiac Anesthesia, New York Hospital, Weill Cornell Medical College, New York, New York

Roman M. Sniecinski, MD
Assistant Professor, Department of Anesthesiology, Emory University School of Medicine, Associate Fellowship Director, Division of Cardiothoracic Anesthesia, Emory University Hospital, Atlanta, Georgia

Claude Tousignant, MD
Assistant Professor, Department of Anesthesia, University of Toronto, Staff, Department of Anesthesia, St. Michael's Hospital, Toronto, Ontario, Canada

William Whitley, MD
Assistant Professor, Department of Anesthesiology, Division of Cardiothoracic Anesthesia, Emory University School of Medicine, Atlanta, Georgia

CONTRIBUTORS

James H. Abernathy III, MD, MPH, FASE
Assistant Professor, Chief, Division of Cardiothoracic Anesthesiology, Medical University of South Carolina, Charleston, South Carolina

Sherif Assaad, MD
Assistant Professor, Department of Anesthesiology, Yale University, New Haven, Connecticut, Attending Anesthesiologist, Department of Anesthesiology, VA Connecticut Healthcare System, West Haven, Connecticut

Edwin G. Avery IV, MD, CPI
Assistant Professor of Anesthesia, Department of Anesthesiology, Harvard Medical School, Assistant Anesthetist, Department of Anesthesia and Critical Care, Massachusetts General Hospital, Boston, Massachusetts

Marc S. Azran, MD
Assistant Professor of Anesthesiology, Cardiothoracic Anesthesiologist, Department of Anesthesiology, Emory University School of Medicine, Atlanta, Georgia

Daniel Bainbridge, MD, FRCPC
Associate Professor, Department of Anesthesiology and Perioperative Medicine, University of Western Ontario, London Health Sciences Centre, London, Ontario, Canada

Daljit K. Birdee, MD
Clinical Fellow, Department of Anesthesiology, Brigham's and Women's Hospital, Harvard Medical School, Boston, Massachusetts

Rebecca Cain, MD
Director of Cardiothoracic Anesthesia, Department of Anesthesiology, Wesley Medical College, Hattiesburg, Mississippi

Robert J.B. Chen, MD, FRCPC
Assistant Professor, Department of Anaesthesia, University of Toronto, Anaesthetist and Intensivist, Department of Anaesthesia and Critical Care, St. Michael's Hospital, Toronto, Canada

Sean J. Dickie, MD, FRCPC
Assistant Professor, Department of Anesthesiology, University of Ottawa, Anesthesiologist, Department of Cardiac Anesthesiology, University of Ottawa Heart Institute, Ottawa, Ontario, Canada

Richard E. Fagley, MD
Assistant Professor, Department of Anesthesiology, Washington University, Saint Louis, Missouri

Jason B. Falterman, MD
Staff Anesthesiologist, Department of Anesthesiology, Division of Cardiothoracic Anesthesiology, Ochsner Health System, New Orleans, Louisiana

Alan C. Finley, MD
Assistant Professor, Department of Anesthesia and Perioperative Medicine, Medical University of South Carolina, Charleston, South Carolina

Sean Garvin, MD
Assistant Professor, Department of Anesthesiology, Weill Cornell Medical College, Assistant Attending, Department of Anesthesiology, New York Presbyterian Hospital, New York, New York

Kathryn Glas, MD, FASE, MBA
Associate Professor, Department of Anesthesiology, Emory University School of Medicine, Atlanta, Georgia

Jason Greenberg, MD
Clinical Fellow, Department of Anesthesiology, Brigham's and Women's Hospital, Harvard Medical School, Boston, Massachusetts

Wendy Gross, MD
Clinical Instructor, Department of Anesthesiology, Brigham's and Women's Hospital, Harvard Medical School, Boston, Massachusetts

George J. Guldan III, MD
Assistant Professor, Department of Anesthesia and Perioperative Medicine, Medical University of South Carolina, Charleston, South Carolina

Jane E. Heggie, MD, FRCPC
Assistant Professor, Department of Anesthesia, University of Toronto, Anesthesiologist, Department of Anesthesia, Toronto General Hospital, University Health Network, Toronto, Ontario, Canada

Mark S. Hynes, MD, FRCPC
Division of Cardiac Anesthesiology, University of Ottawa Heart Institute, Ottawa, Ontario, Canada

Marjan Jariani, MD, FRCPC
Assistant Professor, Department of Anesthesia and Pain Management, University of Toronto, Toronto, Ontario, Canada

Angela Jerath, MD, FANZCA
Clinical Fellow, Department of Anesthesia and Pain Management, University of Toronto, Toronto, Ontario, Canada

Mandisa-Maia Jones-Haywood, MD
Cardiothoracic Anesthesia Fellow, Department of Cardiothoracic Anesthesia, Emory University, Emory University Hospital, Atlanta, Georgia

Paul Kapnoudhis, MD, FRCP(C)
Associate Professor, Department of Anesthesia, University of British Columbia, Member, Department of Anesthesia, Vancouver General Hospital, Vancouver, British Columbia, Canada

Matthew A. Klopman, MD
Chief Fellow, Cardiothoracic Anesthesiology, Department of Anesthesiology, Emory University School of Medicine, Atlanta, Georgia

A. Stephane Lambert, MD, FRCPC
Assistant Professor, Department of Anesthesia, University of Ottawa, Attending Anesthesiologist, Division of Cardiac Anesthesia, University of Ottawa Heart Institute, Ottawa, Ontario, Canada

Jean-Sebastien Lebon, MD, FRCPC, Bpharm
Assistant Professor, Department of Anesthesiology, University of Montreal, Montreal Heart Institute, Montreal, Quebec, Canada

Adam D. Lichtman, MD
Associate Professor of Clinical Anesthesiology, Department of Anesthesiology, Weill Cornell Medical College, Associate Attending Anesthesiologist, Department of Anesthesiology, New York Presbyterian Hospital, New York, New York

Evan T. Lukow, DO
Fellow in Cardiothoracic Anesthesia, Department of Anesthesiology and Perioperative Medicine, Medical University of South Carolina, Charleston, South Carolina

Livia Sofia Marica, MD
Assistant Professor, Department of Anesthesia and Perioperative Medicine, Medical University of South Carolina, Charleston, South Carolina

Wanda C. Miller-Hance, MD
Professor, Departments of Pediatrics (Anesthesiology & Cardiology) and Anesthesiology, Baylor College of Medicine, Attending Physician, Departments of Anesthesiology and Pediatrics (Cardiology), Texas Children's Hospital, Houston, Texas

Michele Mondino, MD
Clinical Fellow, Department of Anesthesia and Pain Management, University of Toronto, Toronto, Ontario, Canada

Fani Nhuch, MD
Clinical Fellow, Department of Anesthesiology, Brigham's and Women's Hospital, Harvard Medical School, Boston, Massachusetts

Donna Nicholson, MD, FRCPC
Assistant Professor, University of Ottawa Heart Institute, Ottawa, Ontario, Canada

Alina Nicoara, MD
Assistant Professor, Department of Anesthesiology, Yale University School of Medicine, New Haven, Connecticut, Attending, Department of Anesthesiology, West Haven VA Hospital, West Haven, Connecticut

Martina Nowak-Machen, MD
Clinical Fellow, Department of Anesthesiology, Brigham's and Women's Hospital, Harvard Medical School, Boston, Massachusetts

Charles Nyman, MBBCh
Clinical Fellow, Department of Anesthesiology, Brigham's and Women's Hospital, Harvard Medical School, Boston, Massachusetts

Albert C. Perrino Jr, MD
Professor, Department of Anesthesiology, Yale University School of Medicine, Attending Anesthesiologist, VA Connecticut Healthcare System, New Haven, Connecticut

Tjorvi Perry, MD
Department of Anesthesiology, Perioperative and Pain Medicine, Brigham and Women's Hospital, Harvard Medical School, Boston, Massachusetts

Scott T. Reeves, MD, MBA, FACC, FASE
The John E. Mahaffey, MD Professor and Chairman, Anesthesia & Perioperative Medicine, Medical University of South Carolina, Charleston, South Carolina

Daryl L. Reust, MD
Instructor, Department of Anesthesia and Perioperative Medicine, Medical University of South Carolina, Charleston, South Carolina

Antoine G. Rochon, MD, FRCPC
Assistant Professor, Department of Anesthesiology, Université de Montréal, Director, Perioperative Echocardiography, Director, Cardiac Anesthesiology Fellowship, Montreal Heart Institute, Montreal, Quebec, Canada

Kathryn Rouine-Rapp, MD
Professor of Clinical Anesthesia and Perioperative Care, University of California, San Francisco, San Francisco, California

Isobel A. Russell, MD, PhD, FACC
Professor, Department of Anesthesia, University of California, San Francisco, Chief, Department of Anesthesia, School of Medicine, San Francisco, California

Benjamin Michael Sherman, MD
Assistant Professor, Department of Anesthesiology, Yale University School of Medicine, New Haven, Connecticut, Attending, Department of Anesthesiology, West Haven VA Hospital, West Haven, Connecticut

Douglas C. Shook, MD
Clinical Instructor, Department of Anesthesiology, Brigham's and Women's Hospital, Harvard Medical School, Boston, Massachusetts

Nikolaos J. Skubas, MD, FASE
Associate Professor, Department of Anesthesiology, Weill Cornell Medical College, Director, Division of Cardiac Anesthesia, New York Hospital, WCMC, New York, New York

Roman M. Sniecinski, MD
Assistant Professor, Department of Anesthesiology, Emory University School of Medicine, Associate Fellowship Director, Division of Cardiothoracic Anesthesia, Emory University Hospital, Atlanta, Georgia

Benjamin Sohmer, MD, FRCPC
Assistant Professor, University of Ottawa Heart Institute, Department of Cardiac Anesthesiology, Ottawa, Ontario, Canada

Scott C. Streckenbach, MD
Lecturer in Anesthesia, Department of Anesthesiology, Harvard Medical School, Assistant Anesthetist, Department of Anesthesia and Critical Care, Massachusetts General Hospital, Boston, Massachusetts

Kenichi Tanaka, MD, MSc
Associate Professor, Department of Anesthesiology, Emory University, Attending Anesthesiologist, Department of Anesthesiology, Emory University Hospital, Atlanta, Georgia

Claude Tousignant, MD
Assistant Professor, Department of Anesthesia, University of Toronto, Staff, Department of Anesthesia, St. Michael's Hospital, Toronto, Ontario, Canada

Annette Vegas, MD, FRCPC
Associate Professor, Department of Anesthesiology, University of Toronto, Staff Anesthesiologist, Department of Anesthesiology, Toronto General Hospital, Toronto, Ontario, Canada

Michael H. Wall, MD, FCCM
Associate Professor of Anesthesiology and Cardiothoracic Surgery, Department of Anesthesiology, Washington University School of Medicine, Clinical Chief of Anesthesiology at Barnes-Jewish Hospital, Department of Anesthesiology, Barnes-Jewish Hospital, St. Louis, Missouri

Marcin Wasowicz, MD
Assistant Professor, Department of Anesthesia and Pain Management, University of Toronto, Toronto, Ontario, Canada

William Whitley, MD
Assistant Professor, Department of Anesthesiology, Division of Cardiothoracic Anesthesia, Emory University School of Medicine, Atlanta, Georgia

Troy S. Wildes, MD
Assistant Professor, Department of Anesthesiology, Washington University School of Medicine, St. Louis, Missouri

Adrienne P. Williams, MD
Assistant Professor, Department of Anesthesiology, Dartmouth Medical School, Dartmouth Medical Center, Lebanon, New Hampshire

PREFACE

We are frequently approached by trainees and established practitioners inquiring "How can I become proficient at perioperative TEE"? Certainly, gaining expertise in the field requires an understanding of the principles of echocardiography and the pathophysiology and management of heart disease. In addition, clinical experience with the essential challenges encountered in perioperative TEE is a must. The National Board of Echocardiography (NBE), as part of the certification process, has established criteria for clinical caseload in echocardiography attesting to the importance of case-based learning. *The Practice of Transesophageal Echocardiography*, a companion to the very successful second edition of *A Practical Approach to Transesophageal Echocardiography*, has been developed to address the need for case-based education in perioperative echocardiography.

In distinction from textbooks and atlases on the subject, *The Practice of Transesophageal Echocardiography* is best described as a clinical casebook. The editors began this project by defining over 100 cases that were felt to be essential to an echocardiographer's training experience. Collectively, these cases represent the foundation for a clinical fellowship in perioperative TEE presented in a highly educational Q&A multimedia format.

The Practice of Transesophageal Echocardiography guides the reader through a series of case presentations covering a wide spectrum of clinical practice. Each case has been condensed to its essence resulting in an easily readable and surprisingly modestly sized casebook. The reader is guided through the physics, principles, and applications of two- and three-dimensional imaging and Doppler modalities for assessing acquired and congenital heart disease in addition to major aortic pathology, ventricular performance, and valve procedures.

To assist the reader the casebook is laid out in a ski resort format with green trails marking the easier material, blue trails for intermediate, and black trails for advanced challenges. Focused references to the companion sections in *A Practical Approach to Transesophageal Echocardiography* and other sentinel publications provide a basis for consolidating understanding of case management.

This casebook offers the reader an insider's view of the echocardiography and case management of renowned experts in the field. It is our hope that readers find these essential cases valuable to accelerate or refresh their clinical training.

Albert C. Perrino, Jr.
Scott T. Reeves
Kathryn E. Glas

ABBREVIATIONS

2D	Two Dimensional
3D	Three Dimensional
ACC	American College of Cardiology
AFib	Atrial Fibrillation
AHA	American Heart Association
AI	Aortic Insufficiency
AL	Anterior Lateral
AS	Aortic Stenosis
ASD	Atrial Septal Defect
AV	Aortic Valve
AVA	Aortic Valve Area
AVR	Aortic Valve Replacement
BSA	Body Surface Area
CABG	Coronary Artery Bypass Graft
CFD	Color Flow Doppler
CHF	Congestive Heart Failure
COPD	Chronic Obstructive Pulmonary Disease
CPB	Cardiopulmonary Bypass
CS	Coronary Sinus
CSept	Coaptation to Septal
CT	Computed Tomography
CVP	Central Venous Pressure
CW	Continuous Wave
Deep TG LAX	Deep Transgastric Long Axis
Desc Ao LAX	Descending Aorta Long Axis
Desc Ao SAX	Descending Aorta Short Axis
DTI	Doppler Tissue Imaging
E	Early
ECG	Electrocardiogram
EDT	Early Deceleration Time
EF	Ejection Fraction
EOA	Effective Orifice Area
ERO	Effective Regurgitant Orifice
EROA	Estimated Regurgitant Orifice Area
FAC	Fractional Area Change
HOCM	Hypertrophic Obstructive Cardiomyopathy
IABP	Intra-Aortic Balloon Pump
ICU	Intensive Care Unit
IVC	Inferior Vena Cava
LA	Left Atrial
LAA	Left Atrial Appendage
LAD	Left anterior descending coronary artery
LAX	Long Axis View
LUPV	Left Upper Pulmonary Vein
LV	Left Ventricle
LVAD	Left Ventricular Assist Device
LVEF	Left Ventricular Ejection Fraction
LVH	Left Ventricular Hypertrophy
LVOT	Left Ventricular Outflow Tract
MAC	Mitral Annular Calcification
ME	Midesophageal
ME 2CH	Midesophageal Two Chamber
ME 4CH	Midesophageal Four Chamber
ME Asc Ao SAX	Midesophageal Ascending Aorta Short Axis
ME Asc Ao LAX	Midesophageal Ascending Aorta Long Axis
ME AV LAX	Midesophageal Aortic Valve Long Axis
ME AV SAX	Midesophageal Aortic Valve Short Axis
ME RV inflow outflow	Midesophageal Right Ventricle inflow-outflow
MR	Mitral Regurgitation
MRI	Magnetic Resonance Imaging
MV	Mitral Valve
OR	Operating Room
PA	Pulmonary Artery
PCWP	Pulmonary Artery Capillary Wedge Pressure
PDA	Patent Ductus Arteriosus
PFO	Patent Foramen Ovale
PHT	Pressure Half Time
PISA	Proximal Isovelocity Surface Area
PM	Posterior Medial
PRF	Pulsed Repetition Frequency
PVF	Pulmonary Venous Flow
PW	Pulsed Wave
RA	Right Atrium
RBBB	Right Bundle Branch Block
RCA	Right Coronary Artery
RIJ	Right Internal Jugular
RV	Right Ventricle
RVOT	Right Ventricular Outflow Track
RWMA	Regional Wall Motion Abnormalities
SAM	Systolic Anterior Motion
SV	Stroke Volume
SVC	Superior Vena Cava
TEE	Transesophageal Echocardiography
TG	Transgastric
TG LAX	Transgastric Long Axis
TG SAX	Transgastric Short Axis
TMF	Transmitral Flow
TR	Tricuspid Regurgitation
TTE	Transthoracic Echocardiogram
TV	Tricuspid Valve
UE Aortic Arch LAX	Upper Esophageal Aortic Arch Long Axis
UE Aortic Arch SAX	Upper Esophageal Aortic Arch Short Axis
V/Q	Ventilation/Perfusion
VSD	Ventricular Septal Defect
VTI	Velocity-Time Integral

Basic

CASE 1

A 65-year-old male undergoes a MV replacement for mitral stenosis, resulting from rheumatic fever. Immediately following separation from CPB, you obtain the images shown in Figures 1.1 and 1.2.

QUESTION 1.1. The echocardiogram is most consistent with the following diagnosis:

A. A normally functioning mechanical bileaflet prosthesis
B. A mechanical bileaflet prosthesis with an immobile leaflet
C. A mechanical bileaflet prosthesis with a paravalvular leak
D. A normally functioning single tilting disc prosthesis

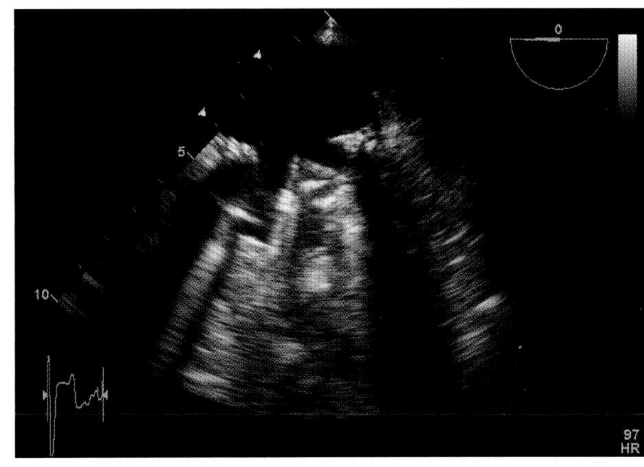

Figure 1.1. ME 4 CH view, 2D, focusing on the MV. See also Video 1.1.

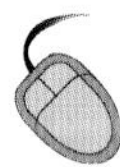

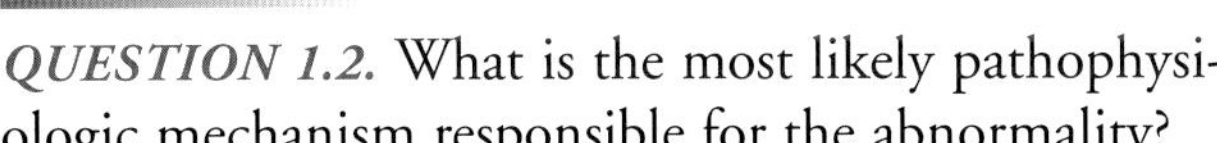

QUESTION 1.2. What is the most likely pathophysiologic mechanism responsible for the abnormality?

A. Acute thrombosis of the valve
B. Acute pannus formation
C. The prosthetic valve was inserted upside down
D. None of the above

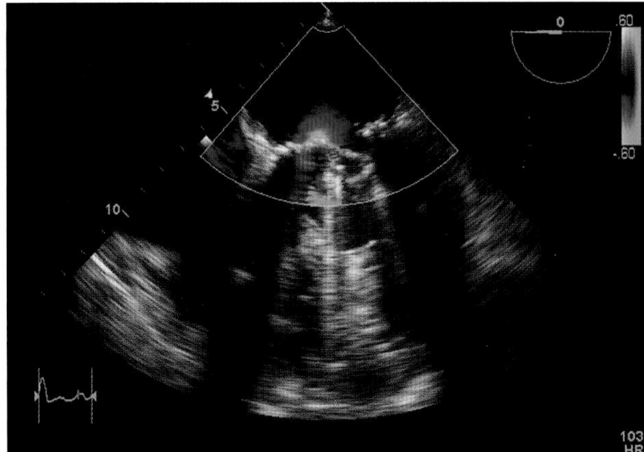

Figure 1.2. ME 4 CH view, CFD, focusing on the MV. See also Video 1.2.

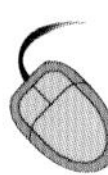

QUESTION 1.3. What is the hemodynamic effect demonstrated in Figure 1.3?

A. It is hemodynamically insignificant
B. Mild mitral stenosis
C. Moderate to severe mitral stenosis
D. Moderate MR

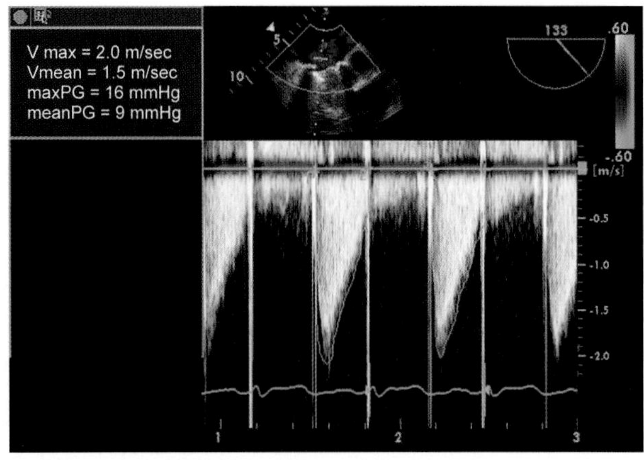

Figure 1.3. CW Doppler of the MV, ME 4 CH view.

QUESTION 1.4. Based on the images in Figures 1.1 and 1.2, and Videos 1.1 and 1.2, what is the orientation of the mechanical MV?

A. Anatomic
B. Antianatomic
C. Pseudoanatomic
D. Para-anatomic

QUESTION 1.5. What is the appropriate course of action, given the above information?

A. Give protamine; this is a normal, well-functioning mechanical valve
B. Return to CPB and rotate the valve
C. Return to CPB and replace the valve with a bioprosthesis
D. Return to bypass, remove the valve, and resect all the chordae tendineae

The surgeon agrees with you that the prosthesis appears to be malfunctioning and returns to CPB. He finds a piece of calcified chordae trapped in one of the prosthetic leaflets, causing it to malfunction. He rotates the valve within its sewing ring and closes the LA. Following separation from bypass, you obtain the images shown in Figures 1.4 to 1.6.

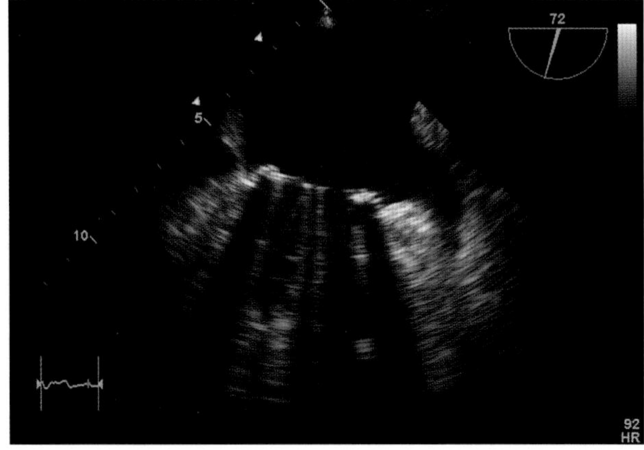

Figure 1.4. ME commissural view of the MV. See also Video 1.3.

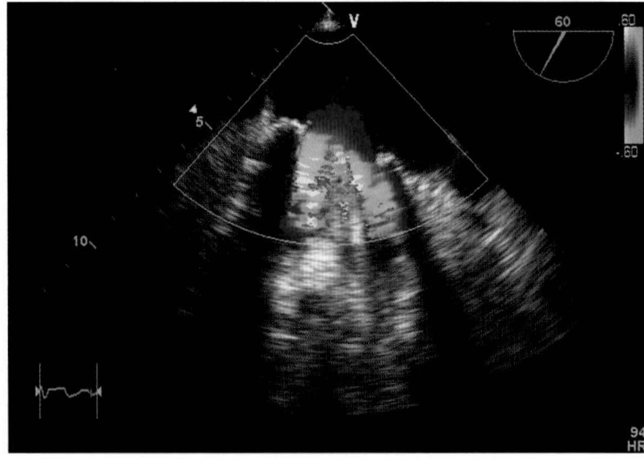

Figure 1.5. ME commissural view of the MV, CFD. See also Video 1.4.

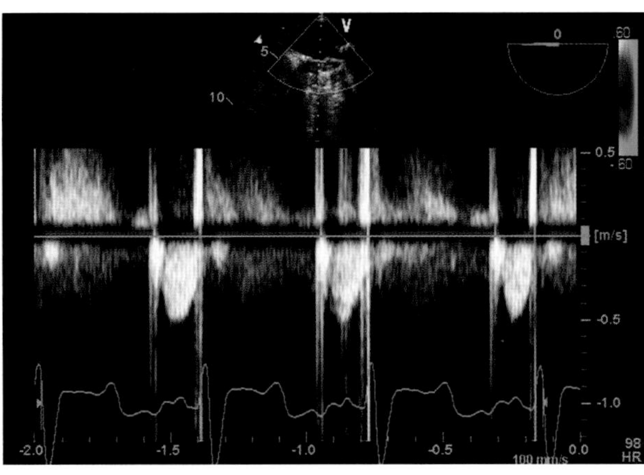

Figure 1.6. CW Doppler of the MV.

QUESTION 1.6. Based on Figures 1.4 to 1.6, what is the best course of action?

A. Give the protamine; this is a successful operation
B. Return to CPB for further adjustment of the valve
C. Return to CPB and replace the valve with a bioprosthesis
D. None of the above

ANSWERS AND DISCUSSION

QUESTION 1.1: The correct answer is B: A mechanical bileaflet prosthesis with an immobile leaflet. The patient has a mechanical bileaflet prosthesis in the mitral position. MV prostheses are reviewed in Ref. 1. This type of prosthesis has become by far the most commonly used mechanical prosthesis, due to its low profile and its favorable flow characteristics. The movement of the leaflets in this type of prosthesis goes from about 30 to 35 degrees, when fully closed, to about 85 degrees in the fully open position. On Figure 1.1 and Video 1.1, one can clearly see that the valve has *two* leaflets (thus answer D is incorrect) but *only one* of the two leaflets (the one most medial) is moving. Sometimes, when the cardiac output is very low, there can be asynchronous opening of the two leaflets (a state referred to as a "lazy" leaflet) but here one of the leaflets clearly fails to open. Figure 1.2 and Video 1.2 also show CFD going down one orifice but not the other. Moreover, one can see a zone of flow convergence (PISA) on the atrial side of the valve, suggestive of restricted diastolic flow. Answer A is incorrect: this is not a normal valve. Answer C is also incorrect: small intravalvular wash jets can be seen but there is no paravalvular leak.

QUESTION 1.2: The correct answer is D: None of the above. Prosthetic heart valves are high-tech pieces of equipment and intrinsic failure of a valve coming "out of the box" is exceedingly rare. The surgeon also inspects the leaflets carefully before implanting the valve to minimize this possibility. By far the most common cause of a prosthetic valve not opening immediately after implantation is a *physical restriction* to opening, usually due to a piece of the subvalvular apparatus. Recent trends have seen surgeons resect a minimum amount of native MV (just enough to seat the prosthesis), in an effort not to distort ventricular geometry. This can result in residual valve tissue (sometimes calcified) that can interfere with prosthetic function. Answer A is incorrect: the malfunction occurs immediately post bypass when the patient is still fully anticoagulated, making thrombosis unlikely. Likewise, answer B is incorrect, since a pannus takes much longer time to develop. Finally, while not unheard of, valves implanted *upside down* would fail to open completely, leading to severe heart failure and inability to wean from CPB. Valve inversion should be recognized on echo *before* separation from bypass is even attempted!

QUESTION 1.3: The correct answer is C: Moderate to severe mitral stenosis. Transmitral gradients are dependent on cardiac output and loading conditions and can be unreliable in the immediate postbypass period. Still they provide a rough estimate of the degree of obstruction of a mitral prosthesis. On Figure 1.3, the peak and mean gradients across the valve are 16 and 9 mm Hg, respectively, corresponding to moderate to severe mitral stenosis. Combined with the aliasing flow of the color Doppler image (Fig. 1.2 and Video 1.2), this suggests a significant degree of flow restriction that should be closely investigated. Answers A and B are incorrect, since this is a significant problem. Answer D is also incorrect: as previously described, there is no abnormal regurgitation through this valve.

QUESTION 1.4: The correct answer is A: Anatomic. The terms *anatomic* and *antianatomic* refer to the orientation of the mechanical bileaflet valve. When the valve is in *anatomic* position, the hinge between the two leaflets is roughly in a *bicommissural* orientation, meaning that the two mechanical leaflets are in the same "anatomic" position as the two native mitral leaflets. *Antianatomic* refers to a position of the valve where the hinge point is roughly perpendicular to the intercommissural line (i.e. in an A2–P2 orientation). Echocardiographically, the orientation of the valve can be determined by placing the MV in the center of the echo screen and rotating the transducer until one obtains an "edge on" view of the valve (i.e. the view in Figs. 1.1 and 1.4 where the imaging plane cuts perpendicular to the valve hinge). Once that view is obtained as perfectly as possible, the angle of rotation of the transducer is noted. A 60-degree angle would be an almost perfect antianatomic position, while 150 degree would correspond to a perfect anatomic position. In this patient, the edge on view is obtained at 0 degree, which is a little off from an anatomic position. Clinically, many surgeons believe that the orientation of these low-profile valves matters little. There is some evidence in the literature that, despite the fact that the valves perform well in any position, the risk of leaflet impingement may be less in the *antianatomic* position.[2] The terms *pseudoanatomic* and *para-anatomic* have no relation to valve orientation.

QUESTION 1.5: The correct answer is B: Return to CPB and rotate the valve. This valve is not functioning properly, with evidence of at least moderate stenosis, and it must be fixed. The easiest solution is to return to CPB and *rotate* the valve within the sewing ring to change its orientation. The advantage of this approach is that it can be done without having to excise the valve and reimplant it. Answer A is obviously incorrect: leaving this valve alone is not acceptable. Answer C is also incorrect: bioprostheses come with their own set of problems and presumably the choice of a mechanical valve was made for a good reason at the onset. Finally, answer D is incorrect: it is possible that the surgeon may ultimately have to resect additional valvular and/or subvalvular tissue, but explanting the valve to resect tissue need only be done if simple rotation is insufficient, or if inspection of the prosthesis reveals a valve defect (exceedingly rare, as mentioned above).

QUESTION 1.6: The correct answer is A: Give the protamine; this is a successful operation. In Figure 1.4 and Video 1.3, one can see both leaflets moving well. Note the angle of transducer rotation on that image: 72 degrees, which is near perpendicular to the initial orientation, and corresponds to an almost perfect antianatomic position. In Figure 1.5 and Video 1.4, one can see nonaliased, laminar CFD going down both orifices of the valve and the peak velocity in Figure 1.6 is about 0.5 cm^2.

TAKE-HOME LESSON:

Recognizing and correctly identifying the cause of acute prosthetic valve dysfunction is critical to patient outcome.

REFERENCES

1. Cheung AT. Prosthetic valves. In: Perrino AC, Reeves ST, eds. *A Practical Approach to Transesophageal Echocardiography*. 2nd ed. Philadelphia: Lippincott Williams & Wilkins; 2008.
2. Laub GW, Muralidharan S, Pollock SB, et al. The experimental relationship between leaflet clearance and orientation of the St. Jude Medical valve in the mitral position. *J Thorac Cardiovasc Surg*. 1992;103(4): 638–641.

CASE 2

A 3-year-child presents to his pediatrician secondary to recurrent colds. A murmur is heard and the child is referred for further evaluation. A TEE is performed to determine whether the patient is eligible for a percutaneous closure device (Fig. 2.1 and Video 2.1).

QUESTION 2.1. What is the diagnosis?

A. Ostium secundum ASD
B. Ostium primum ASD
C. Sinus venosus ASD
D. CS ASD

QUESTION 2.2. Which structure should be closely evaluated for abnormalities in these patients?

A. TV
B. Pulmonic valve
C. AV
D. MV
E. LVOT

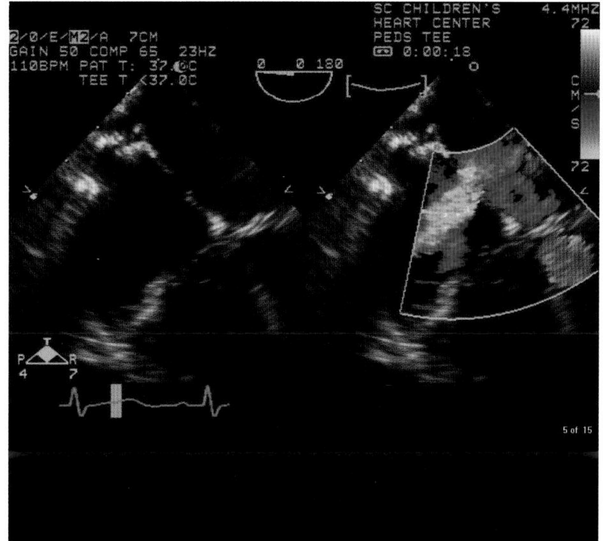

Figure 2.1.

QUESTION 2.3. When determining eligibility for a percutaneous closure device, what TEE finding is most important?

A. Size of the defect
B. Location of the defect
C. Presence of a rim
D. Presence of associated anomalies

QUESTION 2.4. If a percutaneous device is used, a postdeployment TEE examination is necessary to

A. Evaluate for proper seating of the device
B. Evaluate for residual leaks
C. Evaluate for venous in flow obstruction
D. Evaluate for AV valve impairment
E. All of the above

ANSWERS AND DISCUSSION

QUESTION 2.1: The correct answer is A: Ostium secundum ASD. Ostium secundum ASDs are located in the central portion of the interatrial septum. It is the most common ASD accounting for approximately 70% of all ASDs.

ANSWER B: Ostium primum defects accounting for 20% of ASDs are located in the inferior portion of the interatrial septum (Video 2.2).

ANSWER C: Sinus venosus defects occur adjacent to the entrance of the SVC or IVC (Videos 2.3 and 2.4). Videos demonstrate the most common location adjacent to the SVC in the ME bicaval view.

ANSWER D: CS defects result from a communication between the LA and CS and are associated with a persistent left SVC.

QUESTION 2.2: The correct answer is D: MV. While a complete TEE examination is essential to rule out coexisting pathology in all patients with congenital heart disease, associated abnormalities involving MV prolapsed and regurgitation are common in patients with an ostium secundum defect.

QUESTION 2.3: The correct answer is C: Presence of a rim. A preprocedure TEE should be performed in order to evaluate the defect to ensure that the patient is an appropriate candidate for transcatheter closure. The number, size, and location of the defect(s) can be easily determined. Transcatheter closure devices require a *rim* of tissue around the defect in order to anchor the device. This tissue around the defect or "rims" can be measured by TEE to ensure that they are adequate to allow the safe deployment of the device. A comprehensive TEE examination is necessary to evaluate other cardiac structures such as the AV and semilunar valves to ensure that the device will not impinge on their function when it is deployed. Lastly, the structure and function of the heart is examined for other defects or conditions that could be a contraindication to device placement.

QUESTION 2.4: The correct answer is D: All of the above. CFD is utilized after deployment to evaluate for the presence of residual leaks. The AV and semilunar valves are examined for evidence of the device impinging on their function. For an ASD, the pulmonary veins and vena cavae are examined to ensure that the device does not impede venous blood flow.

TAKE-HOME LESSON:

Ostium secundum ASDs are the most common form of ASDs and are located in the central portion of the interatrial septum. They are also the most amendable to percutaneous closure with an occlude device.

SUGGESTED READING

Rouine-Rapp K, Miller-Hance WC. Transesophageal echocardiography for congenital heart disease in the adult. In: Perrino A, Reeves ST, eds. *A Practical Approach to Transesophageal Echocardiography*. 2nd ed. Philadelphia: Lippincott Williams & Wilkins; 2008:372–373.

Basic

CASE 3

I f you don't know what you're looking for, you will never see it!

QUESTION 3.1. Figures 3.1 and 3.2 demonstrate high-velocity jets seen using CW Doppler in the deep TG view of the LV. What is the most likely cause of the changes seen in these two CW velocity envelopes?

A. Respiratory changes in preload filling and SV

B. Envelope A is the velocity of flow in the LVOT. Envelope B represents the velocity of flow across the AV

C. Spectral velocity envelope B represents MR

D. Doppler signal aliasing caused the change in envelope A to envelope B

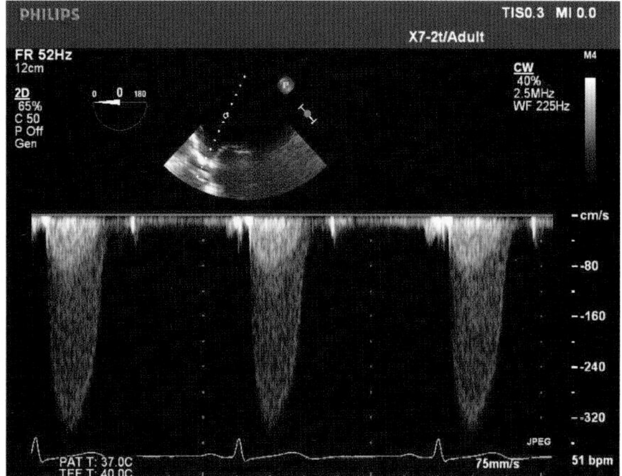

Figure 3.1. Using CW Doppler in the deep TG view, the Doppler velocity envelope A was demonstrated.

QUESTION 3.2. Of the following associated TEE findings, which would support that a Doppler velocity profile is AS and not MR?

A. LV hypertrophy

B. Systolic flow reversal in the pulmonary veins

C. LV RWMAs

D. LA dilatation

E. None of the above

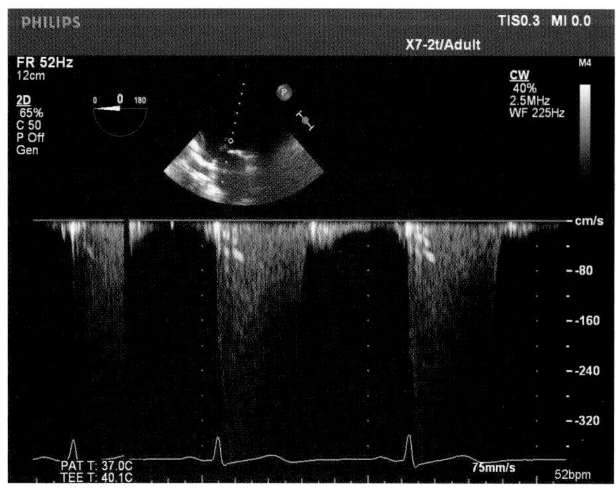

Figure 3.2. A minor adjustment in the aiming of the CW Doppler caused a significant change to the spectral Doppler velocity envelope B.

QUESTION 3.3. Of the following associated TEE findings, which indicates aortic regurgitation rather than mitral stenosis? Choose all correct answers.

A. Fluttering of the MV leaflets during diastole

B. Premature closure of the MV

C. A small LV end diastolic volume

D. Spontaneous echo contrast in left heart

ANSWERS AND DISCUSSION

QUESTION 3.1: The correct answer is C: MR. With suboptimal visualization of the anatomy, misinterpretation of the spectral Doppler flow patterns is possible. It is important to remember the CW Doppler mode lacks depth specificity. Any velocity of blood flow caught within the beam will be displayed. Confusion of MR and AS can easily happen when using Doppler interrogation in the deep TG view or TG LAX view (Fig. 3.3). Both jets are parallel with the transducer and they are immediately adjacent to one another. Both valve pathologies can achieve high velocity flow in systole due to a significant pressure gradient between the heart chambers. Figure 3.4 demonstrates the parallel alignment of the AV and MV in the deep TG view.

MR is holosystolic; AS is not. The first phase of ventricular systole is called isovolumetric contraction. Until the LV pressure exceeds the aortic pressure, there is no blood flow across the AV. This lag time from the QRS to the start of ejection is evident in velocity profile A. Velocity profile B demonstrates the holosystolic, E peaking MR jet. Envelope A is a classic late peaking, double envelope velocity profile for AS (Fig. 3.5).

ANSWER A: Answer A is incorrect. Respiratory variation is possible.

ANSWER B: Answer B is incorrect because CW Doppler lacks depth specificity; both the LVOT and AV velocities are concurrently displayed using CW Doppler in the deep TG view. The acceleration of blood within the LVOT is clearly seen interposed on the higher velocity AV in velocity A (Fig. 3.5).

ANSWER D: Answer D is incorrect. CW Doppler is not susceptible to aliasing artifact. Pulse Wave Doppler is limited by aliasing with high velocity jets and deeper structures such as the AV in the deep TG view.

A

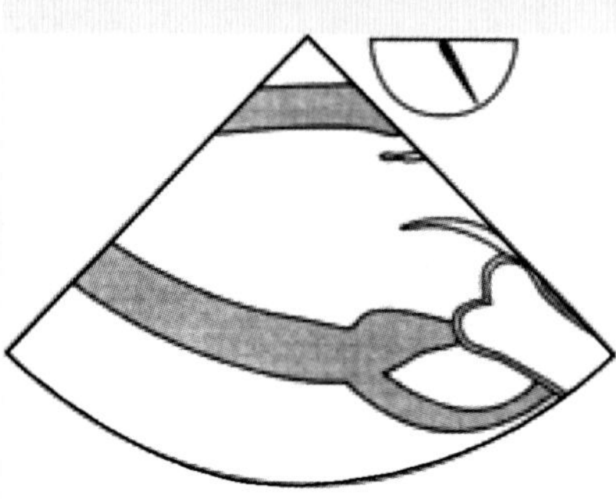

Figure 3.3. **A:** In the exam of a different patient, the TG LAX view with CW Doppler demonstrates the complex velocity profile in systole and diastole. **B:** Sketch of the TG LAX view of the AV.

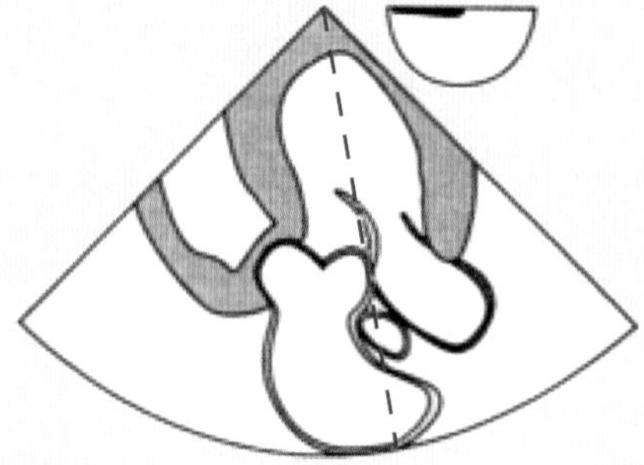

Figure 3.4. Deep TG LAX view of the LV. Note the parallel alignment of the AV and MV in this view.

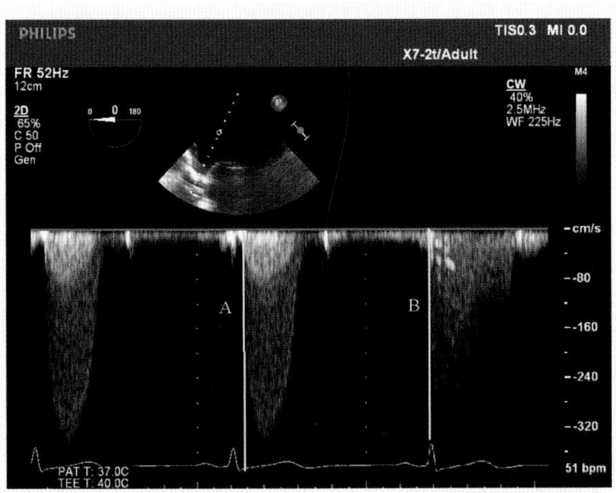

Figure 3.5. Compare the timing of flow of velocity profile. **A:** AS and velocity profile. **B:** MR.

The aliasing makes the velocity envelope difficult to interpret.

QUESTION 3.2: The correct answer is B: LV hypertrophy.

The chronic pressure overload of AS leads to concentric LV hypertrophy. MR is not a pressure overload state, but rather a volume overload state. Chronic volume overload leads to both LA and LV dilation. Systolic flow reversal in the pulmonary veins is consistent with a severe MR jet. Lastly, a LV RWMA is a nonspecific finding. Patients with both AS and MR could have myocardial ischemia leading to a RWMA.

QUESTION 3.3: The correct answers are A and B. Fluttering of the MV leaflets during diastole and premature closure of the MV.

This patient had AS with associated moderate AI. Both the deep TG and TG LAX views allow for good alignment with the AV and reasonable alignment with the MV. Unfortunately, both AI and mitral stenosis will have high velocity, diastolic flow toward the probe. To help distinguish between the two pathologies, using multiple views can be helpful. 2D grayscale and CFD can distinguish the source of flow, especially when multiple views are compared. Associated findings are also clues that can help confirm the correct diagnosis.

An aortic regurgitation jet that is directed toward the MV leaflets will lead to fluttering of the leaflets. Severe aortic regurgitation causes a rapid rise in LV diastolic pressure and premature diastolic closure of the MV. In contrast, the MV leaflets are hypomobile or immobile in advanced mitral stenosis. Fluttering is uncommon and they may appear not to open at all. A low flow state in the LA can induce low-level thrombosis and spontaneous echo contrast (occasionally referred to as SEC or smoke).

Mitral stenosis is associated with a small, chronically under-filled LV. Aortic regurgitation on the other hand is a volume overload state that leads to a high LV end diastolic volume, asymmetric LV hypertrophy, and dilatation.

When MR and AI are both present, spectral and CFD interpretation can be very challenging.

TAKE-HOME LESSON:

CW Doppler lacks depth specificity. The source of the blood flow can be difficult to discern. Timing of the flow and associated findings can be very useful in correct interpretation of the significance of Doppler velocities.

SUGGESTED READING

Perrino AC. Doppler technology and technique. In: Perrino AC, Reeves ST, eds. *A Practical Approach to Transesophageal Echocardiography*. 2nd ed. Philadelphia: Lippincott Williams & Wilkins; 2007:109–124.

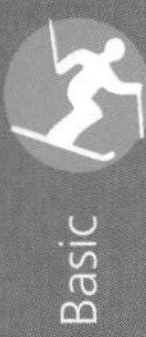

CASE 4

A 49-year-old man with a preoperative EF of 45% is undergoing a mitral and AVR for chronic insufficiency. Immediately after separation from CPB, the patient is hypotensive with a blood pressure of 82/40 mm Hg. Poor visualization of the LV inhibits assessment of the ventricular contractility and preload filling as demonstrated in Figures 4.1 and 4.2.

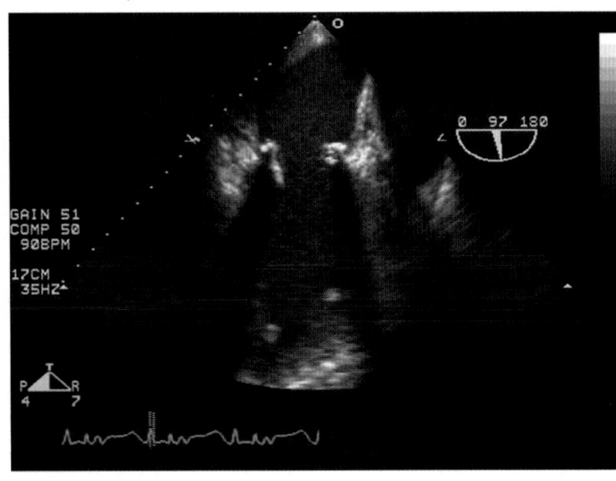

Figure 4.1.

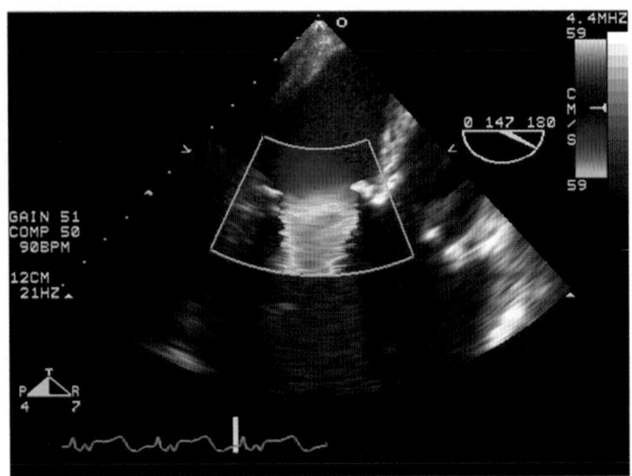

Figure 4.2.

QUESTION 4.1. What is the cause of the poor visualization of the LV?

A. The anterior and inferior walls are parallel to the probe and are poor reflectors of the signal
B. Attenuation of the ultrasound energy due to the prosthetic valves
C. Inadequate amplification of the ultrasound signals deep in sector
D. Probe malfunction of the piezoelectric crystals

QUESTION 4.2. To adequately assess the LV it is necessary to:

A. Use a lower frequency setting on the probe to improve penetration
B. Adjust the time-gain compensation to improve visualization of the deeper ventricular walls
C. Change the visual angle by adjusting the probe depth
D. Inject an ultrasound contrast to improve wall visualization

QUESTION 4.3. You are unable to assess the prosthetic valve for a paravalvular leak with CFD in the aortic position. Appropriate adjustments to interrogate the AV position include:

A. Decrease the Nyquist aliasing limit to accentuate the CFD signal
B. Change the depth of visualization and multiplane angle to see the ME short-axis view of the AV with CFD
C. Change the depth of visualization to see the deep TG view of the AV with CFD
D. Interrogate the AV with pulse wave Doppler in the deep TG view

ANSWERS AND DISCUSSION

QUESTION 4.1: The correct answer is B.

The loss of visual information is due to attenuation of ultrasound energy at the bioprosthetic valve's sewing ring and struts. This is commonly called **Acoustic Shadowing** (Figs. 4.3, 4.4). The shadowing occurs when a strongly reflective medium, such as an artificial heart valve, interrupts the transmission of the ultrasound energy into the deeper tissue structures. Since the sound energy cannot penetrate, there is a loss of information of the true anatomic structures beyond the reflective material. A hypoechoic or anechoic region occurs and is vis-ualized as the same color as a fluid-filled structure or the background. Shadowing commonly occurs with highly calcified tissue, artificial materials such as the plastic or metal, and, ironically, air. The reflectivity of a material or tissue is dependent on the change in impedance as a sound wave moves from one transmission medium to another. The change in acoustic impedance from blood to air is significant enough that nearly total reflection of the ultrasound beam occurs with shadowing deep to the air pocket.

Answer A is incorrect. Although there can be a hypoechoic area due to parallel tissues, this is clearly attenuation due to shadowing. Answer C is also incorrect: The gain seems adequate to visualize the apex of the LV that is not shadowed. Answer D is incorrect.

QUESTION 4.2: The correct answer is C.

Adjusting the angle to an aortic short axis, ME TG, or deep TG approach would allow the ultrasound energy to reach the area of interest at the aortic annulus. It is not possible to improve the LV and LV wall visualization with time-gain compensation or echo contrast, because there is no echo information for the machine to process from this region.

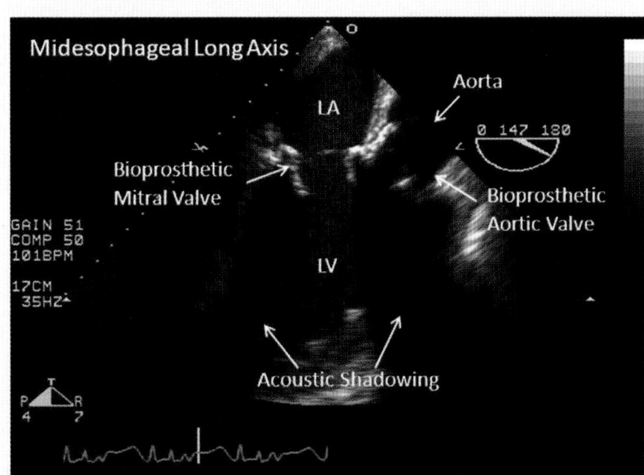

Figure 4.3.

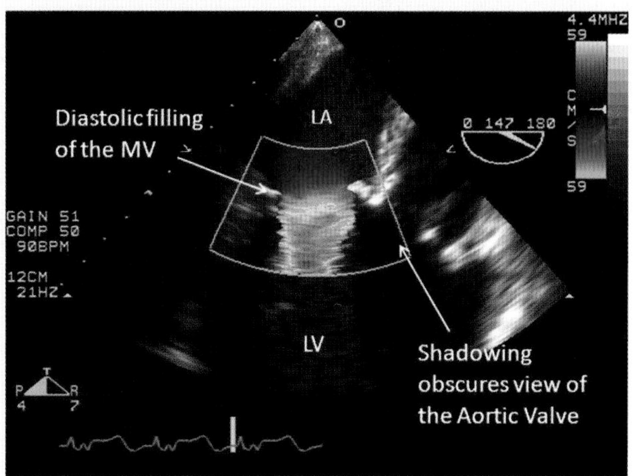

Figure 4.4.

QUESTION 4.3: The correct answers are B, C, and D. Again, there is no echo data deep to the reflector. This affects both 2D grayscale and CFD data. Adjustment of the Nyquist limit will only further obscure the true anatomy. Adjusting the angle to a TG at 120-degree rotation or deep TG approach would allow the ultrasound energy to reach the area of interest at the aortic annulus. CFD or pulse wave spectral Doppler information can be used to look for a paravalvular leak. In this patient CW Doppler potentially would be misleading. CW lacks depth specificity and would detect the acceleration of the mitral inflow in diastole.

Basic

CASE 5

Two patients present to the OR for AVR. You are asked to grade the degree of AI in each patient.

Patient 1: A 51-year-old male who presents for coronary artery bypass surgery has been reported on a preoperative TTE to have at least moderate AI. Further intraoperative clarification is required (Figs. 5.1 and 5.2).

Patient 2: A 65-year-old woman with CHF presents for AVR (Figs. 5.3 and 5.4).

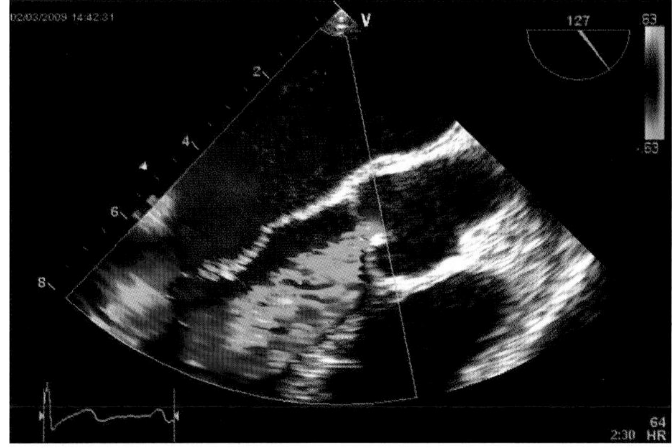

Figure 5.1. ME LAX with CFD. See also Video 5.1.

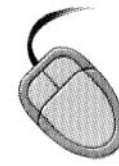

QUESTION 5.1. Which statement is correct?

A. Patients 1 and 2 both have severe AI

B. Patient 2 has severe AI

C. Patient 1 has mild AI

D. Patients 1 and 2 both have moderate AI

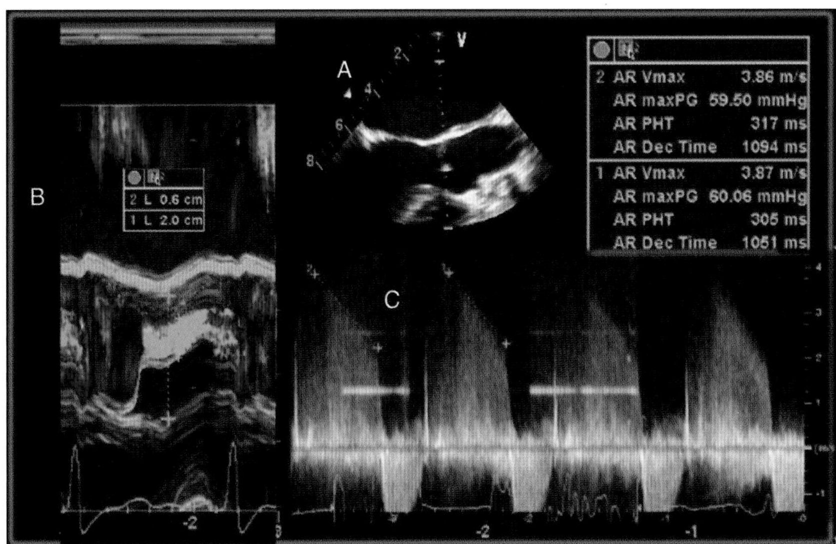

Figure 5.2. **A:** ME LAX with M-mode cursor. **B:** M-mode of AI jet. **C:** CW Doppler of AI jet via TG route.

QUESTION 5.2. Which statement is false regarding AI?

A. An AI PHT shorter than 200 msec denotes severe AI

B. The AI PHT is dependent on the orifice size but is independent of the pressure difference between the aorta and the LV

C. The PHT is the time it takes for the peak velocity to decrease by 30%

D. The larger the RV, the shorter the PHT

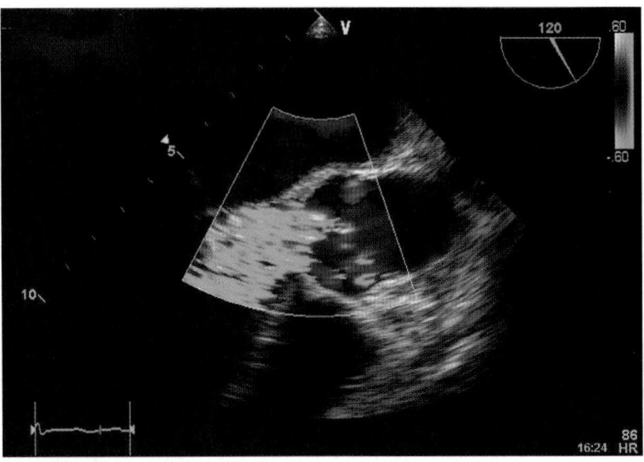

Figure 5.3. ME LAX with CFD. See also Video 5.2.

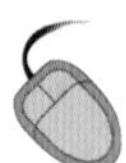

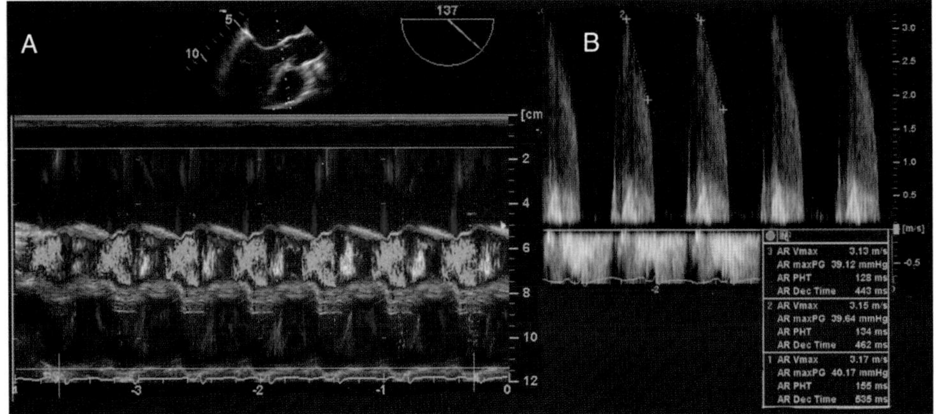

Figure 5.4. **A:** M-mode of AI jet in ME LAX with CFD. **B:** CW Doppler of AI jet using a TG approach.

QUESTION 5.3. From examining Figure 5.5, which statement(s) is/are correct?

A. The Doppler indicates severe AI

B. This image is likely taken from patient 1

C. The associated AI PHT would be >200 msec

D. Both A and C

QUESTION 5.4. On the measurement of severity of AI, which statement is correct?

A. The continuity equation using flow at the mitral and AV can yield a quantitative assessment of AI

B. The quality of the jet in CFD is independent of machine settings and is unaffected by eccentricity

C. The AI RV can be quantitated from aortic Doppler flow reversal

D. The length of the AI jet is a reliable measure of AI severity

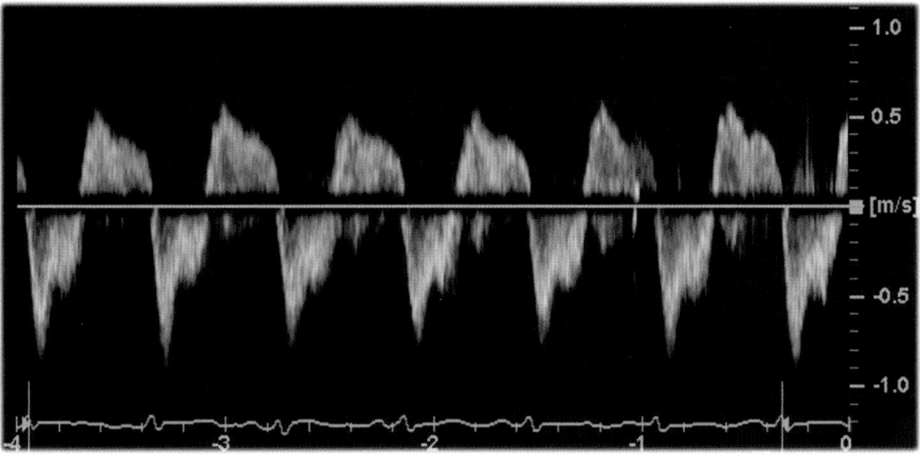

Figure 5.5. PW Doppler of the descending aorta.

ANSWERS AND DISCUSSION

QUESTION 5.1: The correct answer is B: Patient 2 has severe AI.

The severity of AI can be appreciated and graded by observing the color volume in the LVOT and LV. Although this method yields a quick estimate, it is not reliable especially in the presence of eccentric jets. The jet height to LVOT height ratio can be used to grade AI. This is measured using M-mode echocardiography on CFD mapping. The M-mode cursor is placed on the ventricular side of the AV very near the origin of the AI jet such that it transects the LVOT at a 90-degree angle. The ratio of the jet height to the LVOT size can be used to grade the AI such that a jet/LVOT ratio ≥65% denotes severe AI, a ratio <25% denotes mild AI. Continuous Doppler of the AI jet via the TG route may also be used to grade AI. The quality of the Doppler signal can be helpful; a dense envelope is suggestive of severe AI. The PHT of the AI jet (the rate of velocity decline) is helpful in grading AI. In severe AI, the pressure in the aorta will decline rapidly and therefore the AI jet will resolve quickly. A PHT <200 msec denotes severe AI, whereas a PHT >500 msec denotes mild AI (i.e., the pressure gradient between the aorta and the LV is maintained throughout diastole). In patient 1 we observed the following: a central AI jet occupying 30% of the LVOT (Fig. 5.2B) and an AI PHT of 311 msec (Fig. 5.2C). In patient 2 we observed a large AI jet occupying the entire LVOT (Fig. 5.3A) and an AI PHT of 139 msec (Fig. 5.3B).

The AI vena contracta may also be used to assess AI. It is measured as the thinnest neck of AI jet at the valve in CFD in the ME LAX. A vena contracta of 0.3 to 0.6 cm denotes moderate AI (Fig. 5.6).

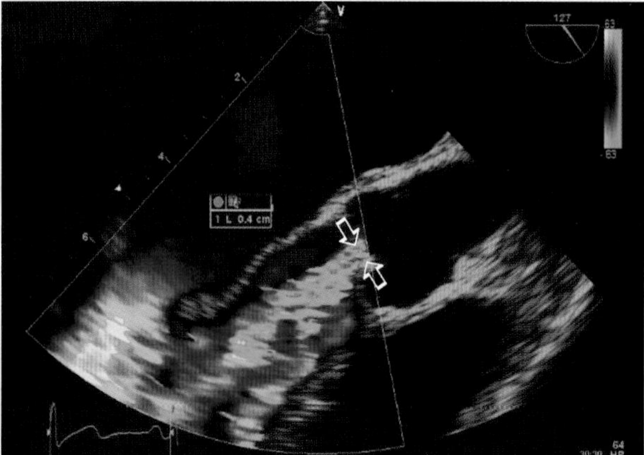

Figure 5.6. ME LAX of AI demonstrating vena contracta (*arrows*) in patient 1.

QUESTION 5.2: The correct answer is B: The AI PHT is dependent on the orifice size but independent of the pressure difference between the aorta and the LV.

The rate of velocity decline of the AI jet measured by CW Doppler is a measure of AI severity and can be expressed as the PHT. PHT depends on the size of the AV defect *and* the pressure gradient between the aorta and the LV. In mild AI where the orifice is very small, the pressure gradient between the aorta and the LV will be maintained and there will be very little velocity decline. In severe AI where the orifice is large, the pressure difference between the aorta and the LV resolves rapidly. This occurs because the LV rapidly becomes full with filling from both the MV and the incompetent AV. The brisk equalization of pressures between the LV and the aorta will result in a more rapid velocity decline through the AV (AI) and therefore a shorter PHT. Answer A is incorrect: a PHT <200 msec denotes severe AI. Answer C is incorrect: the PHT is the *time* it takes for the *pressure gradient* to decline from peak by 50%. When determining the PHT, we do not measure pressure gradients directly; we measure velocity using CW Doppler. The pressure gradient can be expressed as $4V^2$. We need to measure the time interval between peak pressure ($4V^2_{peak}$) and $½P_{peak}$ or $½(4V^2)$. As we actually measure velocities, we need to know the velocity at $½P_{peak}$.

$$P = ½P_{peak}$$
$$4V^2 = ½(4V^2_{peak})$$
$$V^2 = ½V^2_{peak}$$
$$V = \frac{V_{peak}}{\sqrt{2}}$$
$$V = \frac{V_{peak}}{1.4} \text{ or } V_{peak} \times 0.7$$

(the velocity has decreased by 30%)

Answer D is incorrect: the larger the RV, the shorter the PHT as the pressure gradient between the aorta and the LV cannot be maintained for very long.

QUESTION 5.3: The correct answer is A: The Doppler indicates severe AI.

Holodiastolic flow reversal in the descending aorta indicates severe AI. The sample volume in PW Doppler is usually placed just distal to the left subclavian artery. Patient 1 did not have severe AI. The AI PHT in this case would be <200 msec.

QUESTION 5.4: The correct answer is A: The continuity equation using flow at the mitral and AV can yield a quantitative assessment of RV.

In the grading of AI, a RV can be calculated by measuring the systolic flow (i.e., SV) across the MV and the AV. The excess volume transversing the AV when compared to the MV contains the RV. Therefore,

$$\text{Aortic RV} = \text{LVOT flow} - \text{MV flow}$$

$$\text{Aortic RV} = (\text{LVOT}_{AREA} \times \text{VTI}) - (\text{MV}_{AREA} \times \text{VTI}_{MV})$$

RVs <30 mL denote mild AI and RVs >60 mL denote severe AI. Regurgitant fractions, expressed as the ratio of the RV to the total aortic forward flow, can also be used, where an RF <30% is mild and an RF >50% is severe.

The quality of the AI color jet is extremely dependent on machine settings and can be a significant source of error in evaluating AI. Eccentric jets may become entrained along walls and lead to erroneous conclusions. The aortic flow reversal is a qualitative assessment and cannot be used to quantitate AI. Although it is dependent on the severity of AI, it is also dependent on sample location and vessel compliance. The length of the AI jet in CFD is not a reliable measure of severity of AI. It is dependent on the plane of interrogation (AI is a three-dimensional object), the machine settings and is unreliable in the setting of eccentric jets.

TAKE-HOME LESSON:

The use of CFD mapping can be misleading in the assessment of severity of AI. Other modalities such as PHT, vena contracta, and jet height to LVOT height ratio are value-added measures of AI.

SUGGESTED READING

Zoghbi WA, Enriquez-Sarano M, Foster E, et al. American Society of Echocardiography's Nomenclature and Standards Committee and the Task Force on Valvular Regurgitation. American Society of Echocardiography: recommendations for evaluation of the severity of native valvular regurgitation with two-dimensional and Doppler echocardiography. *Eur J Echocardiogr.* 2003;4:237–261.

CASE 6

A 42-year-old male with history of arterial hypertension presented with acute onset chest pain radiating to the back and was admitted to the ICU. He underwent a TEE exam, and the ME ascending aortic LAX is shown in Figure 6.1A and 6.1B.

QUESTION 6.1. What is the diagnosis?

A. Acute, type A aortic dissection

B. Mirror image (linear artifact)

C. Misplaced PA catheter

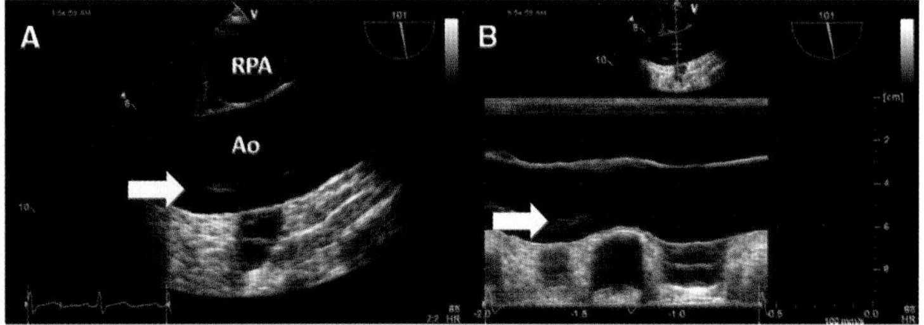

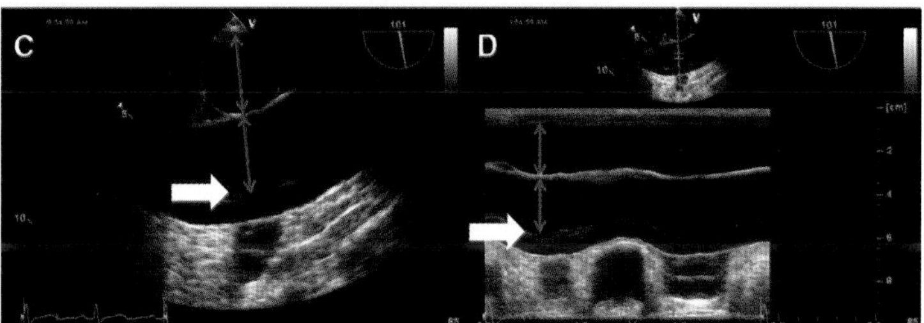

Figure 6.1. Linear artifact of ascending aorta. **A:** ME ascending aortic LAX with a linear structure (*arrow*). **B:** M-mode imaging of right pulmonary artery (RPA), aorta (Ao), and structure (*arrow*). **C:** The interface between the anterior border of RPA and the posterior border of Ao acts as a reflector. The mirror image is positioned inside the lumen of Ao because the diameter of RPA is less than the diameter of Ao. Note that the mirror image is thick (~4 mm). **D:** The mechanism of creation of the mirror image is seen with M-mode. Note that the mirror image is moving parallel to the RPA–Ao interface.

ANSWER AND DISCUSSION

QUESTION 6.1: The correct answer is B: Mirror image (linear artifact).

TEE is considered a first-line diagnostic modality to diagnose acute aortic trauma (dissection or transaction). Intraluminal imaging artifacts, however, limit the diagnostic accuracy of TEE. When ultrasound is reflected off a large surface, lying perpendicular to its transmission path, it will return to the transducer, which will function as an additional reflective surface. Consequently, the ultrasound pulse will propagate once more. This to-and-fro travel of the ultrasound (reverberation) will result in parallel images mirroring the original reflecting surface and positioned away from the transducer (Fig. 6.1C and 6.1D). This form of artifact represents a falsely perceived object, and it was noted in vitro as well as in vivo, in the ascending as well as the descending aorta. These artifacts occur in the ascending aorta when it is dilated >5 cm and is larger than the diameter of the LA, resulting in an aorta-to-atrium ratio of >0.6. Other TEE findings associated with linear artifacts in the ascending aorta are the following: (1) displacement is parallel to aortic walls; (2) location is on a straight line between the transducer and the reflector surface; (3) position is deeper than the reflector surface; (4) similar blood flow velocities are on both sides of the image; (5) angle with the aortic wall is >85 degrees; and (6) thickness is >2.5 mm. A dissection flap has distinct borders, usually displays rapid oscillatory motion, and will interrupt the CFD pattern.

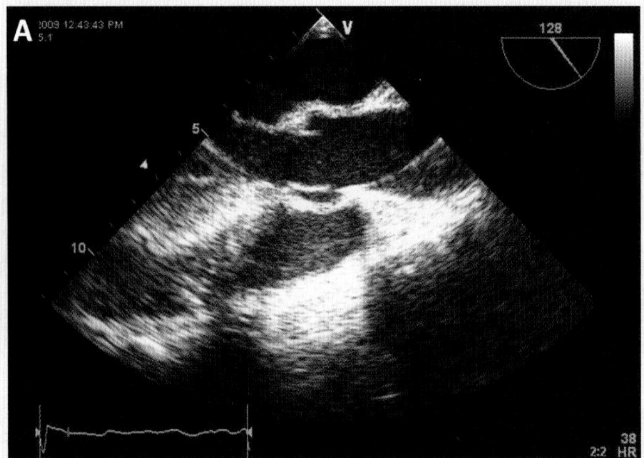

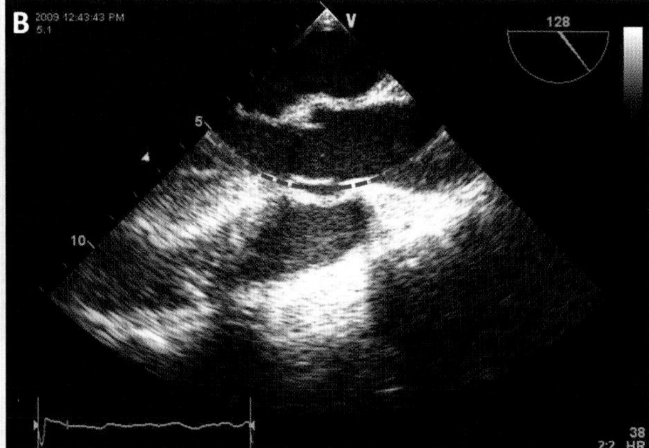

Figure 6.1 A and B demonstrates a mirror artifact within the LVOT and aortic root. The artifact is highlighted in red in Figure 6.B.

TAKE-HOME LESSON:

Ascending aorta dilation may lead to genesis of artifacts mimicking aortic pathology.

SUGGESTED READING

Appelbe AF, Walker PG, Yeoh JK, et al. Clinical significance and origin of artifacts in transesophageal echocardiography of the thoracic aorta. *J Am Coll Cardiol.* 1993;21:754–760.

Vignon P, Spencer KT, Rambaud G, et al. Differential transesophageal echocardiographic diagnosis between linear artifacts and intraluminal flap of aortic dissection or disruption. *Chest.* 2001;119:1778–1790.

CASE 7

An 83-year-old male patient is undergoing elective coronary artery revascularization. His exercise ability is remarkably good and he has NYHA (New York Heart Association) class II functional status. He has a longstanding history of moderate MR but no other valvular disease. Prior to CPB, a comprehensive TEE exam is done and the ME four- and two-chamber views of the LV are shown in Video 7.1.

QUESTION 7.1. An approximate visual estimate of this patient's global LV function is:

A. Normal ([EF] > 55%)

B. Slightly depressed (35% < EF < 55%)

C. Moderately depressed (25% < EF < 35%)

D. Severely depressed (EF < 25%)

A more detailed estimation of the LV function is shown in Figure 7.1.

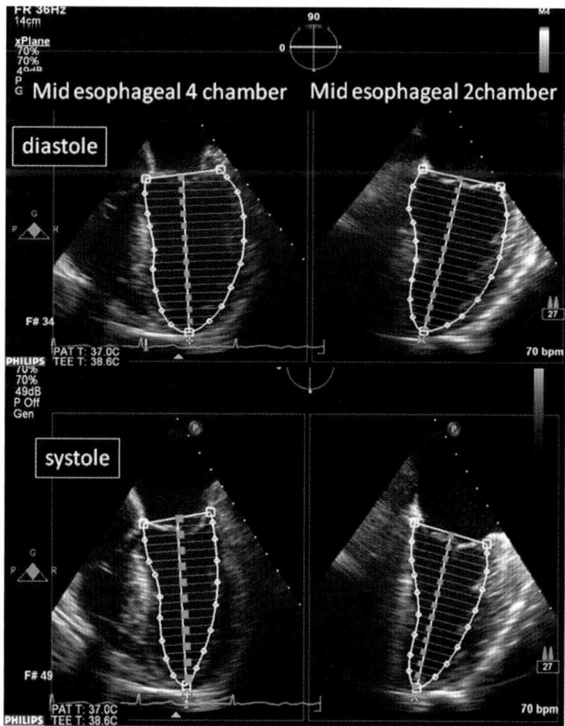

Figure 1
Mid esophageal 4 chamber
Mid esophageal 2chamber
diastole
systole
PHILIPS
PAT T: 37.0C
TEE T: 38.6C
70 bpm
4C
L = 8.69 cm
A = 35.5 cm²
Vol = 119 ml
2C
L = 8.6.5 cm
A = 34.7 cm²
Vol = 115 ml
4C
L = 8.12 cm
A = 22.3 cm²
Vol = 51 ml
2C
L = 7.71 cm
A = 22.1 cm²
Vol = 55 ml

Figure 7.1.

QUESTION 7.2. The technique shown is called:

A. %FAC
B. Method of discs (MOD)
C. Fractional shortening (%FS)
D. Wall motion score index (WMSI)

QUESTION 7.3. Using the numbers obtained in Figure 7.1, what is the SV of the LV?

A. 170 mL
B. 117 mL
C. 64 mL
D. 55 mL

Subsequently, the echocardiographer measures the LV SV using spectral Doppler. A pulsed-wave Doppler is obtained with the sample volume in the LVOT. This tracing is shown in Figure 7.2.

QUESTION 7.4. Assuming that the LVOT cross-sectional area is 2.0 cm², what is the calculated SV?

A. 20.5 mL
B. 41 mL
C. 52 mL
D. 63.5 mL

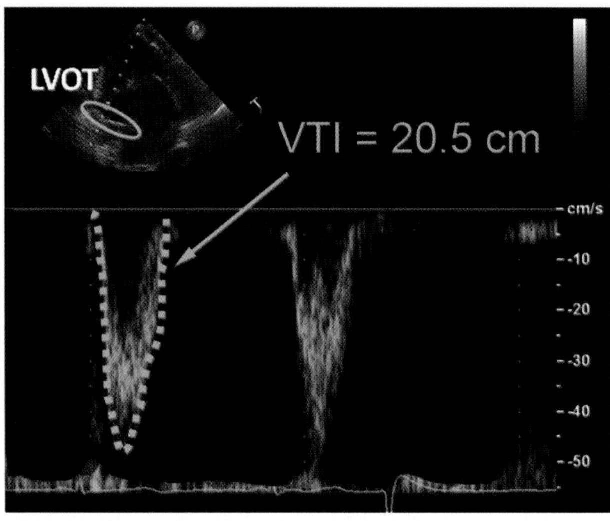

Figure 7.2.

QUESTION 7.5. There is a significant difference between the SV calculated using MOD and the SV calculated using spectral Doppler. This discrepancy is due to:

A. The presence of MR
B. The inaccuracy of the MOD
C. Spectral Doppler's overestimation of forward flow
D. There is no discrepancy; both MOD and spectral Doppler yield the same value

ANSWERS AND DISCUSSION

QUESTION 7.1: The correct answer is B. This patient has slightly depressed (35% < EF < 45%) ventricular function. Global ventricular systolic function is generally described in terms of cardiac output (i.e. SV times heart rate), or EF. Visual estimation of EF relies on determining the degree of myocardial impairment in multiple views. An experienced echocardiographer integrates things such as myocardial thickening, wall movement, and even mitral annular excursion in order to create a mental picture of overall function. Categorizing the EF as normal (>55%), mildly impaired (35%–55%), moderately impaired (25%–35%), or severely impaired (<25%) is useful when using the "eye ball" method, since exact numbers are not very reproducible. The visual estimation of EF is limited by the experience of the echocardiographer, as well as the completeness of the exam. In this particular case, for example, only the ME four- and two-chamber views were given. To view all regions of the ventricle, the ME LAX and the TG mid-SAX views would be needed as well.

QUESTION 7.2: The correct answer is B. The technique shown in Figure 7.1 is MOD. MOD is used to calculate LV volume. It requires the operator to trace the endocardial borders in both systole and diastole in two orthogonally opposite views (usually the ME four and two chambers). The software package then creates a series of discs (usually 20) that have an outer diameter defined by the traced endocardial borders, and are all centered along the long axis of the LV (an imaginary line connecting the center of the mitral annulus to the LV apex). The volume of the LV is obtained by adding the volume of all of the discs together. MOD is one technique recommended by the American Society of

Echocardiography to estimate LV volumes and calculate SV.

FAC, another method to estimate LV systolic function, is based on the relative difference between the end-diastolic and the end-systolic LV areas, measured in the TG mid-SAX view. FS is the relative difference of the end-diastolic and end-systolic diameters, measured with M-mode. WMSI is incorrect since this is a way to evaluate regional ventricular function.

QUESTION 7.3: The correct answer is C. This patient's SV is 64 mL. This is calculated by first averaging the 4C and 2C systolic volumes ([119 + 115]/2 = 117 mL), and diastolic volumes ([51 + 55]/2 = 53 mL). The SV is then the systolic volume minus the diastolic volume (117 − 53 = 64 mL).

QUESTION 7.4: The correct answer is B. The patient's SV as calculated by Doppler is 41 mL. This was obtained by using the formula, cross sectional area (CSA) multiplied by the VTI is equal to the SV. The SV is 2.0 $cm^2 \times 20.5$ cm = 41 mL.

QUESTION 7.5: The correct answer is A. The difference between the SV calculated by spectral Doppler and that calculated by MOD is due to the presence of MR. In this case, MOD SV represents the "total" LV output—both through the LVOT and into the LA. This is larger than the systemic SV (i.e. only that blood going out of the LVOT), which is calculated using spectral Doppler. Such discrepancies are utilized to calculate the RV in the presence of regurgitant lesions or the shunt volume in cases of ASDs or VSDs.

TAKE-HOME LESSON:

Global LV function can be estimated visually or quantified by calculating LV volumes and subsequent EF. The intraoperative echocardiographer should be aware of the different methods of calculation and understand their limitations.

SUGGESTED READING

Lang RM, Bierig M, Devereux RB, et al. Recommendations for chamber quantification: a report from the American Society of Echocardiography's guidelines and standards Committee and the chamber quantification writing group, developed in conjunction with the European Association of Echocardiography, a branch of the European Society of Cardiology. *J Am Soc Echocardiogr*. 2005;18:1440–1463.

Quiñones MA, Otto CM, Stoddard M, et al. Recommendations for quantification of Doppler echocardiography: a report from the Doppler quantification task force of the nomenclature and standards Committee of the American Society of Echocardiography. *J Am Soc Echocardiogr.* 2002;15:167–184.

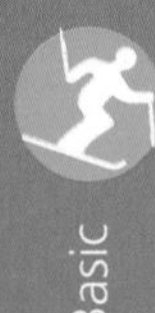

CASE 8

A 48-year-old male presented to his primary care physician with a history of progressive shortness of breath on exertion. During work-up, a TEE was obtained (Fig. 8.1).

QUESTION 8.1. What is the diagnosis?

A. Normal AV
B. Bicuspid aortic valve (BAV)
C. Endocarditis
D. Aortic dissection

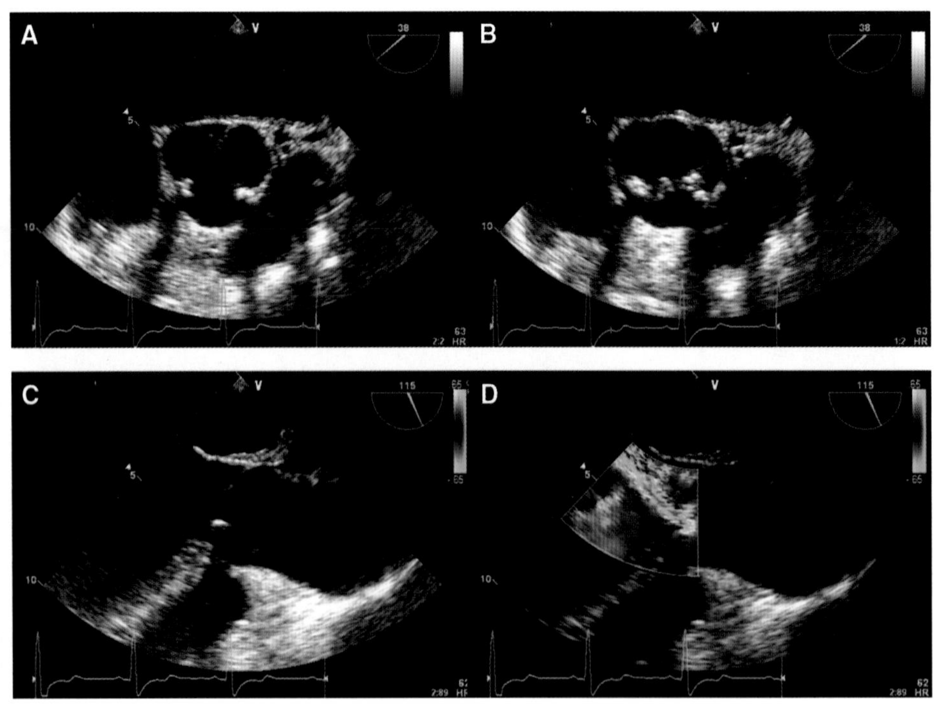

Figure 8.1. ME AV SAX views (**A, B;** Videos 8.1 and 8.2). **A:** Diastole; **(B)** systole; **Video 8.2**: With color. ME AV LAX (**C, D;** Videos 8.3 and 8.4). **C:** Diastole; **(D)** diastole with color; **Video 8.3:** with color and **Video 8.4:** without color.

QUESTION 8.2. Using Figure 8.2, if the left LVOT diameter measures 2.4 cm, what is the calculated AV area?

A. 1.84 cm^2

B. 2.55 cm^2

C. 1.74 cm^2

D. Both A and C

E. None of the above

QUESTION 8.3. What is the diagnosis?

A. Aortic regurgitation

B. Mild AS

C. HOCM

D. Subaortic stenosis

E. Both A and B

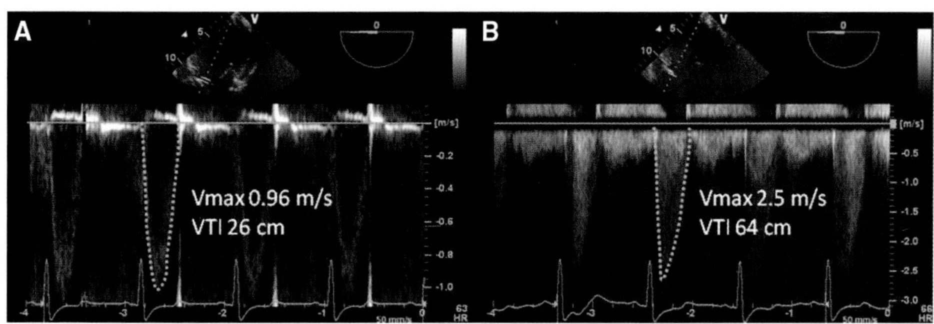

Figure 8.2. Doppler examination of the AV in the deep TG LAX with PW **(A)** and CW Doppler **(B)**.

ANSWERS AND DISCUSSION

QUESTION 8.1: The correct answer is B: BAV.

BAV is the most common form of congenital heart disease diagnosed in adults. It is believed that between 1% and 2% of the population may have BAV and males predominate over females by almost two to one. BAV is asymptomatic in most patients; however, over the course of a patient's life a BAV may develop either AS or, more frequently, AI. In addition, a BAV may be associated with aneurysmal dilatation of the ascending aorta (especially in patients with Marfan syndrome), coarctation of the aorta and a patent foreman ovale. Although most cases of BAV have no genetic basis, there are familial clusters of patients with BAV with up to 10% to 15% occurring in first-degree relatives.

Echocardiographic evaluation of the AV includes determination of the number of valve leaflets, the presence or absence of calcification, and whether AI or stenosis is present. As opposed to the normal trileaflet AV, the BAV has two leaflets or cusps with the larger of the two called the *conjoined leaflet*. In the ME AV SAX view there are only two AV cusps, with the right and the left coronary cusp valves fused into a single one. The fused commissure ("raphe") has increased echogenicity (arrow, Fig. 8.3, Video 8.1), and is appreciated better in a midsystolic view. In diastole, the shape of the BAV orifice may resemble the open mouth of a fish giving a BAV its recognizable shape on echocardiography (Fig. 8.3, Video 8.1). In the ME AV LAX, systolic bowing of the nonfused cusp will result in a "domelike" appearance, while in diastole there is "sagging" of the valve (the cusps prolapsed below the AV annulus) (arrow, Fig. 8.4). Redundancy of the conjoined leaflet may lead to prolapse or aortic regurgitation.

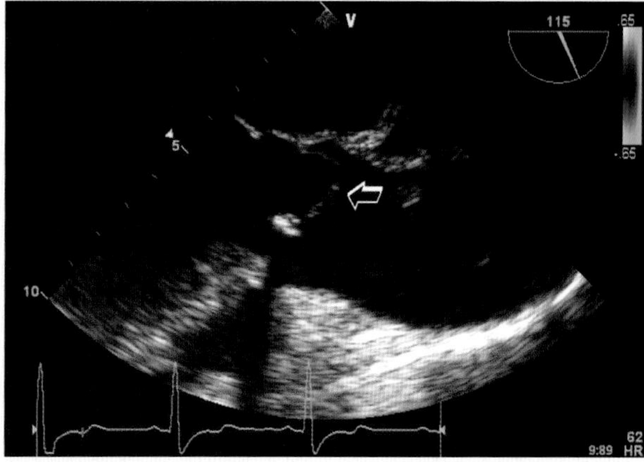

Figure 8.3. ME short-axis view of the bicuspid AV in midsystole with arrow demonstrating raphe.

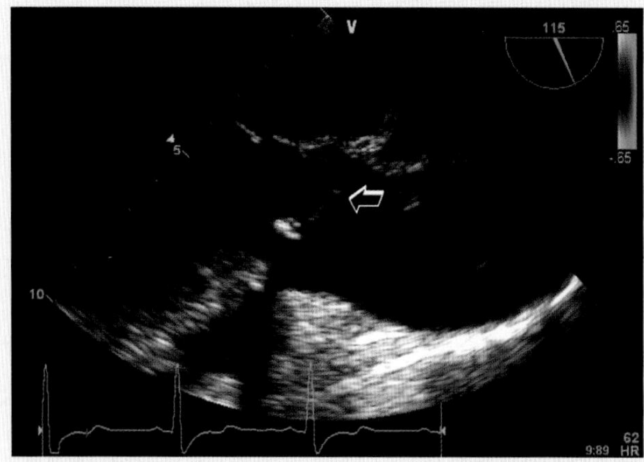

Figure 8.4. ME LAX of the AV with arrow demonstrating "doming" of the bicuspid AV in systole (*arrow*).

If AI is present, it will be detected and graded in the ME LAX using CFD (Fig. 8.1D, Video 8.2). Other associated abnormalities such as dilation or aneurysm of the ascending aorta or arch should also be sought during the exam.

ANSWER A: *Normal AV* is incorrect (see above).

ANSWER C: *Endocarditis* is incorrect. The endocarditis lesions (vegetations) are usually associated with erratic, high-frequency motility, while the "raphe," which may be mistaken for vegetation, is relatively immobile. Endocarditis may affect more than one leaflet as well as involve more than one valve; careful examination of the other valves should be done.

ANSWER D: *Aortic dissection* is incorrect, as it cannot be proven by the images in Figure 8.1, and is not seen in Video 8.4.

QUESTION 8.2: The correct answer is D: Both A and C.

The AVA can be calculated through several methods. It may be calculated using the continuity equation that assumes that flow through the LVOT is equivalent to that across the AV. The current recommendations require the measurements of flow through the LVOT (LVOT area × PW Doppler VTI of the LVOT) and flow through the AV (AVA × CW Doppler VTI). The area of the AV can then be calculated as: AVA = (LVOT area × PW Doppler VTI_{LVOT}) / (CW Doppler VTI_{AoV}) = 1.84 cm^2. The LVOT area is calculated using πr^2 where r is the radius of the LVOT measured by 2D echo. Level 2 recommendations (reasonable when additional information is required) allow for the calculation of the AVA using peak velocities only, assuming that the shape of the velocity contour will be the same in the LVOT and the AV. In this case the calculation becomes: AVA = (LVOT area × PW Doppler peak velocity) / (CW Doppler peak velocity) = 1.74 cm^2. This method is useful when additional confirmation is required, such as situation when tracing the velocity envelope is difficult due to poor contour definition. This latter method, however, is less well accepted.

Answers B and E are incorrect.

QUESTION 8.3: The correct answer is E: Both A and B.

PW (Fig. 8.2A) and CW Doppler (Fig. 8.2B) should be used to interrogate the BAV to determine the degree of AS, if any. In Figure 8.2B, the peak AV velocity is <2.5 m/s and mean pressure gradient is 18 mm Hg, both associated with mild AS. Furthermore, the AVA calculation (see answer to Question 8.2) produced values 1.74 and 1.84 cm^2, also supporting the diagnosis of mild AS. Moderate AS is defined as an AVA of 1.0 to 1.5 cm^2 and severe, <1.0 cm^2. There is also aortic regurgitation as seen in Figure 8.1 and Videos 8.2 and 8.3. You can also note a small portion of the regurgitant velocity profile in Figure 8.2B (above baseline in diastole).

Answers C, HOCM, and D, subaortic stenosis are incorrect, as there is no subvalvular obstruction seen in the two-dimensional images. In HOCM or subaortic stenosis, the LV outflow velocity is increased (usually >1.5–2 m/s). If there is dynamic obstruction, the shape of Doppler spectral velocity may be like a "dagger" (late systolic acceleration).

Due to associated aortic pathology, assessment of the ascending aorta and arch must be performed in concert with that of the BAV. Areas of interest that must be investigated and measured include the diameter of the valve annulus, the sinus of Valsalva, the sinotubular junction, and the size of the ascending aorta and, when possible, the arch. These measurements are especially critical in patients with Marfan syndrome as surgical repair of both the AV and the aorta may be necessary.

TAKE-HOME LESSON:

Surgical repair in BAV is determined by concomitant pathology:

1. **Valve replacement (in significant AS or insufficiency).**
2. **Aortic reconstruction (in diseased aorta).**

SUGGESTED READING

Bauer M, Bauer U, Siniawski H, et al. Differences in clinical manifestations in patients with bicuspid and tricuspid aortic valves undergoing surgery of the aortic valve and/or ascending aorta. *Thorac Cardiovasc Surg.* 2007;55(8):485–490.

Baumgartner H, Hung J, Bermejo J, et al. Echocardiographic assessment of valve stenosis: EAE/ASE recommendations for clinical practice. *J Am Soc Echocardiogr.* 2008;22:1–23.

Bonow RO, Carabello BA, Chatterjee K, et al. Focused update incorporated into the ACC/AHA 2006 guidelines for the management of patients with valvular heart disease: a report of the American College of Cardiology/American Heart Association Task Force on Practice Guidelines (Writing Committee to Revise the 1998 Guidelines for the Management of Patients With Valvular Heart Disease): endorsed by the Society of Cardiovascular Anesthesiologists, Society for Cardiovascular Angiography and Interventions, and Society of Thoracic Surgeons. *J Am Coll Cardiol.* 2008;52(13):e1–e142.

Michelena HI, Desjardins VA, Avierinos JF, et al. Natural history of asymptomatic patients with normally functioning or minimally dysfunctional bicuspid aortic valve in the community. *Circulation.* 2008;117(21):2776–2784.

Sievers HH, Schmidtke C. A classification system for the bicuspid aortic valve from 304 surgical specimens. *J Thorac Cardiovasc Surg.* 2007;133(5):1226–1233.

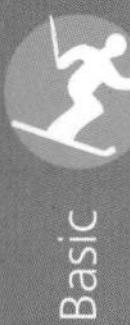

Basic

CASE 9

A 49-year-old man with a LV ejection fraction of 15% undergoes uneventful induction of anesthesia for a cardiac transplant. TEE is performed and the image in Figure 9.1 is obtained.

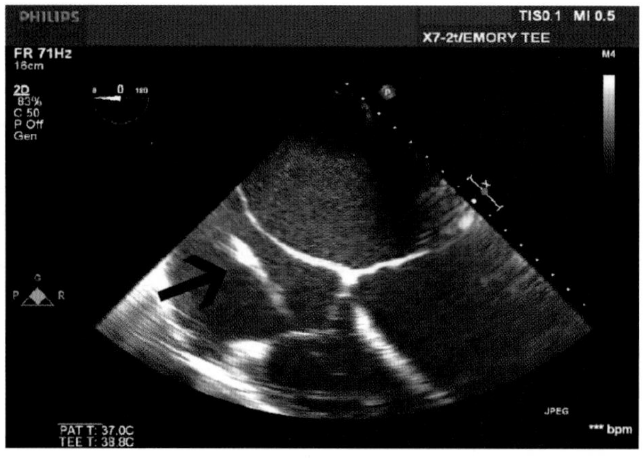

Figure 9.1.

QUESTION 9.1. The object identified by the arrow is

A. ICD defibrillator lead
B. PA catheter
C. Vascular catheter
D. Double-lumen central line

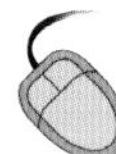

Please review Videos 9.1 and 9.2 prior to proceeding.

QUESTION 9.2. Identify the mobile mass seen in Videos 9.1 and 9.2:

A. Thrombus
B. Vegetation
C. Tumor
D. Unable to determine

ANSWERS AND DISCUSSION

QUESTION 9.1: The correct answer is A: ICD defibrillator lead.

While it is not always possible to discern the specific type of device seen on echocardiography, there are several traits common to certain classes of devices that permit the differentiation of one class from another. The first class of devices likely to be seen as linear opacities in the RA/RV includes catheters. Catheters include single-lumen, multiple lumen, and multifunction (such as PA). The common element seen in catheters is their homogeneous midlevel echogenicity. It is sometimes possible to visualize the lumen of a catheter if caught in cross section and not through the wall. Catheters are typically mobile, vary in position with the cardiac cycle, and can cause side lobe artifact. Continuous cardiac output PA catheters have a characteristic echo signature due to the winding metallic coil along the catheter. The second class of devices likely to be seen in the RA/RV includes pacing and defibrillation leads. Because these leads also contain metal, they are highly echogenic with characteristic appearances. Defibrillation leads are especially echogenic because the mass of metal they contain is much higher than a pacing lead. They are also fixed to a wall of the RA/RV, and many times RA pacing leads are highly coiled in the RA. These devices also produce reverberation artifact.

QUESTION 9.2: The correct answer is D: Unable to determine.

The term "vegetation" should not be confused with mass or thrombus. Its use specifically denotes an organized collection of microorganisms and other material that is adherent to a surface of the heart and is reserved for use during discussions of infective endocarditis (IE). IE is an infection of any structure within the heart including the endocardium, native and prosthetic valves, and any implanted device. It is important to remember that IE is a clinical diagnosis that requires the assessment of patients for several major and minor criteria, including positive blood cultures, fever, and many others. While echocardiographic evidence of endocardial involvement is one of the major criteria, it alone is not sufficient to diagnose definite endocarditis. Furthermore, it is not possible to differentiate a noninfective lesion from a vegetation based on echocardiography alone.

If the patient described above had two sets of positive blood cultures and the echo seen, a diagnosis of definite endocarditis with vegetation would have been appropriate. However, this data was not provided.

The mass seen in the video could also represent a thrombus. Lead-related thrombus is seen commonly after ICD implantation, with some studies reporting an incidence of 25% when examined with TEE. Treatment options for lead-related thrombus include anticoagulation and/or thrombolysis, lead removal, and surgical extraction of the lead(s) and thrombus. The selection of appropriate treatment depends on size of the thrombus, location, presence of a PFO, and patient's condition.

TAKE-HOME LESSON:

Whenever an unexpected mass is encountered on echocardiography, remember that clinical correlation is often required to make an appropriate diagnosis.

SUGGESTED READING

Chow B, Hassan A, Chan KL, et al. Prevalence and significance of lead-related thrombi in patients with implantable cardioverter defibrillators. *Am J Cardiol.* 2003;91:88–90.

Coleman D, DeBarr D, Morales DL, et al. Pacemaker lead thrombosis treated with atrial thrombectomy and biventricular pacemaker and defibrillator insertion. *Ann Thorac Surg.* 2004;78:e83–e84.

Durack D, Lukes AS, Bright DK. New criteria for diagnosis of infective endocarditis: utilization of specific echocardiographic findings. *Am J Med.* 1994;96:200–209.

Otto CM. *Practice of Clinical Echocardiography.* 3rd ed. Philadelphia: Saunders; 2007:502–506.

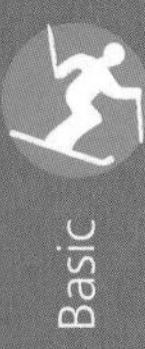

Basic

CASE 10

A 76-year-old male presents for redo AVR and ascending aorta replacement. An arterial line is placed pre-induction, induction and intubation proceed without incident, and you are now preparing to place central venous access under live ultrasound guidance.

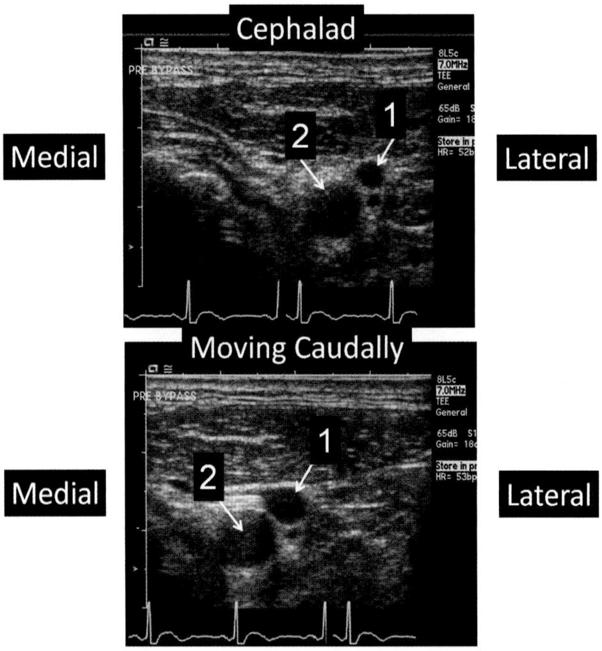

Figure 10.1.

QUESTION 10.1. The ultrasound structures (1 and 2) (Fig. 10.1) show:

A. RIJ vein medial to right carotid artery
B. Right femoral artery medial to right femoral vein
C. An RIJ vein lateral to right carotid artery
D. Left internal jugular vein medial to left carotid artery

QUESTION 10.2. You are now evaluating the left internal jugular vein for possible venous cannulation (see Fig. 10.2). Which of the following are ways of confirming vein versus artery?

A. The jugular vein has no pulsatile flow
B. The artery has pulsatile flow
C. A represents venous flow, B represents arterial flow
D. A represents arterial flow, B represents venous flow

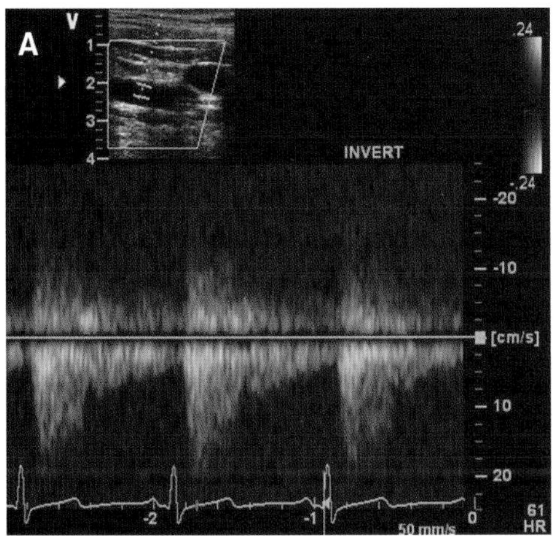

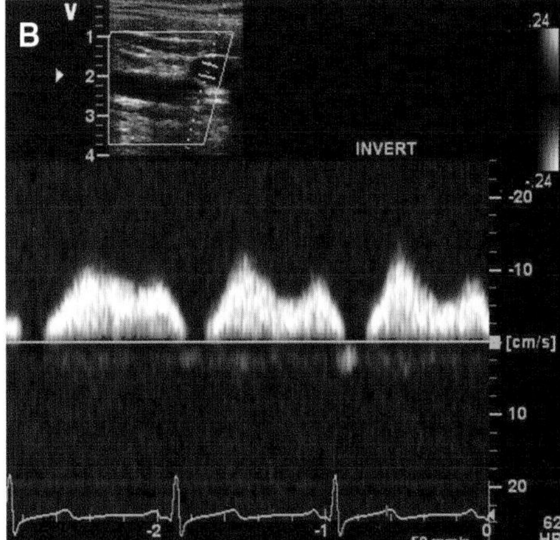

Figure 10.2.

QUESTION 10.3. The images in Figure 10.3 confirm that it is safe to dilate and place the introducer.

True or False?

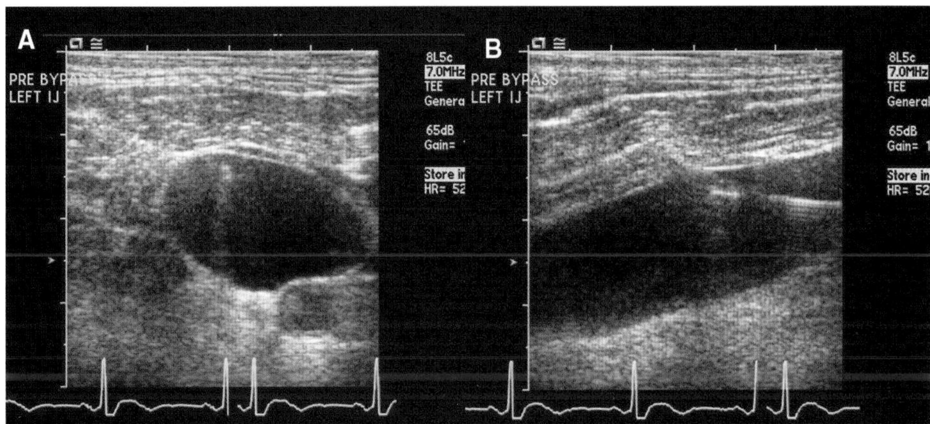

Figure 10.3.

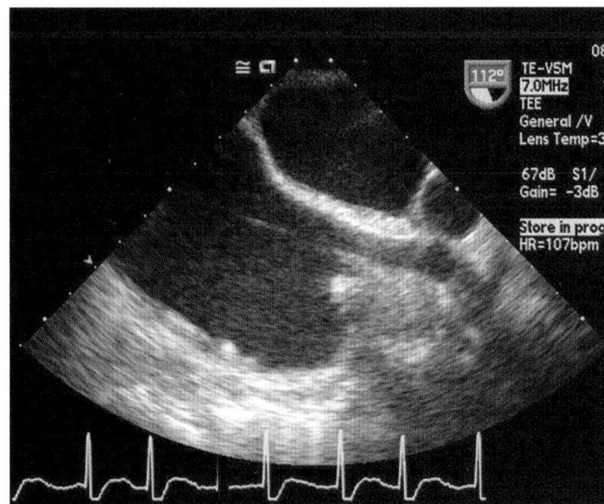

Figure 10.4.

QUESTION 10.4. The combined images in Figure 10.3 and the TEE image in Figure 10.4 confirm that it is safe to dilate and place the introducer.

True or False?

ANSWERS AND DISCUSSION

QUESTION 10.1: The correct answer is C. An RIJ vein lateral to right carotid artery.

The vessels imaged are in the neck. The presence of the sternocleidomastoid muscle (SCM) would be one of the first indicators that we are imaging the neck (Fig. 10.5). The internal jugular vein (v) is lateral and more superficial to the artery (a). The images in Figure 10.1 depict a small RIJ vein (v) tapering down in size as the ultrasound probe is moved caudally.

Answer A is incorrect because it is the left internal jugular vein and carotid artery (a). Answer B is incorrect because it is not the femoral vessels (see above). Answer D is incorrect because the left internal jugular vein is *lateral* to the left carotid artery.

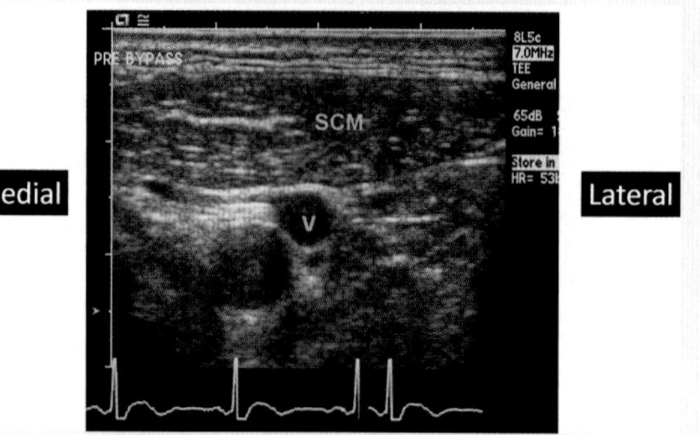

Figure 10.5.

QUESTION 10.2: The correct answer is D: A represents arterial flow, B represents venous flow (Fig. 10.6).

Figure 10.6 is spectral displays, obtained with a PW Doppler sample volume positioned inside the neck vessels (the latter visualized in their long axis). Panel A demonstrates the predominately systolic flow (asterisk) of an artery. Panel B displays the biphasic diastolic flow found in central veins. Similar to the hepatic (or pulmonary) vein flow display, a systolic (S), diastolic (D), and a reversal wave at atrial contraction (rA) are seen. Note that without changing the direction of velocities, the arterial flow is in opposite direction to the venous flow. If the direction of the flow is known, depending on the direction the ultrasound probe is tilted, the opposite direction of the pulsatile flow as well as flow throughout the cardiac cycle can be demonstrated using CFD.

Answers A and B are wrong because either vein or artery will display pulsatile flow. Answer C is wrong (as discussed above).

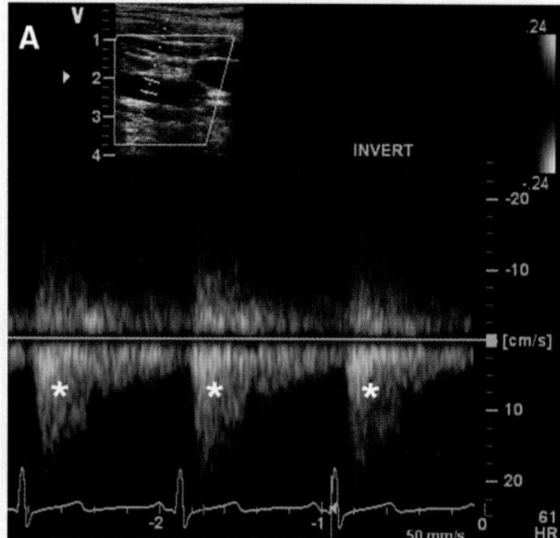

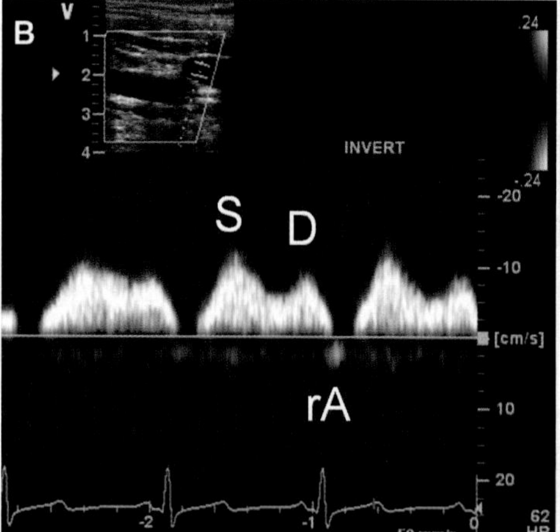

Figure 10.6.

QUESTION 10.3: False.

Although you can see the entry site of the wire into the internal jugular vein (green arrow), you are unable to see if the wire continues to pass through the vein and into the carotid artery. Thus, it is not safe to dilate the vessel without further confirmation (Fig. 10.7).

QUESTION 10.4: True.

By seeing both the wire's entry point (green arrow) and the passage of the wire into the RA (red arrow) via the SVC, it is nearly certain that the carotid artery is not crossed with the guidewire, and thus it is now safe to dilate the vessel (Fig. 10.8).

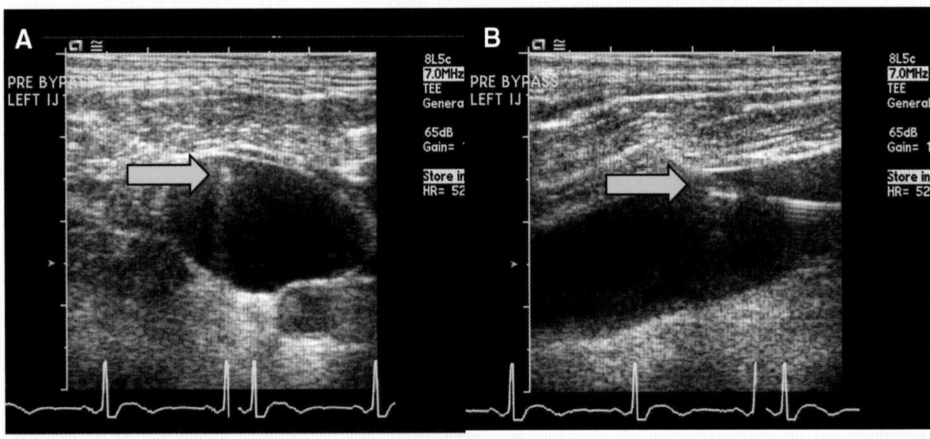

Figure 10.7.

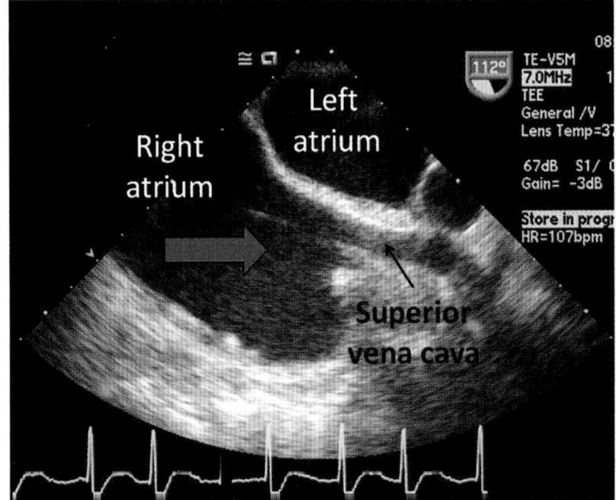

Figure 10.8.

TAKE-HOME LESSON:

Venous structures have a characteristic biphasic flow similar to CVP waveform during the entire cardiac cycle.

The J-tipped guidewire should be imaged inside the RA, entering via the SVC, prior to cannulation with an introducer cannula (when cannulation upper central venous structures).

SUGGESTED READING

Hind D, Calvert N, McWilliams R, et al. Ultrasonic locating devices for central venous cannulation: meta-analysis. *BMJ.* 2003;327:361.

McGee DC, Gould MK. Preventing complications of central venous catheterization. *N Eng J Med.* 2003;348:1123–1133.

Sharma RM, Mohan CVR, Setlus R, et al. Ultrasound guided central venous cannulation. *Methods Med.* 2006;62:371–372.

Stone MB, Nagdev A, Murphy MC, et al. Ultrasound detection of guidewire position during central venous catheterization. *Am J Emerg Med.* 2010;28:82–84.

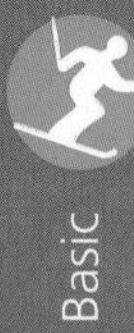

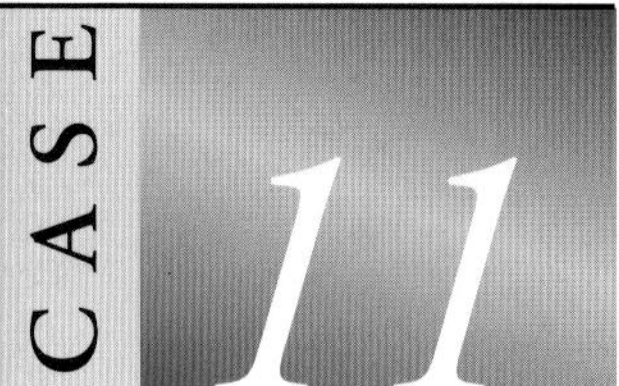

A 29-year-old male with a known bicuspid AV presents with a history of increasing shortness of breath. An outpatient echo performed 1 year ago revealed mild-to-moderate AI with normal LV size and function. The images shown in Figure 11.1 and Video 11.1 are seen on intraoperative TEE.

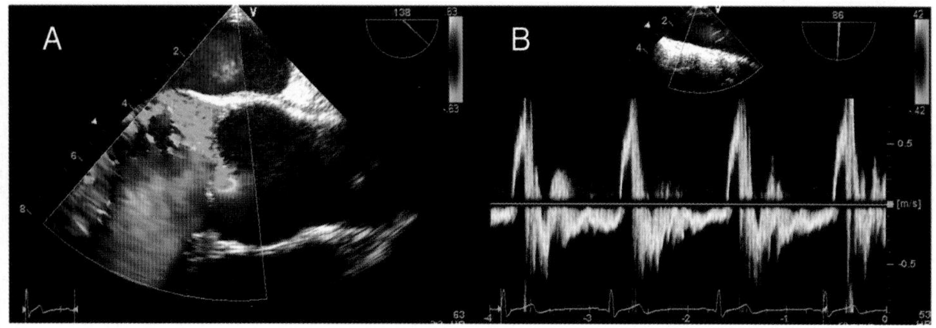

Figure 11.1. ME AV long axis with CFD. See also Video 11.1.

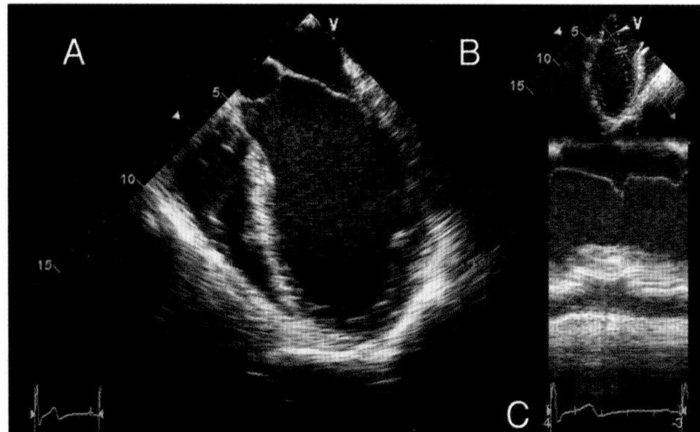

Figure 11.2. **A:** ME 4CH view. See also Video 11.2. **B:** ME LAX with anatomical M-mode cursor (*green*). **C:** M-mode of MV leaflet from B.

QUESTION 11.1. Based on Figure 11.1 and Video 11.1, what is the diagnosis?

A. Severe AI
B. Mild AI
C. Aortic dissection with moderate, eccentric AI
D. AS with AI

QUESTION 11.2. Based on Figure 11.2 and Video 11.2, which statement(s) is/are correct?

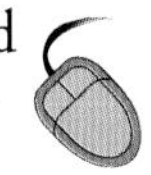

A. Premature closure of MV
B. Concentric LV hypertrophy
C. Dilated LV
D. A and C
E. RV dysfunction

QUESTION 11.3. Based on the LV dimension in Figure 11.3 and on Videos 11.2 and 11.3, what is your conclusion?

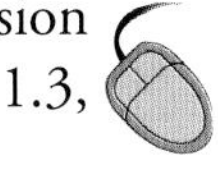

A. Recent myocardial infarction

B. Chronic AI

C. Associated severe MR

D. Acute, severe AI

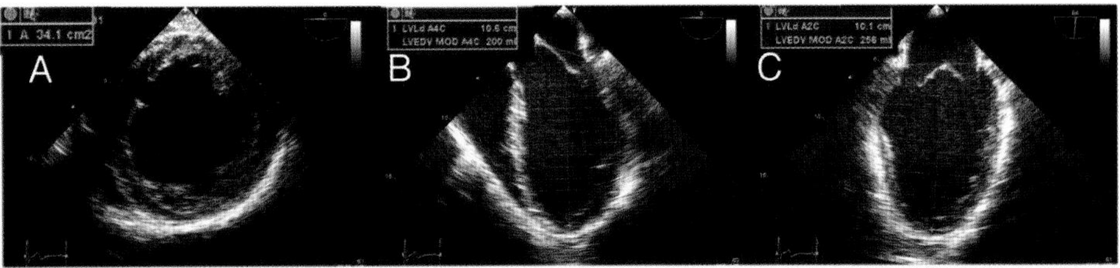

Figure 11.3. **A:** TG SAX view with end diastolic area. **B:** ME 4CH view with end diastolic volume. **C:** ME 2CH view with end diastolic volume. See also Video 11.3 for a TG SAX view of the LV.

ANSWERS AND DISCUSSION

QUESTION 11.1: The correct answer is A: Severe AI.

Figure 11.1 demonstrates severe, eccentric AI. The vena contracta, measured as the narrowest diameter of the AI jet downstream of the convergence point in early to mid-diastole, appears large (~7 mm). The severity of AI based on the vena contracta is graded as mild (<3 mm), moderate (3–6 mm), and severe (≥6 mm). A measurement of the jet height to LV outflow tract diameter ratio can also be used to determine AI severity. A ratio of <25% indicates mild AI, 25% to 64% indicates moderate AI, and >65% indicates severe AI. However, the eccentric course of the jet precludes applicability of this assessment in this particular case. The PHT of the regurgitant jet using CW Doppler can also be used to assess severity (see Case 40). Proper alignment of the Doppler beam with the AI jet can be problematic using TEE. A PHT >500 msec is indicative of mild AI, whereas a PHT less than 200 msec indicates severe AI.

In Figure 11.2B, the PW Doppler pattern demonstrates holodiastolic flow reversal in the proximal descending aorta indicating at least moderate-to-severe aortic regurgitation. Measurements made in the ascending aorta or proximal arch may also show diastolic flow reversal with milder degrees of AI; however, holodiastolic flow reversal in the descending aorta is a clear indication of at least moderate, if not severe, insufficiency.

Answer B is incorrect; the AI is severe based on the holodiastolic flow reversal in the descending aorta. Answers C and D are incorrect; there is no evidence of stenosis and there is no evidence for aortic dissection as no intimal flap is observed in the ascending aorta.

QUESTION 11.2: The correct answer is D: A and C.

A classical finding of acute AI is early MV closure, a result of rapidly increasing LV pressures caused by the severe AI. In Figure 11.2C, the M-mode display demonstrates a very brief opening for the MV as the severe aortic regurgitation causes early closure. Furthermore, when the AI jet is severe and directed toward the anterior MV leaflet, anterior leaflet fluttering may be observed on M-mode (not demonstrated). In Figure 11.2A, the LV appears dilated. Although no particular measurements have been made, we note that the scanning sector is over 15 cm deep and the LV occupies a large portion of the length. Answer B is incorrect; the LV does not demonstrate concentric hypertrophy as wall thickness is normal. The enlarged ventricle is the result of eccentric hypertrophy. Answer E is incorrect; the RV function does not appear depressed and the RV size is normal.

QUESTION 11.3: The correct answer is B: Chronic AI.

The changes to the heart associated with chronic AI include both LV dilatation and LA enlargement. These changes typically take weeks to months to develop. Conversely, acute AI presents with relatively maintained chamber dimensions. Accordingly, quantifying

LV size and LA size provides important clues as to the duration and functional impact of AI. Figure 11.3A shows an enlarged LV end diastolic area of 34 cm^2 (normal adult size: 10–20 cm^2) that suggests that the AI is chronic. Figures 11.3B and 11.3C demonstrate large end diastolic volumes of 200 mL (ME 4CH) and 256 mL (ME 2CH) as calculated using the method of disks. Normal values range from 67 to 155 mL. Measurement of end systolic volumes confirmed an elevated SV as the LV is required to eject the RV in addition to the SV. In this case, the LA was not enlarged.

Answers A and C are incorrect. Ischemic cardiac disease, especially in the presence of previous myocardial infarction, may also result in a dilated LV but this is usually associated with segmental wall motion abnormalities and reduced EF. None of these was observed in this patient (Videos 11.2 and 11.3). Similarly, chronic MR may also result in a dilated LV with or without the presence of AI. There was no evidence for MR (Video 11.1).

Answer D is incorrect. Acute, severe AI would not present with dilated chambers unless there were preexisting conditions that are associated with chamber dilatation.

TAKE-HOME LESSON:

Left heart chamber size provides important clues as to the severity and chronicity of AI.

SUGGESTED READING

Cohen IS. Aortic regurgitation. In: Perrino AC, Reeves ST, eds. *A Practical Approach to Transesophageal Echocardiography*. 2nd ed. Philadelphia: Lippincott Williams & Wilkins, 2008.

Lang RM, Bierig M, Devereaux RB, et al. Recommendations for chamber quantification: a report from the American Society of Echocardiography's Guidelines and Standards Committee and the Chamber Quantification Writing Group, developed in conjunction with the European Association of Echocardiography, a branch of the European Society of Cardiology. *J Am Soc Echocardiogr*. 2005;18: 1440–1463.

CASE 12

A 41-year-old man presents with acute CHF and a new onset of neurologic deficits. A TEE examination study is performed.

QUESTION 12.1. From Figure 12.1 and Video 12.1, what is the most likely diagnosis?

A. LV thrombus
B. AV endocarditis with vegetation
C. Aortic root trauma with valve disruption and prolapse
D. Aortic dissection with prolapsing intimal flap

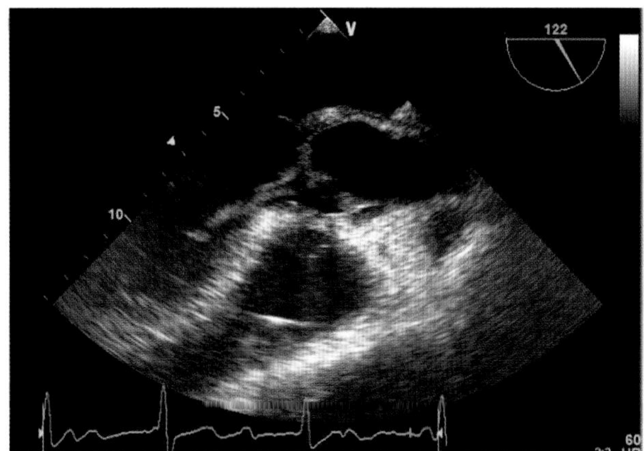

Figure 12.1. ME aortic LAX. See also Video 12.1.

QUESTION 12.2. Examining Figures 12.2 and 12.3, and Videos 12.2 and 12.3, the color Doppler suggests:

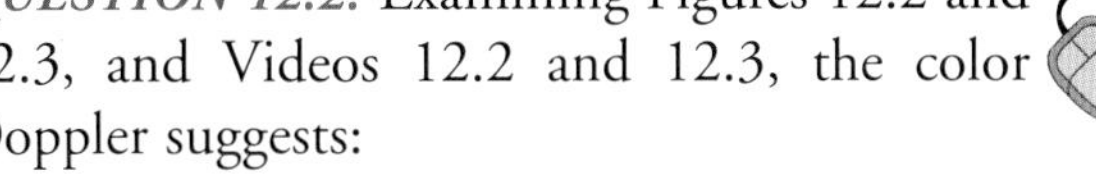

A. Severe aortic regurgitation and aortic root abscess
B. VSD
C. Aortic dissection with severe aortic regurgitation

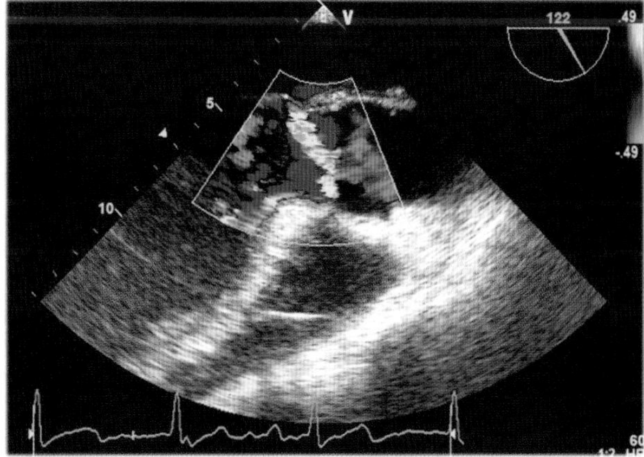

Figure 12.2. ME aortic LAX with color Doppler. See also Video 12.2.

QUESTION 12.3. From Figure 12.4, further CFD examination reveals findings compatible with one of the following:

A. ASD
B. Sinus of Valsalva aneurysm with fistulization
C. Aortic abscess to right atrial fistula
D. Severe tricuspid insufficiency

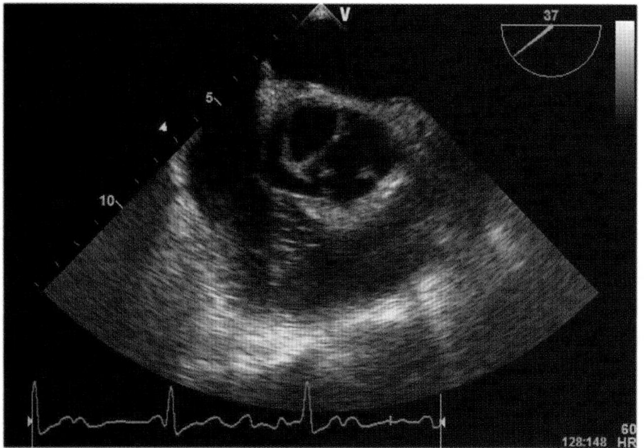

Figure 12.3. ME aortic short-axis view. See also Video 12.3.

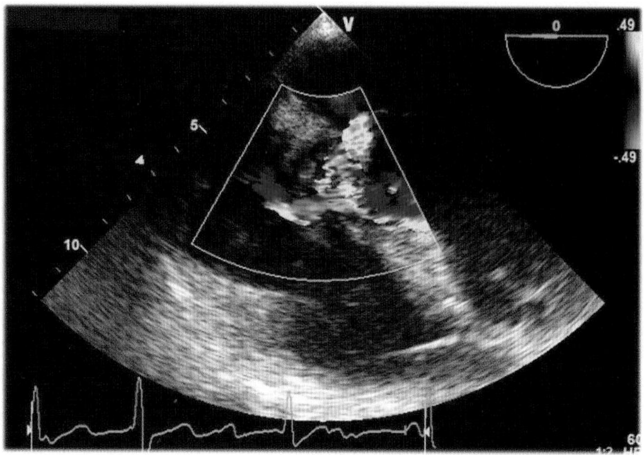

Figure 12.4. ME five-chamber view with color Doppler. See also Video 12.4.

ANSWERS AND DISCUSSION

QUESTION 12.1: The correct answer is B: AV endocarditis with vegetation.

The AV morphology is abnormal as it appears thickened and distorted. There is a large mass compatible with a vegetation prolapsing into the LVOT. An LV thrombus is unlikely as the mass is attached to the AV and is associated with valve pathology. An LV thrombus is most often associated with an LV aneurysm or dilated cardiomyopathy and is more commonly found in the apex. Aortic root trauma with leaflet prolapse is unlikely as the prolapsing structure is too long and there is no associated periaortic or medial hematoma. An aortic dissection is unlikely as an intimal flap is not demonstrated.

QUESTION 12.2: The correct answer is A: Aortic regurgitation with aortic root abscess.

Regurgitation is a common finding with an infected AV. Vegetations may prevent adequate cusp coaptation as well as cause destruction and perforation of the cusps. An aortic root abscess is also visible in the short-axis view at the level of the right coronary cusp. The diastolic color jet's height in the ME aortic LAX is not diagnostic for severe aortic regurgitation. However, as the jets are eccentric, using the jet height to LVOT ratio in the assessment of the severity of AI may be misleading. A pulsed Doppler analysis of the descending aorta shows diastolic flow reversal helping to confirm severe aortic regurgitation (Fig. 12.5).

Measuring the aortic regurgitation jet PHT with CW Doppler in the deep gastric aortic outflow view is frequently difficult and unreliable with eccentric jets. There is no VSD in these images as no systolic jets are

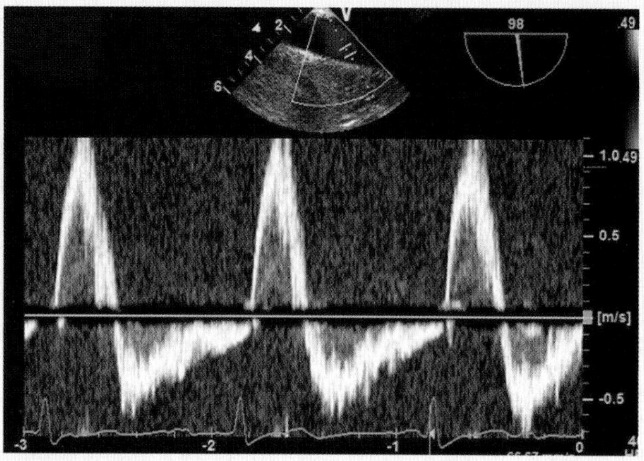

Figure 12.5. PW Doppler of descending thoracic aorta.

observed at the level of the septum. No intimal flap is detected in the ascending aorta.

QUESTION 12.3: The correct answer is C: Aortic abscess to right atrial fistula.

In Figure 12.4 and Video 12.4, there is a diastolic jet that enters the RA. Aortoatrial fistulae are uncommon but well-recognized complications of AV endocarditis, in this case with a root abscess. Fistula formation may involve any of the cardiac chambers and are usually associated with advanced disease and predict a poorer prognosis. This finding underscores the importance of a complete TEE examination as it would not have been apparent if limited to the AV. The interatrial septum is not well visualized in Figure 12.4. A sinus of Valsalva aneurysm may result in fistulization; however, the sinus of Valsalva is not enlarged. TR is unlikely as the jet does not originate at the TV.

TAKE-HOME LESSON:

AV endocarditis usually results in leaflet destruction and may involve the aortic root if frequently associated with aortic regurgitation. A thorough echo examination is essential in detecting associated pathologies such as fistulae seen in this case.

SUGGESTED READING

Lobato EB, Muehlschlegel JD. Transesophageal echocardiography in the intensive care unit. In: Perrino A, Reeves ST, eds. *A Practical Approach to Transesophageal Echocardiography*. 2nd ed. Philadelphia: Lippincott Williams & Wilkins; 2008:354–356.

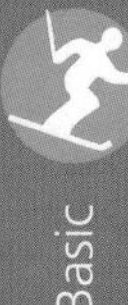

Basic

CASE 13

A 66-year-old male presents to the OR with a history of severe AS and coronary artery disease. Intraoperative echocardiography confirms the AS and normal LV function with no RWMA. No intracardiac shunts were noted on the comprehensive prebypass exam. The patient had an AVR and CABG. After separation from CPB the patient's blood pressure is 104/76 with a normal ECG tracing.

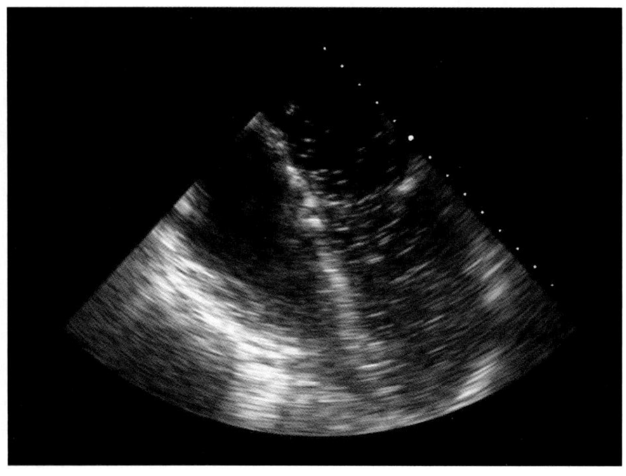

Figure 13.1. ME 4CH view.

QUESTION 13.1. What is the most likely reason for the intracardiac air seen in Figure 13.1 and Video 13.1?

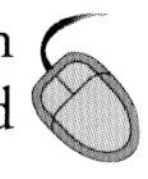

A. CABG
B. Aortotomy
C. PFO
D. Unroofed CS

QUESTION 13.2. What steps can be taken to remove the air from the left side of the heart?

A. Placement of a vent into the aorta
B. Needle aspiration of the LV apex
C. Changing the position of the patient
D. Filling the heart with blood
E. All of the above

QUESTION 13.3. The patient suddenly becomes hypotensive with a blood pressure of 60/40. There are large ST depressions in II, III, and AVF. Protamine has not been given yet. The ME AV LAX and TG SAX views are obtained (Figs. 13.2 and 13.3 and Videos 13.2 and 13.3). What is the most likely reason for the hypotension?

A. Obstruction of the newly placed AV
B. Failure of one of the coronary bypass grafts
C. Air embolism
D. Hypovolemia

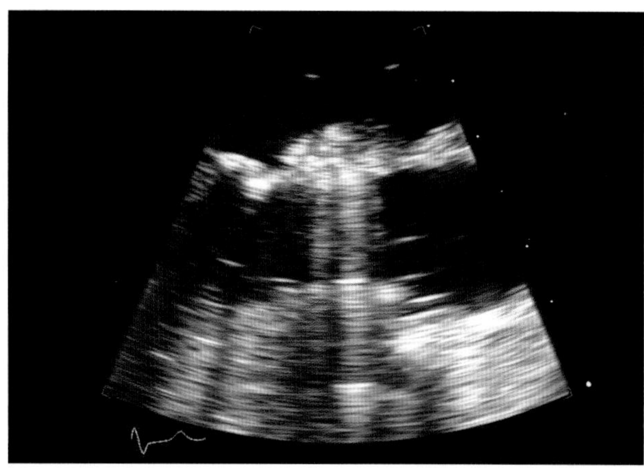

Figure 13.2. ME AV LAX.

QUESTION 13.4. What should be done next to resolve the hypotension?

A. Fluid resuscitation
B. Vasopressors
C. Return to CPB
D. Wait, as the hypotension and ECG changes will likely resolve with time

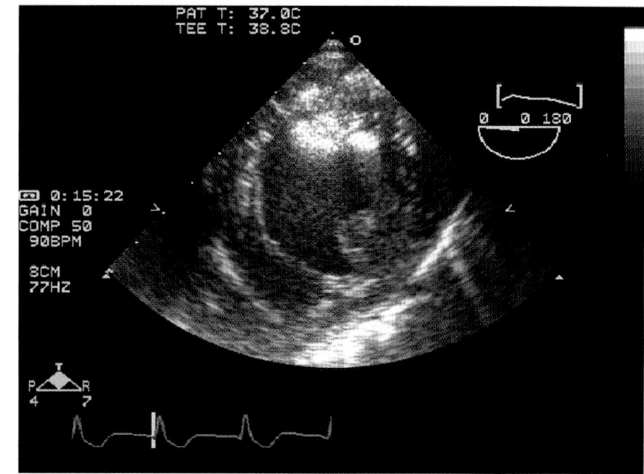

Figure 13.3. TG SAX view.

ANSWERS AND DISCUSSION

QUESTION 13.1: The correct answer is B.

TEE is useful to monitor the amount of intracardiac air present after CPB. It is most common to have intracardiac air after open-chamber cardiac surgery. According to a study by Rodigas et al. in the *American Journal of Cardiology*,[1] the incidence of air is greatest with ASD repairs and LA myxoma resections, followed by valve surgery, with the lowest incidence in patients having coronary artery bypass surgery alone. This patient had an aortotomy performed to replace his AV. Air enters through aortotomy site during the valve replacement and is retained within the left side of the heart after closure of the aorta.

No intracardiac shunts were noted on the comprehensive prebypass exam so air from the venous system is unlikely from a PFO or unroofed CS. If air doesn't clear from the left side of the heart with time, reexamining for intracardiac shunts is necessary.

QUESTION 13.2: The correct Answer is E.

All of the above are ways to remove intracardiac air from the left side of the heart. After the aortotomy is closed, air is trapped within the cardiac chambers and in the pulmonary veins. When the left side of the heart is filled with blood, air pockets then mobilize producing micro air emboli as seen in Figure 13.1 and Video 13.1. Ventilating the lungs helps force air from the pulmonary veins by further augmenting PVF. By filling the left heart with blood and increasing cardiac output the air is mobilized into the aorta. Placing a vent in the ascending aorta allows intracardiac air to escape from the patient. Patients in Trendelenburg position typically have air in the LV apex, as this is the highest portion of the LV. Needle aspiration of the LV apex removes some of this air. It is also possible to place a catheter in the ascending aorta under gentle suction back to the pump. The goal is to entrain air that exits the aorta before it enters the cerebral or coronary circulation and leads to transient ischemic episodes, such as the noted ECG changes. By changing patient position or massaging the heart, air can be further mobilized and removed from the left atrium and ventricle as guided by TEE.

QUESTION 13.3: The correct answer is C.

All of the above answers can be a cause of the patient's hypotension, but air embolism down the RCA is the most likely explanation. In a supine patient, RCA air embolism is more common than left given the superior position of the right ostium in the aortic root. Air will preferentially enter the more superior orifice. In Figure 13.2 and Video 13.2, air can be seen entering the right coronary ostium.

The diagnosis is further confirmed by the inferior and inferoseptal wall dysfunction seen in Video 13.3. In fact, intramyocardial air (hyperechoic spots) can be seen in the distribution of the RCA in Figure 13.3 and Video 13.3. This patient must have right dominant circulation to have this presentation. In a patient with left dominant circulation, inferior wall intramyocardial air and wall dysfunction would be less likely given the more inferior location of the left coronary ostium.

Even though air embolism is the likely diagnosis given the above clinical scenario, proper function of the AV, examination of the bypass grafts, fluid status, and other possible reasons for hypotension should always be considered and ruled out.

QUESTION 13.4: The correct answer is C.

The best answer is return to CPB. No protamine has been given and the hypotension is profound with significant intramyocardial air and regional wall dysfunction noted in the RCA distribution. After returning to CPB, the patient's blood pressure can be elevated to help push the air emboli further distal in the coronary system. Typically, the ST changes and ventricular function improves over 5 to 10 minutes. This will also allow more time to further de-air the left side of the heart.

If the hypotension and amount of air emboli had been less profound, inotropic and vasopressor support could have been instituted to maintain blood pressure and cardiac function until the transient ventricular dysfunction resolves. If the ventricular dysfunction and hypotension do not resolve with these maneuvers, then other causes should be further investigated.

TAKE-HOME LESSON:

Intraoperative TEE is a useful monitor and guide for the management of intracardiac air after CPB.

REFERENCE

1. Rodigas PC, Meyer FJ, Haasler GB, et al. Intraoperative 2-dimensional echocardiography: ejection of microbubbles from the left ventricle after cardiac surgery. *Am J Cardiol.* 1982;50(5):1130–1132.

CASE 14

Consider the upper esophageal, long-axis (UE LAX) image of the aortic arch and proximal descending aorta: See Figure 14.1 and Video 14.1 (short-axis and LAX of the descending aorta).

QUESTION 14.1. The observed CFD pattern is most likely attributed to:

A. Stanford Type A dissection of the aortic arch and descending aorta with retrograde flow in the false lumen
B. Severe AI with flow reversal in diastole
C. Normal CFD pattern in the aorta
D. Inappropriate Nyquist limit setting with aliasing of the aortic flow velocity measurements

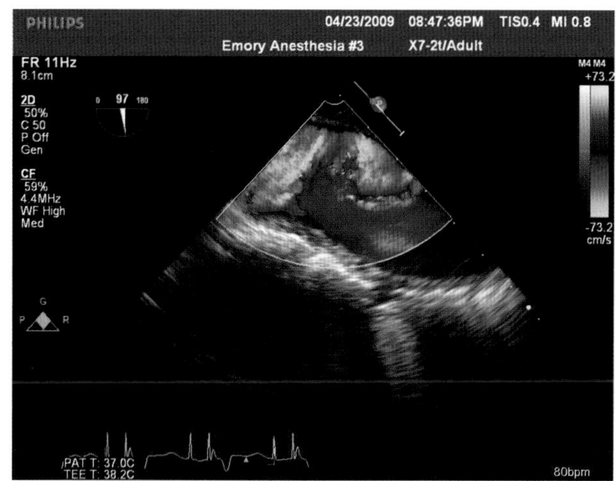

Figure 14.1.

QUESTION 14.2. In the UE LAX of the PA (Fig.14.2), which arrow refers to the Nyquist limit of the CFD sector? See corresponding Video 14.2 (pulm artery).

A. #1
B. #2
C. #3
D. #4

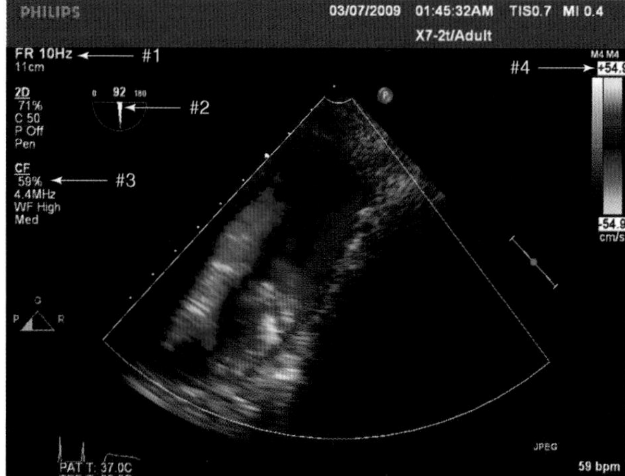

Figure 14.2.

ANSWERS AND DISCUSSION

QUESTION 14.1: The correct answer is C.

This pattern represents the CFD of normal, laminar flow within the aorta. Blood normally flows in a spiraling (helical) pattern throughout the ascending and descending aorta. Doppler shift indicates the velocity. It is important to remember the velocity is vector, which is defined by the two components of speed and directionality. CFD will display the speed and direction of flow using a color bar graph, typically found in the upper left-hand corner of the screen. This example dramatically demonstrates the change in direction of flow in relationship to the Doppler probe. This color display will change from red to blue as evident in this example.

Blood flow within the false lumen is rarely so laminar. Typically, turbulent flow (bright, chaotic CFD display) is seen within the true lumen and the intimal flap is evident. The false lumen can have minimal flow, high-velocity flow at the site of intimal injury, or various stages of thrombosis.

Severe AI can be associated with reversal of flow during diastole, but flow is typically nonlaminar and would not be helical with the CFD pattern shown in this still image.

By convention, the Nyquist limit should be between 50 and 60 mm/s. Inappropriately low Nyquist velocity settings will impede the ability of the ultrasound system to accurately interpret the velocity of flow. In this scenario, the flow will appear artificially turbulent and the CFD display will be more chaotic than this case example.

QUESTION 14.2: The correct answer is D.

With CFD display, the mean velocities of flow are recorded within a pie-shaped sector that is located at the anatomic area of interest. Hundreds of velocities are mapped using a standardized color coding system found in the left-hand corner of the CFD display. This mapping system integrates anatomic location of flow, degree of turbulence, and approximate velocity of flow. Figure 14.2 is the CFD of the main PA. The blue area indicates laminar flow away from the probe. The red is indicative of laminar flow toward the probe.

Aliasing is velocity, above which the system is unable to accurately read the speed and or direction of flow. The Nyquist limit is the blood flow velocity at which aliasing occurs. The aliasing velocity is typically noted associated with the color coding graph in the upper left-hand corner of the display. Any velocity exceeding the Nyquist limit will be seen as reversal of flow or turbulent flow. In this example, the aliasing limit is 54.9 cm/s. This exam is within the target range of 50 to 60 cm/s. Unfortunately as the depth of the sample increases, the maximum Nyquist limit will decrease.

The arrow #1 represents the frame rate (FR). The FR of 10 Hz means the picture is refreshed 10 times every second.

Arrow #2 represents the angle of multiplane. At 90-degree multiplane, the right side of the picture is anatomically superior and the left side is inferior.

Arrow #3 is percentage of CFD gain. The CFD gain affects the amplification of the Doppler signal display and affects the signal-to-noise ratio.

TAKE-HOME LESSON:

The Nyquist limit is the blood flow velocity at which aliasing occurs.

CASE 15

A 58-year-old male has been referred by his primary care physician for shortness of breath and decreasing exercise tolerance over the last several months. He has a systolic murmur on auscultation. Coronary angiography did not reveal any significant coronary artery disease. He is scheduled to undergo MV surgery. After induction of anesthesia, the TEE images shown in Figure 15.1 are obtained.

QUESTION 15.1. Based on Figure 15.1 and Video 15.1, what is the most likely source of the systolic murmur?

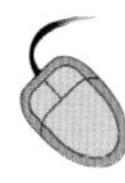

A. SAM of the MV
B. Prolapse of the P2 and P3 scallops
C. Prolapse of the A2 segment
D. Ischemia of posterior papillary muscle

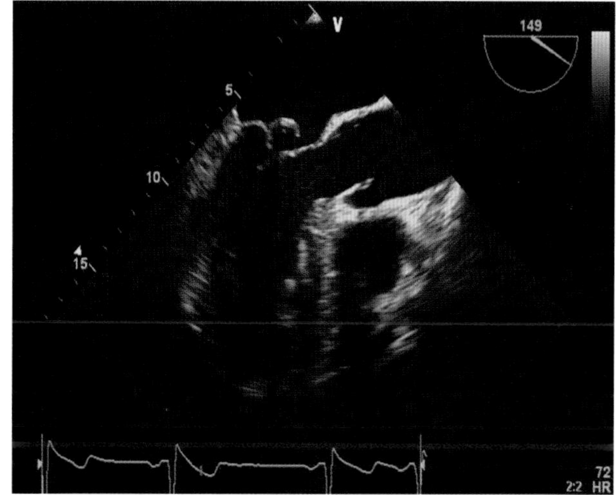

Figure 15.1. ME LAX. See also Video 15.1.

QUESTION 15.2. Based on the Carpentier classification, what type of dysfunction is present in this case?

A. Type 1
B. Type 2
C. Type 3a
D. Type 3b

QUESTION 15.3. Based on Figure 15.2 and Video 15.2, how severe is the MR?

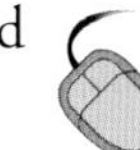

A. Mild MR
B. Moderate MR
C. Severe MR
D. None of the above

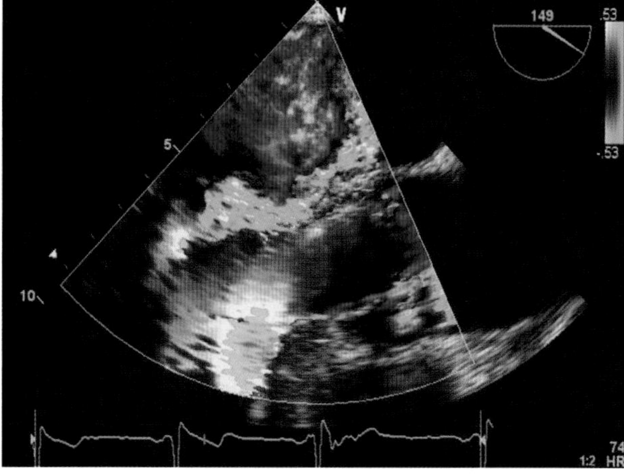

Figure 15.2. ME LAX, with CFD, in systole. See also Video 15.2.

QUESTION 15.4. What is the recommended treatment of this mitral pathology?

A. MV replacement
B. Annuloplasty ring insertion
C. Quadrangular resection of the posterior mitral leaflet and ring insertion
D. Medical management

ANSWERS AND DISCUSSION

QUESTION 15.1: The correct answer is B: Prolapse of the P2 and P3 scallops.

The MV is comprised of two leaflets, a larger semicircular anterior leaflet and a smaller quadrangularly shaped posterior leaflet. The margin of the posterior leaflet has two indentations, which divide it into three functional scallops, referred to as P1, P2, and P3. P1 is the most anterior scallop, P2 the middle scallop, and P3 the most posterior scallop. The corresponding segments of the anterior leaflet are referred to as A1, A2, and A3. Using standard 2D multiplane views of the MV, each of these individual segments of the valve should be imaged to identify pathology. In Figure 15.1, the two posterior mitral scallops extend *above* the mitral annular plane and into the left atrium during systole, a condition termed *prolapse*. When aligned properly, the tomographic plane of the ME LAX usually cuts across the middle posterior scallop (P2) and the middle segment of the anterior leaflet (A2). In this patient, along with P2, there appears to be another prolapsing posterior scallop, a more posterior structure, the medial scallop or P3. Figure 15.3 demonstrates this point. However, to make this diagnosis conclusively additional cross sections of the valve are required. Answer A (*SAM*) is incorrect: there is not anterior motion of the MV leaflets during systole. Answer C (*prolapse of the A2 segment*) is incorrect: the anterior leaflet, on the right of the screen, does not extend above the mitral annulus during systole. Finally, answer D (*ischemic MR*) is incorrect: ischemic heart disease usually results in *functional* MR and does not cause isolated leaflet prolapse. Moreover, this diagnosis is unlikely in a patient with normal coronary arteries.

QUESTION 15.2: The correct answer is B: Type 2.

The Carpentier classification of MR is based on MV leaflet motion. There are three types: In *type 1*, the *leaflet motion is normal,* but there is failure of coaptation because of mitral annular dilatation. In such cases,

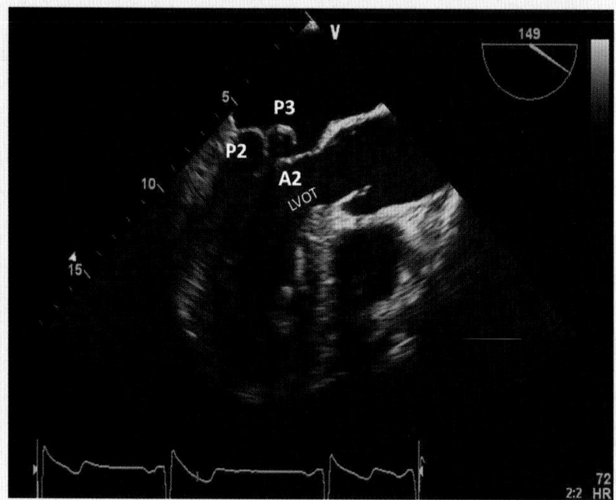

Figure 15.3. ME LAX, in systole, labeling the various MV segments.

the MR jet is usually central. Some cases of leaflet perforation also fall under type 1, although the MR jet can be eccentric in such patients. *Type 2*, as seen in this case, is the result of *excessive leaflet motion*, with the margins of the leaflets extending beyond the level of the annular plane in systole. This can result from elongated or ruptured chordae tendineae, or from a ruptured papillary muscle. In type 2, the MR jet is usually directed *away from* the prolapsing mitral segment. *Type 3* refers to *restricted leaflet motion*, and is subdivided into two subgroups, 3a and 3b: In type 3a, the MV is restricted in both systole and diastole, as is seen in rheumatic valve disease, while in type 3b the valve is restricted predominantly in systole, usually from tethering of the leaflets by an apically and posteriorly displaced papillary muscle, as is often seen in chronic ischemic heart disease. Answers A (type 1), C (type 3a), and D (type 3b) are all incorrect.

QUESTION 15.3: The correct answer is C: Severe MR.

In Figure 15.2 there is a large jet of MR, directed anteriorly, away from the prolapsing posterior leaflet and tracking along the anterior LA wall. In valvular prolapse the affected leaflet segment acts as a trap door directing blood *away from* the involved leaflet. CFD usually demonstrates a jet entering the left atrium in systole. Note that general anesthesia by virtue of its effects on inotropy and loading conditions results in underestimation of the severity of MR. In general, an eccentric jet that "hugs" the atrial wall is considered severe until proven otherwise. See Case 23 for a detailed discussion of this topic.

QUESTION 15.4: The correct answer is C: Quadrangular resection of the posterior mitral leaflet and ring insertion. This is a surgical technique whereby the prolapsing mitral segment is resected and the remaining parts of the leaflet are brought together to reduce the size of the valve and improve the coaptation between the leaflets. The mitral annular ring then supports the repair and prevents further dilatation of the mitral annulus. Answer A (*MV replacement*) is incorrect: MV repair is widely viewed as preferable to MV replacement, whenever it is feasible. Middle posterior scallop prolapse in expert hands has a very high success rate with very low complications. The benefits of preservation of the native anatomic structures include lower reoperation rates, lower complication rates and no need for long-term anticoagulation. Answer B (*annuloplasty ring insertion*) is incorrect, as it is more often reserved for annular dilatation or functional MR. Answer D (*medical management*) is incorrect. While it may help symptoms, medical management will not correct this problem because the MR is due to a structural abnormality (prolapsing posterior scallop).

TAKE-HOME LESSON:

Understanding the functional causes of MR provides invaluable information to the surgeon when MV repair is planned.

SUGGESTED READING

Amirak E, Chan KM, Zakkar M, et al. Current status of surgery for degenerative mitral valve disease. *Prog Cardiovasc Dis*. 2009;51(6):454–459.

Lambert AS. Mitral regurgitation. In: Perrino AC, Reeves ST, eds. *A Practical Approach to Transesophageal Echocardiography*. Philadelphia: Lippincott Williams & Wilkins; 2008.

O'Gara P, Sugeng L, Lang R, et al. The role of imaging in chronic degenerative mitral regurgitation. *JACC Cardiovasc Imaging*. 2008;1(2):221–237.

Zoghbi WA, Enriquez-Sarano M, Foster E, et al. Recommendations for evaluation of the severity of native valvular regurgitation with two-dimensional and Doppler echocardiography. *J Am Soc Echocardiogr*. 2003;16(7):777–802.

CASE 16

A patient is undergoing a TEE examination. A ME 4CH view is demonstrated in Videos 16.1 to 16.3.

QUESTION 16.1. The control is being manipulated in Videos 16.1 to 16.3?

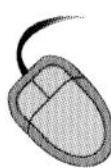

A. Reject
B. Compression
C. System gain
D. Time-gain compensation

QUESTION 16.2. The ME 4CH view shown in Videos 16.4 to 16.6 have been produced by manipulating which of the following ultrasound control?

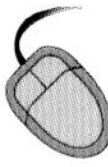

A. Frequency
B. Compression
C. System gain
D. Time-gain compensation

QUESTION 16.3. Which of the two videos (Video 16.7 or 16.8) has a higher "reject"?

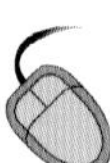

ANSWERS AND DISCUSSION

QUESTION 16.1: The correct answer is C: System gain.

Returning ultrasound signals have reduced energy (amplitude) compared to transmitted signals. This is due to ultrasound energy being lost as a consequence of refraction and reflection during interaction with tissues (Video 16.1). In order to optimize the displayed image, the returning electric signals frequently need to be amplified before it can be further processed. The amplification is produced by the system's "gain" control. By increasing the gain, all returning signals are amplified. Compared to Video 16.1 that demonstrates the gain settings set too low, excessive gain will make the image brighter and structures appear more obvious, but at the expense of image resolution (Video 16.2). Gain is set at an appropriate level if fluid and blood appear totally black. The myocardium ideally should demonstrate shades of gray. Gain should be added in increments until imaging is optimized as shown in Video 16.3. Figure 16.1 is a composite of Videos 16.1 to 16.3 demonstrating the effects of adjustments of the gain setting.

QUESTION 16.2: The correct answer is B: Compression.

Unfortunately, current echocardiography monitors are unable to adequately display the tremendous range of returning amplitudes obtained from tissues. This monitoring limitation is partially corrected through the use of compression. Compression limits the difference between the highest and the lowest echo amplitudes by fitting them into a grayscale range that the echocardiographic monitor can display. Increasing the compression produces an image with more shades of gray and the appearance of smearing of tissue borders (Video 16.4). Decreasing the compression provides an image with high contrast and strong white and black components (Video 16.5). The appropriate degree of compression is set in a stepwise fashion (Video 16.6). Figure 16.2 is a composite of Videos 16.4 to 16.6 demonstrating the effects of adjustments of the compression setting.

QUESTION 16.3: The correct answer is Video 16.7.

Reject is another ultrasound control that allows the echocardiographer to select the amount of returning low-amplitude signals that are eliminated, rejected. This tool can be useful to eliminate background noise but is also useful when evaluating low signals such as tissue Doppler. An image with low reject setting will display more "noise" than a high reject display. Video 16.7 has a higher reject setting than Video 16.8. Figure 16.3 is a composite of Videos 16.7 and 16.8 demonstrating the effects of adjustments of the reject setting.

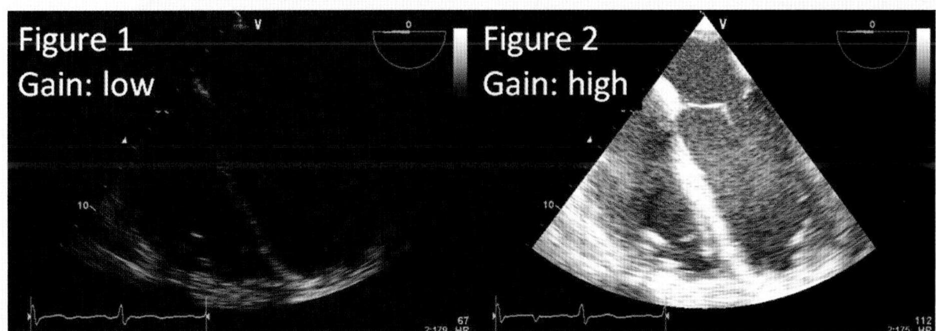

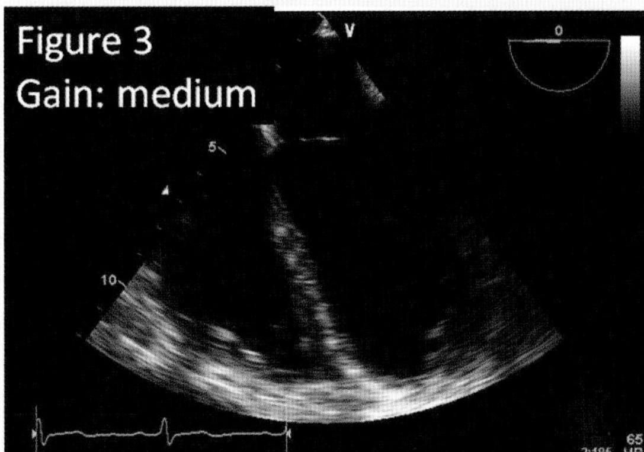

Figure 16.1.

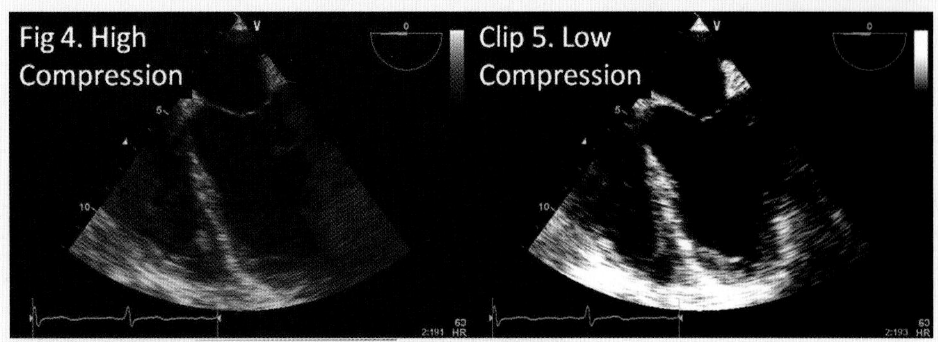

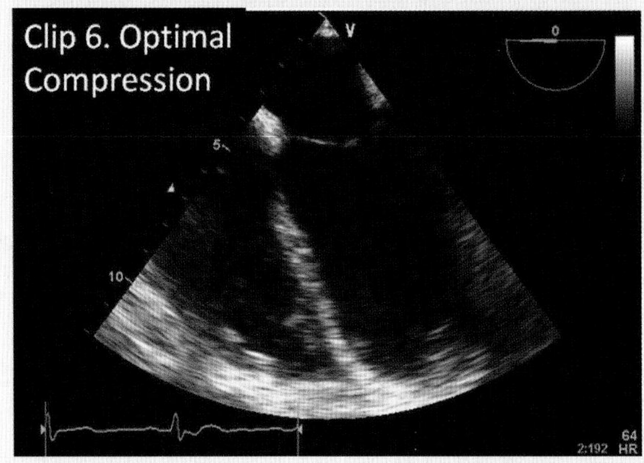

Figure 16.2.

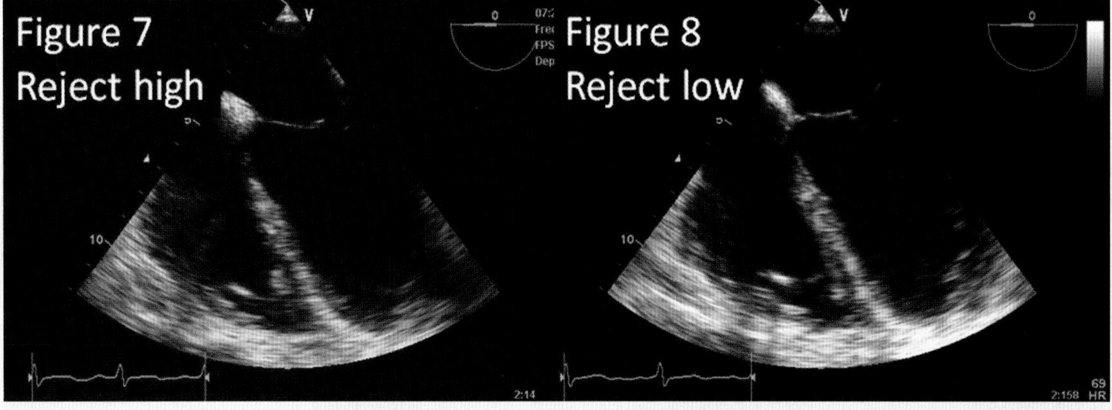

Figure 16.3.

TAKE-HOME LESSON:

The quality of the displayed image is dependent on manipulation of the returning echocardiographic signals. The echocardiographer has the ability to adjust the gain, compression, and reject settings, just to name a few.

SUGGESTED READING

Forsberg E, Adams D. Understanding ultrasound system controls. In: Mathew JP, Ayoub CM, eds. *Clinical Manual and Review of Transesophageal Echocardiography*. New York: McGraw Hill; 2005:16–18.

Malsow A, Perrino AC, Jr. Principles and technology of two-dimensional echocardiography. In: Perrino AC Jr, Reeves ST, eds. *A Practical Approach to Transesophageal Echocardiography*. 2nd ed. Philadelphia: Wolters Kluwer/Lippincott Williams & Wilkins; 2008:17.

CASE 17

An intraoperative TEE in an adult patient prior to elective AVR for AS revealed presence of MR. The MR jet occupied a large area of the left atrium (Fig. 17.1).

QUESTION 17.1. Based on Figure 17.1, what is the diagnosis?

A. Moderate-to-severe MR

B. Mild MR

C. MR is overestimated because of AS

D. CFD gain inappropriate

Further manipulation of CFD settings resulted in a different MR jet (Fig. 17.2).

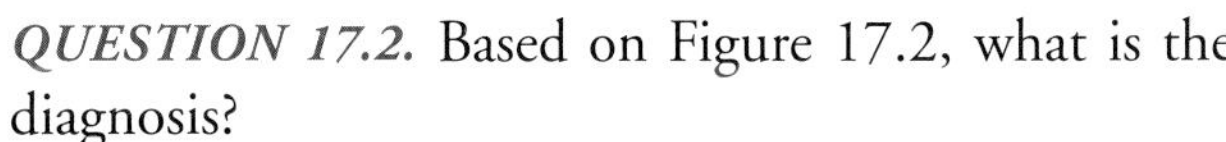

QUESTION 17.2. Based on Figure 17.2, what is the diagnosis?

A. MR is the same

B. MR is worse than before

C. MR is overestimated because of variance mapping

D. MR is accompanied by acceleration of blood in the LVOT

After an uneventful AVR, and following weaning off CPB, CFD of the MV revealed the image shown in Figure 17.3.

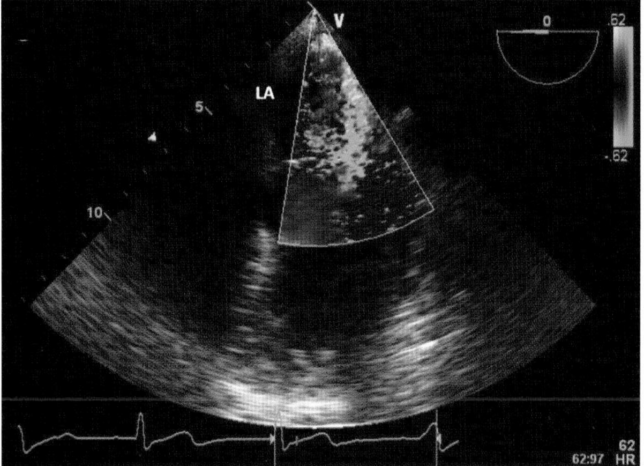

Figure 17.1.

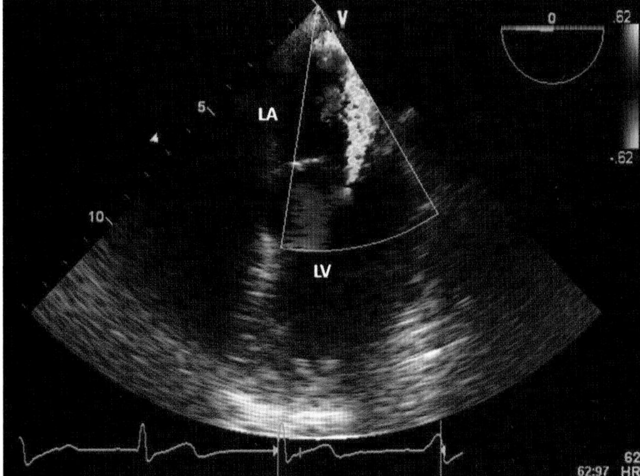

Figure 17.2.

QUESTION 17.3. What is the diagnosis and proper intervention?

A. New MR—return to CBP to address it

B. MR is overestimated because of erroneous CFD scale—continue with protamine

C. MR jet occupies less than 30% of LA volume—leave it alone

D. MR is due to LV outflow obstruction—attempt pharmacologic intervention

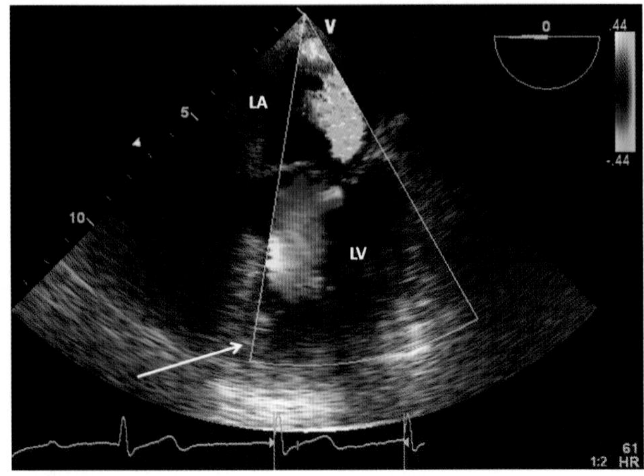

Figure 17.3.

ANSWERS AND DISCUSSION

QUESTION 17.1: The correct answer is D: CFD gain inappropriate.

The MV is evaluated with CFD in the ME 4CH view in Figure 17.1. Proper evaluation with CFD requires the scale to be set at approximately ±60–70 cm/s (here at ±62 cm/s). To optimize imaging, the gain should be increased until color pixels appear within the tissue. Then, CFD gain should be reduced one or two clicks until there are no longer color pixels evident within tissue (Fig. 17.4). Excessive gain (Fig. 17.1) will increase the jet area and result in overestimation of the degree of MR. If the gain is set too low, an underestimation of the degree of regurgitation may occur (Fig. 17.5). Answer C is incorrect; irrespective of AV disease, CFD can be used to evaluate the function of MV. Answers A and B are incorrect because of inappropriate CFD setting.

QUESTION 17.2: The correct answer is A: MR is the same.

The only difference between Figures 17.1 and 17.2 is the presence of variance mapping in the CFD scale. In the CFD, direction is coded with blue if moving away from and red if toward the echocardiographic transducer. The shade of color indicates the velocity (with lighter shades allocated to higher velocities). As demonstrated in Figure 17.6, the addition of green color in the CFD scale allows imaging of blood turbulence, usually associated with increased velocity. When using CFD, the echocardiographer can choose from a variety of color maps, and subsequent exams during the intraoperative course should be performed with the same color map for ease and accuracy of comparison.

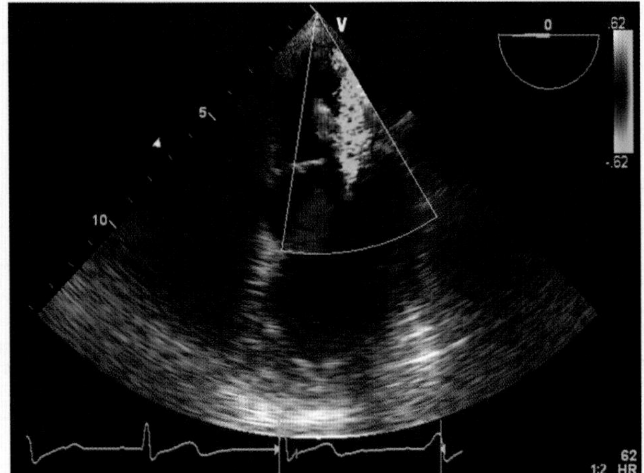

Figure 17.4.

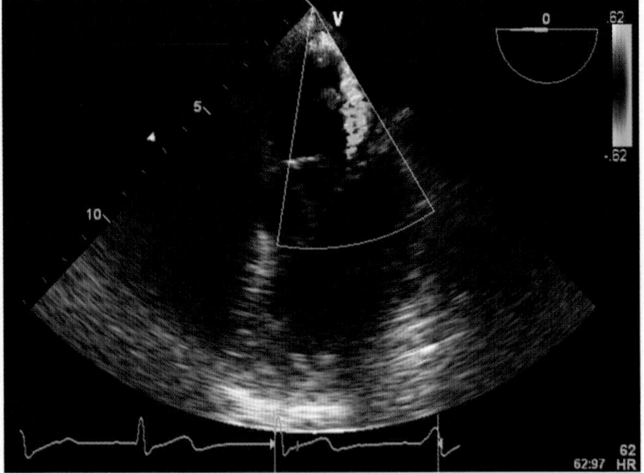

Figure 17.5.

QUESTION 17.3: The correct answer is B: Erroneous CFD setting.

CFD is PW Doppler mode and subjected to the same constraints as conventional PW Doppler: limit of peak velocity and low frame rate. The Nyquist limit (usually in the range of ±60–70 cm/s) is the limit of CFD velocity in either direction. When the sampled velocity exceeds this limit, the color shows "aliasing" and will change to a color shade of the opposite direction (blue shades will turn to red and red shades to blue). Aliasing will misrepresent the direction and magnitude of the velocity. The CFD scale is reduced as the CFD sector increases in size. Here, the CFD sector (arrow) is positioned over a large area and resulted in a decreased Nyquist limit (±42 cm/s). Answer A is incorrect for the above reasons: too low CFD scale. Answer C is incorrect, because the LA size cannot be imaged in its entirety (because it lies in the near field); therefore the comparison between MR jet and LA area is inaccurate. Answer D is incorrect; the red color inside the LV is the result of low CFD scale. Even more, it is resolved without aliasing, which means it is of low velocity, that is laminar flow.

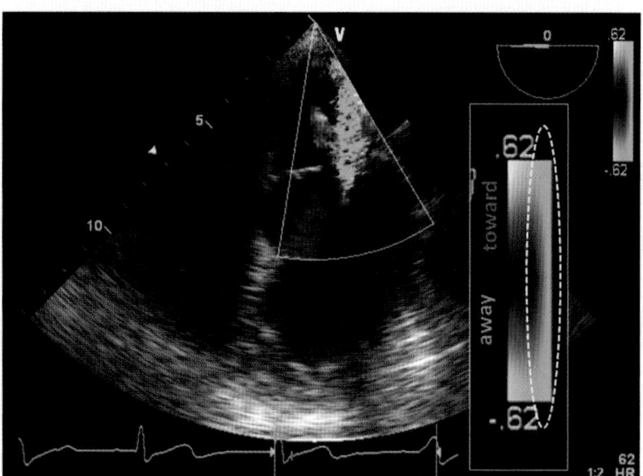

Figure 17.6.

TAKE-HOME LESSON:

Special care must be taken when setting the color Doppler scale to avoid under- or overestimating the degree of regurgitation jets.

CASE 18

A 68-year-old male undergoes CABG for severe three-vessel coronary artery disease. Past medical history is positive for diabetes mellitus, hypertension, CHF, and peripheral vascular disease. On separation from CPB, increasing doses of inotropes are given to manage low cardiac output and blood pressure. A decision is made to insert an IABP. You are asked by the surgical team to assist in positioning the IABP.

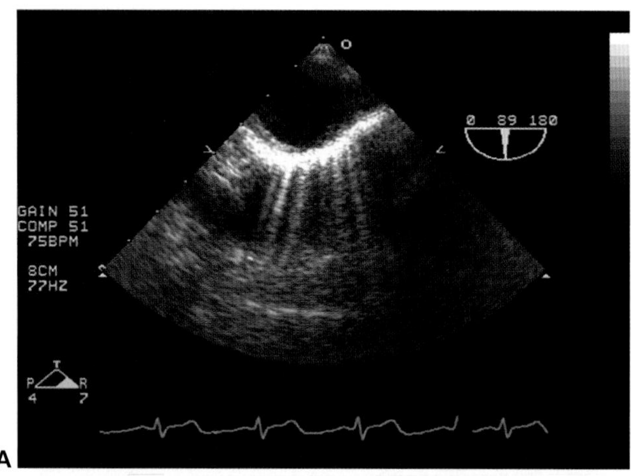

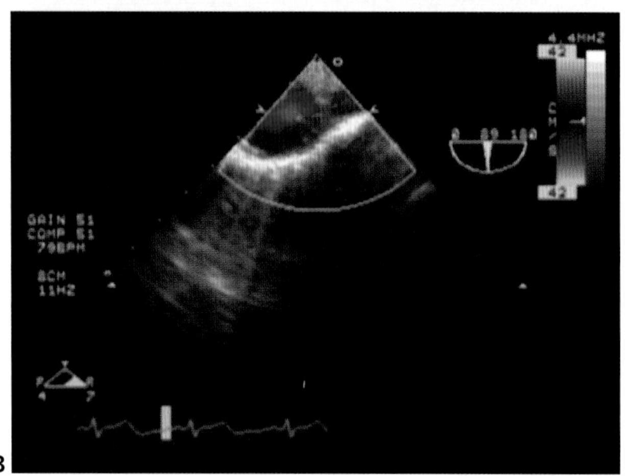

Figure 18.1. **A:** 2D Upper esophageal aortic arch view. **B:** Upper esophageal aortic arch with CFD. (See also Video 18.1.)

QUESTION 18.1. Which TEE imaging level is used to assist positioning of an IABP?

A. Upper esophageal level
B. ME level
C. TG level
D. All of the above

QUESTION 18.2. Which vessel(s) is/are visible in Figure 18.1 and Video 18.1?

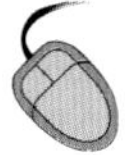

A. Innominate artery
B. Aortic arch
C. Ascending aorta
D. Left subclavian artery
E. Both B and D

The surgeon advances a guide wire through the left femoral artery (Fig. 18.2 and Video 18.2).

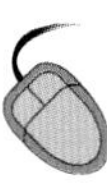

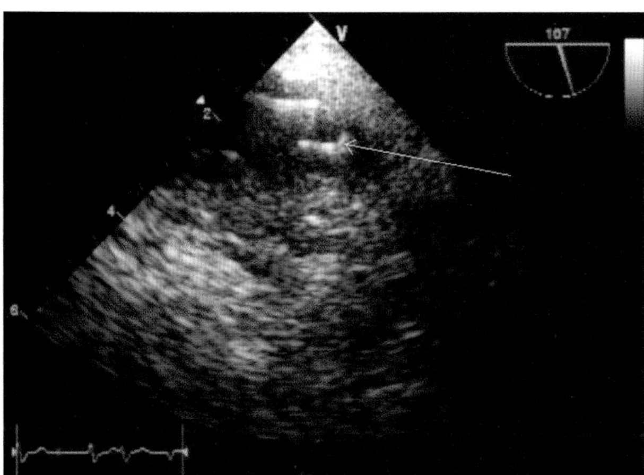

Figure 18.2. LAX of the descending aorta showing a J-wire. (See also Video 18.2.)

QUESTION 18.3. At which aortic location is the guide wire position considered optimal?

A. Aortic arch
B. Immediately proximal to the left subclavian artery
C. Immediately distal to the left subclavian artery
D. Descending aorta

The IABP is inserted as illustrated in Figures 18.3 and 18.4, and Videos 18.3 and 18.4.

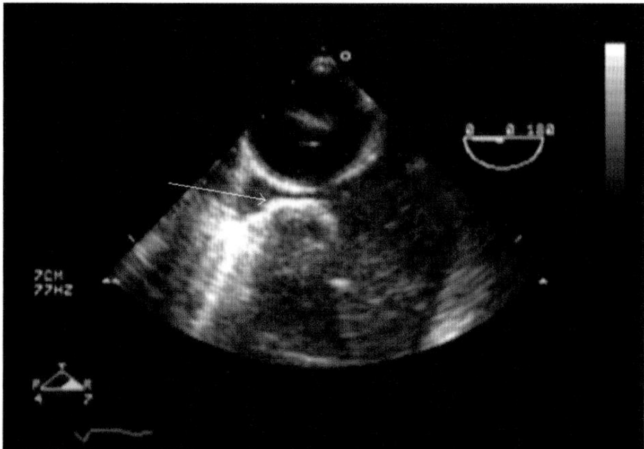

Figure 18.3. Short-axis view of the descending aorta with IABP. (See also Video 18.3.)

QUESTION 18.4. The structure identified by the arrow in Figures 18.3 and 18.4 represents:

A. Mirror image of the IABP
B. Flap of aortic dissection
C. Chest tube
D. Atherosclerosis

QUESTION 18.5. At this point (Fig. 18.5), you would communicate to the surgeon that:

A. The IABP is in the correct position
B. The IABP needs to be advanced
C. The IABP needs to be withdrawn
D. There is an intramural aortic hematoma

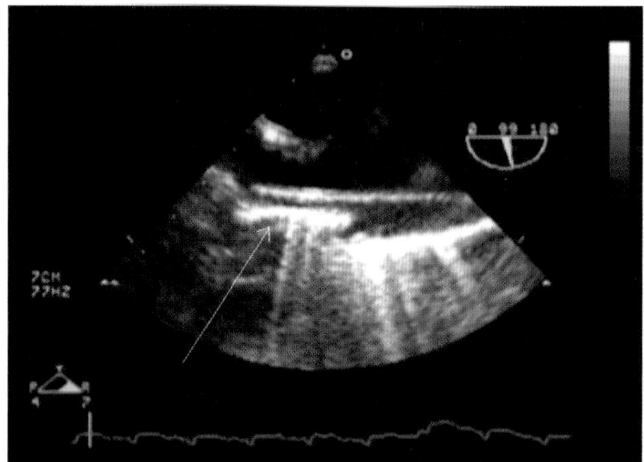

Figure 18.4. LAX of the descending aorta with IABP. (See also Video 18.4.)

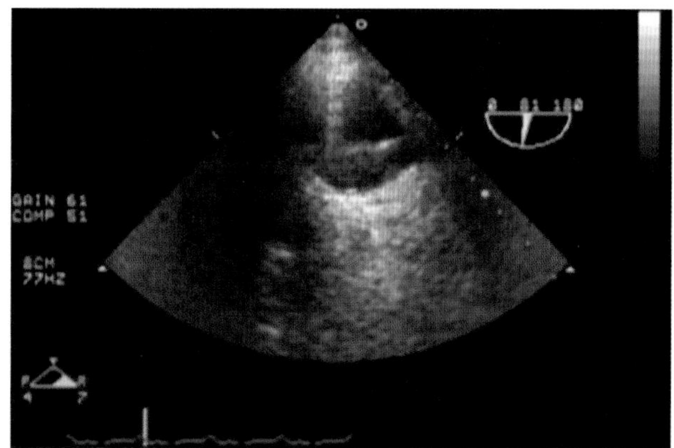

Figure 18.5. 2D aorta with inserted IABP. (See also Video 18.5.)

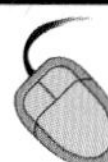

ANSWERS AND DISCUSSION

QUESTION 18.1: The correct answer is D: All of the above.

A full examination of the aorta at all the three levels is of an utmost importance. Examination of the aorta at the upper esophageal level identifies the aortic arch and the left subclavian artery, the ME level examines the ascending and descending aorta, and the TG level examines the descending aorta. Prior to the insertion of the IABP, it is important to diagnose aortic disease, such as the degree of atherosclerosis and the presence of mobile plaques. Presence of severe atherosclerotic disease, aortic dissection, or aneurysm may preclude insertion of the IABP. During the insertion of the guide wire, full examination is required to visualize the intraluminal presence of the wire and to rule out aortic dissection, and to determine the anatomic location of the IABP in relation to major cerebral vessels to ensure proper positioning.

QUESTION 18.2: The correct answer is D: Aortic arch and left subclavian artery.

Figure 18.1 and Video 18.1 show a short-axis view of the aortic arch with the take off of the left subclavian artery seen at the 2 o'clock position with red CFD. The left carotid artery and the innominate arteries are rarely visualized with TEE secondary to the interposition of the air-filled trachea between these structures and the TEE probe.

QUESTION 18.3: The correct answer is C: Immediately distal to the left subclavian artery.

The proper positioning of the IABP is 2 to 4 cm distal to take off of the left subclavian artery. As illustrated in Figure 18.2, the J-wire has been advanced in the descending aorta from the distal (left side of screen) to the proximal (right side of screen). The IABP is optimally placed between the left subclavian artery and the renal arteries to achieve the most benefit on coronary perfusion and afterload reduction. More distal placement can compromise renal blood flow. Placement of the IABP proximal to the left subclavian artery in the aortic arch increases the risk of embolization to the cerebral vessels and occlusion of the left subclavian artery.[1]

QUESTION 18.4: The correct answer is C: Chest tube.

Answer A, mirror image of the IABP, is incorrect because the IABP and the structure at the arrow are not at equidistant from each other. A mirror image is an artifact that occurs when strong echoes are reflected from the transducer itself. The reflection then travels back to the same target, where it is echoed a second time back toward the transducer. This results in an artifact that appears at double the distance of the reflecting structure from the transducer.[2] An example of a mirror artifact from the strongly reflective IABP is shown in Figure 18.6. Answers B and D are incorrect because the structure shown lies outside the lumen of the aorta.

QUESTION 18.5: The correct answer is C. The IABP needs to be withdrawn.

This is an upper esophageal view of the aortic arch with reverberation artifact from the trachea. Reverberations are caused by the repeated back-and-forth reflections of an ultrasound wave between two strong specular reflectors.[2] Presence of the IABP at that level is not optimal as it increases the risk of cerebral embolization and occlusion of the arch vessels.

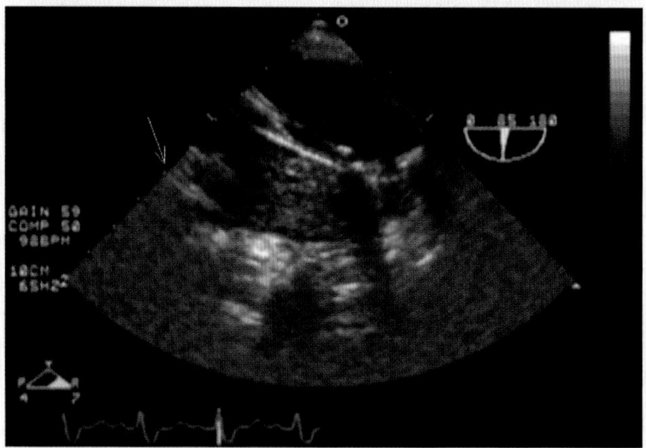

Figure 18.6. LAX of the descending aorta with IABP. The arrow is pointing to a mirror image of the highly reflective IABP. (See also Video 18.6.)

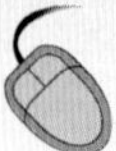

TAKE-HOME LESSON:

TEE examination of the aorta assists in the placement of an IABP by identifying potential aortic pathology and injury as well as by confirming proper positioning. The optimal positioning of the tip of the IABP is 2 to 4 cm distal to the take off of the left subclavian artery.

REFERENCES

1. Miller JP, Perrino AC Jr, Hillel Z. Man and machine. In: Perrino A, Reeves S, eds. *A Practical Approach to Transesophageal Echocardiography*. 2nd ed. Philadelphia: Lippincott Williams & Wilkins; 2007.
2. Kim JT, Lee JR, Kim JK, et al. The carina as a useful radiographic landmark for positioning the intra-aortic balloon pump. *Anesth Analg*. 2007;105(3):735–738.

CASE 19

A 65-year-old female presented with chest pain, new-onset seizure activity, and pulmonary edema. After a negative coronary work-up, a TTE was done showing a large mass in the left atrium attached to the septum and posterior wall. Prior to surgical resection, intraoperative TEE evaluation of this mass was performed (Fig. 19.1 and Videos 19.1 and 19.2).

QUESTION 19.1. What is seen in the left atrium?

A. Thrombus in the LAA
B. ASD
C. Chiari network
D. A large myxoma

QUESTION 19.2. Where is the most likely site for the mass's attachment?

A. Posterior LA wall
B. Interatrial septum
C. Lateral MV annulus
D. Coumadin ridge

QUESTION 19.3. LA myxomas can be composed of what type of tissue?

A. Cardiac muscle
B. Lipomatous tissue
C. Mucopolysaccharide matrix
D. Calcium deposits

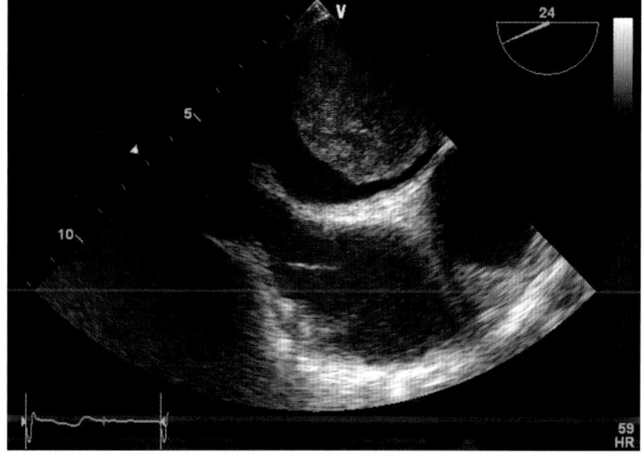

Figure 19.1. ME 4CH view.

QUESTION 19.4. A patient with LAA myxoma typically present with:

A. Dyspnea
B. Syncope
C. CHF
D. All of the above

ANSWERS AND DISCUSSION

QUESTION 19.1: The correct answer is D: A large myxoma. In this ME 4CH view, a large LA mass, most likely a myxoma is seen without any specific attachment sites.

QUESTION 19.2: The correct answer is B: Interatrial septum. After a thorough exam of the mass from multiple views and varying scan planes, it appears that this atrial myxoma has a broad-based attachment to the interatrial septum.

QUESTION 19.3: The correct answer is C: Mucopolysaccharide matrix. Myxomas contain a mucopolysaccharide myxoid matrix with an inhomogeneous configuration of channels, cystic areas, hemorrhage, and calcification.

QUESTION 19.4: The correct answer is D: All of the above. A typical triad of symptoms result from embolization, obstruction, and constitutional symptoms such as dyspnea, positional-related palpitations, syncope, CHF, and sudden death. Emboli can cause acute coronary and cerebrovascular events. Myxomas that are very mobile, attached by a pedicle can actually create a "ball-valve" effect (see Videos 19.1 and 19.2), occluding MV in flow resulting in syncope.

TAKE-HOME LESSON:

Determination of the attachment site of the myxoma is important to designing the appropriate surgical plan for resection of any intracardiac mass.

SUGGESTED READING

Jadbabaie F. Cardiac masses and embolic sources. In: Perrino A, Reeves ST, eds. *A Practical Approach to Transesophageal Echocardiography*. 2nd ed. Philadelphia: Lippincott Williams & Wilkins; 2008:401–402.

Basic

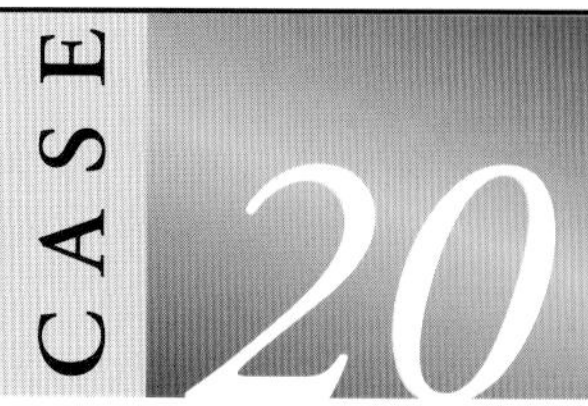

CASE 20

A 62-year-old woman undergoes cardiac surgery to fix her severe MR. Immediately after separation from CPB, you obtain the images seen in Figure 20.1 and Video 20.1.

QUESTION 20.1. What operation was performed on the patient's MV?

A. A mitral repair and prosthetic ring was inserted
B. A bioprosthetic MV was inserted
C. A tilting disc mechanical MV was inserted
D. A bileaflet mechanical MV was inserted
E. No operation was performed on the MV

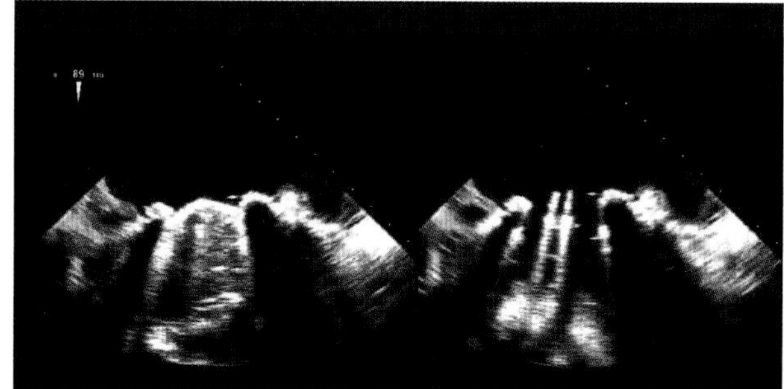

Figure 20.1. ME 4CH view of the MV in systole (left) and in diastole (right). See also Video 20.1.

QUESTION 20.2. Video 20.2 shows a color compare view of the patient's MV. What finding does the CFD show?

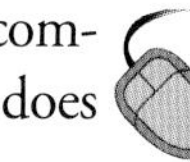

A. CFD shows abnormal severe MR
B. CFD suggests significant mitral stenosis
C. CFD shows a normal amount of MR
D. CFD does not show any MR
E. CFD shows a significant paravalvular leak

QUESTION 20.3. Spectral Doppler interrogation of the patient's valve yields the tracing shown in Figure 20.2. What does the green arrow point to?

A. A normal finding
B. An indication of severe stenosis
C. An abnormal regurgitation jet
D. A significant paravalvular leak
E. A sign of valve dehiscence

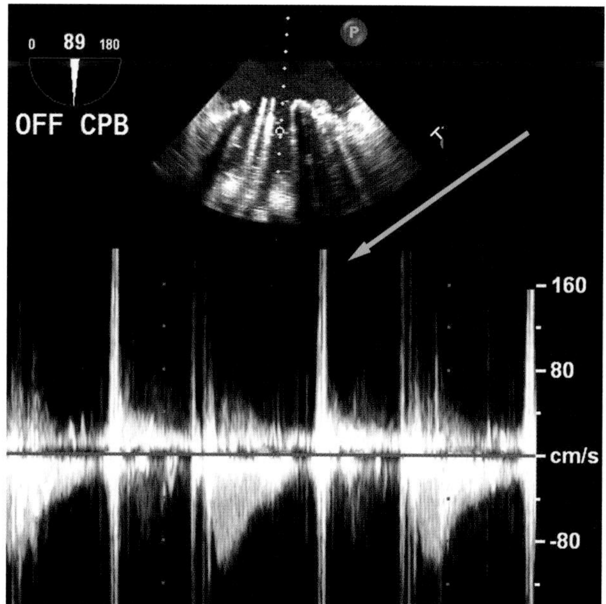

Figure 20.2. CW Doppler of the MV.

QUESTION 20.4. To estimate the mean diastolic pressure gradient across the MV involves:

A. Doppler measurement of peak velocity of diastolic transvalvular flow
B. Tracing of diastolic transmitral velocity envelope
C. Calculation of PHT
D. Estimation of LA pressure
E. Continuity equation

QUESTION 20.5. A mean gradient of 4.5 mm Hg is obtained by tracing out the mitral VTI from the spectral Doppler tracing in Figure 20.1. The next appropriate thing to do is:

A. Inform the surgeon that one of the leaflets is stuck
B. Administer thrombolytics to try to dissolve the occluding thrombus
C. Replace the valve with a larger-sized prosthesis
D. Examine the valve again for a paravalvular leak
E. Administer protamine since interrogation of the valve is normal

ANSWERS AND DISCUSSION

QUESTION 20.1: The correct answer is D: A bileaflet mechanical valve was inserted in this patient. This type of valve consists of two rigid leaflets attached to a carbon ring at recessed hinge points. Figure 20.1 and Video 20.1 clearly demonstrate *two* leaflets opening and closing. The leaflets pivot open to about 80 degrees, creating two lateral orifices and a central one. The normal closing angle of the leaflets is about 30 to 35 degrees from the horizontal. By contrast, a tilting disc valve (answer C) consists of a single large disc that travels along a central strut, creating two orifices. A stented bioprosthetic valve (answer B) consists of a semi-flexible frame, which provides support for the valve leaflets. These can be made from pig valves or bovine pericardium. Because the leaflets are made of tissue, they are clearly visible on TEE, while the struts of the support frame create shadowing artifact. Examples of both a tilting disc mechanical valve and a stented bioprosthetic valve are shown in Figure 20.3. If a mitral repair had been done (answer A), the patient would still have her native leaflets.

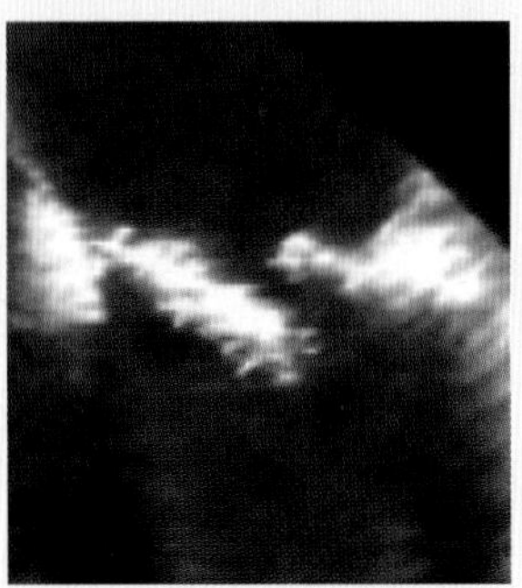

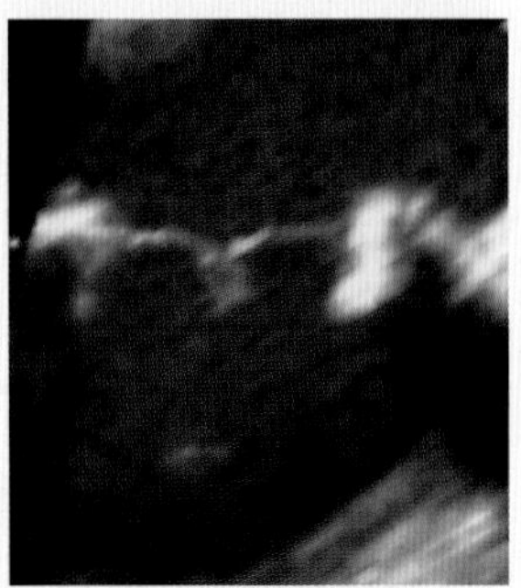

Figure 20.3. Example of a single tilting disc mechanical valve (left) and a bioprosthetic valve (right).

QUESTION 20.2: The correct answer is C. The CFD panel demonstrates a normal amount of MR.

Every modern mechanical valve allows a small amount of regurgitation around the leaflets to reduce the risk of thrombus formation. These normal "wash jets" are typically located at the hinge points and can be seen as small, discrete, wisps of color when the valve closes. They tend to be low velocity and do not extend more than a centimeter or so into the left atrium. A typical small wash jet is pointed out by the arrow in Figure 20.4. It would be unusual to see absolutely no regurgitation coming from a mechanical valve. It is important to remember that these normal regurgitation jets originate from inside the sewing ring and they

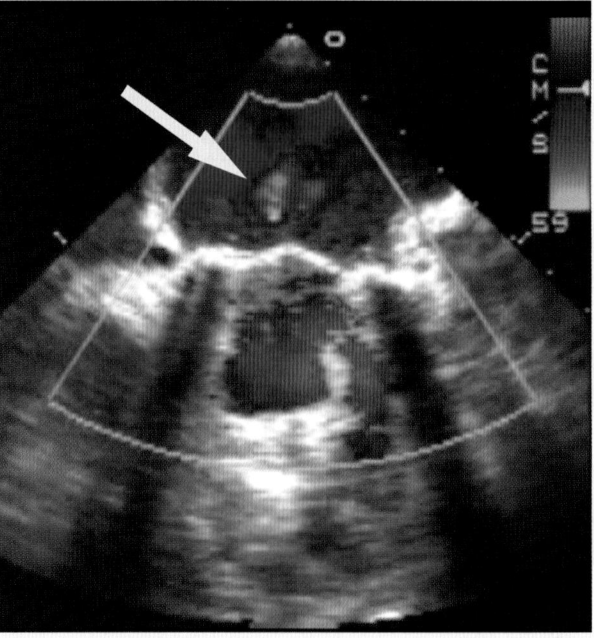

Figure 20.4. ME 4CH view with CFD, showing the normal wash jets of the MV prosthesis.

should not be confused with paravalvular leaks. Paravalvular leaks are abnormal and they originate from outside of the sewing ring. This patient does not have any regurgitant jet outside the sewing ring. Finally, the CFD in this patient does not suggest significant stenosis.

QUESTION 20.3: The correct answer is A. The arrow points to a normal finding. This very high amplitude signal, commonly referred to as a valve "click," can often be seen during opening and closing of a mechanical valve leaflet (more pronounced when the valve closes). An ultrasound transducer is a very sophisticated listening device and the same clicking sound that can be heard with a stethoscope can also be displayed graphically on the spectral Doppler signal. The actual sound can be made audible by turning on the echo machine's volume while performing a spectral Doppler interrogation. There is nothing pathologic about this signal.

QUESTION 20.4: The correct answer is B: Tracing of the diastolic transmitral velocity envelope.

As the mean pressure gradient represents the average of the instantaneous pressure gradients throughout diastole a tracing of the complete diastolic velocity profile is required. Doppler measurement of peak velocity of diastolic transvalvular flow (answer A) is thus not sufficient. Calculation of PHT (answer C) is also used to determine severity of mitral stenosis and is used to estimate valve area, not pressure gradient. Answers D and E are incorrect as estimation of LA pressure is not required as the pressure gradient is estimated by the Bernoulli equation, where pressure gradient is calculated as four times the square of transvalvular blood velocity.

QUESTION 20.5: The correct answer is D. The next step should be to administer protamine since interrogation of the valve is normal. Spectral Doppler should be performed on all prosthetic valves as part of a complete valve evaluation. Unusually high gradients can be a warning sign of a valve obstruction and must be investigated closely. Valve gradients, however, should always be interpreted with caution in the immediate post-CPB period, since many factors can lead to higher than normal flows across the valve. These factors include the administration of inotropes, changes in loading conditions, and a hyperdynamic state following separation from CPB. Thus, a prosthetic valve gradient must be interpreted in light of the cardiac output and loading conditions at the time of the measurement. As a general rule, smaller valves produce higher gradients, but in the mitral position, a mean gradient <10 mm Hg is expected for just about any type and size of prosthetic valve. A summary of the expected Doppler findings for various types and sizes of prosthetic heart valves is found in the suggested reading section below.

TAKE-HOME LESSON:

There are several types of mechanical prosthetic valves on the market. Each has a particular appearance and Doppler flow characteristics on echo. After mechanical MV replacement, a detailed echo examination will allow early diagnosis of prosthetic valve dysfunction and establish a baseline, with which future examinations can be compared.

SUGGESTED READING

Appendix D: Valve Prostheses. In: Perrino AC, Reeves ST, eds. *A Practical Approach to Transesophageal Echocardiography.* 2nd ed. Philadelphia: Lippincott Williams & Wilkins, 2008:457–464.

Rosenheck R, Binder T, Maurer G, et al. Normal values for Doppler echocardiographic assessment of heart valve prosthesis. *J Am Soc Echocardiogr.* 2003;16:116–127.

CASE 21

A 75-year-old male with long-standing history of hypertension and dyspnea on exertion is scheduled to undergo elective coronary revascularization. He has a systolic ejection murmur best audible over the cardiac apex and is diagnosed with MR.

QUESTION 21.1. The TMF pattern, recorded with a PW Doppler sample positioned between the tips of the MV, is seen in Figure 21.1. The best way to resolve the spectral signal (asterisk) is to:

A. Increase the Doppler velocity scale
B. Switch to CW Doppler
C. Move the zero velocity baseline
D. Switch to a different view

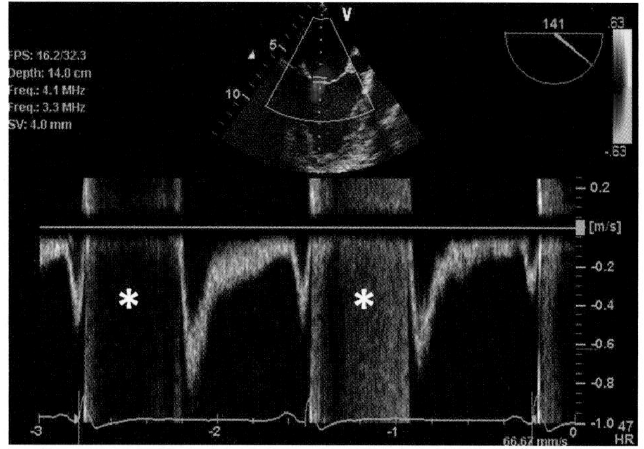

Figure 21.1. Intraoperative TEE with CFD reveals a central MR jet (Video 21.1). Manipulation of the settings results in a different MR jet (Video 21.2).

QUESTION 21.2. The different appearance of MR jet is due to a change of:

A. Frequency of transducer
B. Nyquist scale
C. Nyquist baseline
D. Sector depth

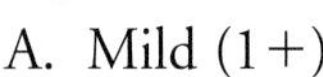

QUESTION 21.3. As seen in Video 21.1 and Figure 21.2, the MR is graded as:

A. Mild (1+)
B. Mild-to-moderate (2+)
C. Moderate-to-severe (3+)
D. Severe (4+)

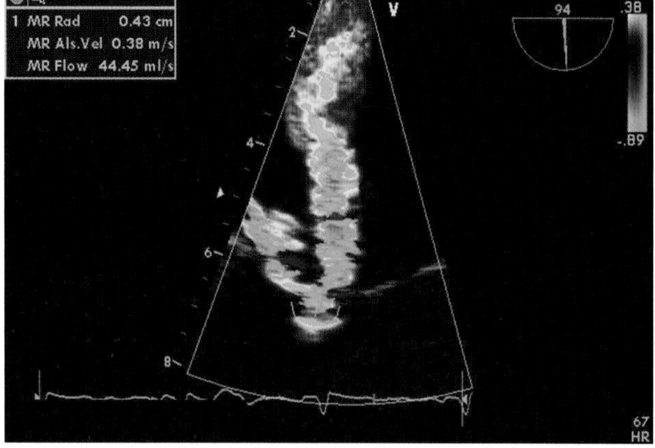

Figure 21.2.

ANSWERS AND DISCUSSION

QUESTION 21.1: The correct answer is B: Switch to CW Doppler.

Switching to CW Doppler will resolve the peak velocity (Fig. 21.3). The loss of spatial resolution can be compensated for by the 2D imaging on the top of the spectral display, which reveals that the velocity is due to MR.

Answer A—increasing the Doppler velocity scale—is incorrect. PW Doppler cannot resolve velocities faster than 1.5 m/s. The peak of the recorded systolic velocity is not apparent in the spectral display and will probably not resolve even if the PW Doppler is increased from 1.25 to 1.5 m/s. Answer C—moving the zero baseline—is also incorrect. The peak velocity is far too fast to be "fitted" in either the top or the bottom of the zero velocity baseline. Switching to a different view (answer D) will not correct the problem as the problem may be encountered again.

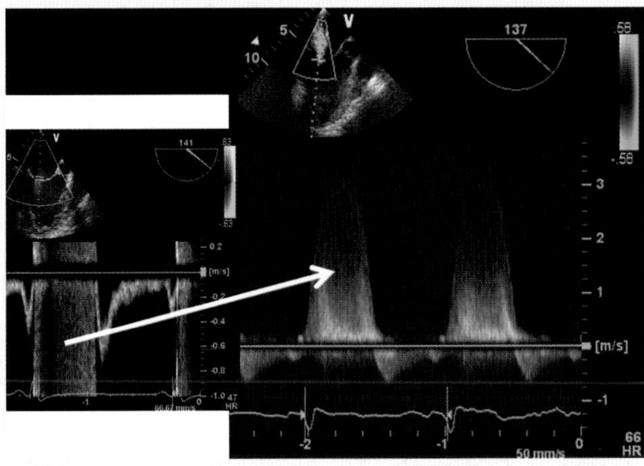

Figure 21.3.

QUESTION 21.2: The correct answer is C: Nyquist baseline.

In Video 21.2, the Nyquist baseline has been shifted upward. Now, the range of resolvable velocities is not the same: velocities up to 38 cm/s can be resolved if directed toward the transducer, and up to 89 cm/s if directed away from the transducer. Adjusting the transducer frequency will result in a change of frame rate of the moving image only (temporal resolution and frequency are inversely related). The upper and lower limits in Video 21.1 are +64 cm/s and −64 cm/s, respectively, for an absolute velocity scale of 128 cm/s. The upper and lower limits in Video 21.2 are +38 cm/s and −89 cm/s, for an absolute velocity scale of 127 cm/s. The Nyquist scale in either video is the same (128 cm/s vs. 127 cm/s). As can be seen in the left side of the sector, depth remains unchanged at 8 cm.

QUESTION 21.3: The correct answer is A: Mild (1+).

In MR, the Nyquist baseline shift is utilized to make the upward moving velocities (from the LV to the left atrium) alias early. In this way, the velocity "front" is easier to identify, and its radius can be measured. Assuming that MR occurs on the flat underside of the LV side of the mitral annulus, the measured radius (r) is used to estimate the ERO of the incompetent MV: ERO = $r^2/2$. This is based on the premise that the average MR jet has a velocity of 5 m/s. The measured radius is 0.4 cm, and the estimated ERO is 0.08 cm (<0.2 cm), which characterizes the MR jet as mild.

TAKE-HOME LESSON:

PW Doppler cannot resolve velocities faster than 1.5 m/s and hence CW Doppler must be used.

SUGGESTED READING

Dyal HW, Frith MD, Reeves ST. Techniques and tricks for optimizing transesophageal images In: Perrino AC Jr, Reeves ST, eds. *A Practical Approach to Transesophageal Echocardiography*. 2nd ed. Philadelphia: Wolters Kluwer/Lippincott Williams & Wilkins; 2008:435–450.

CASE 22

A 67-year-old woman was scheduled for MV surgery. A PW Doppler sample volume was placed in the LVOT (deep TG LAX). The spectral display is shown in Figure 22.1. There are systolic (1) and diastolic (2) velocities.

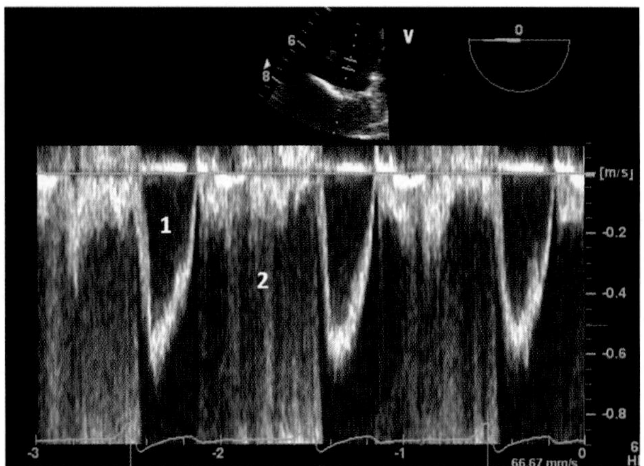

Figure 22.1.

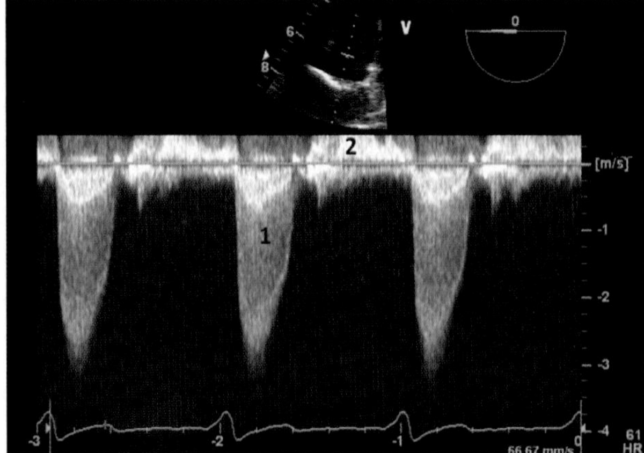

Figure 22.2.

QUESTION 22.1. Which of the following is correct?

A. There is no AS

B. There is MR

C. There is aortic regurgitation

D. There is subvalvular AS

QUESTION 22.2. What are the necessary adjustments in order to improve imaging?

A. Switch to CW Doppler

B. Decrease the velocity scale

C. Shift the velocity scale downward

D. Decrease the Doppler gain

Following adjustments, the spectral display is shown in Figure 22.2. There are systolic (1) and diastolic (2) velocities.

QUESTION 22.3. What are the necessary adjustments in order to improve imaging of both (1) and (2) velocities?

A. Switch to PW Doppler

B. Increase the velocity scale

C. Shift the velocity baseline downward

D. Decrease the Doppler gain

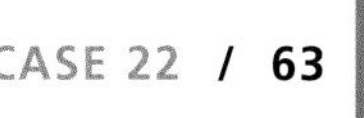

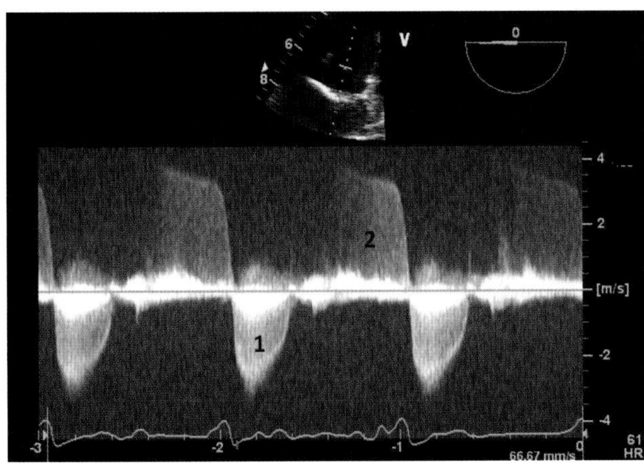

Figure 22.3.

Following further adjustments, the spectral display is shown in Figure 22.3.

ANSWERS AND DISCUSSION

QUESTION 22.1: The correct answer is C: There is aortic regurgitation.

In the deep TG LAX view, the sample volume is just proximal to the AV. The velocities displayed arise from within the sample volume. Velocities away from the transducer are displayed below the zero velocity baseline, while those moving toward the transducer will be displayed above the zero velocity baseline. Velocity (2) is diastolic, but cannot be resolved within this velocity range—0.2 to 1.0 m/s. Nevertheless, it arises from the LV outflow area, and is suspicious for aortic regurgitation.

ANSWER A: *There is no AS* is incorrect. Presence or absence of AS depends on maximum transaortic valve peak velocity, mean gradient, and AVA. Neither of these is present in Figure 22.1.

ANSWER B: *There is MR* is incorrect. The sample volume is not within the mitral annulus, and neither velocity is associated with MR.

ANSWER D: *There is subvalvular AS* is incorrect. If that was the case, the velocity envelope should have a gradually accelerating upslope and peak velocity should have been higher. Systolic velocity (1) has a peak velocity of 0.7 m/s. Using the simplified Bernoulli equation (pressure gradient = 4 V^2_{max}), the pressure gradient in the LVOT has a value of <4 mm Hg. This is not consistent with subvalvular stenosis.

QUESTION 22.2: The correct answer is A: Switch to CW Doppler.

Velocity tracing (1) has a well-delineated, thin modal velocity, and is directed downward. Velocity tracing (2) is too high for the Doppler scale, exceeds the Nyquist limit (the velocity scale is set from +10 cm/s to −90 cm/s), and neither peak velocity nor direction can be visualized. As a result, it appears to "wrap-around" itself. This inability of PW Doppler to accurately describe peak velocity and direction is called "aliasing." Switching to CW Doppler will increase the maximum recordable velocity and will resolve both direction and peak velocity of signal (2).

ANSWER B: *Decrease the velocity scale* is incorrect. Obviously, decreasing the velocity will further worsen imaging, as aliasing will affect velocity (1) as well.

ANSWER C: *Shift the velocity scale downward* is incorrect. Shifting the velocity baseline will sometimes resolve the velocity ambiguity due to spectral Doppler aliasing if the peak velocity minimally exceeds the Nyquist limit. In this example, shifting the baseline will not resolve the velocities, as the velocity range (0–100 cm/s) will remain the same and wrap around of the velocity will still occur.

ANSWER D: *Decrease the Doppler gain* is incorrect. The velocity envelopes are thin and crisp, which means that the Doppler gain is set right.

QUESTION 22.3: The correct answer is B: Increase the velocity scale.

This will increase the range of velocities that can be resolved and will be able to display both systolic (1) and diastolic (2) velocities.

ANSWER A: *Switch to PW Doppler* is incorrect, as the maximum scale in PW Doppler is usually <1.5 m/s.

ANSWER C: *Shift the baseline downward* is incorrect. This may display diastolic velocity (2) but will result in aliasing of systolic velocity (1).

ANSWER D: *Decrease the Doppler gain* is incorrect. This will change only the appearance of the displayed velocities, leaving the velocity range unaffected.

TAKE-HOME LESSON:

PW Doppler offers spatial resolution but is limited to a maximum velocity of ≤1.5 m/s. Switching to CW Doppler will increase the maximum velocity resolved but without spatial resolution.

SUGGESTED READING

Quiñones MA, Otto CM, Stoddard M, et al. Recommendations for quantification of Doppler echocardiography: a report from the Doppler Quantification Task Force of the Nomenclature and Standards Committee of the American Society of Echocardiography. *J Am Soc Echocardiogr.* 2002;15:167–184.

CASE 23

A 70-year-old man with severe AS presents for AVR. During the intraoperative transesophageal echocardiographic examination you perform Doppler interrogation of the blood flow across the AV.

QUESTION 23.1. Figure 23.1 was obtained by using CW Doppler in the deep TG LAX view. The Doppler spectra above the baseline represent:

A. AI

B. MR

C. TMF

D. Mitral stenosis

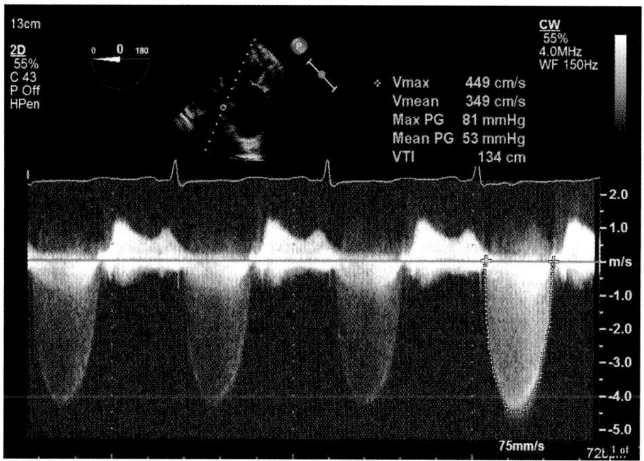

Figure 23.1. CW Doppler display.

QUESTION 23.2. What spectral Doppler display is shown in Figure 23.2?

A. CW Doppler

B. PW Doppler

C. PW Doppler with aliasing

D. High pulse repetition frequency Doppler

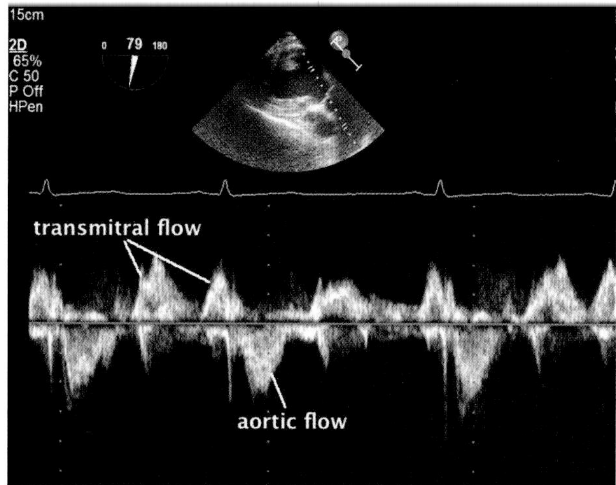

Figure 23.2. Doppler interrogation in the TG LAX view.

ANSWERS AND DISCUSSION

QUESTION 23.1: The correct answer is C: TMF.

CW Doppler echocardiography uses two transducers, one to continuously transmit and the second to continuously receive ultrasound signals. This approach avoids the limitation in maximal velocity measurements seen with PW Doppler techniques. However, CW Doppler introduces range ambiguity as it measures all velocities encountered along the ultrasound beam path. Thus it provides no information on the specific location from where each velocity occurs.

By applying CW Doppler in the deep TG LAX view through the AV, the ultrasound beam will intercept the flow through the AV as well as the TMF, which crosses the beam path as it enters the LV cavity (Fig. 23.3).

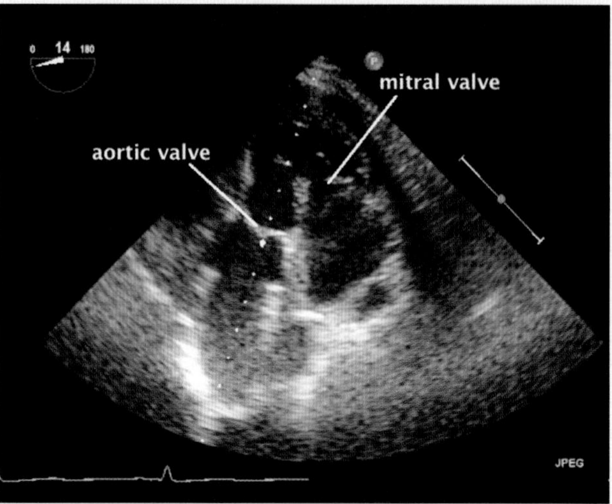

Figure 23.3. Deep TG LAX view with the cursor placed across the AV and the LVOT.

The CW Doppler spectrum biphasic envelope seen in diastole corresponds to the E and A wave of the early and late diastolic TMF. AI, answer A, can also present during diastole on the CW spectral display. However, AI would be distinguished by its much higher velocities and Doppler profile lacking a biphasic appearance (Fig. 23.4). MR interrogated by CW Doppler in the deep TG LAX view would appear as a negative velocity envelope (below the baseline due to blood flowing away from the transducer) at much higher velocities and occurring during systole. Mitral stenosis profile would be similar to the TMF profile with fused E and A waves and higher velocities.

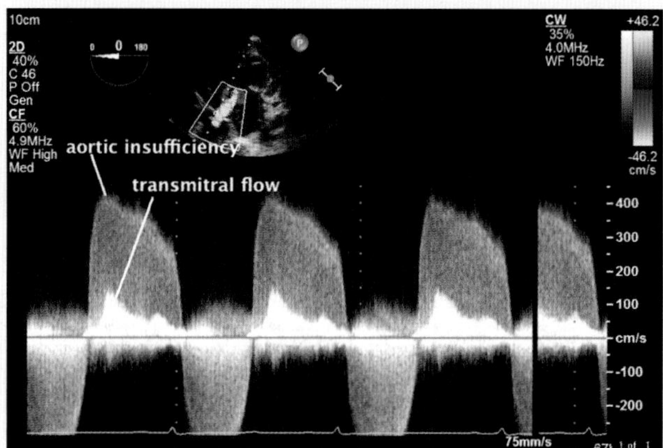

Figure 23.4. CW Doppler in the deep TG LAX view in a patient with AI.

Range ambiguity of CW Doppler can frequently present diagnostic challenges to the echocardiographer. For example, in the TG LAX view, the CW Doppler ultrasound beam applied through the AV may also intercept flow through the MV (Figs. 23.5 and 23.6). In the ME 4CH view in patients with LVAD, the CW Doppler ultrasound beam will intercept both the flow through the LVAD cannula placed in the LV apex and the flow through the MV. In these situations, when employing CW Doppler, the clinician should be aware of the location generating the highest velocities along the Doppler beam or should measure the velocities in an imaging view where the Doppler beam is not intercepting blood flow from various sources.

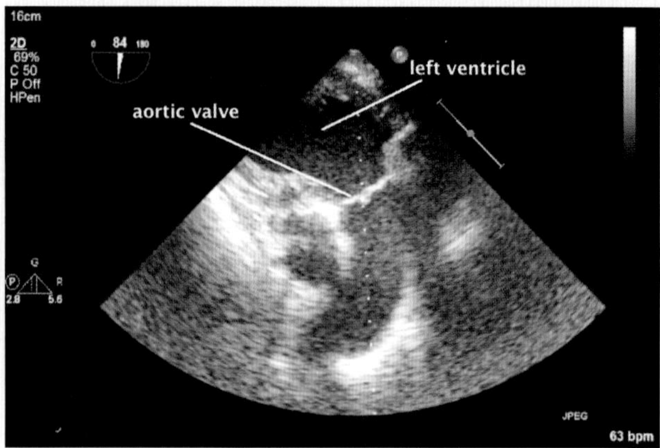

Figure 23.5. TG LAX axis view with the cursor placed across the AV and the LVOT.

QUESTION 23.2: The correct answer is D: High pulse repetition frequency Doppler as Figure 23.2 shows two sample volumes (gates) along the Doppler beam measuring velocities: the distal gate positioned in the target of interest, which is the ascending aorta and resulting in the velocity envelope below the baseline in the spectral display, and the second gate (proximal gate) that lies in the LV and intercepts TMF seen as the biphasic velocity envelope above the baseline in the spectral display.

High pulse repetition frequency Doppler is selected in situations where the PRF with standard PW Doppler is too low to measure the target velocity. When the sample volume is placed far from the transducer, the PRF is low and the Nyquist limit leads to aliasing. Inadequate PRF occurs in this situation because the aorta lies in the far field and the blood flow velocities are high. To avoid this limitation high pulse repetition frequency Doppler was selected. The principle of high pulse repetition frequency Doppler is to emit a second or third pulse signal before the first signal has returned. In this way the PRF is doubled or tripled; however, it introduces additional sample volumes proximal to the target that introduces range ambiguity as the operator is not sure whether the velocities are sampled at the intended location or at more proximal locations. In this case, the timing of flow and the distinctive profiles allow the echocardiographer to interpret the spectral display correctly and avoid misdiagnosis.

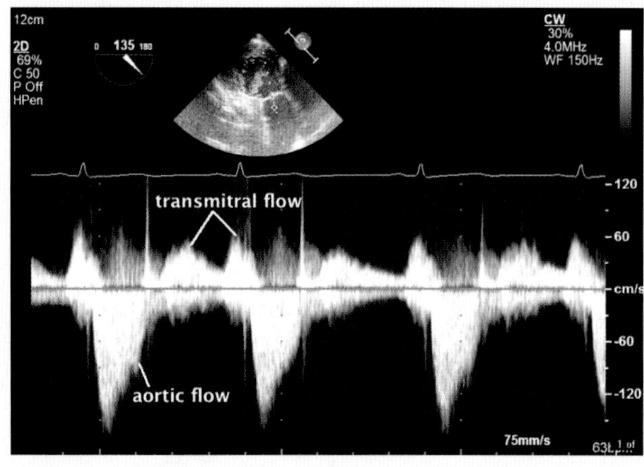

Figure 23.6. CW Doppler spectral display in the TG LAX view.

TAKE-HOME LESSON:

Range ambiguity of CW Doppler can frequently present diagnostic challenges to the echocardiographer.

Basic

CASE 24

A 58-year-old woman with a history of rheumatic fever presented to the hospital with a chief complaint of dyspnea. Rheumatic heart disease was suspected and she underwent a TEE, which yielded the images seen in Figures 24.1 and 24.2 and Videos 24.1 and 24.2.

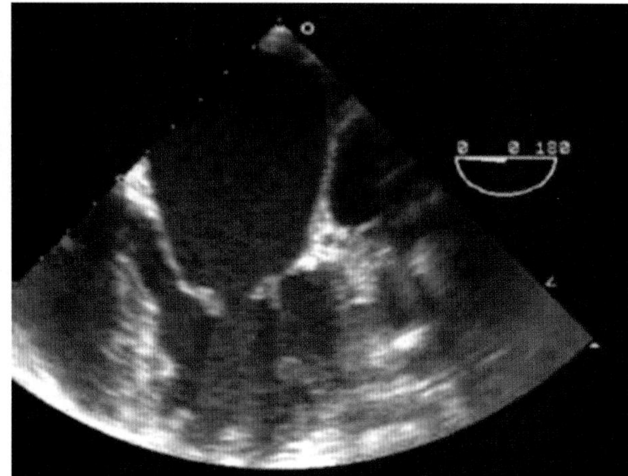

Figure 24.1. ME 4CH view, 2D. See also Video 24.1.

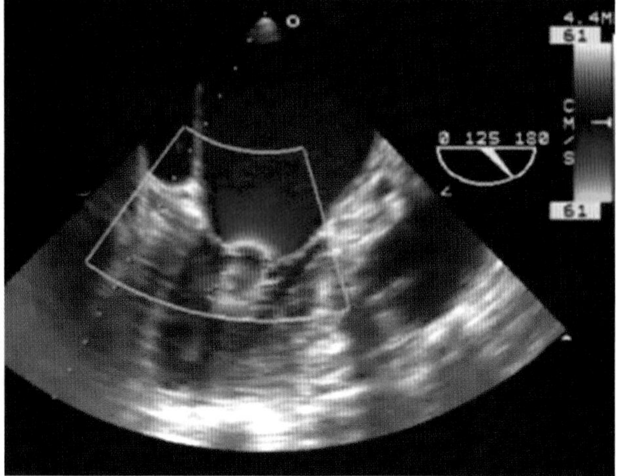

Figure 24.2. ME 4CH view, color Doppler. See also Video 24.2.

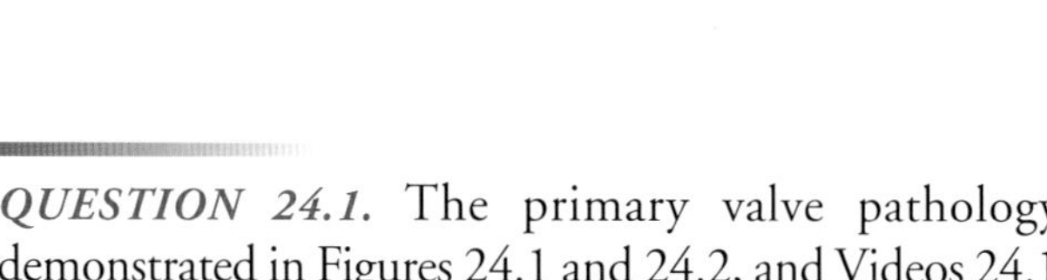

QUESTION 24.1. The primary valve pathology demonstrated in Figures 24.1 and 24.2, and Videos 24.1 and 24.2, is

A. MR
B. Mitral stenosis
C. Cleft MV
D. MV mass
E. None of the above

QUESTION 24.2. The leaflet deformity pointed out by the blue arrow in Figure 24.3 and Video 24.1 is caused by

A. A severe regurgitant jet
B. Congenital malformation
C. Commissural fusion and leaflet tethering
D. Thrombus formation
E. Surgical intervention

QUESTION 24.3. The following TEE findings are commonly associated with this patient's pathology *except*

A. An enlarged left atrium
B. Thrombus in the LAA
C. A high gradient between the RV and the RA
D. TR
E. Coarctation of the descending aorta

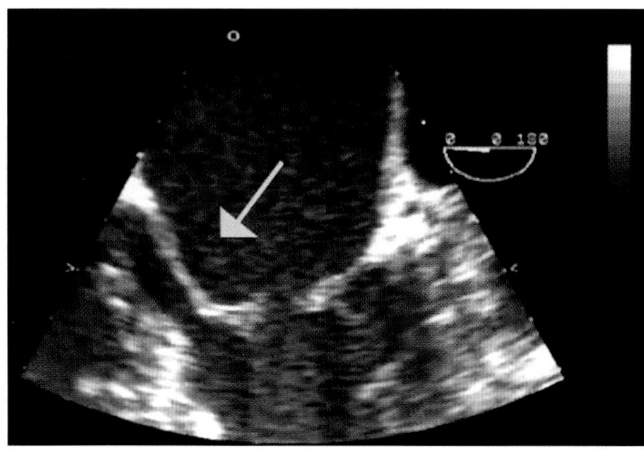

Figure 24.3. ME 4CH view, zooming on the MV. See also Video 24.1.

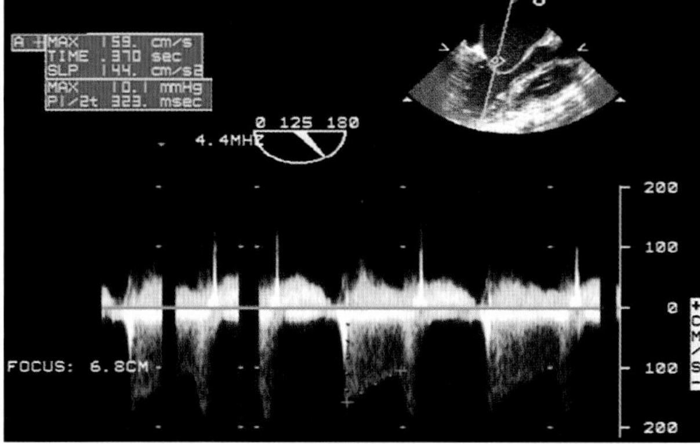

Figure 24.4. CW Doppler of the MV.

QUESTION 24.4. Based on the spectral Doppler tracing obtained in Figure 24.4, what is this patient's estimated MV area?

A. 0.33 cm^2
B. 0.68 cm^2
C. 1.38 cm^2
D. 1.46 cm^2
E. 2.52 cm^2

QUESTION 24.5. Which of the following conditions typically makes the measurement of mitral PHT unreliable?

A. The patient has a mechanical MV
B. Moderate or severe aortic regurgitation is present
C. Mitral valvuloplasty was just performed
D. The patient has a restricted cardiomyopathy
E. All of the above statements are true

QUESTION 24.6. Based upon the TEE findings presented above, this patient should

A. Undergo MV surgery
B. Be placed on long-term antibiotics
C. Be given aspirin and nitroglycerin
D. Undergo mass excision
E. Receive radiation therapy

ANSWERS AND DISCUSSION

QUESTION 24.1: The primary valve pathology demonstrated in Videos 24.1 and 24.2 is B: Mitral stenosis. It is the most frequent valvular complication of rheumatic fever. While other cardiac valves may be affected in addition to the MV, sparing of the MV is extremely rare. Videos 24.1 and 24.2 display the hallmark characteristics of rheumatic valves: limited leaflet mobility, leaflet thickening, and calcification of both the leaflets and subvalvular apparatus. The CFD in Video 24.2 also shows flow convergence on the LA side of the valve, indicating a narrowing of the valve orifice. Answer A—MR—is incorrect: in MR, one would see a jet entering the left atrium in systole and the flow convergence would be seen on the ventricular side of the valve. Answer C—cleft MV—is also incorrect, as one would likely have an associated MR. Finally, although the mitral leaflets are thickened, there is no discrete visible mass on this valve. Therefore, answer D is also incorrect.

QUESTION 24.2: The correct answer is C. Commissural fusion and leaflet tethering cause loss of leaflet mobility and restricted MV opening. The blue arrow in Figure 24.3 and Video 24.1 points toward the body of the anterior MV leaflet, which displays the characteristic "hockey stick" deformity (also referred to as "doming" of the valve). Answer B—congenital mitral stenosis—is incorrect: it typically involves the subvalvular apparatus, not the commissures, and does not result in this appearance. As discussed in Question 24.1, this patient does not have MR or a mass on the leaflet. A similar appearance (*doming* or *hockey stick*) can be seen as a result of an edge-to-edge MV repair ("Alfieri" stitch). However, such a repair is typically combined with a valvuloplasty ring, which is not present in this patient.

QUESTION 24.3: The correct answer is E. Coarctation of the descending aorta is not associated with mitral stenosis. Obstruction of flow into the LV results in increased LA pressures and dilatation of the LA chamber. As a result of this LA enlargement, there is often stagnant blood flow (seen as spontaneous contrast in the LA), which can lead to thrombus formation. Careful inspection of the LAA is required to rule out the presence of clot. High LA pressures may eventually lead to pulmonary hypertension, indicated by a high RV to right atrial gradient (RVSP) on echocardiography. Patients with longstanding mitral stenosis and pulmonary hypertension often have an enlarged RV and a significant TR.

QUESTION 24.4: The correct answer is B: 0.68 cm^2. The MV area can be quickly calculated using the PHT method:

$$MVA = \frac{220}{PHT}$$

(where MVA = MV area in cm^2 and PHT = PHT measured in milliseconds). The PHT is the time it takes for the peak diastolic transmitral pressure gradient to decrease by half. It is obtained by placing a spectral Doppler signal (usually CW for measuring high velocities) through the stenotic orifice. The caliper function is then used to obtain the slope of the E wave, as shown in Figure 24.5. The software package on the machine then converts this to PHT (denoted as "P1/2t 323 msec" in Fig. 24.5). Using the above formula, this patient's MVA = 220/323 = 0.68 cm^2.

QUESTION 24.5: The correct answer is E: All of the above statements are true.

The PHT method of calculating MV area has several limitations. It should *not* be applied to mechanical

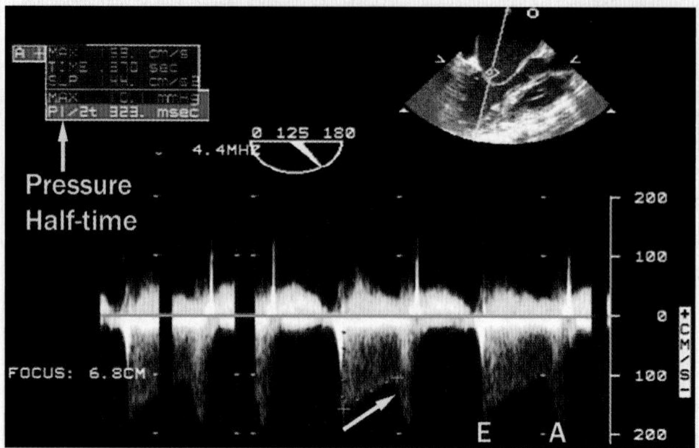

Figure 24.5. CW Doppler of the MV, demonstrating the PHT technique.

valves or immediately following balloon valvuloplasty. Moderate aortic regurgitation causes the LV pressure to rise more quickly (independently of mitral inflow), thus falsely shortening the PHT and leading to an underestimation of the mitral stenosis severity. Severe aortic regurgitation may also impair opening of the anterior mitral leaflet, thus further affecting the pressure half-time. Finally, the pressure gradient that drives mitral inflow is also a function of LV compliance and the PHT method should not be used when that compliance is significantly impaired, such as in a restricted cardiomyopathy.

QUESTION 24.6: The correct answer is A: Undergo MV surgery.

With severe mitral stenosis and dyspnea, this patient is likely a candidate for either balloon commissurotomy or open surgical replacement. Mild mitral stenosis is classified as a valve area >1.5 cm^2 and moderate stenosis is classified as an area between 1.5 and 1.0 cm^2. Severe mitral stenosis exists with a valve area <1.0 cm^2. The decision to proceed to MV surgery involves many factors, including symptoms and the severity of pulmonary hypertension. Bonow et al., 2006 presents a more in-depth discussion of this topic. Answers B, C, D, and E are not recommended treatments for mitral stenosis.

TAKE-HOME LESSON:

Mitral stenosis is most commonly rheumatic in origin. It usually presents with calcified restricted MV leaflets, commissural fusion, and calcification of the subvalvular apparatus. Increased diastolic gradients and PHT across the valve are also seen. Surgical treatment is indicated in cases of severe stenosis.

SUGGESTED READING

Baumgartner H, Hung J, Bermejo J, et al. Echocardiographic assessment of valve stenosis: EAE/ASE recommendations for clinical practice. *J Am Soc Echocardiogr*. 2009;22:1–23.

Bonow RO, Carabello BA, Chatterjee KA, et al. ACC/AHA 2006 guidelines for the management of patients with valvular heart disease: a report of the American College of Cardiology/American Heart Association task force on practice guidelines. Developed in collaboration with the Society of Cardiovascular Anesthesiologists; Endorsed by the Society for Cardiovascular Angiography and Interventions and the Society of Thoracic Surgeons. *Circulation*. 2006;114:e84–e231.

Wilkins GT, Weyman AE, Abascal VM, et al. Percutaneous balloon dilatation of the MV: an analysis of echocardiographic variables related to outcome and the mechanism of dilatation. *Br Heart J*. 1988;60: 299–308.

Moderate

CASE 25

A 4-kg boy becomes increasingly cyanotic 2 days after birth.

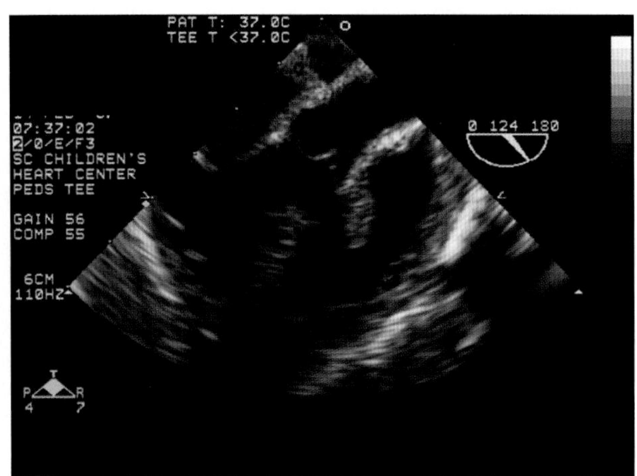

Figure 25.1.

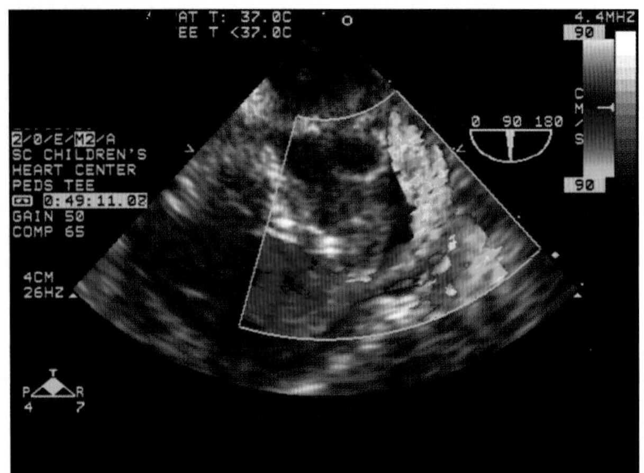

Figure 25.2.

QUESTION 25.1. The following congenital cardiac conditions result in cyanosis *except*

A. Tetralogy of Fallot
B. Transposition of the great arteries
C. Hypoplastic left heart syndrome
D. ASD

Surgical correction is scheduled. The intraoperative TEE images are shown (Figs. 25.1 and 25.2, and Videos 25.1 to 25.4).

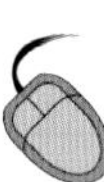

QUESTION 25.2. What is the most likely diagnosis?

A. Pulmonary stenosis
B. VSD
C. Tetralogy of Fallot
D. Transposition of the great vessels

QUESTION 25.3. Tetralogy of Fallot consists of all the following *except*

A. ASD
B. RVOT obstruction
C. Aortic override
D. VSD

QUESTION 25.4. Figure 25.1 demonstrates what type of VSD?

A. Perimembranous

B. Muscular

C. Inlet

D. Subarterial

QUESTION 25.5. TEE is useful post repair to evaluate for all the following except?

A. RVOT obstruction

B. Pulmonary insufficiency

C. Evaluation of RV to PA conduct

D. Presence of coarctation

ANSWERS AND DISCUSSION

QUESTION 25.1: The correct answer is D: ASD. The classical cyanotic congenital heart lesions include tetralogy of Fallot, transposition of the great arteries, hypoplastic left heart syndrome, pulmonary stenosis, tricuspid atresia, truncus arteriosis, and total anomalous pulmonary venous return.

QUESTION 25.2: The correct answer is C: Tetralogy of Fallot. The collection of videos and images demonstrates the classic findings in tetralogy of Fallot. They include a perimembranous VSD and overriding aorta (Fig. 25.1), RVOT obstruction (Fig. 25.2), and RV hypertrophy (Video 25.1) (Fig. 25.3). Approximately, one third of cases have an ASD but it is not part of the tetralogy.

QUESTION 25.4: The correct answer is A: Perimembranous. Tetralogy of Fallot patients classically have large unrestrictive perimembranous VSDs. The degree of ventricular right-to-left shunting accounts for the degree of cyanosis. Video 25.5 is surgical footage of a neonatal tetralogy (TET) repair. First, the extensive RV hypertrophy is resected. Second, the subpulmonic and pulmonic stenoses are addressed. Finally, the perimembranous VSD is closed with a pericardial patch.

QUESTION 25.5: The correct answer is D: Presence of coarctation. All the other answers are common conditions that need to be evaluated following separation from postcardiopulmonary bypass. Coarctation of the aorta is not an associated condition with tetralogy of Fallot. The anterior position of the air-filled trachea relative to the esophagus limits the TEE examination of the distal ascending aorta and proximal aortic arch, thereby making this a difficult lesion to examine by TEE.

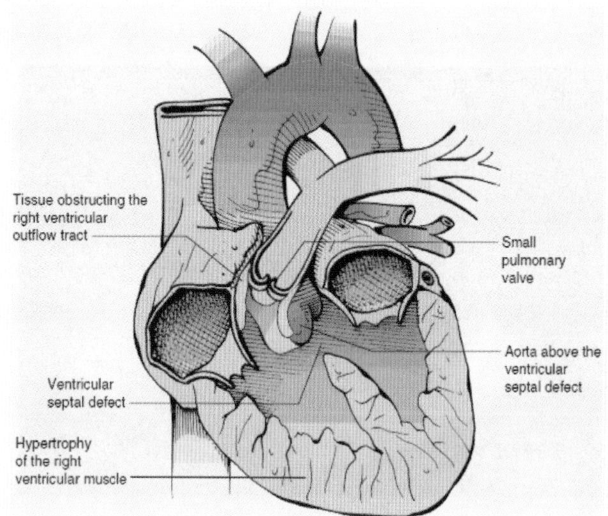

Figure 25.3. Tetralogy of Fallot. Characteristics of this lesion include a VSD, RVOT obstruction, RV hypertrophy, and aortic override, that is the aortic position is above the VSD. Note the tissue below the pulmonary valve in this figure; it contributes to the RVOT obstruction. The pulmonary valve can be small and dysplastic. (From Perrino A, Reeves ST, eds. *A Practical Approach to Transesophageal Echocardiography.* 2nd ed. Philadelphia: Lippincott Williams and Wilkins; 2008, with permission.)

TAKE-HOME LESSON:

Tetralogy of Fallot includes a perimembranous VSD and overriding aorta (Fig. 25.1), RVOT obstruction (Fig. 25.2), and RV hypertrophy (Video 25.1). Approximately, one third of cases have an ASD but it is not part of the tetralogy.

SUGGESTED READING

Rouine-Rapp K, Miller-Hance WC. Transesophageal echocardiography for congenital heart disease in the adult. In: Perrino A, Reeves ST, eds. *A Practical Approach to Transesophageal Echocardiography.* 2nd ed. Philadelphia: Lippincott Williams & Wilkins; 2008:387–389.

Moderate

CASE 26

A 48-year-old female is in the cardiac catheterization lab for elective closure of an ASD. She presented after a murmur was heard on her physical exam, and the ASD diagnosed during a transthoracic echocardiography exam. She has complaints of increased fatigue and occasional palpitations.

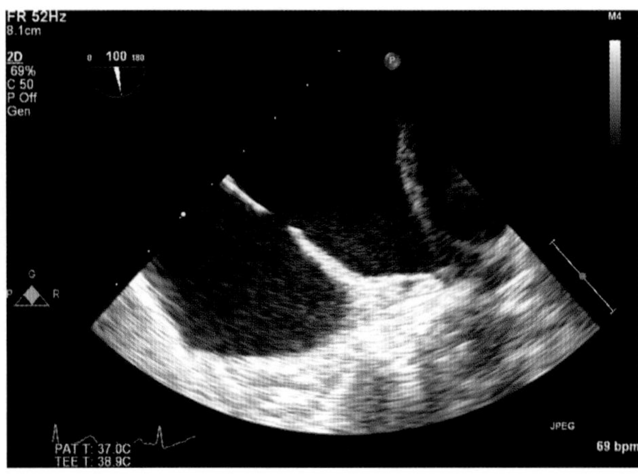

Figure 26.1. Image of atrial septum.

QUESTION 26.1. What lesion is commonly associated with this type of defect (Fig. 26.1) (see Video 26.1)?

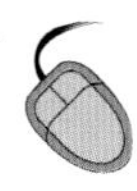

A. Cleft MV
B. Anomalous pulmonary veins
C. MV prolapse
D. Persistent left SVC
E. Pulmonary valve stenosis

QUESTION 26.2. Which of the following ASD can be closed using a percutaneous technique in the cardiac catheterization lab?

A. Primum ASD
B. Secundum ASD
C. Sinus venosus ASD
D. CS septal defect

QUESTION 26.3. What is considered an adequate atrial septal rim for the placement of an atrial septal occluder device?

A. No rim is needed
B. 3–5 mm
C. 5–7 mm
D. 7–10 mm
E. 10–12 mm

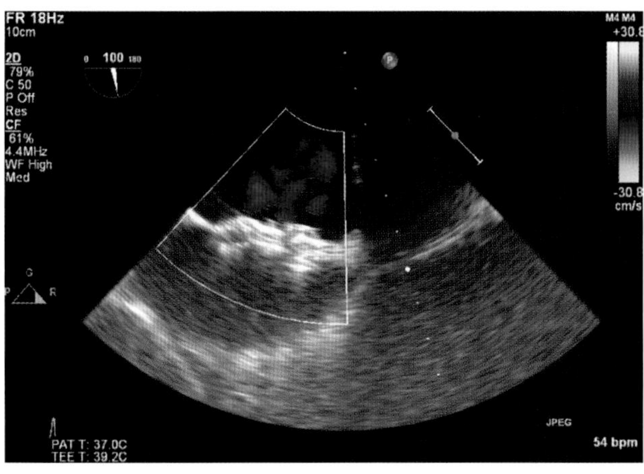

Figure 26.2. Septal occluder device in place.

QUESTION 26.4. After device placement, the position of the occluder is confirmed. There is minimal residual flow across the atrial septum by CFD (Fig. 26.2 and Video 26.2) and after bubble testing with Valsalva. What additional echocardiographic information should be obtained prior to leaving the cardiac catheterization lab?

A. Rule out thrombus formation
B. Evaluate for venous flow obstruction
C. Evaluate the function of the tricuspid, mitral, and aortic valves
D. Rule out pericardial effusion
E. All of the above

ANSWERS AND DISCUSSION

QUESTION 26.1: The correct answer is C. This patient has a secundum ASD. All patients with congenital cardiac pathology should have a comprehensive echocardiographic exam to rule out other associated congenital abnormalities. MV prolapse is commonly associated with secundum ASD.

ANSWER A: Answer A is incorrect. A cleft anterior mitral leaflet is most commonly associated with primum ASD. This is best visualized in the TG basal short-axis view.

ANSWER B: Answer B is incorrect. Anomalous pulmonary venous return is frequently associated with sinus venosus defects and must always be thoroughly examined in patients with this type of defect.

ANSWER D: Answer D is incorrect. A persistent left SVC is associated with CS septal defects and may also have anomalous pulmonary venous return.

ANSWER E: Answer E is incorrect. Pulmonic stenosis is associated with ASD, but more frequently there is increased flow across the pulmonary valve due to the increased right-sided flow from the ASD with the typical left to right shunt.

QUESTION 26.2: The correct answer is B. The only septal defect amenable to percutaneous closure in the cardiac catheterization lab is the secundum defect. The other defects can only be repaired surgically. Secundum defects with a large septal aneurysm or multiple fenestrations may not be amenable to percutaneous closure (Fig. 26.3 and Video 26.3).

QUESTION 26.3: The correct answer is C. A rim of 5 to 7 mm is considered enough septal tissue to hold the device in place. The septal occluder device is

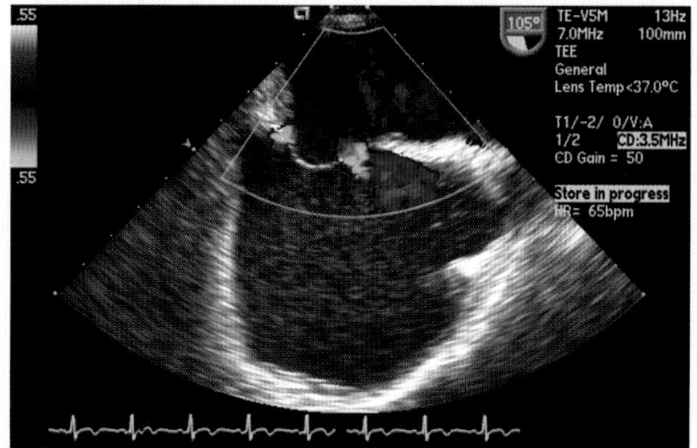

Figure 26.3. Fenestrated aneurysmal atrial septum.

composed of two discs that project on each side of the atrial septum. There must be enough septal tissue between the two discs to prevent the occluder from embolizing.

QUESTION 26.4: The correct answer is E. At the end of any procedure a comprehensive exam should be performed. Placing foreign devices into the heart is thrombogenic. Although the patient is heparinized, there is always the possibility that thrombus could form in the heart during the procedure. The occluder device could impinge venous inflow from the vena cava, CS, and right pulmonary veins. Each of these structures needs to be evaluated to assure that there is no flow acceleration after device placement. The discs of the occluder device can reach the mitral and TV. In addition, the device can impinge on the aortic root causing AV dysfunction. Finally, the catheters used to place the device may perforate the myocardium. Hence, the comprehensive exam must also rule out pericardial effusion or cardiac tamponade.

TAKE-HOME LESSON:

The only ASD amenable to percutaneous closure in the cardiac catheterization lab is the secundum defect. An adequate atrial septal rim of 5 to 7 mm is necessary for the placement of the occluder device to assure stabilization.

SUGGESTED READING

Reeves ST, Shanewise J, eds. *Fundamental Applications of Transesophageal Echocardiography*, SCA 2005 Monograph on DVD. Philadelphia: Lippincott Williams & Wilkins; 2005.

Rouine-Rapp K, Miller-Hance WC. Transesophageal echocardiography for congenital heart disease in the adult. In: Perrino A, Reeves ST, eds. *A Practical Approach to Transesophageal Echocardiography*. 2nd ed. Philadelphia: Lippincott Williams & Wilkins; 2008:372–374.

CASE 27

A 42-year-old female with a longstanding history of a heart murmur presents with increasing dyspnea and chest pain on exertion. She is a smoker with a strong family history of coronary artery disease. Further investigations reveal that she has significant three-vessel coronary artery disease. A TTE demonstrates severe MR but the mechanism is not clear. After induction of anesthesia, one obtains the TEE images shown in Figures 27.1 and 27.2.

QUESTION 27.1. Based on Figures 27.1, 27.2 and Videos 27.1, 27.2, what is the most likely *mechanism* of MR?

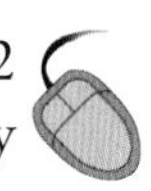

A. Anterior mitral leaflet prolapse
B. Posterior mitral leaflet restriction
C. LVOT obstruction and SAM causing MR
D. None of the above

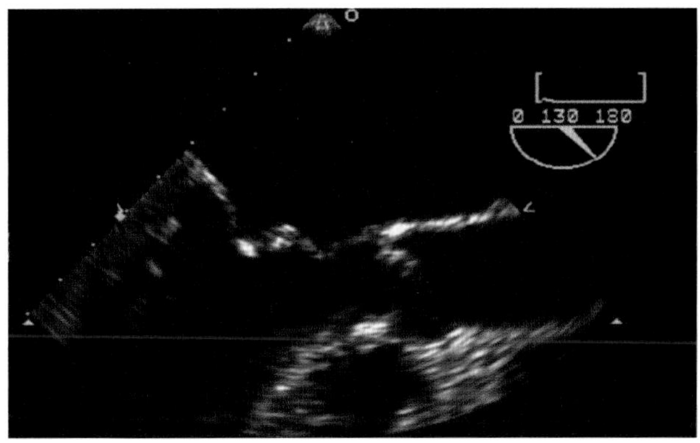

Figure 27.1. ME LAX view of the MV, 2D. See also Video 27.1.

QUESTION 27.2. Based on Figure 27.3 and Video 27.3, what is the cause of the MR?

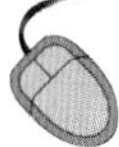

A. Moderate MAC
B. Cleft anterior MV leaflet
C. Endocarditis with perforation of the anterior mitral leaflet
D. Parachute MV

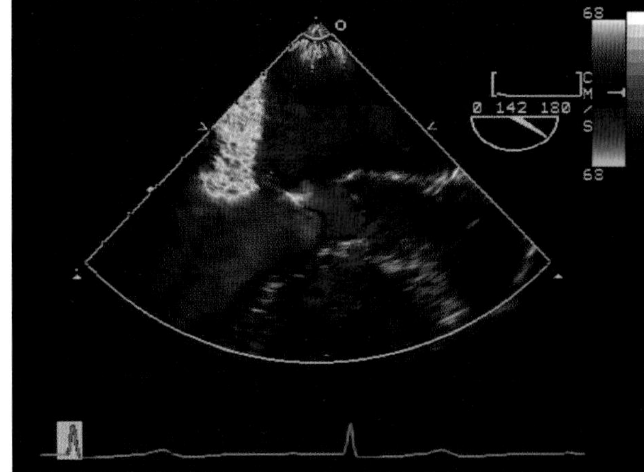

Figure 27.2. ME LAX view of the MV with CFD. See also Video 27.2.

QUESTION 27.3. You determine that the patient has a cleft anterior MV leaflet. What other congenital lesion is *most often* associated with a cleft MV?

A. Bicuspid AV

B. Anomalous pulmonary venous drainage

C. Muscular type VSDs

D. Ostium primum type ASDs

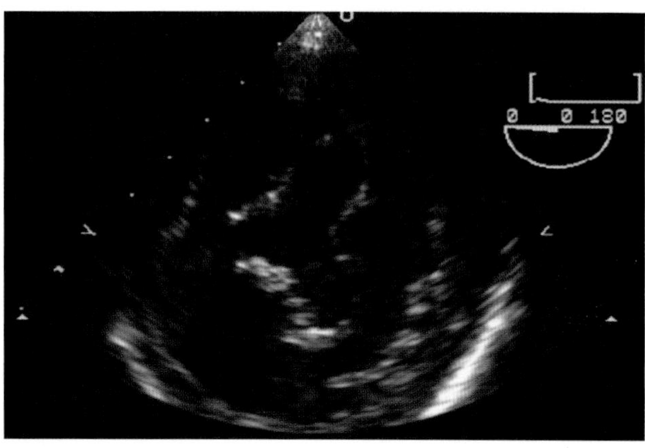

Figure 27.3. TG basal SAX view of the MV. See also Video 27.3.

After a complete TEE examination, it is determined that the patient has an isolated cleft mitral valve (ICMV). This is confirmed by direct inspection of the valve. The surgeon determines that MV repair would be the best option for this patient and he performs a complex MV repair.

QUESTION 27.4. Based on Figure 27.4 and Video 27.4, what type of mitral repair has been performed?

A. Closure of the cleft with a pericardial patch and an Alfieri suture

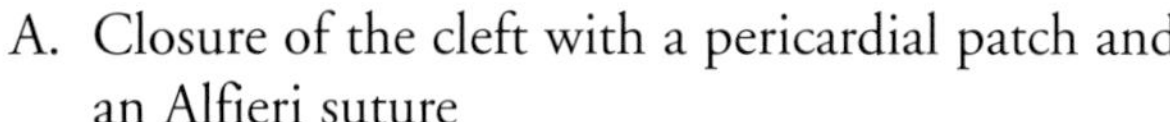

B. Quadrangular A2 resection with sliding annuloplasty

C. Primary suturing of the anterior mitral leaflet cleft

D. Isolated cleft closure with a pericardial patch

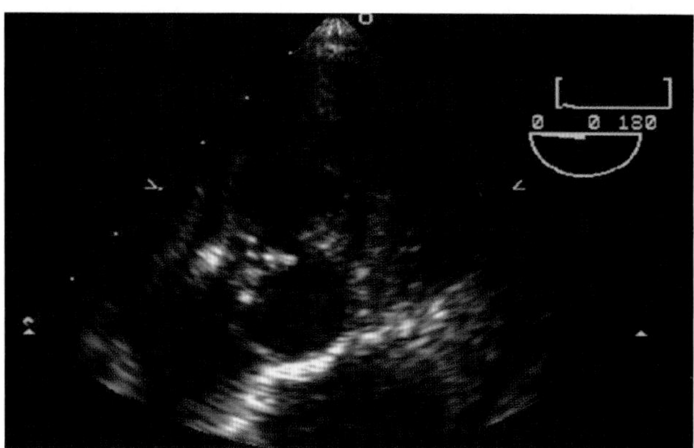

Figure 27.4. TG basal SAX view of MV *post repair*. See also Video 27.4.

The MV repair consisted of pericardial patch closure of the anterior mitral leaflet cleft and an Alfieri suture to minimize anterior leaflet prolapse post repair.

QUESTION 27.5. Upon further TEE interrogation (Figures 27.5 and 27.6 and Videos 27.5 and 27.6), what can you conclude about the status of the repaired MV?

A. There is mild residual MR and no evidence of mitral stenosis

B. There is no residual MR but there is a mild mitral stenosis

C. There is no residual MR or mitral stenosis

D. There is no residual MR but there is severe mitral stenosis

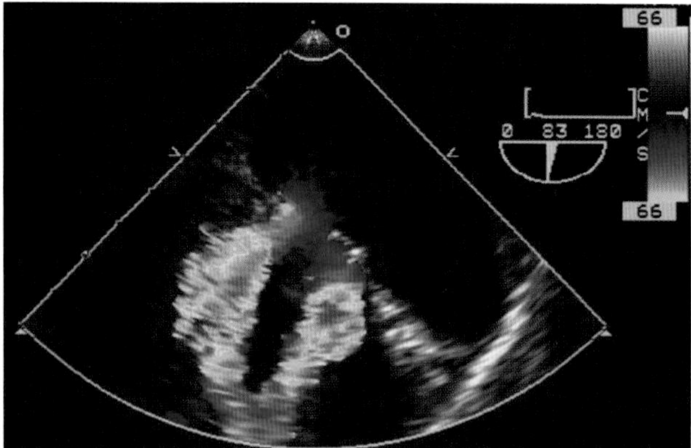

Figure 27.5. ME 2CH view of the MV with CFD, in diastole. See also Video 27.5.

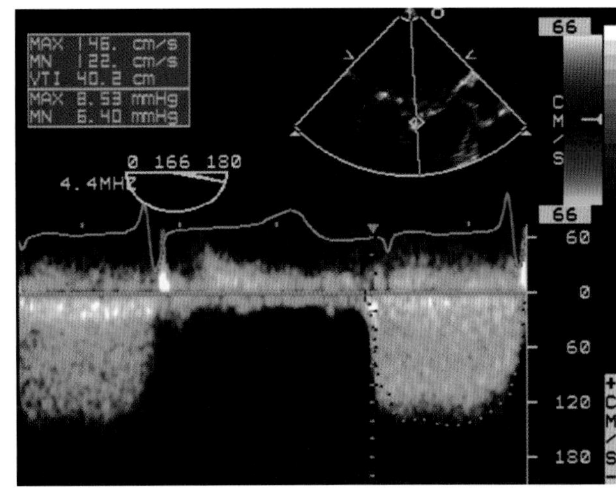

Figure 27.6. CW Doppler of the mitral inflow.

ANSWERS AND DISCUSSION

QUESTION 27.1: The correct answer is D: None of the above. Close inspection of the coaptation between the anterior and the posterior leaflets does not reveal an obvious defect but there is clearly a broad-based, posteriorly directed MR jet originating near that area. Also, there is a smaller high velocity jet between the left atrium and the LVOT that seems to pass through the body of the anterior mitral leaflet. One should strongly suspect a defect within the anterior leaflet itself, the nature of which cannot be conclusively determined with these images alone. Answer A (*anterior leaflet prolapse*) is incorrect: the anterior mitral leaflet clearly does not prolapse above the MV annulus. Answer B (*posterior leaflet restriction*) is also incorrect: the posterior mitral leaflet does not appear significantly restricted. Finally, answer C (*SAM causing MR*) is incorrect: although SAM typically generates a posteriorly directed MR jet with turbulent LVOT flow, there is no 2D evidence of SAM of the anterior leaflet or subvalvular apparatus. By process of elimination, D is the correct answer.

QUESTION 27.2: The correct answer is B: Cleft anterior MV leaflet. Cleft MV is a rare form of congenital MR. A recent review of adult patients found that congenital causes accounted for 2.1% of adult MR patients and that the preoperative diagnosis was often incorrect. In this case, the cleft can be seen on the short-axis view, extending toward the ventricular wall (Fig. 27.3 and Video 27.3). There is significant thickening and fibrosis along the edges of the cleft, the extent of which usually correlates with the age of the patient. Figure 27.7 demonstrates the position of the cleft in the anterior mitral leaflet. The cleft points toward the LVOT, which is often the case in ICMVs. Answer A (*moderate MAC*) is incorrect: Although the edges of the cleft are thickened and calcified, there is no MAC. Furthermore, severe isolated MAC tends to be associated with mitral stenosis rather than MR. Answer C (*endocarditis*) is incorrect: Erosive endocarditis can be a cause of acquired mitral leaflet cleft, but this lesion appears to be chronic, both by history (longstanding murmur) and by echocardiographic appearance. Finally, answer D (*parachute MV*) is incorrect: A parachute MV is another rare congenital MV disorder, characterized by the presence of a single papillary muscle in the LV. The leaflets are generally dense, with restricted motion in most patients.

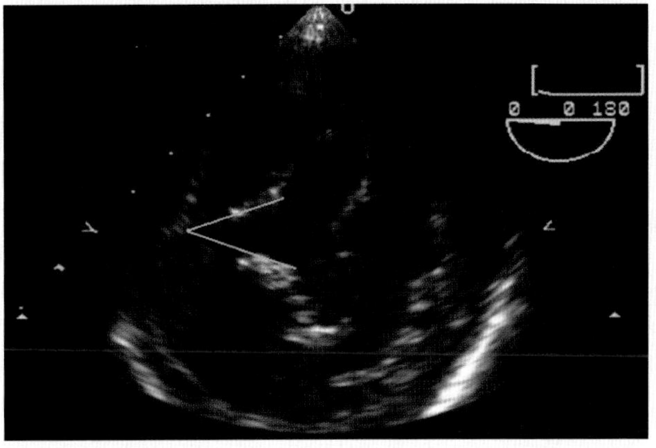

Figure 27.7. Short axis of the MV demonstrating the cleft in the anterior leaflet.

QUESTION 27.3: The correct answer is D: Ostium primum type ASD. A cleft MV can exist by itself or in combination with an ostium primum ASD, in which case it is part of a spectrum of defects called *atrioventricular septal defects* (AVSDs). As AVSDs are more prevalent than ICMVs, ostium primum ASD is the lesion *most commonly associated with a cleft MV*. This patient, however, has an ICMV. In a large review, ICMVs accounted for 1.2% of all congenital structural heart defects. Other findings associated with cleft MV include perimembranous VSD, accessory chordal attachments, AS and, depending on whether the conus arteriosus is involved, tetralogy of Fallot, transposition of the great arteries, double outlet RV, and tricuspid atresia.

Distinguishing between an ICMV and an AVSD is important perioperatively, as it helps predict the ability to perform successful MV repair surgery. Important morphological differences exist between an ICMV and an AVSD: the presence of a discrete atrioventricular junction supporting the cleft leaflet and a mural leaflet comparable in size to the normal MV suggest an ICMV. Moreover, the orientation of the cleft is often determined by the presence of an ostium primum ASD or a large membranous VSD. The orientation of the cleft in ICMV is directed toward the LVOT. This is in contrast to AVSDs and ICMV with membranous VSD, where the cleft is directed toward the ventricular septum. Another distinguishing feature between ICMV and AVSD is the position of the papillary muscles: in ICMV, the papillary muscles assume the typical orientation, whereas in AVSD they are rotated counterclockwise.[1] Answers A and B are incorrect: there is no association between cleft MV and bicuspid aortic valves and/or anomalous pulmonary venous drainage. Answer C is also incorrect: both AVSD and ICMV are more likely to be associated with perimembranous VSD rather than muscular-type VSD.

QUESTION 27.4: The correct answer is A: Closure of the cleft with a pericardial patch and an Alfieri suture. Most surgical repairs of ICMVs occur early in childhood. When undertaken early, the surgical repair can be as simple as suturing the free edges of the cleft together. With time, the leaflet edges thicken and fibrose, as is the case in this patient, making a simple cleft suture repair almost impossible in adult patients. Therefore, leaflet repair with a pericardial patch after resecting the fibrotic edges is often required in adult patients. In this patient, the surgeon felt that the reconstructed anterior mitral leaflet was too large and might prolapse into the left atrium. Hence an Alfieri suture was performed. Answer B (*quadrangular A2 resection*) is incorrect: the anterior mitral leaflet was actually augmented with a patch rather than reduced as would occur with a quadrangular resection. Furthermore, sliding annuloplasty is generally performed on the posterior mitral leaflet not on the anterior leaflet. Answers C (*primary suturing of the cleft*) and D (*isolated patch*) are incorrect: in addition to the previously cited reasons for not performing a simple cleft suture, the presence of a double orifice on the short-axis MV view (Fig. 27.4 and Video 27.4) demonstrates that this is neither a simple cleft suture nor a simple patch closure of the cleft.

QUESTION 27.5: The correct answer is B: There is no residual MR but there is mild mitral stenosis. The thickened leaflets with reduced excursion are expected considering the pericardial patch and Alfieri suture. However, the degree of aliasing flow through the two MV orifices is exaggerated. The mean transvalvular gradient is measured at 6.4 mm Hg, possibly reflecting some mild degree of mitral stenosis. Some sources quote a gradient ≤8 mm Hg as acceptable for an Alfieri repair. As with any other repair, one must keep in mind the loading conditions at the time of the assessment: a high flow state after separation from CPB may overestimate the degree of stenosis. As such, this would represent at most mild stenosis and a very acceptable repair. There is no residual MR on the images provided.

TAKE-HOME LESSON:

A cleft MV can exist by itself or in combination with an ostium primum ASD, in which case it is part of a spectrum of defects called AVSDs.

REFERENCE

1. Perrier P, Clausnizer B. Isolated cleft mitral valve: valve reconstruction techniques. *Ann Thorac Surg.* 1995;59: 56–59.

SUGGESTED READING

Anderson R, Zuberbuhler J, Penkoske PA, et al. Of clefts, commissures, and things. *J Thorac Cardiovasc Surg.* 1985;90:605–610.

Banerjee A, Kohl T, Silverman NH, et al. Echocardiographic evaluation of congenital mitral valve anomalies in children. *Am J Cardiol.* 1995;76:1284–1291.

Di Segni E, Edwards J. Cleft anterior leaflet of the mitral valve with intact septa: a study of 20 cases. *Am J Cardiol.* 1983;51:919–926.

Kohl T, Silverman N, et al. Comparison of cleft and papillary muscle position in cleft mitral valve and atrioventricular septal defect. *Am J Cardiol.* 1996;77:164–169.

Sigfuson G, Ettedgui J, Silverman NH, et al. Is a cleft anterior leaflet of an otherwise normal valve an atrioventricular canal malformation? *J Am Coll Cardiol.* 1995;26:508–515.

Van Praagh S, Porras D, Oppido G, et al. Cleft mitral valve without ostium primum defect: anatomic data and surgical considerations based on 41 cases. *Ann Thorac Surg.* 2003;75:1752–1762.

Zegdi R, Amahzoune B, Ladjali M, et al. Congenital mitral valve regurgitation in adult patients. A rare, often misdiagnosed but repairable, valve disease. *Eur J Cardiothorac Surg.* 2008;34:751–754.

CASE 28

A 68-year-old male presented to the emergency department with a 1-week history of increasing shortness of breath and chest pain. His SpO_2 is 88% on room air and he could not lie flat. He required endotracheal intubation and mechanical ventilation for respiratory support. A chest x-ray was unremarkable and subsequently TEE was performed.

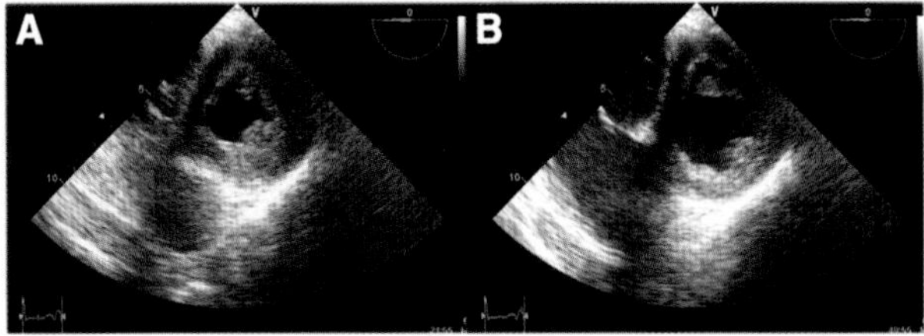

Figure 28.1. TG midpapillary short-axis views (TG mid SAX) in systole (**A**) and diastole (**B**). See also Video 28.1.

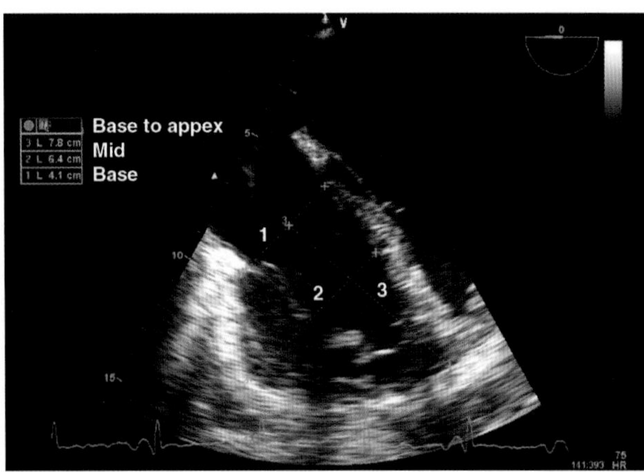

Figure 28.2. ME 4CH view with measurements of RV dimensions. See also Video 28.2.

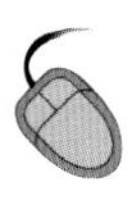

QUESTION 28.1. The images in Figure 28.1, Video 28.1 support which of the following findings?

A. Eccentricity index in systole suggests RV pressure overload

B. Volume overload of the RV

C. Septal infarct

D. LV volume overload

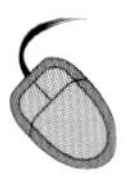

QUESTION 28.2. From Figures 28.1 and 28.2 and Videos 28.1 and 28.2, which diagnosis is the most likely?

A. Tricuspid endocarditis

B. RV infarct

C. Pulmonary embolus

D. Both B and C

QUESTION 28.3. From the Doppler findings in Figure 28.3A, B, which statement is correct?

A. The PA systolic pressure is normal

B. The pulmonary Doppler is consistent with pulmonary hypertension

C. The RV systolic pressure (RVSP) is normal

D. The pulmonary Doppler is consistent with acute RV infarction

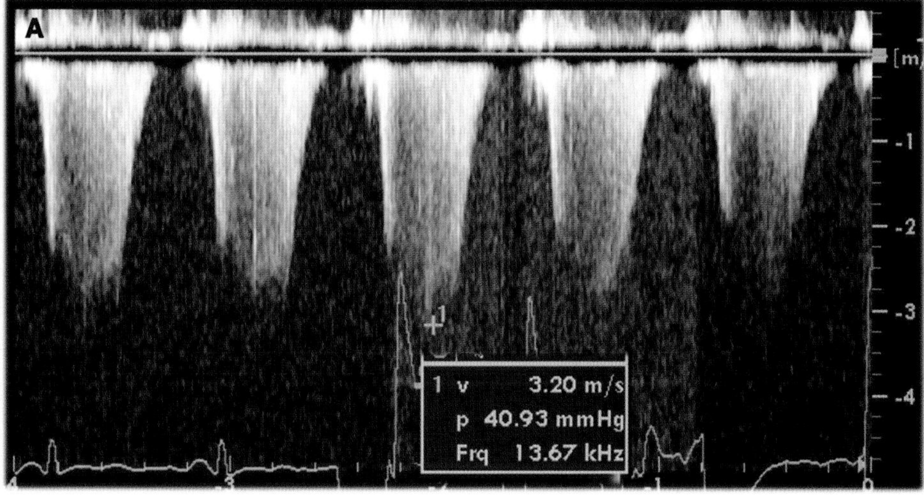

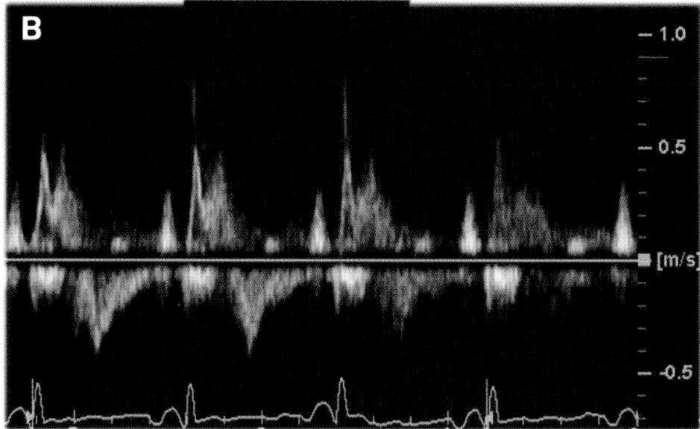

Figure 28.3. **A:** CW Doppler of the tricuspid regurgitant jet via a modified TG RV inflow–outflow view was performed to assess the RVSP generated by the dilated RV. **B:** PW Doppler of the proximal main PA via upper esophageal aortic short axis.

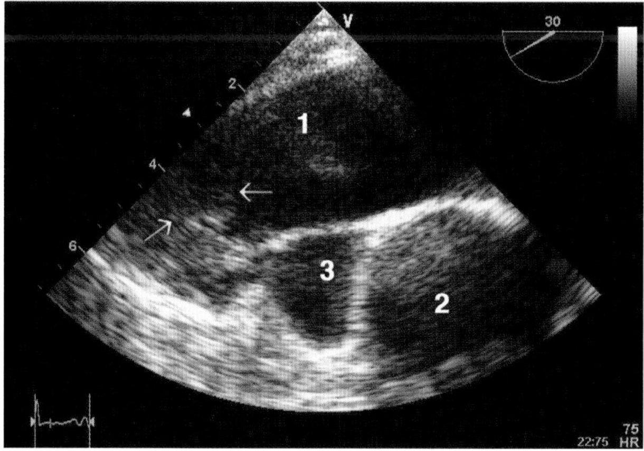

Figure 28.4. ME ascending aortic short-axis view was obtained to examine the more distal pulmonary vasculature. See also Video 28.3.

QUESTION 28.4. Using Figure 28.4 which statement(s) is(are) *incorrect?*

A. Item 3 demonstrates the right upper pulmonary vein

B. Item 1 is the right main PA

C. Item 2 is the ascending aorta

D. The arrows indicate thrombus in the left main PA

QUESTION 28.5. Using Figure 28.5 which statement is incorrect?

A. The RV strain pattern is consistent with McConnel sign

B. The strain pattern demonstrates apical dyskinesis

C. The RV lateral wall strain pattern is consistent with infarction

D. A negative strain value denotes shortening

QUESTION 28.6. Which is the most likely diagnosis in this patient?

A. RV infarction

B. Pulmonary embolus

C. Pericardial tamponade

D. Tricuspid stenosis

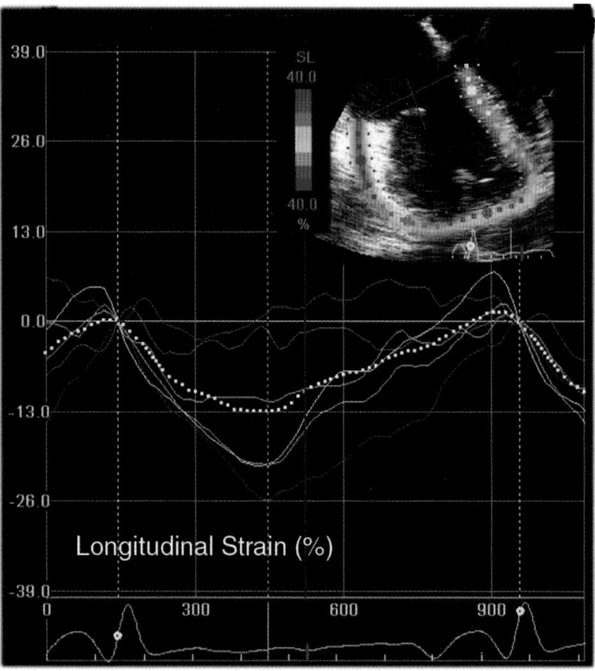

Figure 28.5. In order to more clearly delineate the RV wall motion abnormalities, a ME 4CH view of RV with speckle tracking analysis of longitudinal strain (%). Inset: four-chamber view with color-coded peak systolic strain. Each color trace represents a particular wall; red: basal-lateral, blue: midlateral, pink: apical-lateral, and green: apical-septal. The white dotted line represents global strain.

ANSWERS AND DISCUSSION

QUESTION 28.1: The correct answer is B: Volume overload of the RV. There is diastolic indentation (flattening) of the interventricular septum toward the LV in diastole (Fig. 28.1A and Video 28.1). In patients without heart disease the LV appears circular in shape when viewed in short axis during both systole and diastole. The diastolic flattening of the septal wall seen in this patient (giving a "D" shaped appearance to the LV) is a subtle indicator of volume overload on the right side. Afterload strain may also cause septal flattening; however, this will occur in systole. Systolic septal flattening may not be observed in cases of acute afterload increases. The eccentricity index is a geometric index of septal shifting which may help in distinguishing between pressure and volume overload in the RV. It is measured from LV dimensions in the TG mid short-axis (SAX) view as the ratio of the inferoanterior internal diameter to the septolateral diameter measured at both end systole and end diastole. A ratio >1 at end systole indicates RV pressure overload, whereas a ratio >1 at end diastole indicates volume overload. The index need not be calculated as it can be appreciated without making measurements. A ratio >1 would give the LV a characteristic "D" shape. This is easy to appreciate in this patient in diastole (Fig. 28.1B); therefore, answer A is incorrect. Septal infarcts or bundle branch blocks may also cause abnormal septal motion. Answer C, septal infarct, is unlikely to be correct given the clinical presentation, the shifting of the septum in diastole and the large RV (Fig. 28.1B and Video 28.1). In a septal infarct, the shifting would occur in systole, toward the RV and would likely be associated with other segmental wall motion abnormalities. Answer D is incorrect. The LV does not appear dilated based on the scale in the two-dimensional image. The internal inferoanterior diameter appears to be ~5 cm in diastole (Fig. 28.1B); the normal range is 3.5 to 6.0 cm in the adult.

QUESTION 28.2: The correct answer is D: Both B and C. Figure 28.2 demonstrates a grossly dilated RV (diastole) with the following measurements: basal diameter 4.1 cm; mid-diameter: 6.4 cm; and base to apex (major axis diameter): 7.8 cm. The RV is considered severely enlarged when the basal diameter exceeds 3.9 cm, the mid-diameter exceeds 4.2 cm, and the base to apex length is above 9.2 cm. Multiple factors may result in gross dilatation including RV infarct, pulmonary embolism, and other causes of pulmonary hypertension as well as valvular disease or cardiac shunts. In Video 28.2, we note that the RV is grossly dilated, the systolic function appears depressed, and there are significant wall motion abnormalities. These findings are consistent with both pulmonary embolism and RV infarct. Wall motion abnormalities are seen in both RV infarct and pulmonary embolisms. There is insufficient information at this time to differentiate between RV infarct and pulmonary embolism. Tricuspid endocarditis is unlikely as no vegetations are seen on the TV (Video 28.2).

QUESTION 28.3: The correct answer is B: The PA Doppler tracing is consistent with pulmonary hypertension. Figure 28.3B is a pulsed-wave Doppler trace of the proximal main PA. In this trace we note a sharp triangular velocity pattern with rapid velocity development. This is consistent with pulmonary hypertension. A normal velocity pattern is more rounded or "domed." In this case, there is also midsystolic notching (Fig. 28.6, arrow). This notching pattern, first described by Kitabatake, is also seen in pulmonary hypertension; however, it is not necessarily related to severity. Prominent "A" or atrial velocity waves detected in the PA Doppler throughout the respiratory cycle may be indicative of restrictive RV physiology as a result of gross dilatation. These were observed in this patient (Fig. 28.6); however, the patient was mechanically ventilated making this sign less reliable. Answer A, the PA systolic pressure is normal, is incorrect for the reasons above. Answer C, the RVSP is normal, is incorrect: based on the tricuspid regurgitant jet velocities (Fig. 28.3A), the systolic pressure gradient between the RV and the RA is 40 mm Hg. If the CVP is estimated to be at least 15 mm Hg, this predicts an RVSP exceeding 55 mm Hg. Answer D is incorrect: an RV infarct would not likely

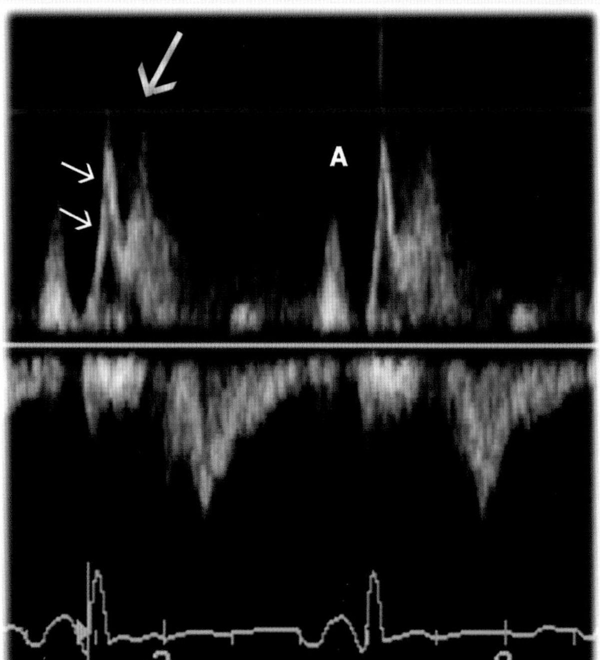

Figure 28.6. PW Doppler of proximal PA with large arrow demonstrating midsystolic notching and double arrows demonstrating velocity acceleration. *A* indicates atrial contraction wave.

produce evidence of increased RVSP and PA systolic pressure that were demonstrated here. Furthermore, pulmonary velocity acceleration (Fig. 28.6, double arrows) is not increased in the presence of an RV infarct.

QUESTION 28.4: Answers A and D are incorrect. Item 3 (Fig. 28.4, Video 28.3) demonstrates the SVC, not the right upper pulmonary vein. Although the arrows in Figure 28.4 indicate a thrombus (seen better in Video 28.3), it is lodged in the right main PA, not the left. Answer B is correct: Item 1 is the right main PA. Answer C is correct: Item 2 is the ascending aorta.

QUESTION 28.5: The incorrect answer is B: The strain pattern demonstrates apical dyskinesis. The apical segments strain demonstrated by the pink and green traces do not cross the zero value (positive strain, stretching) in systole (Fig. 28.5). In fact, the blue and pink traces (midlateral and apical-lateral) are akinetic. Answer A is correct: the RV strain pattern is consistent with McConnel sign. McConnell described RV systolic wall motion abnormalities associated with pulmonary embolism involving mostly the midlateral and apical-lateral regions of the RV free wall (McConnell sign). This can be seen in Figure 28.5: the blue and pink traces where the midlateral and apical-lateral segments are akinetic and there is relative sparing of the basal-lateral wall. The apical-septal segment is depressed. Answer C is correct: the RV lateral wall strain pattern is consistent with infarction. The basal free wall strain is normal (red trace, Fig. 28.5); however, the midlateral and apical-lateral walls (Fig. 28.5; blue and pink traces) demonstrate akinesis. This is consistent with infarction. Answer D is correct: a negative strain value denotes shortening.

QUESTION 28.6: The correct answer is B: Pulmonary embolus. There is a thromboembolic mass inside the right PA (Fig. 28.4, Video 28.3), consistent with a diagnosis of pulmonary thromboembolism. Masses may be present inside the main and left PAs as well; however, the latter is difficult to visualize as the interposition of the air-filled bronchial tree between the esophagus and the pulmonary vessel obstructs the imaging. You will also note on careful examination of Video 28.2 that there is mobile embolic material in the RA. Answer A—RV infarct—is incorrect. Although the dilated and hypokinetic RV may be the result of pulmonary embolism or RV infarct, the latter is less likely in the presence of Doppler evidence of increased pulmonary and RV pressures. Furthermore, the detection of thromboembolic material in the PAs makes a diagnosis of pulmonary embolus more likely. Answer C—pericardial tamponade—is incorrect as there is no evidence of a pericardial collection in this patient. Answer D—tricuspid stenosis—is incorrect. The TV does not appear stenotic (Fig. 28.2, Video 28.2).

TAKE-HOME LESSON:

The diagnosis of pulmonary embolism by echocardiography is problematic. RV wall motion abnormalities in acute pulmonary embolism and RV infarction may appear similar. In the absence of evidence of thromboembolic material, Doppler evidence of elevated RV and PA pressures may be helpful in establishing a diagnosis.

SUGGESTED READING

Haddad F, Couture P, Tousignant C, et al. The right ventricle in cardiac surgery, a perioperative perspective: I. Anatomy, physiology, and assessment. *Anesth Analg.* 2009;108:407–421.

Haddad F, Couture P, Tousignant C, et al. The right ventricle in cardiac surgery, a perioperative perspective: II. Pathophysiology, clinical Importance, and management. *Anesth Analg.* 2009;108:422–433.

Kitabatake A, Inoue M, Asao M, et al. Noninvasive evaluation of pulmonary hypertension by a pulsed Doppler technique. *Circulation.* 1983;68:302–309.

Lang RM, Bierig M, Devereux RB, et al. Recommendations for chamber quantification: a report from the American Society of Echocardiography's Guidelines and Standards Committee and the Chamber Quantification Writing Group, developed in conjunction with the European Association of Echocardiography, a branch of the European Society of Cardiology. *J Am Soc Echocardiogr.* 2005;18:1440–1463.

McConnell MV, Solomon S, Rayan ME, et al. Regional right ventricular dysfunction detected by echocardiography in acute pulmonary embolism. *Am J Cardiol.* 1996;78:469–473.

Naeije R, Torbicki A. More on the noninvasive diagnosis of pulmonary hypertension: Doppler echocardiography revisited. *Eur Respir J.* 1995;8:1445–1449.

Redington AN, Penny D, Rigby ML. Antegrade diastolic pulmonary artery blow as a marker of right ventricular restriction after complete repair of pulmonary atresia with intact ventricular septum and critical pulmonary valve stenosis. *Cardiol Young.* 1992;2:382–386.

Ryan T, Petrovic O, Dillon JC, et al. An echocardiographic index for separation of right ventricular volume and pressure overload. *J Am Coll Cardiol.* 1985;5:918–927.

CASE 29

A 77-year-old male with CHF presents for redo AVR because of AI on a previous stentless valve. On an earlier echo, his LVEF was reported to be 20% to 30% with a moderate degree of TR and pulmonary hypertension. His angiogram did not reveal any coronary artery disease.

QUESTION 29.1. From Figures 29.1 and 29.2 what is the diagnosis?

A. Moderate TR
B. Ebstein anomaly with severe TR
C. Severe functional TR
D. TV prolapse with severe regurgitation

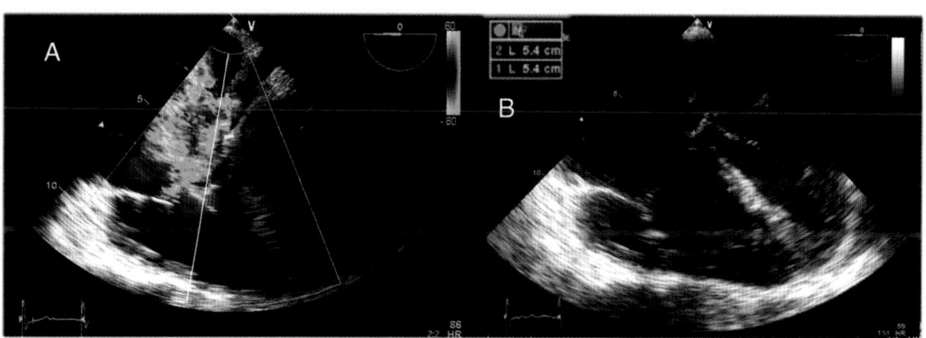

Figure 29.1. **A:** ME 4CH view in systole with CFD and VC (*arrows*) measuring 0.7 cm. **B:** ME 4CH view with RV cavity dimensions: 5.4 cm for both basilar and midcavity dimensions.

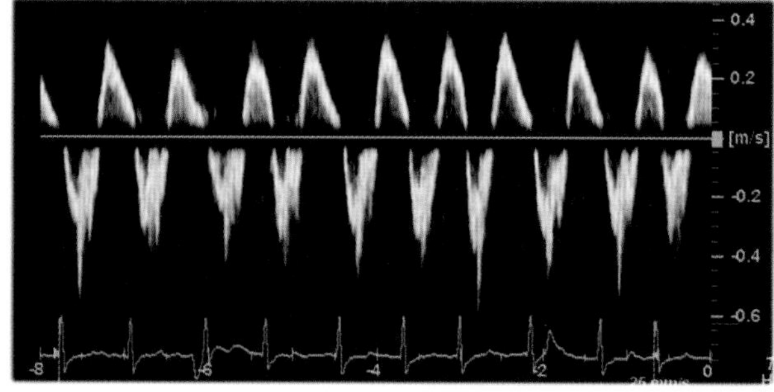

Figure 29.2. Hepatic vein Doppler (PW Doppler with flow toward the RA above the baseline).

QUESTION 29.2. The estimated pulmonary systolic pressure (PAP) from the TR jet was 35 mm Hg (20 mm Hg + CVP 15 mm Hg). After examining Figure 29.3, which of the following statements is *incorrect* regarding RV systolic function?

A. The systolic function by tricuspid annular plane systolic excursion (TAPSE) is underestimated in the presence of severe TR
B. The systolic function estimated by TAPSE is overestimated
C. The PAP may reflect poor RV function
D. Poor LV function decreases TAPSE

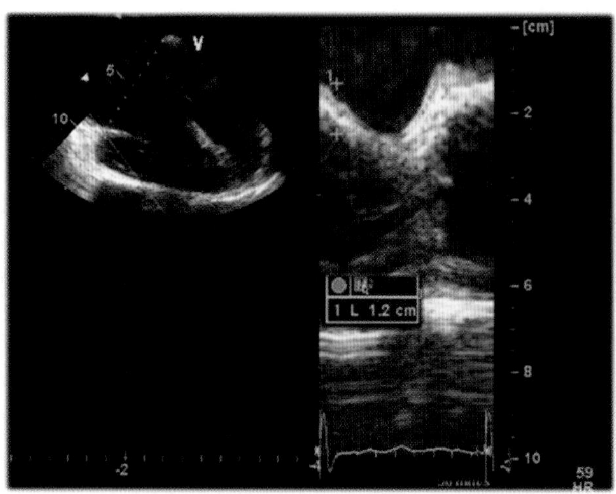

Figure 29.3. TAPSE using anatomical M-mode.

QUESTION 29.3. Regarding management options for this patient, which statement is *not* correct?

A. Do nothing, correcting the left-sided pathology will resolve the TR
B. TV replacement with a prosthetic valve offers a poorer survival than TV repair
C. TV valve repair is the recommended option
D. Recurrent TR is frequent following TV repair when associated with severe leaflet tethering

ANSWERS AND DISCUSSION

QUESTION 29.1: The correct answer is C: Severe functional TR. The TR jet area is a quick and easy screening tool to assess for TR. Jet areas exceeding 34% of the RA are consistent with severe TR while areas of 20% to 34% are consistent with moderate TR. In this case, although the RA is not seen in its entirety, the jet area appears large and appears to occupy over 50% of the visible RA meeting initial criteria for severe TR. To confirm the diagnosis of TR, a vena contracta (VC) and hepatic vein blood flow were measured. A VC >6.5 mm is indicative of severe TR and, in this case, the measurement of 7 mm confirms the diagnosis of severe TR. Hepatic vein Doppler normally demonstrates three waves; the forward S and D waves and the reversed A wave representing flow reversal during atrial contraction. The S wave represents forward flow toward the RA during systole when the ventricle empties and creates space within the pericardium allowing blood to fill the RA. The D wave is a result of TV opening and the drop in RA pressure as blood fills the RV. This allows for venous flow into the empty RA. Blunting of the S wave may occur in moderate TR. In Figure 29.2, the PW Doppler of hepatic venous flow shows marked flow reversal in systole (below the baseline) indicative of severe TR.

The 2D exam reveals that the RV and annular dimensions are enlarged (5.4 cm, Figure 29.1B). The upper limits of normal for the basilar and mid diameter dimensions are 2.8 cm and 3.3 cm, respectively. This is a significant factor that contributes to functional TR where distraction of the TV leaflets by the subvalvular apparatus causes poor leaflet coaptation in systole. The most common causes of functional TR include left-sided heart or valvular disease and pulmonary hypertension. Organic TR is a result of multiple causes including rheumatic valve disease, prolapse, carcinoid disease, and Ebstein anomaly. There is no evidence from the echocardiographic exam for these conditions.

ANSWER A: Answer A, moderate TR, is incorrect; the TR is clearly severe meeting criteria of jet area, VC, and hepatic vein flow pattern.

ANSWER B: Answer B is incorrect. Ebstein anomaly is a cause of organic TR. The embryonic origins of the TV are derived from the RV wall. In Ebstein anomaly, the leaflets do not completely separate from the underlying myocardium and this abnormality is present most commonly in the septal and posterior leaflets. The TV is atrially displaced resulting in a small "atrialized" RV. Most notably, however, the leaflets are tethered and there is significant TR (Fig. 29.4). There is no evidence for Ebstein anomaly in the echo exam of this patient.

ANSWER D: Answer D is incorrect. There is no evidence for prolapse of the TV.

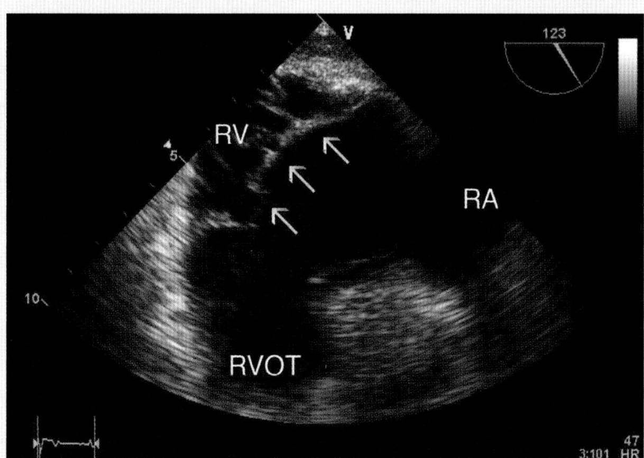

Figure 29.4. Modified TG RV inflow view demonstrating the apical, tethered inferior tricuspid leaflet (*arrows*) of Ebstein anomaly.

QUESTION 29.2: The *incorrect* answer is A: The systolic function by TAPSE is underestimated in the presence of severe TR and poor LV function. The TAPSE is a measure of RV systolic function. It is the tricuspid annular descent during the ejection phase. It is influenced by the RV systolic function, the SV, and the PA pressure. Its normal value measured in the ME 4CH view is approximately 24 mm. In the presence of TR, ejection will occur into both the PA and the low resistance RA, thereby increasing the TAPSE and overestimating the RV systolic function. The LV function also affects the TAPSE value as the LV can be a significant contributor to RV function via the shared septum and superficial myocardial fibers. A normal TAPSE in the presence of LV dysfunction measures approximately 20 mm.

Answer B is correct; the RV function by TAPSE is overestimated.

Answer C is correct. In cases of marked RV dysfunction and/or severe TR, the PA pressure may be reduced in a patient who otherwise had antecedent elevated PA pressures. This is a result of a failing RV.

Answer D is correct as discussed above.

QUESTION 29.3: The incorrect answer is A: Do nothing, correcting the left-sided pathology will improve the TR. Correcting left-sided heart disease without addressing severe TR is associated with significant late morbidity and mortality. In the presence of moderate-to-severe TR, a dilated tricuspid annulus (>4.0 cm) in association with left-sided valve disease,[1] the TV should be addressed. Furthermore, survival is improved in patients who receive an adequate TV repair when compared to a TV replacement. However, in cases of severe TR, there is a higher risk of recurrence following a repair. This may be the result of RV dilatation and distraction of the leaflets by the subvalvular apparatus (as in our case). Indeed, undersizing the tricuspid annulus during repair does not guarantee freedom from recurrence. It is also preferable to repair TR prior to the development of RV dysfunction. In the case above, the RV function was already significantly depressed, thereby increasing mortality following a TV repair. In this patient, it was considered too high a risk to perform a TV annuloplasty following the AVR. Unfortunately, the patient succumbed to severe RV failure 2 weeks postoperatively.

TAKE-HOME LESSON:

Appreciating tricuspid dysfunction and addressing it at the time of surgery impacts on outcome.

REFERENCE

1. Messika-Zeitoun D, Thomson H, Bellamy M, et al. Medical and surgical outcome of tricuspid regurgitation caused by flail leaflets. *J Thoracic Cardiovasc Surg*. 2004;128:296–302.

SUGGESTED READING

Chang BC, Lim SH, Yi G, et al. Long-term clinical results of tricuspid valve replacement. *Ann Thorac Surg.* 2006;81:1317–1324.

Fukuda S, Gillinoy MA, McCarthy PM, et al. Echocardiographic follow-up of tricuspid annuloplasty with a new three-dimensional ring in patients with functional tricuspid regurgitation. *J Am Soc Echocardiogr.* 2007;20:1236–1242.

McCarthy PM, Bhudia SK, Rajeswaran J, et al. Tricuspid valve repair: durability and risk factors for failure. *J Thoracic Cardiovasc Surg.* 2004;127:674–685.

Raja SG, Dreyfus GD. Surgery for functional tricuspid regurgitation: current techniques, outcomes and emerging concepts. *Expert Rev Cardiovasc Ther.* 2009;7(1):73–84.

Shiran A, Sagie A. Tricuspid regurgitation in mitral valve disease. *J Am Coll Cardiol.* 2009;52:401–408.

Singh S, Tang GHL, Maganti MD, et al. Midterm outcomes of tricuspid valve repair versus replacement for organic tricuspid disease. *Ann Thorac Surg.* 2006;82:1735–1741.

CASE 30

A 51-year-old man with severe MR undergoes a MV replacement with a bileaflet mechanical valve. After successful separation from CPB, a mobile, echogenic structure is noted in the LV using the ME 4CH view seen in Figure 30.1. (See the arrow in Fig. 30.1 and refer to Video 30.1.)

Thorough examination of the LV in the TG SAX and TG LAX views did not demonstrate a mobile structure in the LV (Fig. 30.2).

QUESTION 30.1. What is the most likely cause of the mobile structure seen in the ME views of the left heart?

A. Side-lobe artifact of the PA catheter

B. Ruptured papillary muscle after implantation of the mechanical MV

C. SAM of the residual MV leaflets in the LV

D. Mirroring artifact of the mechanical MV leaflets in the LV

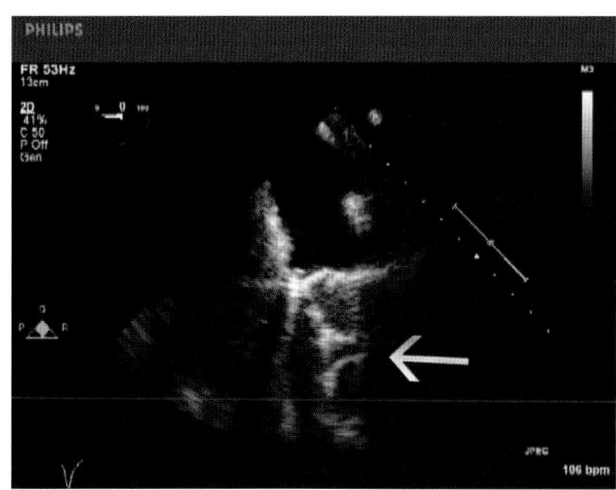

Figure 30.1. ME 4CH view post-CPB for mechanical MV replacement. (Please refer to Video 30.1.)

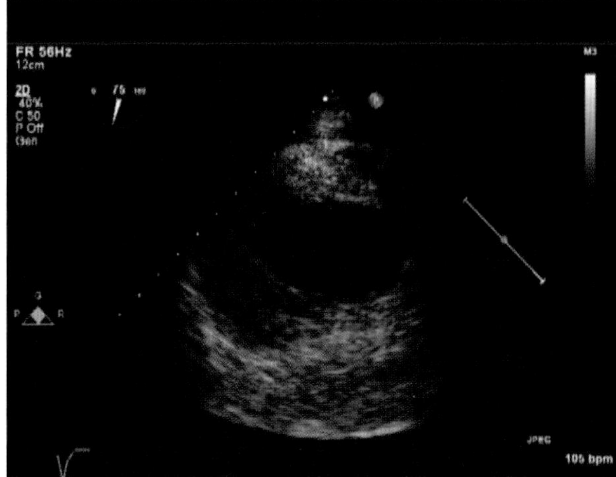

Figure 30.2. TG LAX view of the LV. (Please refer to Video 30.2.)

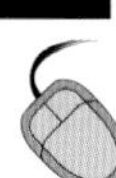

ANSWERS AND DISCUSSION

QUESTION 30.1: The correct answer is D.

This is a good example of mirror image artifact, a common cause for misrepresentation of the position of a reflective structure in the heart. There are several assumptions made by the ultrasound (US) machine as it processes the reflected US pulses and formulates a two-dimensional picture. A basic assumption is that sound travels in a straight line and is reflected directly back to the probe. It is very common that US pulses will "ping-pong" within the heart prior to returning to the probe. The extra time of flight of the pulse will cause the machine to misinterpret the true depth of the reflectors and often a second, deeper structure is seen. This is seen very commonly when examining the descending aorta and with strong reflectors such as mechanical valves. This type of artifact can be seen with calcified, native valves as well (see Video 30.3).

This phenomenon also causes multiple false copies of the true reflective structure seen at progressive depth. A reverberation artifact will appear as a step ladder evenly spaced reflectors is a parallel line to the axis of the beam (Fig. 30.3). When the reflectors are very close to each other, the ladder may appear as a fused, bright line known as a Comet tail.

A side-lobe artifact (answer A) violates the assumption that the reflector arises from the main axis of the US beam. The physics of US beam generation causes multiple weaker beams to propagate outward at oblique angles to the main beam. If one of these beams strikes a strong reflector, the structure may be falsely perceived within the main axis of the US beam (Fig. 30.4). As the main axis of the beam sweeps left or right, a lateral artifact is falsely perceived at a consistent depth with the true reflector.

Answer B is incorrect. A ruptured papillary muscle should be evident in the TG SAX and TG LAX views. Typically, one of the mitral leaflets will be flail, with a mobile structure moving into the left atrium in systole and significant MR.

Answer C is incorrect. SAM of the MV is abnormal movement of the anterior leaflet into the LVOT during systole. A variable amount of MR is associated depending on the leaflet pathology and the dynamic state of the heart. SAM is most commonly seen after MV repair. It is not associated with MV replacement. In a MV replacement, the residual leaflet structure is typically tucked behind the sewing ring and is not very mobile.

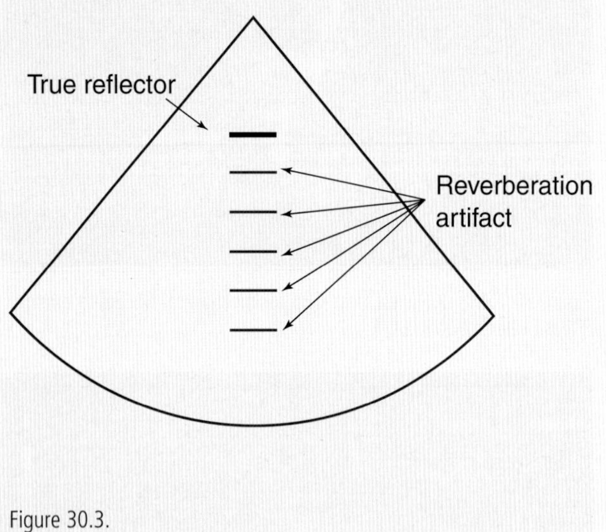

Figure 30.3.

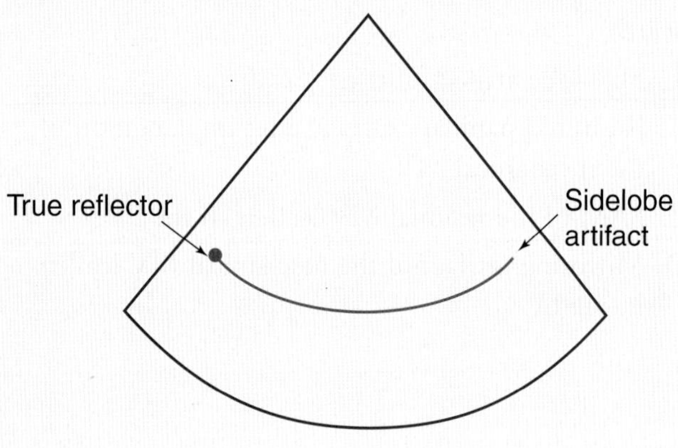

Figure 30.4.

TAKE-HOME LESSON:

Artifacts can be caused by missing or falsely perceived structures. It is important to integrate multiple image planes to rule out artifacts. Reverberation of echo is a common cause of falsely perceived structures.

SUGGESTED READING

Edelman SK. *Understanding Ultrasound Physics.* 3rd ed. Woodlands, TX: ESP Inc.; 2004.

Heller LB, Aronson S. Imaging artifacts and pitfalls. In: Savage RM, ed. *Comprehensive Textbook of Intraoperative Transesophageal Echocardiography.* 1st ed. Philadelphia: Lippincott Williams & Wilkins; 2005:39–47.

CASE 31

A comprehensive TEE exam is performed. Match the numbers (or letters) in each view with the correct anatomic structure(s). For each question, please choose from the following answer bank. An answer can be used more than once.

AL papillary muscle
PM papillary muscle
Chordae tendinae first order
Chordae tendinae second order

QUESTION 31.1. Figure 31.1 shows a partial ME five-chamber view. Identify the structures labeled 1, 2, and 3.

QUESTION 31.2. Figure 31.2 shows a ME 4CH view. Identify the structures labeled 1 and 2.

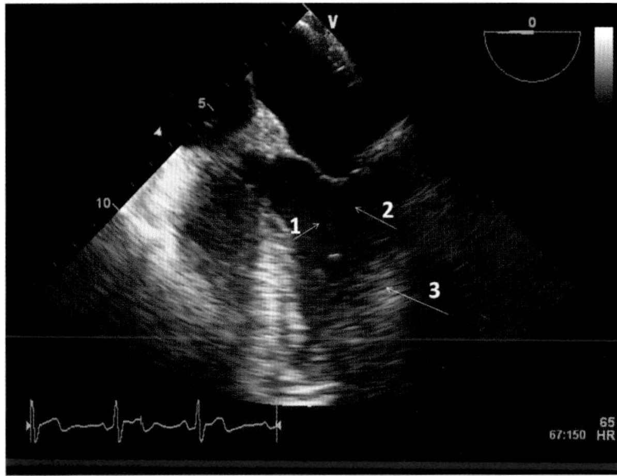

Figure 31.1.

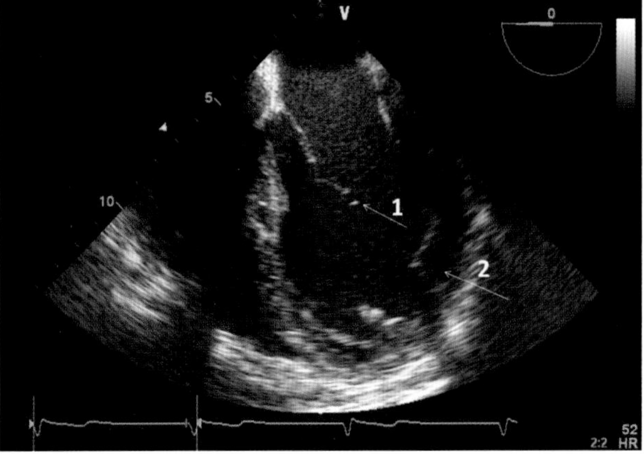

Figure 31.2.

QUESTION 31.3. For the images in Figure 31.3, identify numbers 1 to 7.

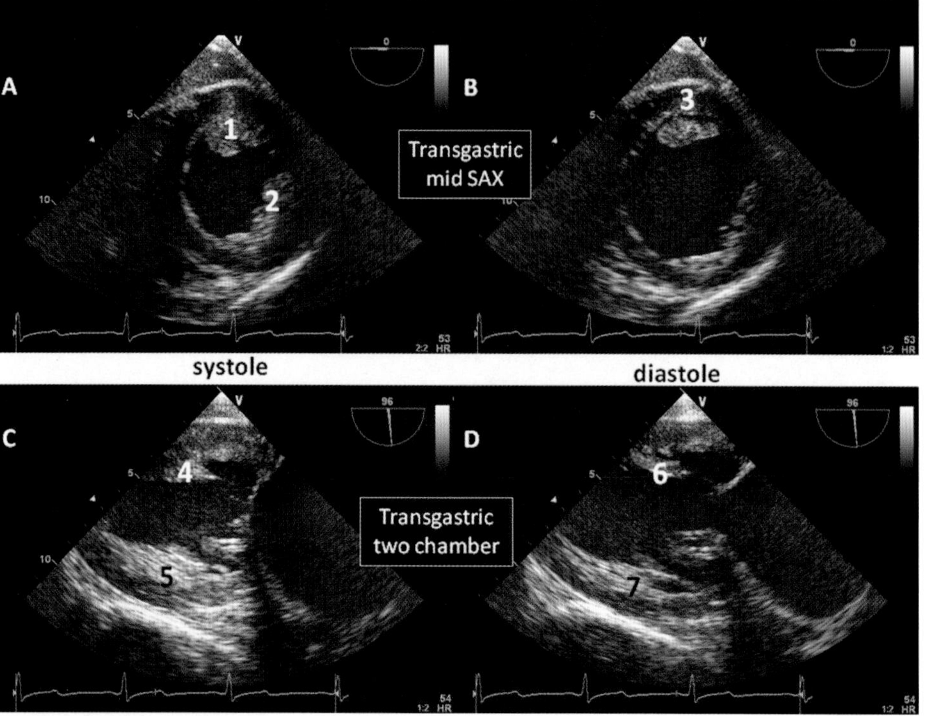

Figure 31.3.

QUESTION 31.4. In the TG two-chamber view in Figure 31.4, identify the structures labeled 1, 2, and 3.

QUESTION 31.5. In the TG two-LAX view in Figure 31.5, identify the structures labeled 1, 2, and 3.

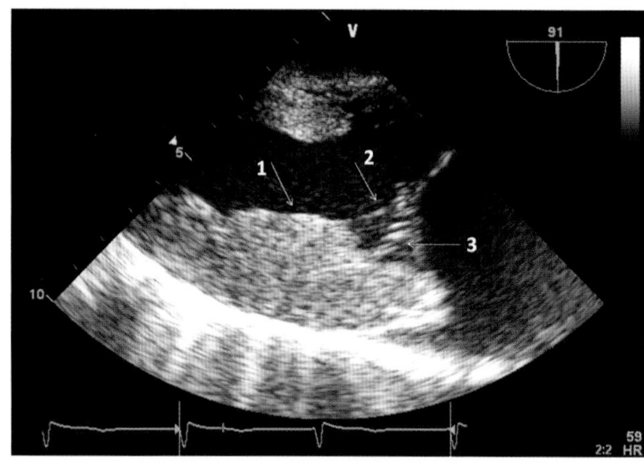

Figure 31.4.

QUESTION 31.6. In the TG two-chamber view in Figure 31.6, identify the structures labeled 1, 2, and 3.

QUESTION 31.7. In the TG two-chamber view in different stages of systole in Figure 31.7, identify the structures labeled a, b, and c.

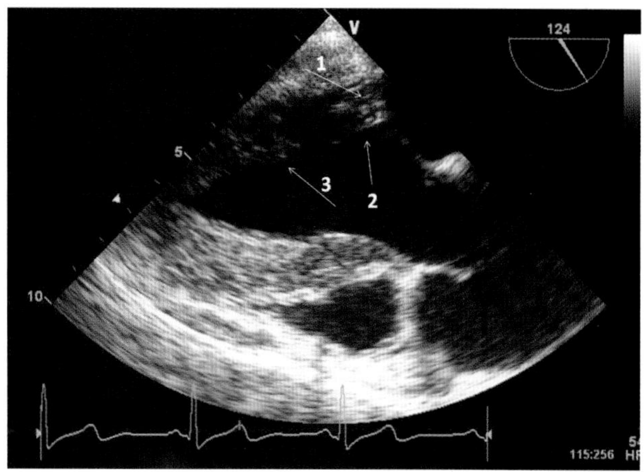

Figure 31.5.

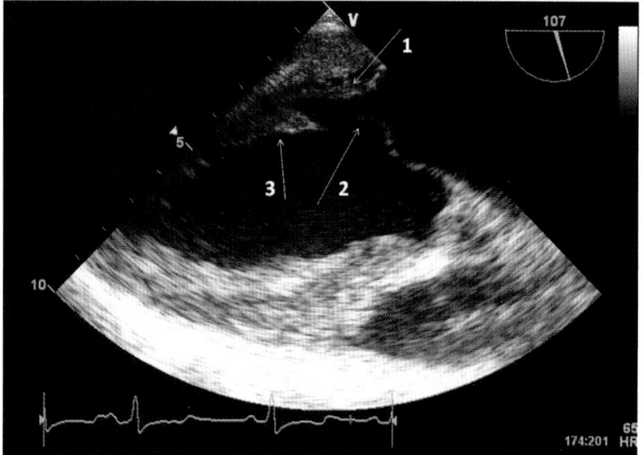

Figure 31.6.

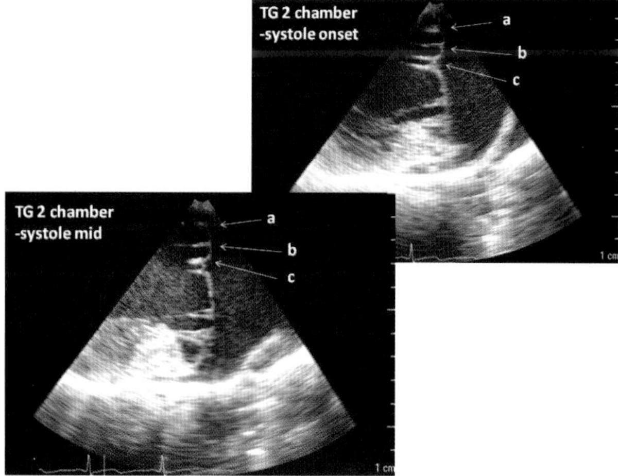

Figure 31.7.

ANSWERS AND DISCUSSION

QUESTION 31.1

1 = Chordae tendinae first order
2 = Chordae tendinae first order
3 = AL papillary muscle

QUESTION 31.2

1 = Chordae tendinae first order
2 = AL papillary muscle

QUESTION 31.3

1 = PM papillary muscle
2 = AL papillary muscle
3 = PM papillary muscle
4 = PM papillary muscle
5 = AL papillary muscle
6 = PM papillary muscle
7 = AL papillary muscle

QUESTION 31.4

1 = AL papillary muscle
2 = Chordae tendinae first order
3 = Chordae tendinae second order

QUESTION 31.5

1 = Chordae tendinae second order
2 = Chordae tendinae first order
3 = PM papillary muscle

QUESTION 31.6

1 = Chordae tendinae first order
2 = Chordae tendinae first order
3 = PM papillary muscle

QUESTION 31.7

a = Chordae tendinae second order
b = Chordae tendinae second order
c = Chordae tendinae first order

The MV apparatus consists of annulus, leaflets, and components of the subvalvular apparatus, which are the papillary muscles and the chordae tendinae.

Chordae tendinae are fibrous strings radiating from the LV papillary muscles or the ventricular free wall (for the posterior leaflet only) and attaching to the mitral leaflets. The majority of the leaflets branch either soon after leaving the papillary muscle or before insertion into the leaflet. First-order chordae tendinae attach on the free margin of the leaflet. Second-order chordae tendinae insert anywhere from a few to several millimeters away from the free edge of the leaflet. Third-order chordae tendinae travel from the ventricular wall and insert into the base of the posterior leaflet only.

It has recently been appreciated that there are two relatively stronger chordae tendinae for each leaflet that have increased tensile strength and are called "stay" chordae. They attach to the medial aspect of each leaflet.

TAKE-HOME LESSON:

First-order chordae tendinae attach on the free margin of the leaflet, second-order chordae tendinae insert away from the free edge of the leaflet, and third-order chordae tendinae travel from the ventricular wall and insert into the base of the posterior leaflet only.

SUGGESTED READING

Bollen B, Duran C, Savage RM. Surgical anatomy of the heart: correlation with echocardiographic-imaging planes. In: Savage RM, Aronson S, eds. *Comprehensive Textbook of Intraoperative Transesophageal Echocardiography*. 1st ed. Philadelphia: Lippincott Williams & Wilkins; 2005:69–74.

Degandt AA, Weber PA, Saber HA, et al. Mitral valve basal chordae: comparative anatomy and terminology. *Ann Thorac Surg*. 2007;84:1250–1255.

Kumar N, Kurmar M, Duran CMG. A revised terminology for recording surgical findings of the mitral valve. *J Heart Valv Dis*. 1995;4:70–75.

Lam HJC, Ranganathan N, Wigle ED, et al. Morphology of the human mitral valve. II. The valve leaflets. *Circulation*. 1970;41:449–458.

CASE 32

A 75-year-old female presents to the OR for an AVR. After an uncomplicated induction of anesthesia and bioprosthetic AVR, the patient was easily weaned from CPB. The initial hemodynamics and cardiac indices were reassuring but 5 minutes after weaning from bypass, the patient develops hypotension and low cardiac output. You obtain the TEE images shown in Figures 32.1 and 32.2

QUESTION 32.1. What is the most likely etiology for the acute drop in blood pressure?

A. Coronary artery air embolism
B. Coronary artery entrapment by prosthetic valve annular sutures
C. Stunned myocardium
D. Coronary dissection

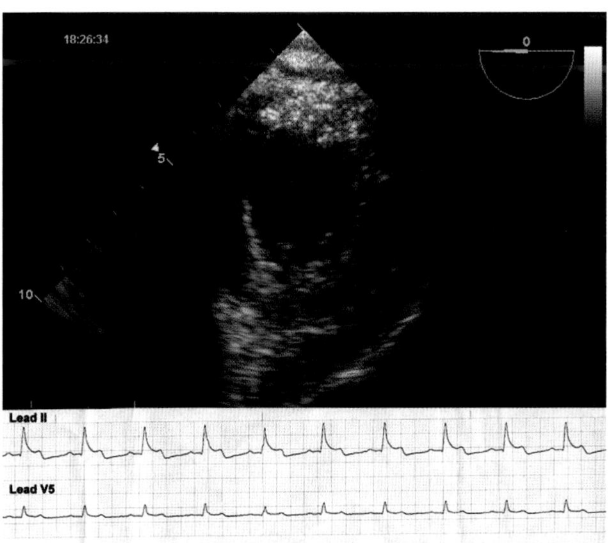

Figure 32.1. TG SAX of the LV (see also Video 32.1), with ECG strip of leads II and V5 while the images were captured.

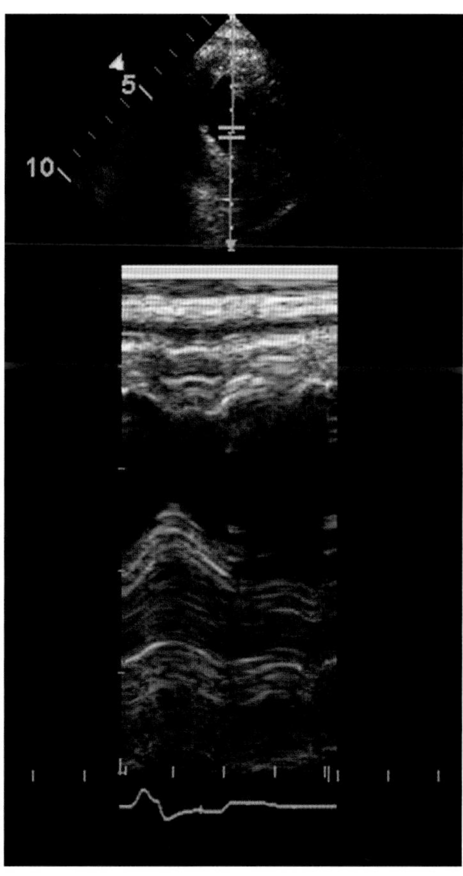

Figure 32.2. M-Mode of the TG SAX view of the LV at the time of the event.

QUESTION 32.2. Which coronary vessel has most likely been embolized?

A. Left main

B. LAD

C. RCA

D. Circumflex coronary artery

QUESTION 32.3. Potential treatment options include all of the following *except*

A. Aspirating residual air from the LV

B. Increasing the blood pressure to increase coronary perfusion

C. Returning to CPB

D. Beta blockade

The patient improves over the next few minutes and the TEE images shown in Figures 32.3 and 32.4 are obtained.

QUESTION 32.4. What typical TEE findings are consistent with intracoronary air embolism?

A. Increased brightness and RWMAs of the affected myocardial segment(s)

B. Persistent RWMAs that do not improve with time

C. RWMAs that only occur in the RCA territory

D. Shadowing of the affected myocardial segment(s)

E. All of the above

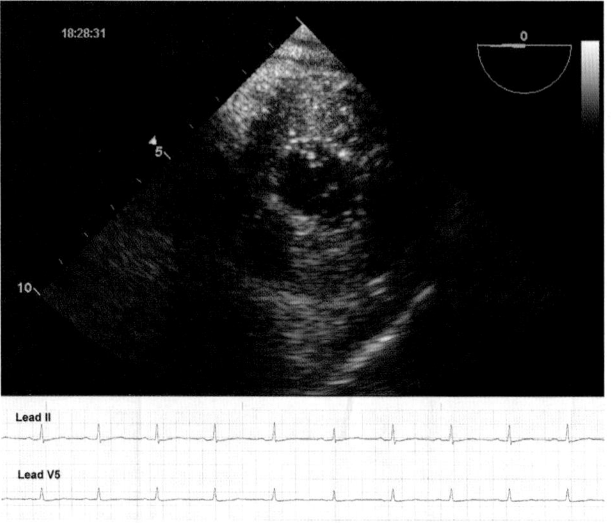

Figure 32.3. TG SAX view of the LV a few minutes later (see also Video 32.2), with ECG strip of leads II and V5 while the images were captured.

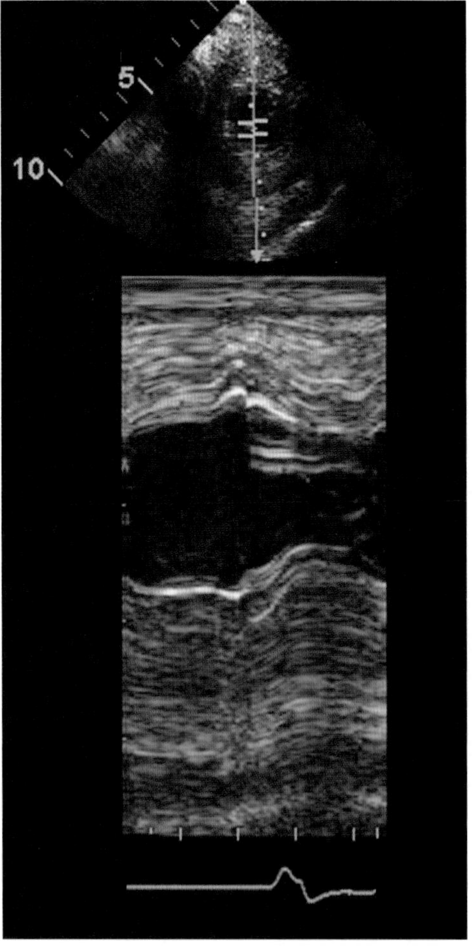

Figure 32.4. M-Mode, TG SAX view of the LV a few minutes later.

ANSWERS AND DISCUSSION

QUESTION 32.1: The correct answer is A: Coronary artery air embolism. Intracoronary air embolism is a common complication of open heart surgery. Intracavitary air tends to rise against gravity, making the anteriorly located RCA ostium most susceptible to air embolism. The corresponding area of myocardium that is most commonly affected is the inferior LV wall, with or without associated RV dysfunction. In this patient, the increased brightness of the LV inferior wall along with the associated acute onset and rapidly resolving hypotension support this diagnosis. Typically, this brightness is associated with a *transient* RWMA (seen in Fig. 32.2 and in Video 32.1). Note also the ST segment elevation in lead II in Figure 32.1, which resolves a few minutes later (Fig. 32.3). Answer B—coronary artery entrapment by prosthetic valve annular sutures—is incorrect: Coronary artery entrapment can occur during valve surgery, but it would not result in increased myocardial *brightness* nor would the RWMA improve with time. Answer D—coronary dissection—is incorrect for the same reasons. Finally, answer C—stunned myocardium—is incorrect: stunned myocardium is unlikely to cause an abrupt deterioration following an easy wean from CPB. Rather, one would expect some difficulty separating from bypass.

QUESTION 32.2: Which coronary vessel has most likely been embolized?

The correct answer is C: RCA. In Figure 32.1 and Video 32.1, the TG short-axis view of the LV demonstrates an increased brightness of the *inferior wall*, which corresponds to the *right coronary* distribution. By contrast, the anterior, anteroseptal, septal (*LAD distribution*), lateral, and inferolateral (*circumflex distribution*) walls of the LV appear homogenous. In Figure 32.2, the M-mode demonstrates the same increased brightness of the inferior wall, along with a significant hypokinesis, compared to the anterior wall.

Figure 32.5 demonstrates an example of air accumulating near the RCA ostium in the aortic root of a different patient.

QUESTION 32.3: The correct answer is D: Beta blockade.

Myocardial dysfunction secondary to intracoronary air is usually *transient*. It is often associated with ST segment elevation in the affected territory and can lead to hemodynamic instability. Ideally, careful cardiac deairing should be performed *before* separating from bypass. Still, air can accumulate in the pulmonary veins and only come out after full separation from CPB (i.e. when there is flow through the pulmonary vasculature). If air

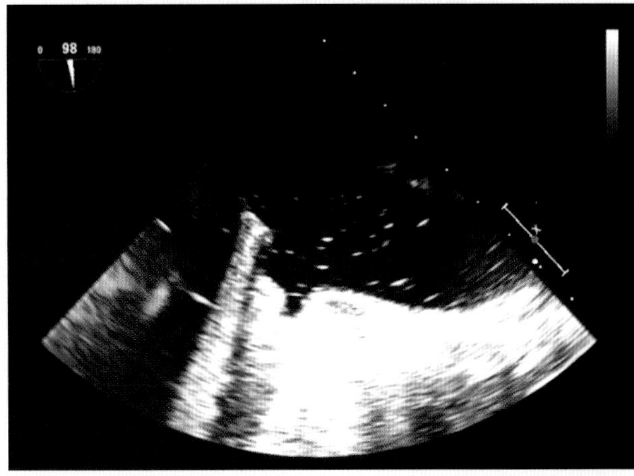

Figure 32.5. Upper esophageal LAX of the ascending aorta: note the air bubbles in the aortic root, which appear to be entering the RCA.

embolism occurs post bypass, the management is usually supportive, and aims at eliminating the air and preventing further embolization. This would include placing the bed in Trendelenburg position to trap the air in the LV apex, *vasopressor support* to increase coronary perfusion pressure (which may help "push" the air through the coronary vasculature), *aspirating residual air* from the heart (or opening the aortic root vent if still in place) to minimize further escape of air emboli into the systemic and coronary circulation, and *maintaining adequate systemic forward flow* (inotropes may be needed or, in extreme cases, return to CPB). Beta blockade would *not* be beneficial in this situation and may be detrimental if it results in a drop in blood pressure.

QUESTION 32.4: The correct answer is A: Increased brightness and RWMAs in the affected myocardial segment(s). Air has high acoustic impedance and embolized air in the coronary circulation typically results in an *increased brightness* of the myocardium in the distribution of the affected coronary artery. Additionally, the air causes transient myocardial dysfunction, seen as RWMAs in the associated segments. Answer D (*acoustic shadowing*) is incorrect: *large* collections of air inside the heart can cause acoustic shadowing, but this is not the case with tiny air bubbles in the coronary system. Answer C (*RWMA only in the RCA territory*) is also incorrect: the RCA, by virtue of the fact that its ostium is located anteriorly, tends to be affected *most often*. However, air emboli can occur anywhere in the myocardium, especially when coronary bypass grafts are anastomosed to the anterior ascending aorta. Finally, answer B (*persistent RWMA*) is incorrect: as stated above, air emboli typically cause transient RWMAs, as illustrated in Figures 32.1 to 32.4 and Videos 32.1 and 32.2. A persistent RWMA would suggest a more serious problem, like embolization of solid material, coronary dissection, or inadvertent entrapment of a coronary vessel by a suture.

TAKE-HOME LESSON:

If coronary air embolism occurs post bypass, the management is usually supportive, and aims at eliminating the air and preventing further embolization.

SUGGESTED READING

Chandraratna A, Ashmeg A, Pasha HC. Detection of intracoronary air embolism by echocardiography. *J Am Soc Echocardiogr*. 2002;15:1015–1017.

CASE 33

Following an aortic root replacement for prosthetic AV endocarditis, a 62-year-old male presents with LV dilation and severe functional MR. MV surgery is performed via a right thoracotomy and the TEE images shown in Figures 33.1 to 33.3 are obtained.

QUESTION 33.1. What type of MV surgery has been performed?

A. Quadrangular resection of the posterior leaflet
B. Alfieri edge-to-edge repair with mitral annuloplasty
C. Insertion of bileaflet mechanical prosthesis
D. Annuloplasty ring only

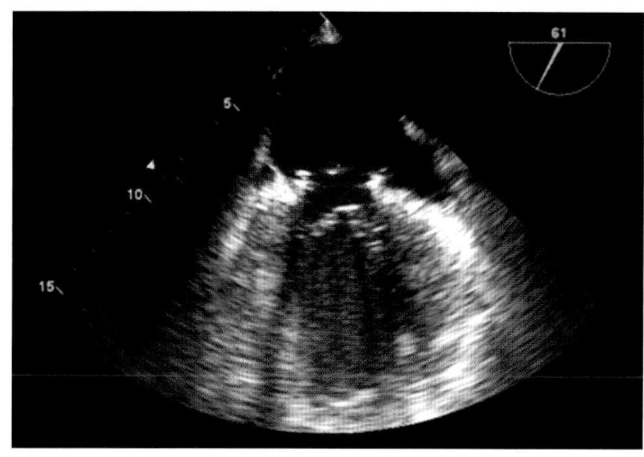

Figure 33.1. ME mitral commissural view, 2D, in diastole. See also Video 33.1.

QUESTION 33.2. How should this type of surgery be interrogated to assure adequacy?

A. CFD evaluation
B. PISA calculation of the EROA
C. PW Doppler of the TMF velocities
D. All of the above

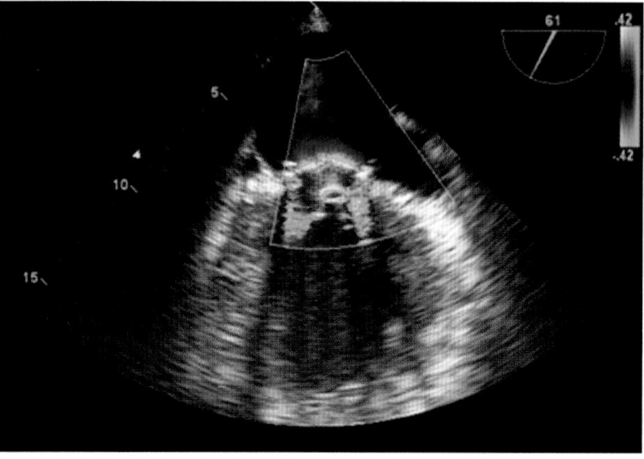

Figure 33.2. ME mitral commissural view with CFD of mitral inflow. See also Video 33.2.

QUESTION 33.3. Which of the following complications is of particular importance with this form of surgery?

A. SAM of the anterior mitral leaflet
B. AFib
C. Mitral stenosis
D. Prevalence of endocarditis

QUESTION 33.4. What other type of MV surgery could result in a similar CFD pattern in the ME 4CH view?

A. Starr–Edwards valve in the mitral position
B. Bileaflet mechanical valve in the mitral position
C. Bioprosthetic MV
D. Mitral annuloplasty ring

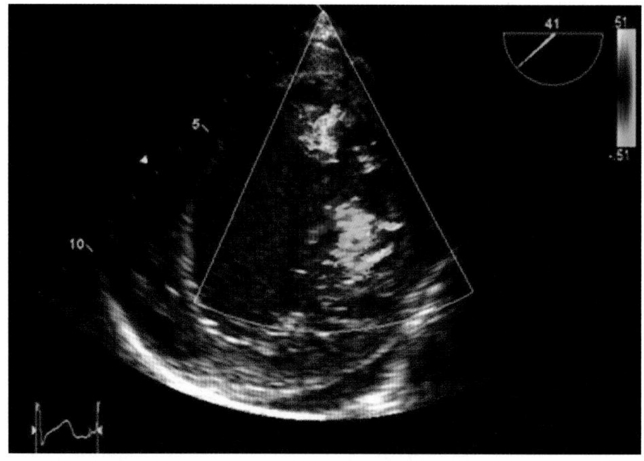

Figure 33.3. TG basal short-axis view of the MV, with CFD, in diastole. See also Video 33.3.

ANSWERS AND DISCUSSION

QUESTION 33.1: The correct answer is B: Alfieri edge-to-edge repair with mitral annuloplasty. In addition to a MV annuloplasty, an Alfieri stitch was placed to limit the amount of MR. This procedure involves attaching the free edges of the midportion of the anterior leaflet and the posterior leaflet, forming a double orifice MV. Figure 33.1 shows the area where A2 and P2 were surgically attached and Figure 33.2 shows CFD entering the LV on either side of the suture. Figure 33.3 demonstrates the two separate mitral orifices in short axis (an appearance often referred to as *double-barrel* MV). This type of repair has been shown to be useful in MR caused by leaflet prolapse and has been utilized when the effect of a MV annuloplasty is deemed suboptimal. Answer A (*quadrangular resection*) is incorrect: quadrangular resection is a MV repair technique used in cases of severe leaflet prolapse. In such cases, a segment of leaflet is resected and the remaining segments are sewn together. This type of repair does not produce a double orifice MV. Answer C is incorrect as there are no hallmarks of an implanted mechanical prosthesis.

QUESTION 33.2: The correct answer is A: CFD evaluation. Although there is no consensus on the single best way to evaluate an Alfieri MV repair, a complete postrepair exam should be performed using multiple echocardiographic modalities. A complete 2D evaluation demonstrates adequate opening and closure of the valve, and planimetry can be performed to document the area of each orifice. CFD interrogation of the valve is done to show laminar flow in each orifice, with minimal regurgitation during systole. CW spectral Doppler is then used to assess the gradient across the valve. Answer B (*PISA calculation of EROA*) is incorrect: PISA calculations are generally felt to be unreliable in Alfieri repairs, due to the double orifice nature of these valves (unless PISA was done on each orifice separately). Answer C (*PW Doppler*) is also incorrect: spectral Doppler interrogation of valve stenosis requires the use of *CW Doppler*, since placing the PW sampling gate at the wrong level may miss the true gradient across the orifice and lead to underestimation of the pressure gradient. Finally, each orifice may be of different caliber, further complicating the hemodynamic analysis of the repair. For these reasons, some authors advocate planimetry of each mitral orifice as a means to confirm adequate valve area following an Alfieri repair.

QUESTION 33.3: The correct answer is C: Mitral stenosis. Because an Alfieri repair turns one large mitral orifice into two separate channels, the particular concern with this type of repair is the conversion of MR into mitral stenosis. Significant aliasing of diastolic CFD through one or both orifices should prompt further investigation. Spectral Doppler interrogation of each orifice is performed to determine the success of the repair. Though no definitive study has verified what constitutes normal gradients through an Alfieri repair, mean gradients of less than 8 mm Hg are considered appropriate under typical hemodynamics and loading conditions. Figure 33.4 demonstrates a CW Doppler interrogation of both orifices after the repair, showing mean gradients less than 8 mm Hg for each. Answer A (*SAM of the anterior leaflet*) is incorrect: edge-to-edge repair is actually one of the *treatments for SAM* complicating other types of mitral repair. Answer B (*AFib*) and answer D (*endocarditis*) are also incorrect:

Atrial fibrillation and endocarditis are no more likely to occur than after any other type of MV repair.

QUESTION 33.4: The correct answer is A: *Starr–Edwards valve in the mitral position:* The Starr–Edwards mechanical valve has a "ball in cage" design which, when placed in the mitral position, creates the *appearance* of a double orifice mitral inflow. On some ME views, it can resemble the double-barrel appearance of an Alfieri repair. The TG short-axis view, however, is completely different. Also, because of its bulky structure, a Starr–Edwards valve causes prominent acoustic shadowing, which is not seen with an edge-to-edge repair. These differences emphasize the need to evaluate structures using multiple cross sections from multiple transducer locations. Answer B (*bileaflet mechanical valve*) is incorrect: Valves of this type have a characteristic appearance, with two tilting hemi-discs and washing jets. Answer C (*bioprosthetic valve*) is also incorrect: a mitral bioprosthetic valve has thin leaflets, characteristic struts on the ventricular side, and a single orifice. Finally, answer D (*annuloplasty ring*) is incorrect: although this patient does have an implanted ring, it does not in itself cause a double orifice and it is placed on the atrial side of the valve.

Figure 33.5 shows an example of a Starr–Edwards valve.

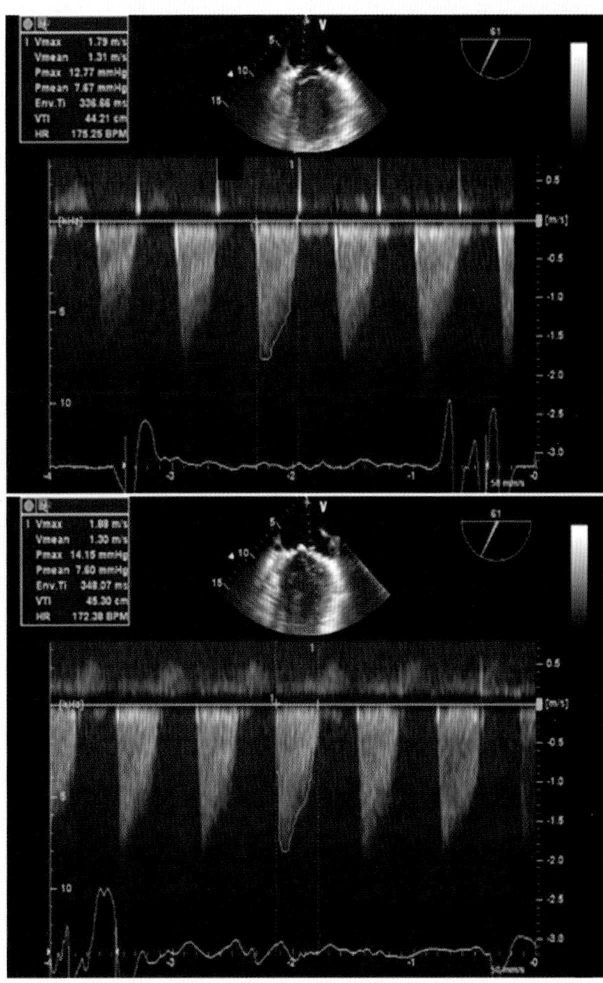

Figure 33.4. ME mitral commissural view with CW Doppler tracings of the two mitral orifices, showing mean gradients less than 8 mm Hg.

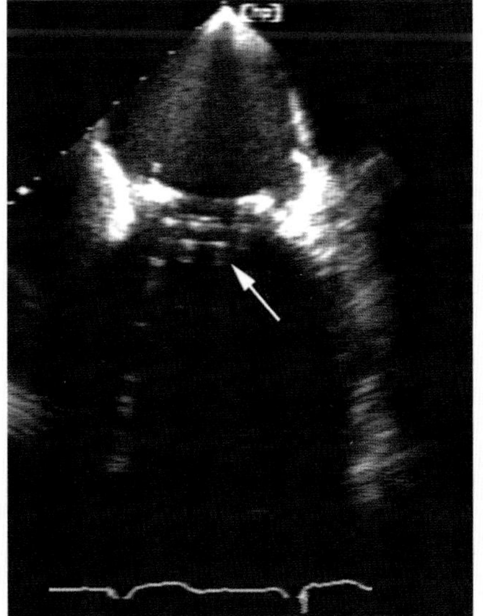

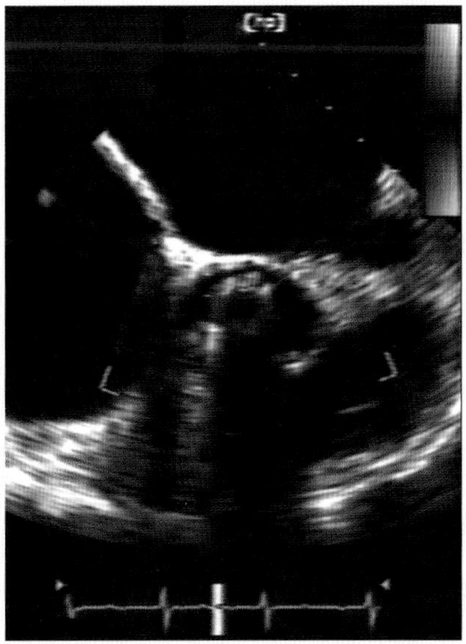

Figure 33.5. Starr–Edwards valve. Adapted from Perrino AC, Reeves ST. *Practical Approach to Transesophageal Echocardiography*. 2nd ed. Philadelphia: Lippincott Williams & Wilkins, 2008.Copyright LWW 2008.

TAKE-HOME LESSON:

An edge-to-edge Alfieri MV repair is a quick and effective way to repair certain types of MV regurgitation. It produces a typical "double barrel" appearance on echo, and its assessment can be difficult because of the double orifice. A good 2D examination is paramount.

SUGGESTED READING

Alfieri O, Maisano F, De Bonis M, et al. The double-orifice technique in mitral valve repair: a simple solution for complex problems. *J Thorac Cardiovasc Surg.* 2001;122:674–681.

Bhudia SK, McCarthy PM, Smedira NG, et al. Edge-to-edge (Alfieri) mitral repair: results in diverse clinical settings. *Ann Thorac Surg.* 2004;77:1598–1606.

Maisano F, Torracca L, Oppizzi M, et al. The edge-to-edge technique: a simplified method to correct mitral insufficiency. *Eur J Cardiothorac Surg.* 1998;13(3):240–245.

Moderate

CASE 34

A 78-year-old female with a long-standing history of shortness of breath, systemic arterial hypertension, and a diastolic murmur is scheduled for an aortic procedure. She underwent a comprehensive TEE exam in the prebypass period.

QUESTION 34.1. The ME ascending aortic short-axis view is shown in Figure 34.1. What is the correct diagnosis?

A. Type I Crawford aortic aneurysm
B. Ascending aortic dissection
C. Ascending aortic aneurysm
D. Aortic root dilation

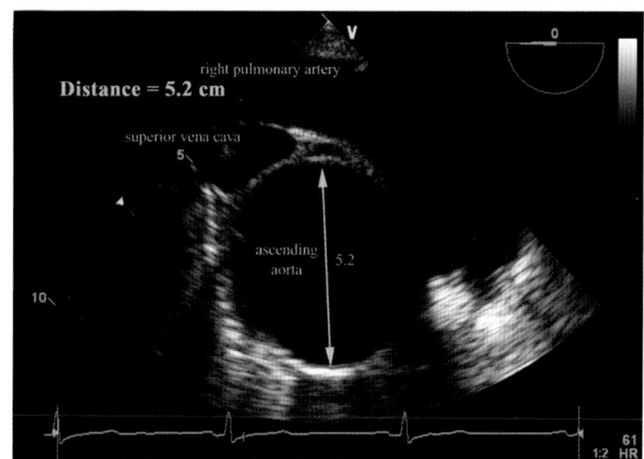

Figure 34.1. ME ascending aortic short-axis view.

QUESTION 34.2. The ME ascending aorta and AV LAX with and without CFD are shown in Figure 34.2. What is the indicated surgical procedure?

A. Bentall procedure for AS and ascending aortic aneurysm
B. Bentall procedure for AI and ascending aortic aneurysm
C. Graft replacement of ascending aortic aneurysm only
D. Graft replacement of aortic root and ascending aorta

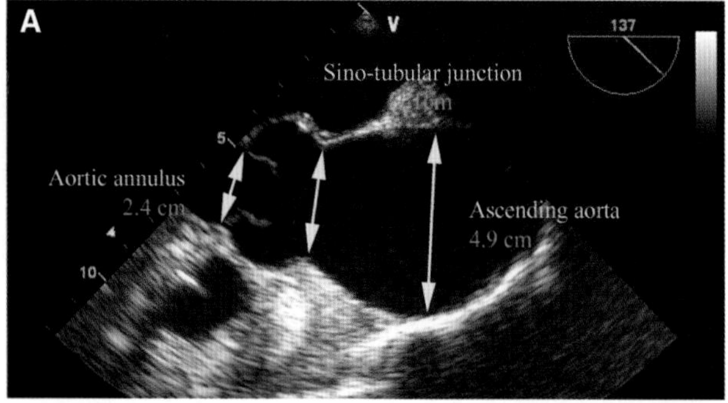

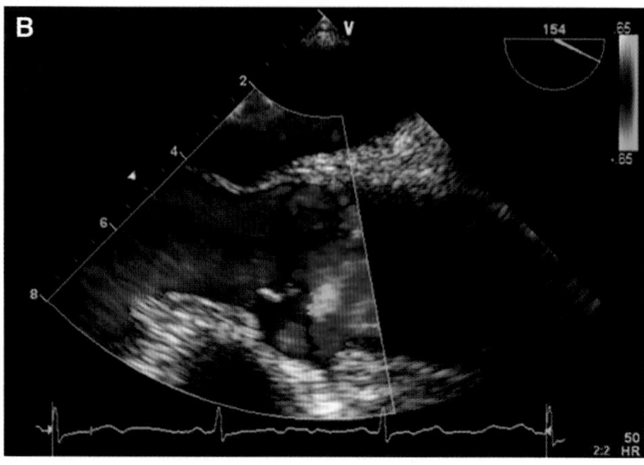

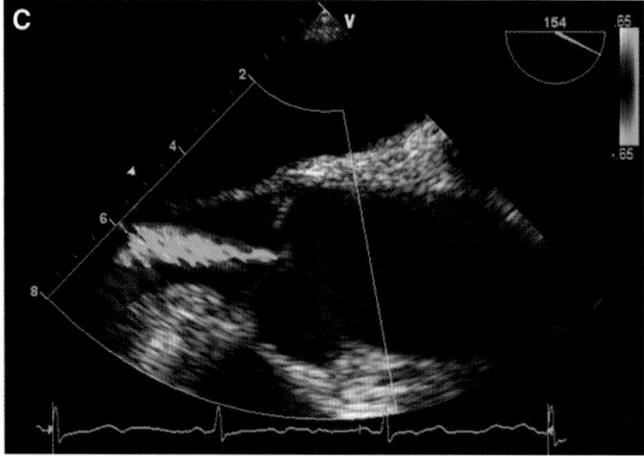

Figure 34.2. ME aorta and AV LAX. **A:** Measurements. **B:** CFD in systole. **C:** CFD in diastole.

ANSWERS AND DISCUSSION

QUESTION 34.1: The correct answer is C: Ascending aortic aneurysm.

An aortic aneurysm is a dilation of the aortic lumen beyond 4 cm in diameter. Aneurysms of the aorta can occur at any of its parts: ascending, arch, or descending. An aortic aneurysm is called fusiform if the entire aortic circumference is involved and saccular when dilation is localized only in part of the aortic circumference. In either case, the dilated aortic wall contains all three layers, and the aortic lumen is intact (there is no intimal flap as in aortic dissection, where the aortic lumen is divided into false and true lumens). An ascending aortic aneurysm requires surgical repair if the aortic diameter measures >4 cm (or >6 cm if it is located in the descending aorta). An aortic aneurysm should be differentiated from a pseudoaneurysm (false aneurysm); the latter is essentially a contained rupture of the aortic wall that involves all the layers. Containment of rupture is by the adventitia or via formation of adhesions and fibrosis with the neighboring anatomic structures. The only treatment is surgical excision and repair of the aortic wall, irrespective of the size of the aortic diameter.

ANSWER A: Type I Crawford aortic aneurysm is the wrong answer, as the Crawford classification pertains to aneurysms of the descending thoracic and abdominal aorta.

ANSWER B: Ascending aortic dissection is the wrong answer, because no dissection flap is imaged. However, it would be wrong not to scan the entire aorta (arch and descending) in search of a dissection (intimal) flap with 2D as well as CFD ultrasound.

ANSWER D: Aortic root dilation is the wrong answer. This can be verified (or excluded) with imaging of the ascending aorta and AV in long axis.

QUESTION 34.2: The correct answer is C: Graft replacement of ascending aortic aneurysm only.

The type of surgical repair of an ascending aortic aneurysm depends on the presence of associated anatomic lesions of the AV/aortic root, sinuses of Valsalva, and sinotubular junction. If the AV is diseased, it needs to be replaced (AS) or repaired (in some cases of AI). The presence of dilation of the sinuses of Valsalva or the sinotubular junction means that there is no "anchoring area" for the proximal graft anastomosis. In this case, the AV is replaced along with the ascending aorta (Bentall procedure), and the two coronary arteries are reattached to the graft either directly or via another, smaller tube graft (Cabrol procedure). Alternatively, the

AV can be "spared" and reattached inside the aortic graft (AV resuspension). In the case presented, AI is mild, based on the narrow proximal AI jet and the ratio of the jet to the diameter of the LVOT measuring <30%.

ANSWER A: Bentall procedure for AS and ascending aortic aneurysm is wrong because there is no AV stenosis. Figure 34.2B shows laminar flow in the LVOT and through the normally opposed AV cusps.

ANSWER B: Bentall procedure for AI and ascending aortic aneurysm is wrong, based on the findings shown in Figure 34.2C.

ANSWER D: Graft replacement of aortic root and ascending aorta is wrong. The diameters of aortic root, sinuses of Valsalva, and sinotubular junction are within normal.

TAKE-HOME LESSON:

In aortic aneurysms, inspect the AV, sinuses of Valsalva, and sinotubular junction to determine the extent of disease and appropriate surgical therapy.

SUGGESTED READING

Lang RM, Bierig M, Devereux RB, et al. Recommendations for chamber quantification. *J Am Soc Echocardiogr*. 2005;18:1440–1463.

Leverich A, Johnston C, Stiles B, et al. Cabrol composite graft for aortic root replacement: echocardiographic imaging. *Anesth Analg*. 2009;108:1107–1109.

Moderate

CASE 35

A 45-year-old executive with a history of a systolic murmur for 20 years presents for evaluation of dyspnea during a recent golf tournament. A preoperative echo indicates MV disease, and MV surgery is scheduled. Pre-bypass the TEE images shown in Figures 35.1 to 35.4 are obtained.

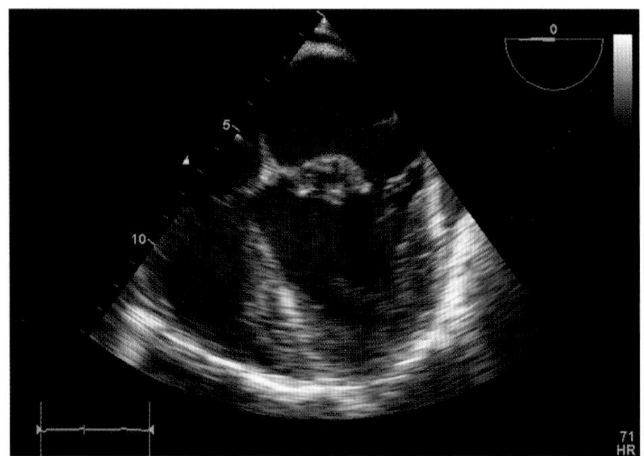

Figure 35.1. ME 4CH view, 2D, in systole. See also Video 35.1.

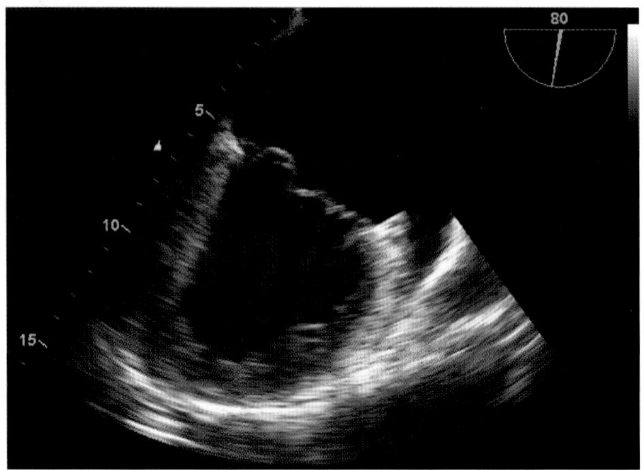

Figure 35.2. ME commissural view, 2D, in systole. See also Video 35.2.

QUESTION 35.1. Describe the pathology of the anterior mitral leaflet:

A. Anterior leaflet billowing
B. Anterior leaflet prolapse
C. Anterior leaflet flail
D. Anterior leaflet perforation

QUESTION 35.2. In the ME commissural view (Fig. 35.2, Video 35.2) the prolapsed segment is

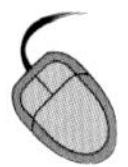

A. A1
B. A2
C. P2
D. P3

QUESTION 35.3. The MV pathology demonstrated in the TEE images is most consistent with:

A. Barlow syndrome
B. Taku-Tsubo heart disease
C. Ebstein anomaly
D. Cleft MV

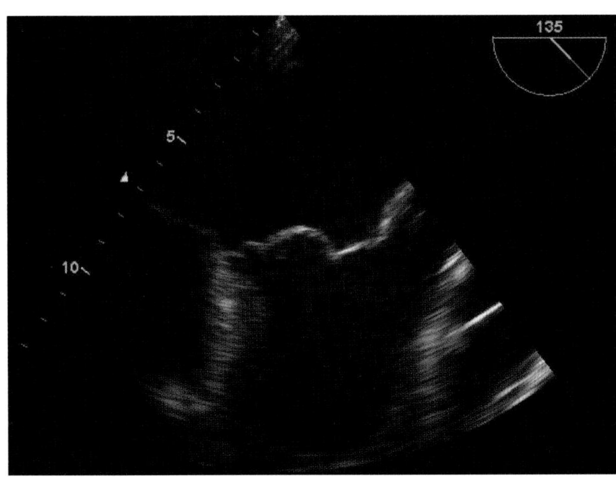

Figure 35.3. ME LAX, 2D, in systole. See also Video 35.3.

QUESTION 35.4. Which of the following would be a surprising finding in this patient?

A. Graves disease

B. Female gender

C. Eosinophilia

D. Mother died of sudden death

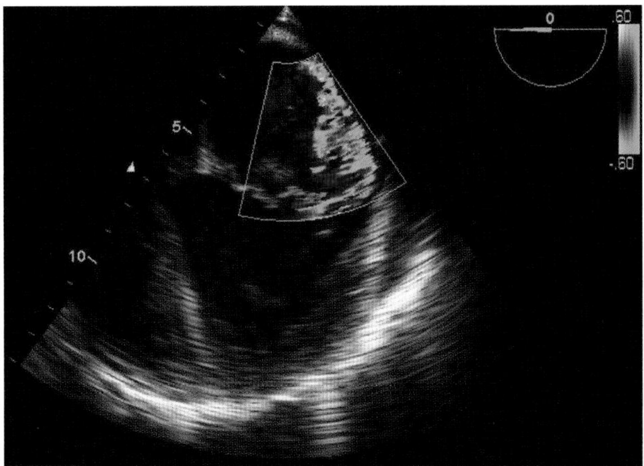

Figure 35.4. ME 4CH view, with color Doppler, in systole. See also Video 35.4.

ANSWERS AND DISCUSSION

QUESTION 35.1: The correct answer is B: Anterior leaflet prolapse.

Billowing (or scalloping) refers to a situation where part of a mitral leaflet projects above the annulus in systole, but the coaptation point remains below the mitral annulus. Thus, answer A is incorrect. *Prolapse* is used to describe the excursion of a leaflet tip above the level of the mitral annulus during systole, causing regurgitation that is directed away from the prolapsed leaflet. Figures 35.1 and 35.3 demonstrate the prolapse of the anterior leaflet and Figure 35.4 (CFD) shows the expected posteriorly directed eccentric jet. Answer C (*flail leaflet*) is incorrect: the term flail is reserved for a situation where a leaflet edge is flowing freely into the left atrium in systole, as a result of one or more ruptured *chordae tendinae*. Answer D (*leaflet perforation*) is also incorrect: with a perforation, the origin of the color jet is typically seen in the body of a leaflet, rather than at the point of coaptation, as regurgitant blood passes *through* the defect in the valve leaflet. In large leaflet perforation, the defect would be observed in the 2D echo exam as well as the color Doppler images.

QUESTION 35.2: The correct answer is B: A2 segment. In the ME commissural view (Fig. 35.2), this segment of the anterior leaflet is typically seen between the more posteriorly located P3 scallop and the more anteriorly located P1 scallop. Note the separation of the A2 segment from both P1 and P3 during the diastolic frames of Video 35.2, confirming that the segment is not part of the posterior leaflet. Importantly, this diagnosis is strengthened by consideration of the additional ME images (Figures 35.1, 35.3,

35.4 and Videos 35.1, 35.3, 35.4), which confirm the presence of severe A2 prolapse.

QUESTION 35.3: The correct answer is A: Barlow syndrome or MV prolapse syndrome. The findings of a late systolic murmur, redundant mitral leaflet with prolapse and MR are hallmarks of this disorder. Answers B and C are incorrect: Taku-Tsubo heart disease is a form of cardiomyopathy and Ebstein anomaly is an abnormality of the *TV*, not the mitral. Answer D, cleft MV, is incorrect: a cleft is a defect within the leaflet leading to regurgitation. It can present by itself or as part of the spectrum of endocardial cushion defects. Redundant leaflets and prolapse are not associated findings with cleft MV disease.

QUESTION 35.4: The correct answer is C: Eosinophilia. Heart disease with eosinophilia presents as subendocardial fibrosis and in some cases MR due to valve restriction (Carpentier class 3). Answer A (*Graves disease*) is known to be associated with MV prolapse syndrome. Answer B (*female gender*) is also known to be associated with *MV prolapse syndrome*. MV prolapse appears in two distinct patient populations. Patients presenting with MV prolapse at less than 40 years of age are more often female and the disease follows an autosomal dominant inheritance with variable penetration. This group is often referred to as *MV prolapse syndrome*. In contrast, males predominate in older patients presenting with MV prolapse. These older patients typically exhibit more severe disease including significant MR, thickened leaflets with myxomatous degeneration, and chordal rupture. The more specific term *myxomatous MV disease* is often applied to this second group of patients. There is a clear relationship between MV prolapse and arrhythmias and sudden death. Consequently, given the inheritance pattern of the disease a family history reporting a mother with sudden death (*answer D*) would not be surprising.

SUGGESTED READING

Otto, C (ed.). Mitral valve prolapse. In: *Valvular Heart Disease*. 2nd ed. Philadelphia: Saunders; 2004.

CASE 36

A 75-year-old female presents to the OR for urgent CABG following an angiogram that showed isolated tight left main coronary artery disease. Following induction of anesthesia you insert a TEE probe as part of your routine intraoperative management (Fig. 36.1 and Video 36.1).

QUESTION 36.1. Which of the following would be *least* useful in further evaluating the aorta?

A. CFD evaluation of the ascending aorta
B. CW Doppler of the ascending aorta
C. Short-axis examination of the aortic root
D. M-mode examination of the ascending aorta

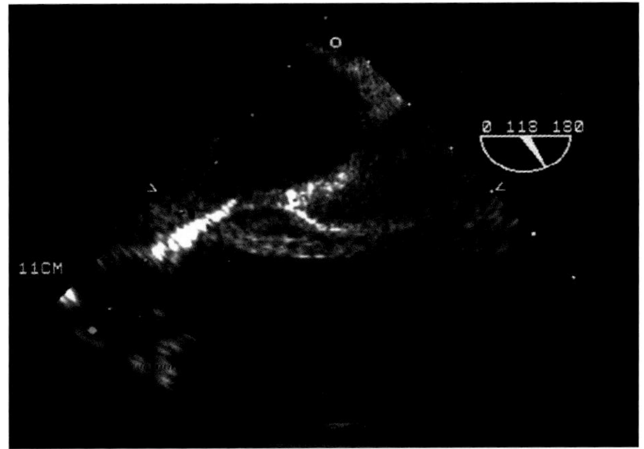

Figure 36.1. ME LAX of ascending aorta (see also Video 36.1).

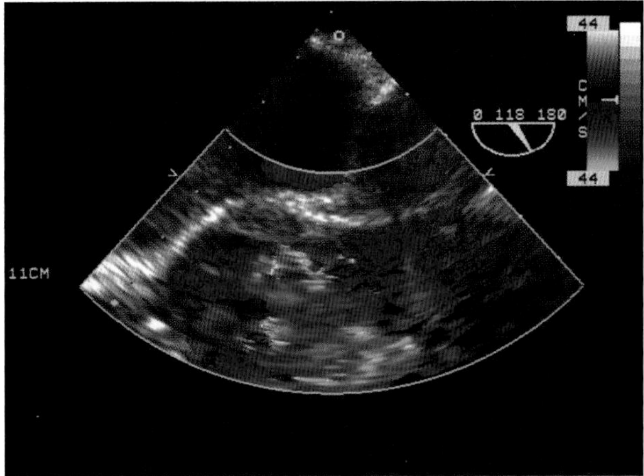

Figure 36.2. ME LAX of ascending aorta with CFD (see also Video 36.2).

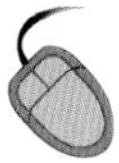

QUESTION 36.2. The echocardiographic findings are most consistent with (Figs. 36.2–36.5 and Videos 36.2–36.4)

A. Acute aortic dissection
B. Intramural hematoma (IMH)
C. Normal anatomy
D. Arterial thrombus

QUESTION 36.3. How does IMH differ from acute aortic dissection?

A. The section of the aorta where the pathology is located
B. In IMH, there is no direct communication between the true and the false lumen
C. The benign nature of IMH
D. The clinical presentation of IMH and Aortic Dissection (AD) are different

QUESTION 36.4. How do treatment options for IMH differ from acute dissection?

A. Conservative (i.e., nonsurgical) treatment of an ascending IMH is an acceptable management plan in selected cases
B. IMH of the descending aorta is best treated surgically
C. The natural history of IMH suggests that surgical intervention is inevitable
D. There is no role for endovascular stent grafts

QUESTION 36.5. Echocardiographic criteria for IMH include

A. An aortic wall thickness of 3 mm
B. Presence of Doppler flow in the thickened aortic wall
C. Thrombus-like consistency and layered appearance
D. Lateral displacement of the intimal calcification

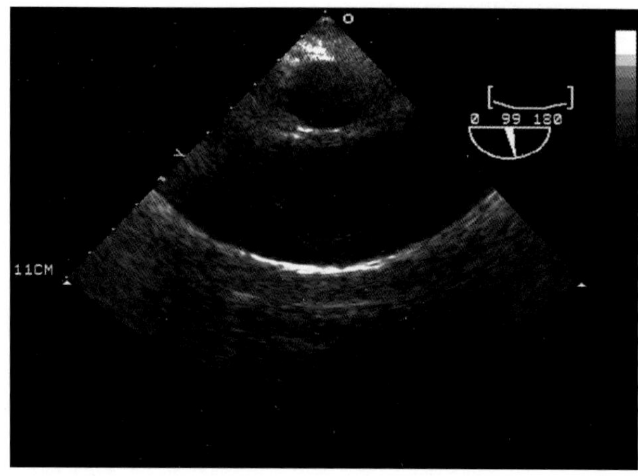

Figure 36.3. Upper esophageal LAX of ascending aorta.

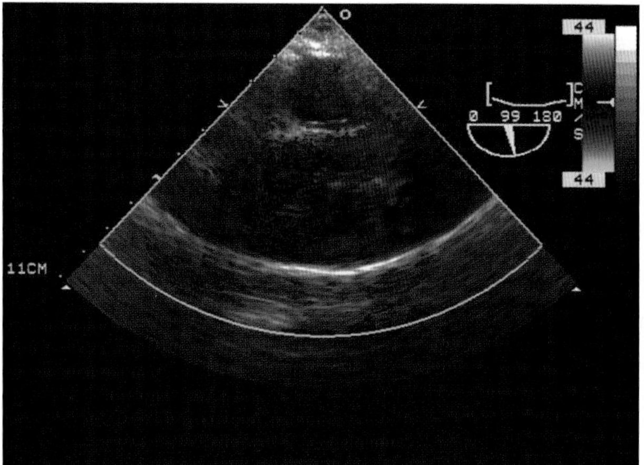

Figure 36.4. Upper esophageal long-axis color Doppler of ascending aorta (see also Video 36.3).

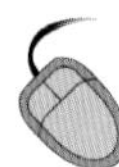

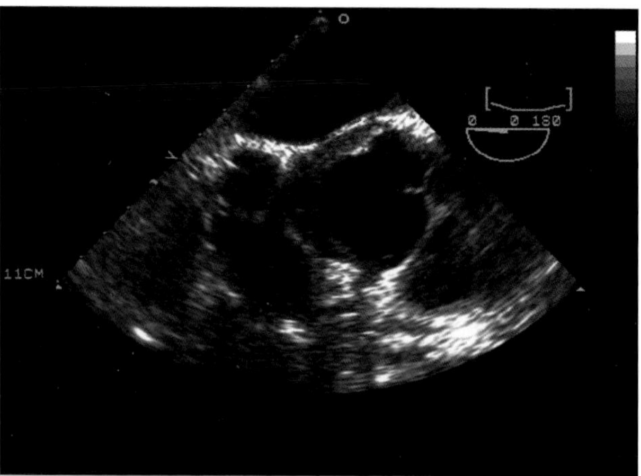

Figure 36.5. ME 4CH view with anteflexion and zoom to focus on the proximal aorta (see also Video 36.4).

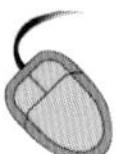

ANSWERS AND DISCUSSION

QUESTION 36.1: The correct answer is D: M-mode examination of the ascending aorta. M-mode uses a single scan line directed toward various structures in the heart. This mode is characterized by very rapid sampling rate and therefore is good at evaluating rapidly moving structures. However, since M-mode is limited to a single line as opposed to a sector, evaluating the extent of anatomical or pathological structures can be more difficult. Detecting the presence of a false lumen in the aorta or an IMH, while not impossible with M-mode, would likely be difficult. Answer A—CFD evaluation of the ascending aorta—is incorrect. CFD *is* useful for identifying blood flow into or out of an aortic false lumen and possibly finding a communication between the true and the false lumen. Answer B—CW Doppler of the ascending aorta—is incorrect. CW Doppler of the aorta may be useful for evaluating complications of aortic disease, including AI. Answer C—Short-axis examination of the aortic root—is incorrect. Short-axis evaluation is necessary to evaluate the location and extent of an IMH.

QUESTION 36.2: The correct answer is B: IMH. Note how, in Figures 36.1 and 36.5, there is an apparent separation between the intima and the adventitia, creating a false lumen. However, in Figure 36.2, no flow can be seen entering or exiting the false lumen. Answer A—Aortic dissection—is incorrect. Echocardiographically, an acute dissection of the aorta would reveal an intimal flap separating the true and the false lumen, often with different Doppler CFD patterns in each lumen. This intimal flap is often (but not always) mobile, typically showing systolic expansion of the true lumen and contraction of the false lumen. No such flap is visible in this case (Figures 36.1, 36.3, and 36.5). In this patient, the phenomenon is localized to proximal 3 cm of aorta and there is no apparent flap or communication between the true and the false lumen. Answer C—Normal anatomy—is incorrect. There is an obvious echolucent thickened area in the posterior aortic root that shouldn't be there. Answer D—Arterial thrombus—is incorrect. In Figures 36.1 and 36.5, one can see a layer of intima between the "mass" and the true lumen of the aorta. An arterial thrombus (as can be seen within an aneurysm) would be located in the true aortic *lumen* (rather than the aortic wall) and may be mobile. Other clues that make a thrombus unlikely in this setting are the smoothness of the mass (because it is covered with endothelium, the surface of an intraluminal thrombus tends to be less regular) and the high flow area in which it is located.

QUESTION 36.3: The correct answer is B: Absence of direct communication between the true and the false lumen. IMH is believed to be a hemorrhage within the aortic wall, resulting in localized separation of the layers of the aortic wall in the absence of an intimal tear (i.e., no direct communication between the thrombus in the false lumen and the true lumen of the aorta). It can be caused by the spontaneous rupture of aortic *vaso vasora* (blood vessels within the aortic wall), by localized trauma from percutaneous catheter manipulations, insertion of IABP or hemorrhage within an atherosclerotic plaque. Answer A—The section of the aorta where the pathology is located—is incorrect. Both aortic dissection and IMH have been described in both the ascending (type A) and descending aorta (type B). Answer C—The benign nature of IMH—is incorrect. The acute mortality rate of IMH involving the ascending aorta has been reported to be as high as 8%.[1] Answer D—The clinical presentation of IMH and acute dissection are different—is incorrect. Clinically, IMH and aortic dissection can be indistinguishable.[2]

QUESTION 36.4: The correct answer is A: Conservative (i.e., non surgical) treatment of an ascending IMH is an acceptable management plan in selected cases.

Because there is no communication between the true and the false lumen of the aorta, a nonoperative expectant approach may be taken to IMH involving the ascending aorta.[3] In both type A and type B IMH, the thickness of the hematoma and the aortic diameter are reported to be important predictors of outcome. Although not universally agreed upon, observation with serial TEEs or CT scans has been advocated by some authors. Answer B—IMH of the descending aorta is best treated surgically—is incorrect. IMH in that location is generally treated nonoperatively as one would treat a type B dissection. Answer C—The natural history of IMH suggests that surgical intervention is inevitable—is incorrect. The natural history of IMH is variable with complete resolution of IMH in as many as 50% of patients. Answer D—There is no role for endovascular stent grafts—is incorrect. In fact, given the segmental nature of IMH, this disease entity may be ideally treated with endovascular stenting. Long-term survival and success of endovascular stenting has yet to be determined; however, this treatment modality appears very promising.[4]

QUESTION 36.5: The correct answer is C: Thrombus-like consistency and layered appearance.

Answer A—An aortic wall thickness of 3 mm—is incorrect. That is the maximum normal thickness of the aorta. The classic definition of IMH includes a wall thickness >7 mm extending 1 to 20 cm longitudinally along the thoracic aorta. Recently, some authors suggest that a thickness >5 mm is enough to entertain the diagnosis.[3] Answer B—Presence of Doppler flow in the thickened aortic wall—is incorrect. There can be *no* evidence of Doppler flow: a diagnosis of IMH requires that there be no intimal tear or communication between the true lumen and the false lumen of the aorta. Answer D—Outward displacement of the intimal calcification—is incorrect. The aortic intimal displacement is typically directed *inward* into the lumen of the aorta by an IMH.

TAKE-HOME LESSON:

Aortic dissection and IMH can be distinguished by the presence or absence of blood flow in the periaortic area that looks like a false lumen.

In some instances an ascending aortic IMH does not require immediate surgical intervention.

Echocardiographically, IMH has a thrombus-like consistency and layered appearance.

REFERENCES

1. Coady MA, Rizzo JA, Elefteriades JA. Pathologic variants of thoracic aortic dissections. Penetrating atherosclerotic ulcers and intramural hematomas. *Cardiol Clin*. 1999;17:637–657.
2. Evangelista A, Mukherjee D, Mehta RH, et al. Acute intramural hematoma of the aorta. A mystery in evolution. *Circulation*. 2005;111:1063–1070.
3. Grabenwoger M, Fleck T, Czerny M, et al. Endovascular stent graft placement in patients with acute thoracic aortic syndromes. *Eur J Cardiothorac Surg*. 2003;23:788–793.
4. Song JK, Kim HS, Song JM, et al. Outcomes of medically treated patients with aortic intramural hematoma. *Am J Med*. 2002;113:181–187.

Moderate

CASE 37

An asymptomatic 60-year-old male with mildly reduced LV function is scheduled to undergo an elective three-vessel CABG.

QUESTION 37.1. During the intraoperative TEE exam a mass was seen on the AV in the ME LAX (Fig. 37.1 and Video 37.1). Choose the answer that best describes the mass seen:

A. It is expected to rapidly increase in size and cause symptoms of heart failure
B. It is highly vascularized and CFD is crucial for the diagnosis
C. It is typically located on the AV
D. It can typically be found at multiple locations in the heart
E. It is an example of Lambl excrescences (LE)

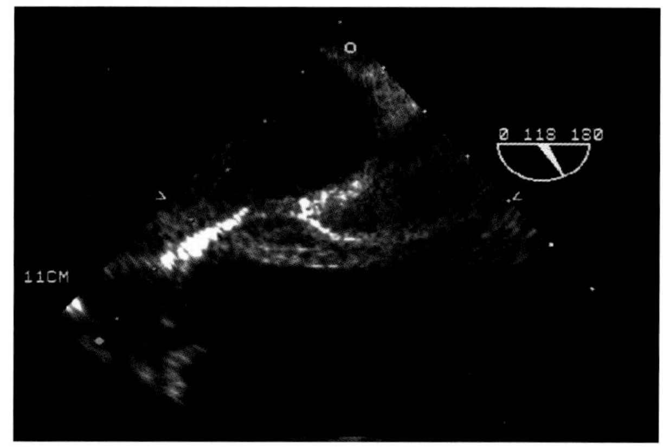

Figure 37.1. ME long-axis AV view.

QUESTION 37.2. Choose the answer that best describes the characteristics of the mass seen in the above patient:

A. Has a female predominance
B. Occurs most often in the third through fourth decade of life
C. Can metastasize to cardiac and extracardiac locations
D. Typically has a heterogeneous appearance on echo caused by hemorrhagic and cystic areas
E. Is frequently a coincidental finding

QUESTION 37.3. Choose the best answer from the choices below:

A. Mobility of the tumor as seen on echo is an independent predictor of death or nonfatal embolization

B. TEE and transthoracic echocardiography (TTE) are equally sensitive in diagnosing this tumor

C. The most common clinical presentation of patients with this tumor is syncope

D. There is a strong correlation between bacterial endocarditis and formation of this tumor

E. The tumor has a high recurrence rate after surgical resection

QUESTION 37.4. After a comprehensive TEE exam, the following action would be most appropriate:

A. The mass should be removed from the AV

B. The AV should be replaced

C. The mass should be left untouched and the patient closely monitored since he has been asymptomatic

D. The mass should be left untouched and the patient closely monitored and systemically anticoagulated

E. A filter should be placed in the ascending aorta via percutaneous femoral access and the AV should be left untouched.

ANSWERS AND DISCUSSION

QUESTION 37.1: Answer C is correct. Cardiac papillary fibroelastomas (CPF) are the most common benign primary cardiac valve tumors, although they represent less than 10% of all cardiac tumors. Fibroelastomas arise most commonly from the AV cusps (44.5%) and MV leaflets (36.4%). Most commonly, they arise from the atrial side of atrioventricular valves or from either side of semilunar valves. Attachment to the ventricular septum or the LVOT has been described. Ninety-five percent of fibroelastomas are located within the left side of the heart.

Typically, fibroelastomas remain small in size, with a range of 1 to 15 mm in diameter. Fibroelastomas can rapidly increase in size when thrombotic material adheres to its surface, but this is not typical of its evolution. Echocardiography usually demonstrates a small, mobile, pedunculated or sessile mass, which on many occasions flutters or prolapses into the cardiac chambers. Patients presenting with CPF are usually asymptomatic, but life-threatening complications such as stroke, acute valve dysfunction, embolism, and sudden death can occur. Fibroelastomas are avascular tumors and the diagnosis cannot be made with CFD. They typically appear as a solitary mass, with a 7% incidence of multiple lesions. LEs typically originate as small filamentous strands on endocardial surfaces where the valve margins make contact. "Giant LE" results from the adherence of multiple adjacent excrescences that grow large and can present like a fibroelastoma morphologically. LEs should be monitored closely. If there is evidence of a cerebrovascular accident in a patient with LEs, anticoagulation is advised. Any suggestion of a second such episode should lead to operative removal.

QUESTION 37.2: Answer D is correct. Fibroelastomas are often asymptomatic and usually found on autopsy or as an incidental finding on echo. They have a slight male predominance (55%), and a higher incidence of appearance between the fourth and the eighth decades of life. Myxomas, not fibroelastomas, contain a mucopolysaccharide myxoid matrix and have the described heterogeneous appearance on echo. CPF may appear speckled with echolucencies and a stippled pattern near the edges, which correlated with the papillary projections on the surface of the tumor.

QUESTION 37.3: Answer A is correct. Tumor mobility is the only independent predictor of CPF-related death or nonfatal embolization. TEE represents an excellent tool to describe tumor mobility. TEE is superior to TTE because of its close proximity to the heart for diagnosing small structures such as fibroelastomas. In patients with MV fibroelastomas, stroke is the most common clinical presentation, whereas in patients with AV fibroelastomas, sudden death and myocardial infarction are the leading clinical signs. CPFs are asymptomatic in most patients. Remnants of cytomegalovirus on specimens sent to pathology suggest a possibility of a virus-induced tumor, therefore evoking the concept of a chronic form of viral endocarditis as an underlying mechanism of CPF formation. Recurrence is rare after surgical resection.

QUESTION 37.4: Answer A is correct. In this case the tumor should be surgically resected because of its mobile nature and the associated risk of death and embolization. Surgical excision of CPF is curative and in most cases the tumor can be easily dissected off of the AV because of its pedunculation. The AV should not be replaced unless the removal of the tumor causes damage to the valve leaflets resulting in aortic regurgitation. Asymptomatic patients with nonmobile tumors could be followed up closely with periodic clinical evaluation and echocardiography, and they receive surgical intervention when symptoms develop or the tumor becomes mobile. Symptomatic patients who are not surgical candidates can be offered long-term systemic anticoagulation. Our patient does not fall into this category. There are no commercially available aortic filters.

TAKE-HOME LESSON:

It is common to discover new echocardiographic findings during an intraoperative exam. In this case, knowledge of the different types of AV masses including their pathophysiology is integral to guiding intraoperative decision-making and treatment for the patient.

SUGGESTED READING

Basso C, Valente M, Poletti A, et al. Surgical pathology of primary cardiac and pericardial tumors. *Eur J Cardiothorac Surg*. 1997;12:730–738.

Cohn LH. *Surgery in the Adult*. 3rd ed. New York: McGraw Hill Medical; 2008:170–171.

Dehnee AE, Brizendine S, Herrera CJ. Recurrent strokes in a young patient with papillary fibroelastoma: a case report and literature review. *Echocardiography*. 2006;23(7):592–595.

Sun JP, Asher CR, Yang XS, et al. Clinical and echocardiographic characteristics of papillary fibroelastomas: a retrospective and prospective study in 162 patients. *Circulation*. 2001;103(22):2687–2693.

Moderate

CASE 38

A 66-year-old African American male, status post AVR, is now in acute heart failure with a new holodiastolic murmur that radiates along the left sternal border. He also has a fever greater than 38°C.

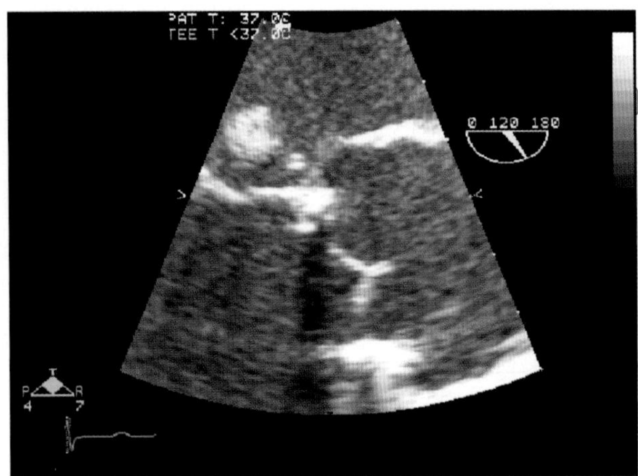

Figure 38.1. Zoom of ME AV LAX.

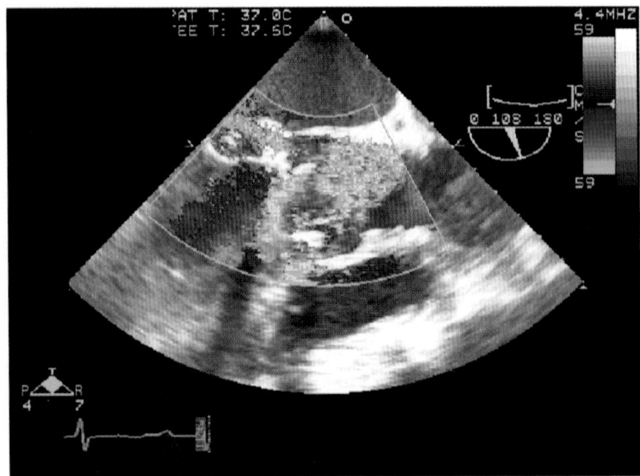

Figure 38.2. ME AV LAX with CFD.

QUESTION 38.1. After reviewing Figure 38.1 and Video 38.1, what is your echocardiographic finding?

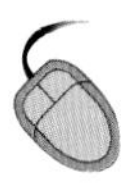

A. Lambl excrescences
B. Reverberation artifact
C. Echodense mass consistent with vegetation
D. Normal image

QUESTION 38.2. Upon further evaluation of Figure 38.2 and Video 38.2, the following pathology is identified:

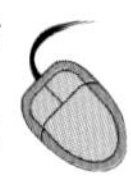

A. Dehiscence of prosthetic valve
B. Periannular abscess
C. Aorta to left atrium fistulae
D. All of the above

QUESTION 38.3. In suspected infective endocarditis (IE) the following is (are) major criteria in the Duke clinical criteria for diagnosis of IE:

A. Mobile, echodense masses attached to valvular leaflets
B. Periannular abscesses
C. Dehiscence of a valvular prosthesis
D. All of the above

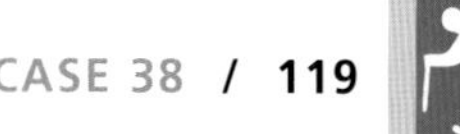

QUESTION 38.4. In Figures 38.3 and 38.4, the echocardiograms demonstrate

A. CW Doppler
B. Normal flow patterns
C. Diastolic flow reversal
D. Blunting of the diastolic component of the Doppler wave pattern

QUESTION 38.5. Optimal management of this patient included

A. Immediate surgical intervention
B. Surgical intervention after completion of antibiotic treatment
C. AVR with an aortic homograft
D. AVR with a prosthetic valve
E. Answers A and C
F. Answers B and D

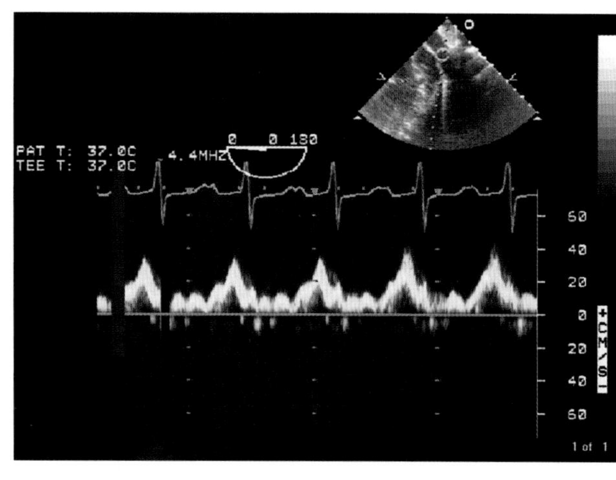

Figure 38.3. PW Doppler tracing of pulmonary vein blood flow.

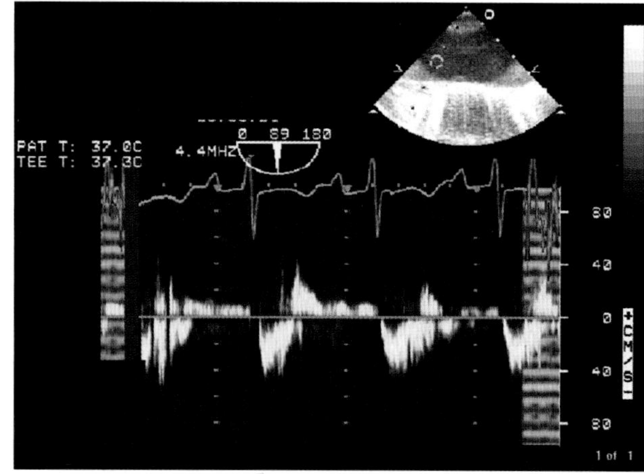

Figure 38.4. Descending AO LAX with PW Doppler.

ANSWERS AND DISCUSSION

QUESTION 38.1: The correct answer is C: Echodense (mobile) mass consistent with vegetation. Answer A is incorrect. Lambl excrescences are characterized as fine filamentous strands, which originate on the endocardial surfaces where the valve margins make contact and appear to be "wear-and-tear" lesions most commonly of the AV. Answer B is incorrect. The artifact demonstrated is acoustic shadowing. Acoustic shadowing occurs when the ultrasound beam meets an interface of two structures that differ greatly in acoustic impedance such as the struts of bioprosthetic valves, mechanical valves, or heavily calcified valves. Answer D is incorrect. This is definitely not a normal image.

QUESTION 38.2: The correct answer is D: All of the above. The patient had received a bioprosthetic AV. Following an episode of endocarditis, the patient experienced a perivalvular abscess that resulted in valve dehiscence and the formation of an aorta to left atrium fistula.

QUESTION 38.3: The correct answer is D: All of the above.

Echocardiography is part of the major criteria in the Duke clinical criteria for diagnosis of IE. Within the definition of major criteria for evidence of endocardial involvement, major diagnostic weight is given to only three typical echocardiographic findings: mobile, echodense masses attached to valvular leaflets or mural endocardium; periannular abscesses; or new dehiscence of a valvular prosthesis. Although TTE is rapid, noninvasive, and has a 98% specificity for vegetations >2 mm located on right-sided valves, its overall sensitivity is <60%. Its views may also be inadequate in up to 20% of adult patients. It has been shown that, in experienced hands, TEE has >90% specificity and sensitivity, for detection of intracardiac lesions associated with IE.

Complications of IE such as periannular abscess, perforation, fistulae, mycotic aneurysm, and new dehiscence of a prosthetic valve are best determined by TEE. Any patient at risk for perivalvular extension of IE requires prompt evaluation. Unfortunately, the sensitivity of TTE to detect perivalvular abscess is low (18% in prospective to 63% in retrospective studies). Sensitivity and specificity of defining periannular extension of IE is greatly improved by using TEE 76% to 100% and 95%, respectively. TEE spectral and CFD can demonstrate distinctive flow patterns of both pseudoaneurysms and fistulae as well as rule out communications from unruptured abscess cavities. Hence, TEE has become the modality of choice for the initial assessment of patients at risk of perivalvular extension.

QUESTION 38.4: The correct answer is C: Diastolic flow reversal. Figure 38.4 demonstrates holodiastolic flow reversal by pulse wave Doppler in the descending aorta consistent with severe AI. Answer A is incorrect. Both of the images show pulse wave Doppler that utilizes a single crystal as both the emitter and the receiver of ultrasound waves and uses a process known as *time gating*, in which only those signals associated with a specific depth or location are selected for evaluation. In turn, this allows the echocardiographer to evaluate a volume of blood at a specific location. Answer B is incorrect. The volume of blood being evaluated in Figure 38.3 is that of a pulmonary vein that shows systolic flow blunting. Hence both Doppler patterns are abnormal. Answer D is incorrect. It is the systolic component of the pulmonary vein flow, which is blunted, not the diastolic component. Flow in the pulmonary vein is forward in both systole and diastole with a small wave of reversal, which correlates with atrial systole. Blunting of the systolic component is seen in conditions of elevated left atrium pressure and decreased LV compliance.

QUESTION 38.5: The correct answer is E: Immediate surgical intervention and AVR with an aortic homograft is the most common surgical treatment. This patient presented in acute heart failure due to both the dehiscence of his prosthetic valve and the intracardiac lesion (aorta to left atrium fistulae) that developed as an extension of his periannular abscess. In IE it is heart failure that has the most impact on prognosis (regardless of management), coupled with the fact that the fistulae won't heal with medical management alone that precipitates the need for urgent surgical intervention. The surgical approach in this patient would be to replace the valve, drain any remaining abscess, debride necrotic tissue, and close the fistulae tract. An aortic homograft would accomplish the replacement of the valve as well as the repair of the aorta and is commonly used in these situations. Figure 38.5 and Video 38.3 demonstrate a properly placed aortic homograft without any AI in this patient.

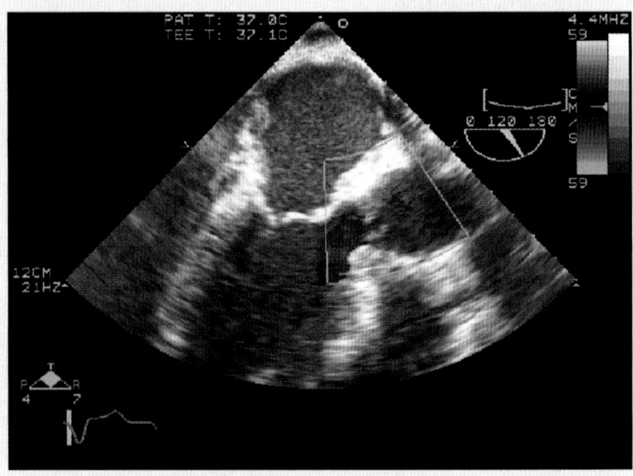

Figure 38.5. ME LAX with CFD.

TAKE-HOME LESSON:

The use of TEE is superior to TTE in the diagnosis of IE. It is particularly valuable in patients who are difficult to image with TTE, have the possibility of prosthetic valve IE, or have an intermediate-to-high suspicion clinically of IE.

SUGGESTED READING

Lobata EB, Muehsclegel JD. Transesophageali echocardiography in the intensive care unit. In: Perrino A, Reeves ST, ed. *A Practical Approach*. 2nd ed. Philadelphia: Lippincott Williams & Wilkins, 2008:354–356.

A 75-year-old male with aortic regurgitation is scheduled for AVR (Fig. 39.1A). His LV function moderately decrease (EF <43%). During the intraoperative TEE exam, TMF, Fig. 39.1B and PVF, Fig. 39.1C are recorded with PW Doppler.

QUESTION 39.1. From the Doppler traces in Figure 39.1, what is the grade of diastolic dysfunction of the LV?

A. Impaired relaxation

B. Pseudonormal pattern

C. Restrictive pattern

D. Not sure

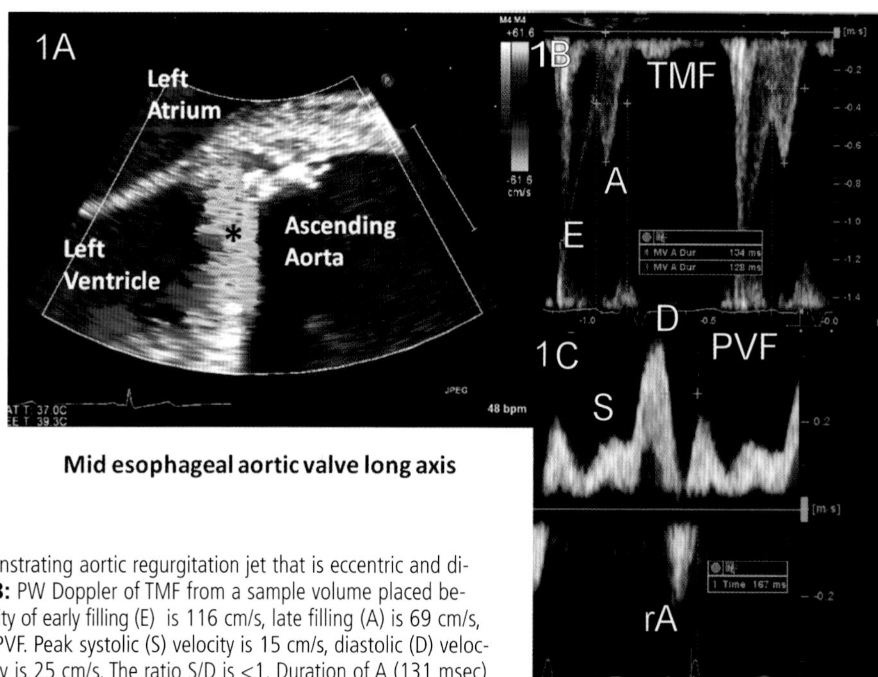

Figure 39.1. **A:** ME AV LAX with CFD demonstrating aortic regurgitation jet that is eccentric and directed toward the interventricular septum. **B:** PW Doppler of TMF from a sample volume placed between the tips of the MV leaflets. Peak velocity of early filling (E) is 116 cm/s, late filling (A) is 69 cm/s, and the E/A ratio is 1.7. **C:** PW Doppler of PVF. Peak systolic (S) velocity is 15 cm/s, diastolic (D) velocity is 40 cm/s, and atrial reversal (rA) velocity is 25 cm/s. The ratio S/D is <1. Duration of A (131 msec) is shorter than rA (167 msec).

Following replacement of the incompetent AV, the TMF and PVF shown in Figure 39.2 were obtained with PW Doppler.

QUESTION 39.2. Based on the Doppler displays in Figure 39.2, what conclusions can be drawn with respect to diastolic filling of the LV?

A. Impaired relaxation
B. Insufficient information to diagnose the state of diastolic function
C. Pseudonormal pattern
D. Reduction in filling pressures from pre-op
E. B and D

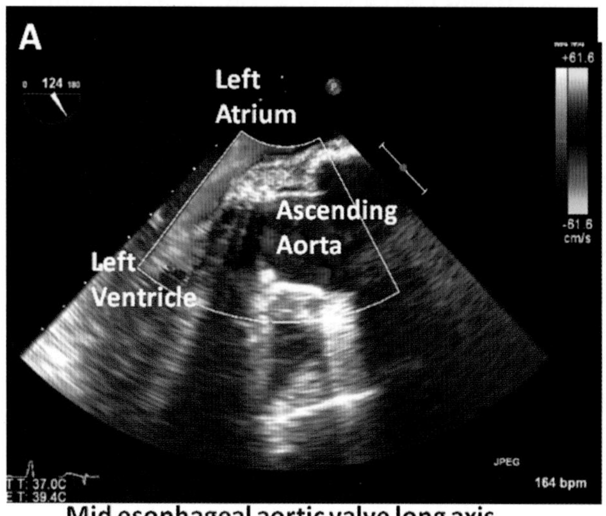

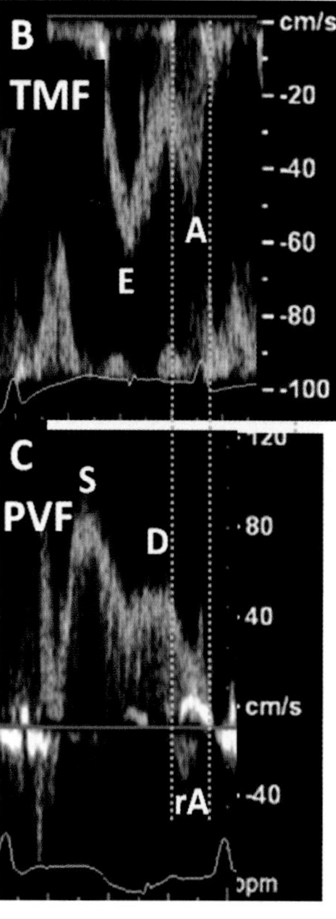

Figure 39.2. **A:** ME AV LAX with CFD in diastole; no aortic regurgitation is detected. **B:** PW Doppler of TMF. Mitral inflow shows a peak E velocity of 85 cm/s, peak A velocity of 70 cm/s, and E/A of 1.2. **C:** PW Doppler of PVF. PVF shows peak S velocity of 120 cm/s, peak D velocity of 80 cm/s, and rA of 20 cm/s. The S/D ratio is 1.5. The rA now appears slightly shorter than the A.

ANSWERS AND DISCUSSION

QUESTION 39.1: The correct answer is D: Not sure. As LV filling is augmented by aortic regurgitation, an assessment of the state of diastolic function is precluded.

Assessment of LV diastolic function and estimation of filling pressures are considered integral components of a comprehensive TEE exam. This is done with the combination of TMF and PVF velocity spectral displays. Diastolic dysfunction occurs when the LV is incapable of accommodating at normal pressures a volume of blood sufficient to maintain an adequate cardiac output. Diastolic function is related to myocardial relaxation, passive LV properties as well as external factors (pericardial) altering chamber compliance. TMF velocities are recorded by placing the pulsed-wave Doppler sample volume between the tips of MV. Two distinct waves are observed: E (early) and A (atrial or late). Measurements derived from these two waves include E and A velocities, the E/A ratio, the E deceleration time (EDT), and the duration of the A waves. These parameters are modulated by the pressure gradient between the LA and the LV. As a result, an E/A ratio 0.75 to 1.5 can be found in both normal diastolic function and impaired relaxation with an associated compensatory increase in filling pressures. PW Doppler with the sample volume inside the orifice of a pulmonary vein is used to record the systolic (S), the diastolic (D), and flow reversal velocities during atrial contraction (rA). The evaluation of the PVF pattern is helpful in determining whether a normal E/A pattern represents normal diastolic function or rather the result of an increased LA pressure in the presence of diastolic dysfunction (pseudonormal pattern). A depressed S/D ratio generally means an increase in LA pressure. However, it may on occasion be misleading; for example, a healthy young athlete with normal ventricular function will have a depressed S/D ratio due to vigorous relaxation (high D velocity).

In healthy adults, E/A ratios are usually above 1 and decrease with age (0.75 to 1.5). A depressed E/A ratio suggests relaxation abnormalities, whereas a ratio above 2 suggests restrictive physiology. These ratios may be misleading as a patient with relaxation abnormalities may have a normal E/A ratio as a result of an increase in left atrial pressure (LAP). The PVF is helpful in determining the preload. In adults, an S/D ratio inferior to 1 is reflective of increased LAP.

Further enhancements to the estimation of LAP are feasible by comparing the mitral A wave duration (Adur) and the pulmonary vein flow rA duration (rAdur). As the LV diastolic pressure increases, atrial contraction causes an increase in the proportion of retrograde pulmonary blood flow when compared to forward flow into the LV. Therefore, in a patient in sinus rhythm, an rAdur – Adur > 30 msec is consistent with an increased LV end-diastolic pressure (Fig. 39.1).

In this patient, aortic regurgitation results in a "dual-source" for diastolic LV filling: "orthodromic" via the MV and "retrograde" via the AV. As the increase in LV diastolic pressure is the result of aortic regurgitation, standard TMF and PVF measurements do not reflect myocardial properties and cannot be used to determine the stage of diastolic dysfunction.

Answers A, B, and C are all incorrect based on the above.

QUESTION 39.2: The correct answer is E: B and D. There is insufficient information to diagnose the state of diastolic dysfunction and there is a reduction in filling pressures from pre-op.

Following AVR, the E/A ratio has decreased from 1.7 before replacement to just slightly above 1. The E velocity is slightly reduced at approximately 90 cm/s. The S/D ratio has changed from <1.0 to >1.0. There is now a slightly shorter rA duration when compared to that of A, indicating a reduction in filling pressures compared to pre-op.

Although the reduction in E/A indicates a reduction in filling pressures, a diagnosis of pseudonormal diastolic dysfunction remains elusive. Unfortunately, a large number of combinations of filling pressures and degrees of relaxation abnormalities will give the same E/A ratio. An independent evaluation of myocardial relaxation is required, such as tissue Doppler of the mitral annulus. Surrogate measures of filling pressures must be utilized in order to determine whether the patient has elevated filling pressures as a result of diastolic dysfunction, such as the ratio of mitral E velocity to the tissue Doppler mitral annular *e* (*e*′). This was not provided in this case. A maneuver that transiently decreases LV preload such as a Valsalva can be employed to unmask a pseudonormal pattern. During Valsalva, a pseudonormal LV filling pattern will revert to one of impaired relaxation. This was not performed.

The new guidelines for grading of diastolic function require assessment of a plethora of factors: Doppler velocity of the myocardium, change in TMF velocities with Valsalva, and comparison of durations between transmitral A and pulmonary vein flow rA, among others. It requires a fundamental understanding of filling physiology and how this relates to myocardial properties. Postoperatively, the now-competent AV has eliminated LV retrograde diastolic filling, thereby reducing significantly the LV filling pressure. Information on myocardial relaxation is missing, thereby making further comments on diastolic dysfunction very difficult.

Answers A and C are incorrect based on the above stated reasons.

TAKE-HOME LESSON:

In aortic regurgitation, the LV fills from both the MV and the incompetent AV. Because of the atypical filling pattern, determination of LV diastolic function with traditional indices is precluded.

SUGGESTED READING

Recommendations for the evaluation of left ventricular diastolic function by echocardiography. *J Am Soc Echocardiogr*. 2009;22:107–134.

Moderate

CASE 40

A 75-year-old male with a history of hypertension, ischemic heart disease, and myocardial infarction presents for urgent revascularization for triple vessel disease and unstable angina.

QUESTION 40.1. What wall motion abnormality is present in Video 40.1?

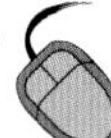

A. No wall motion abnormalities
B. Mild hypokinesia of the midanteroseptal wall
C. Hypokinesia of the inferoseptal wall
D. Dyskinesia of the inferoseptal wall

QUESTION 40.2. What is the visually estimated EF in Video 40.1?

A. 55%
B. 45%
C. 35%
D. Don't know

QUESTION 40.3. Given the additional information in Videos 40.2, 40.3, and 40.4, how will your estimation of the EF change?

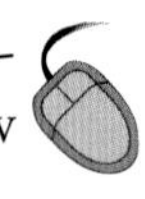

A. It will not change
B. 25%–35%
C. 45%–55%
D. Don't know

QUESTION 40.4. The following wall motion abnormalities are present in Video 40.2 *except:*

A. Basal inferoseptal akinesia
B. Apical septal akinesia
C. Apical lateral hypokinesia
D. Apical cap akinesia

QUESTION 40.5. What artifact, identified by the arrow, interferes with wall motion evaluation in Figure 40.1?

A. Comet tail

B. Ghosting

C. Shadowing

D. Enhancement

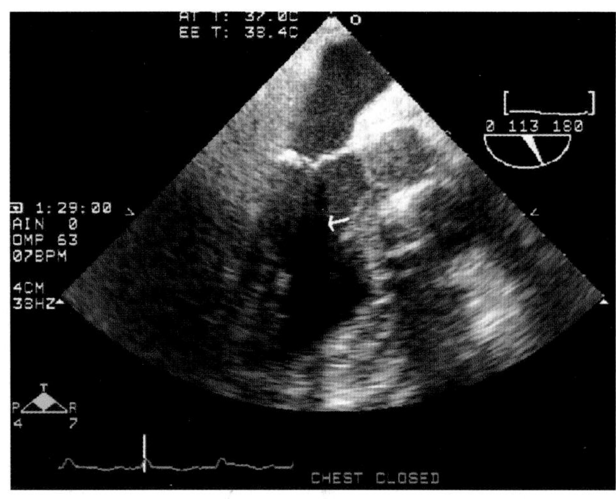

Figure 40.1. ME LAX view.

ANSWERS AND DISCUSSION

QUESTION 40.1: The correct answer is B: Mild hypokinesia of the midanteroseptal wall. The view shown in Video 40.1 is the TG midsax view in which one can evaluate the wall motion of the anterior, anteroseptal, inferoseptal, inferior, and anterolateral walls at the midpapillary level. Wall motion in the septal segments might be slightly problematic to interpret in the TG basal SAX view because of the vicinity with the membranous part of the septum that might be erroneously interpreted as wall motion abnormality.

QUESTION 40.2: The correct answer is D. EF, a volumetric measurement defined as the ratio of SV to end-diastolic volume cannot be reliably estimated from the single 2D imaging plane provided in Video 40.1. This is especially relevant given this patient's history of ischemic heart disease and the potential for RWMA. In such cases accurate estimates of LVEF benefit from multiple cross-sectional views, including the basal, mid, and apical segments.

QUESTION 40.3: The correct answer is B: 25%–35%. After reviewing Videos 40.2, 40.3, and 40.4 it is apparent that global systolic function is substantially more impaired than observed in Video 40.1. While Video 40.1 shows normal wall motion in all but one segment at the midpapillary level, Video 40.2 shows severe hypokinesia/akinesia in the apical septal and lateral walls, Video 40.3 shows severe hypokinesia/akinesia in the apical anteroseptal segment, and Video 40.4 shows severe hypokinesia/akinesia in the apical anterior and inferior walls. Therefore, assessing LVEF only by Video 40.1 would have resulted in an overestimation. In Figures 40.2 and 40.3 it can be observed that while there is a change in the internal diameter of the LV at the midpapillary level between diastole and systole, the internal diameter of the LV remains relatively unchanged at the apical level.

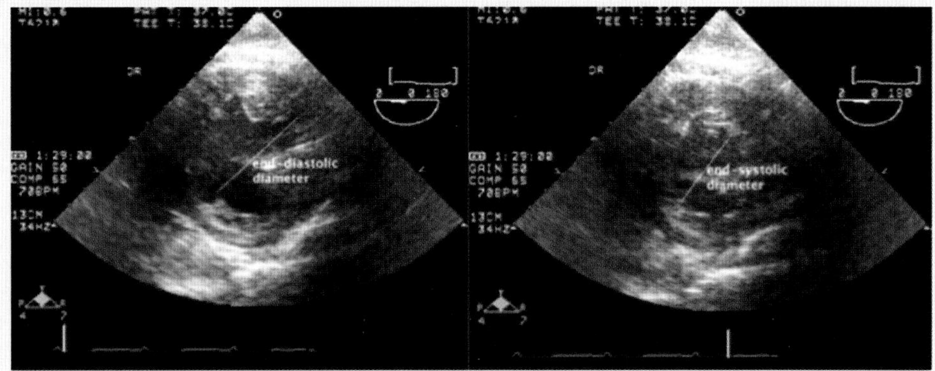

Figure 40.2. TG mid-SAX view

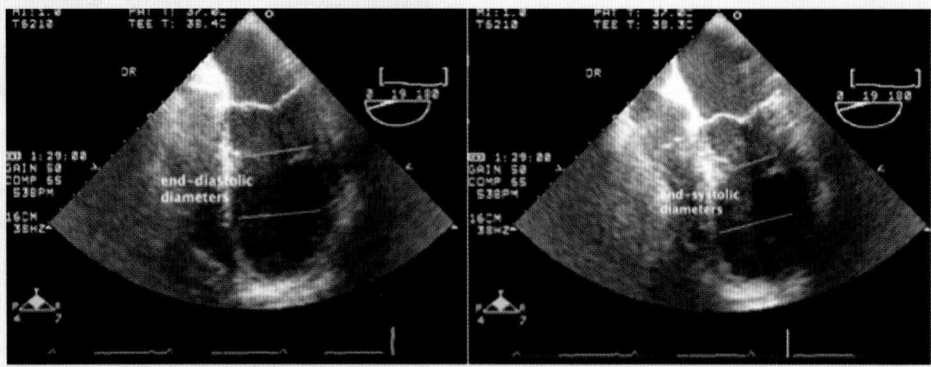

Figure 40.3. ME 4CH view.

QUESTION 40.4: The correct answer is A: Basal inferoseptal akinesia.

While the apical segments show little or no thickening or endocardial inward motion during systole, the basal segments show relatively normal motion.

QUESTION 40.5: The correct answer is C: Shadowing. The artifact that interferes with wall motion evaluation in Figure 40.1 is shadowing probably originating from mitral annulus calcifications.

TAKE-HOME LESSON:

Multiple imaging planes are necessary to make an accurate visual assessment of LVEF.

SUGGESTED READING

London MJ. Diagnosis of myocardial ischemia. In: Perrino A, Reeves ST, eds. *A Practical Approach to Transesophageal Echocardiography*. 2nd ed. Philadelphia: Lippincott Williams & Wilkins, 2008:87–97.

CASE 41

After undergoing an elective bioprosthetic AVR for severe AS (peak gradient 75 mm Hg, AVA 0.7 cm^2), a postreplacement TEE was performed on a 62-year-old female (Fig. 41.1).

QUESTION 41.1. This view of the left atrium demonstrates

A. A large, mobile thrombus in the LAA
B. Atrial myxoma
C. Pulmonary embolus
D. Atrial trabeculation

QUESTION 41.2. What is the best view(s) to image the LAA?

A. ME bicaval view
B. ME 4CH- and ME 2CH views
C. ME RV inflow–outflow view
D. TG LAX view

QUESTION 41.3. What additional Doppler interrogation should be done to further reassure no thrombus formation in the LAA?

A. CW Doppler velocity of 50 cm/s
B. CFD with a Nyquist limit of 0.56
C. PW Doppler velocity greater than 0.4 m/s
D. PW Doppler velocity of 10 cm/s

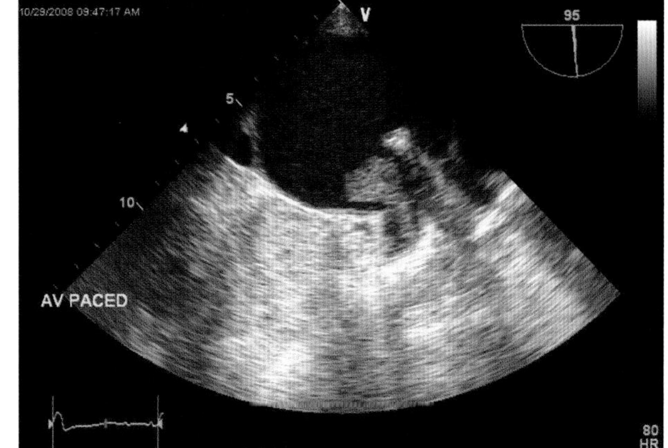

Figure 41.1. ME 2CH view (modified) and Video 41.1.

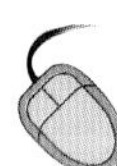

ANSWERS AND DISCUSSION

QUESTION 41.1: The correct answer is A: A large, mobile thrombus in the LAA. This TEE image after AVR (Fig. 41.1) shows a large, mobile thrombus in the LAA. This post-CPB finding is a dreaded event and presents the anesthesiologist and cardiac surgeon with a complicated dilemma: should CPB be reinstituted and the thrombus extracted or should the clot be treated with anticoagulation after a major cardiac procedure. In this case, after extensive deliberation, the patient received postoperative heparin with eventual conversion to Coumadin therapy with no untoward events.

QUESTION 41.2: The correct answer is B: ME 4CH and ME 2CH views. The LAA arises from the superior lateral portion of the left atrium and separated from the LUPV by the *Coumadin ridge*, a normal band of LA tissue that can be mistaken for thrombus. Because of its location, the LAA is best visualized in the ME 4CH and ME 2CH views, and appears as a triangular chamber below the LUPV, with the apex pointing toward the RV. Withdrawing the probe and turning the probe to the left may help optimize its visualization. A scan through the multiplane angle with the LAA in focus will allow for a complete evaluation of this accessory chamber and help identify any thrombus.

QUESTION 41.3: The correct answer is C: PW Doppler velocity greater than 0.4 m/s.

Peak velocities greater than 0.4 m/s in the LAA and normal sinus rhythm can reassure the echocardiographer that the LAA has normal flow conditions sufficient to prevent stasis and thrombus formation within the LAA (Fig. 41.2).

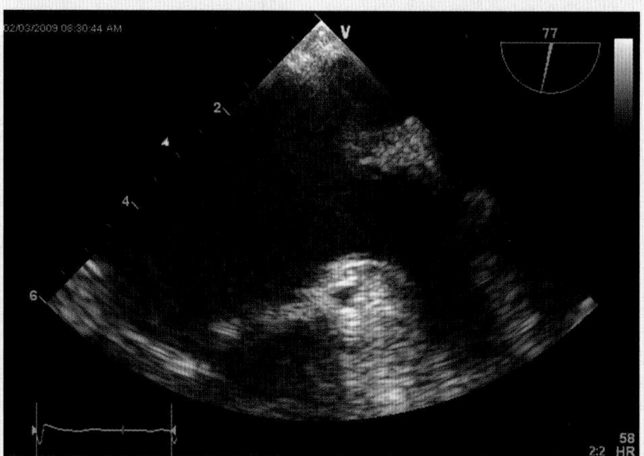

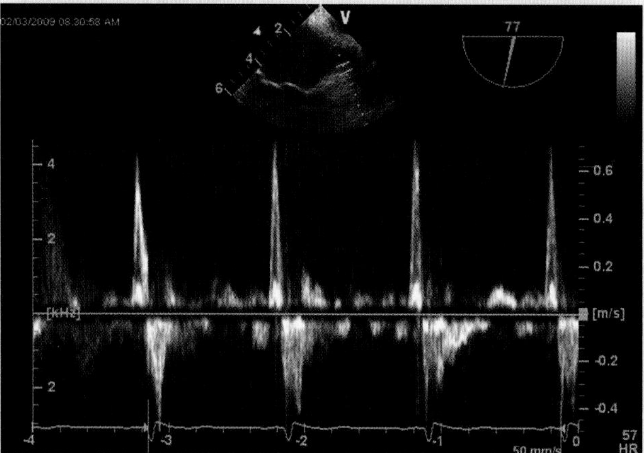

Figure 41.2. ME 2CH view. **Top:** 2-D image of LAA free of thrombus. **Bottom:** PW Doppler tracing with peak velocities greater than 0.6 m/s consistent with **NO** thrombus formation.

TAKE-HOME LESSON:

Multiple viewing angles of the LAA will help to elucidate thrombus. PW Doppler velocities greater than 0.4 m/s make the conditions unfavorable for the presence of spontaneous echo contrast and/or thrombus within the LAA.

SUGGESTED READING

Miller JP. Two-dimensional examination. In: Perrino A, Reeves ST, eds. *A Practical Approach to Transesophageal Echocardiography.* 2nd ed. Philadelphia: Lippincott Williams & Wilkins, 2008:39.

CASE 42

A 52-year-old female presents with symptoms of CHF and the recent diagnosis of cancer. A TEE is performed for diagnosis and management (Figs. 42.1 to 42.5).

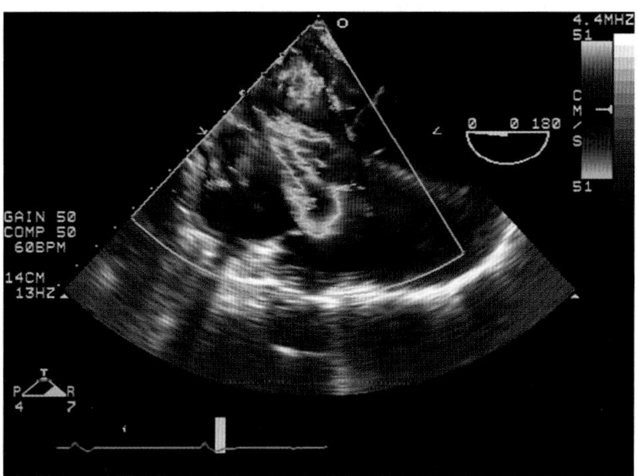

Figure 42.1. ME 4CH view with CFD. See also Video 42.1.

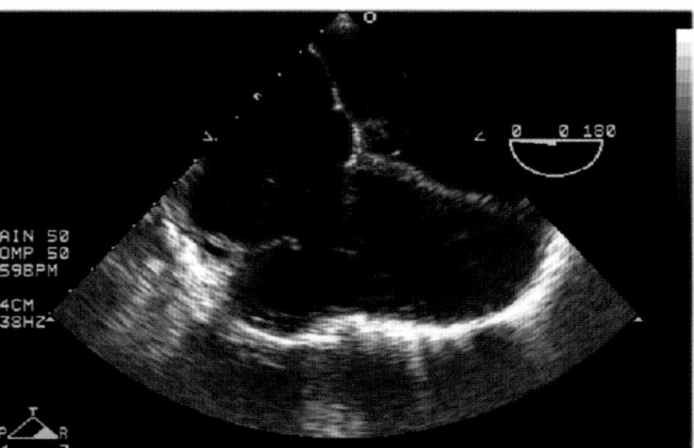

Figure 42.2. ME 4CH view. See also Video 42.1.

QUESTION 42.1. Considering the above TEE data, what is the most likely diagnosis?

A. TV consistent with Ebstein anomaly
B. Carcinoid heart disease
C. Chronic pulmonary embolism
D. ASD
E. Primary pulmonary hypertension

QUESTION 42.2. In Figure 42.3, what does the PW Doppler indicate?

A. Normal hepatic vein flow
B. Retrograde systolic flow consistent with TR
C. Doppler "cross-talk" artifact
D. Diastolic dysfunction of the RV
E. Retrograde diastolic flow associated with low systemic vascular resistance

QUESTION 42.3. What views are appropriate to assess the function of the PV?

A. UE Aortic Arch SAX view
B. ME RV inflow–outflow
C. ME Asc Ao SAX view
D. A and B
E. All of the above

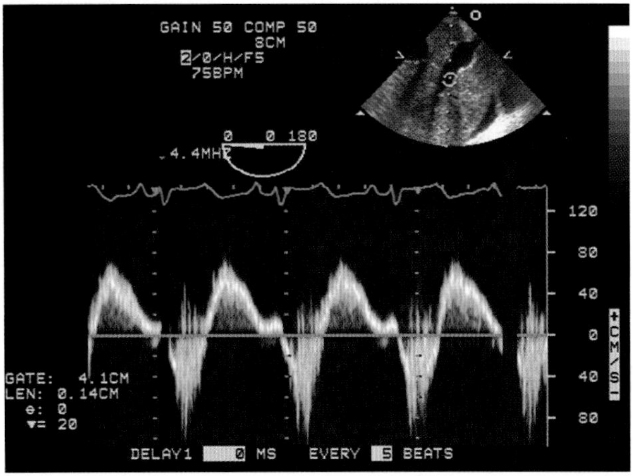

Figure 42.3. PW Doppler of hepatic veins.

QUESTION 42.4. In this patient a finding of MV stenosis and insufficiency would warrant a further investigation for

A. PFO

B. Elevated sedimentation rate

C. Marfan syndrome

D. Graves disease

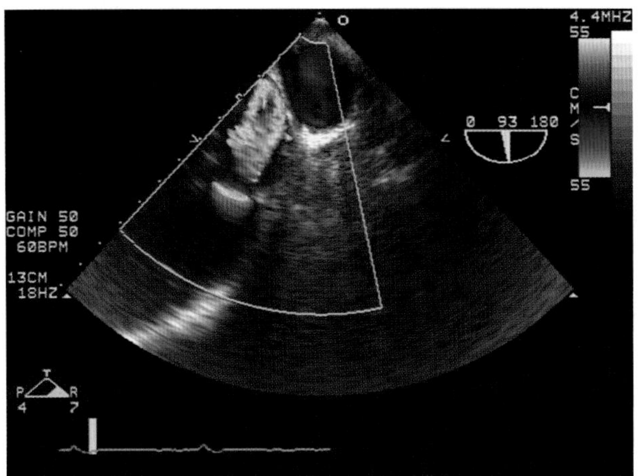

Figure 42.4. Upper esophageal view of PA and SAX of ascending aorta with CFD. See also Video 42.2.

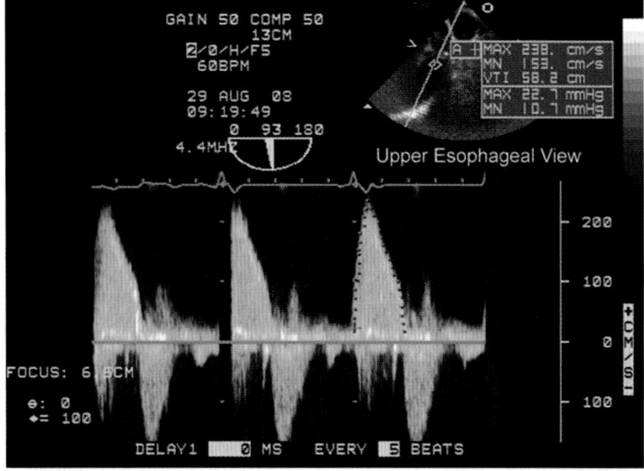

Figure 42.5. Upper esophageal CW Doppler of pulmonary valve (PV).

ANSWERS AND DISCUSSION

QUESTION 42.1: The correct answer is B: Carcinoid heart disease.

These images represent a patient with a dilated RV, TR, and pulmonary stenosis (PS). These echardiographic findings are consistent with carcinoid heart disease. Chronic secretion of vasoactive substances such as serotonin from the carcinoid tumor results in thick, pearly white plaques deposited on the surfaces of the right-sided valves and cardiac chambers. The valve leaflets become retracted and hypomobile. Significant TR and PS can occur. Longstanding TR and PS result in volume overload of the RV.

In Ebstein anomaly, one or two of the three TV leaflets are adherent to the wall of the RV and do not move normally. This can result in TR and a dilated RA. It is not, however, associated with PS. Chronic pulmonary embolism and primary pulmonary hypertension may result in RV pressure overload and TR. ASDs result in right-sided volume overload and can eventually lead to annular dilatation and TR. None of the options, other than carcinoid, is associated with PS.

QUESTION 42.2: The correct answer is C: Retrograde systolic flow consistent with severe TR.

Figure 42.3 demonstrates retrograde systolic flow in the hepatic vein consistent with severe TR. Compare Figure 42.3 with the normal hepatic flow pattern example in Figure 42.6.

Normal hepatic blood flow consists of three distinct waves (Fig. 42.6). The A wave occurs during atrial systole and results in retrograde flow in the IVC. The S wave occurs during ventricular systole and results from atrial relaxation and apical movement of the TV during ventricular contraction. The D wave occurs during ventricular diastole and results from a drop in atrial pressure due to ventricular filling. The ECG helps to correctly identify the timing of each wave.

Excessive Doppler gain while performing wither, a PW Doppler or CW Doppler exam may lead to Doppler "cross-talk" artifact. This condition results from overflow background noise (leakage from one channel to another) in the opposite direction appearing as a waveform with flow both toward and away from the probe in the same phase of the cardiac cycle. Doppler echocardiography of the hepatic vein is not used to either measure the diastolic function of the RV or determine low systemic vascular resistance.

QUESTION 42.3: The correct answer is E. The PV can be imaged using all of these views (Fig. 42.7).

The ME RV inflow–outflow view is a good window to place CFD over the PV to asses for pulmonary regurgitation, but the leaflets themselves are not clearly seen.

The ME Asc Ao SAX view offers a good window to assess the proximal PA for pathology.

Lastly, the upper esophageal aortic arch view can be used to assess for PS. In this view, the blood flowing across the PV is well aligned with the probe making this an ideal window for measuring pressure gradients.

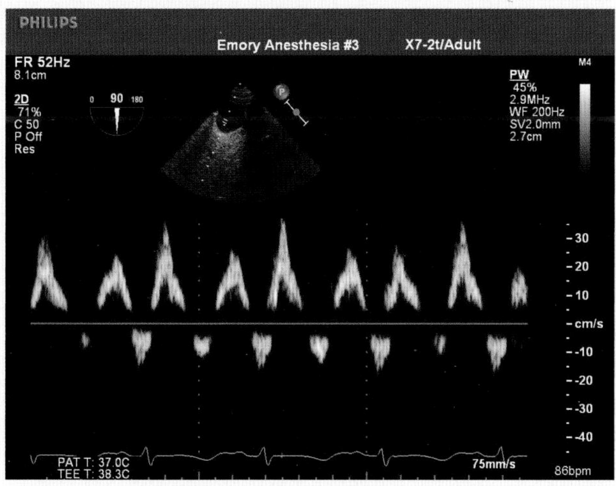

Figure 42.6. Normal PW Doppler of hepatic vein flow.

QUESTION 42.4: The correct answer is A: PFO.

Carcinoid affects primarily the right heart structures as the secreted vasoactive substances are spread via venous blood flow and cleared in the pulmonary circulation. Left heart valve abnormalites are thus uncommon and their appearance suggests right-to-left flow across the interatrial or interventricular septum. Thus a PFO should be ruled out. Carcinoid with left-sided heart disease does not suggest diseases such as Marfan's or Grave's, and assessing the sedimentation rate is not indicated.

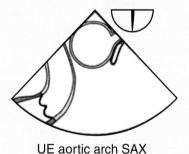

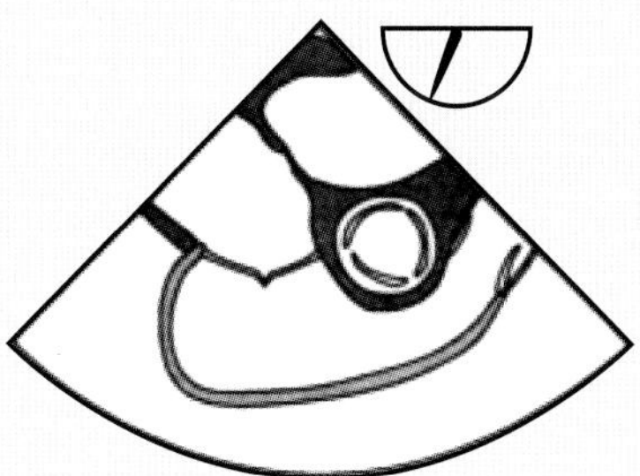

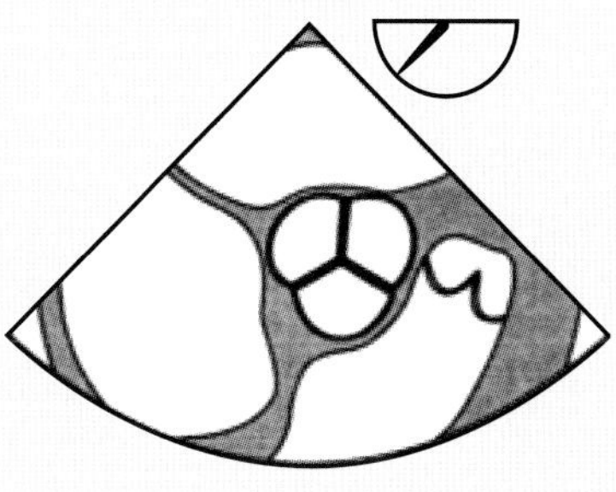

UE aortic arch SAX

Figure 42.7.

TAKE-HOME LESSON:

Carcinoid disease typically will affect all right heart structures. The combination of TR and PS is classic for this disease. The appropriate diagnosis requires a thorough exam and interrogation using multiple different TEE views.

SUGGESTED READING

Abi-Saleh B, Schoondyke JW, Abboud L, et al. Tricuspid valve involvement in carcinoid heart disease. *Echocardiography.* 2007;24:439–442.

Mizuguchi KA, Fox AA, Burch TM, et al. Tricuspid and mitral valve carcinoid disease in the setting of a patent foramen ovale. *Anesth Analg.* 2008;107(6):1819–1821.

Pellikka PA, Tajik J, Khandheria BK, et al. Carcinoid heart disease: clinical and echocardiographic spectrum in 74 patients. *Circulation.* 1993;87:1188–1196.

CASE 43

A 72-year-old male suffered a recent myocardial infarction. His past medical history was significant for a long history of stable angina and hypertension. No other significant cardiac medical history was noted. Preoperative transthoracic echocardiography showed normal cardiac function and no other significant abnormalities. The patient had a TEE probe placed for a three-vessel CABG.

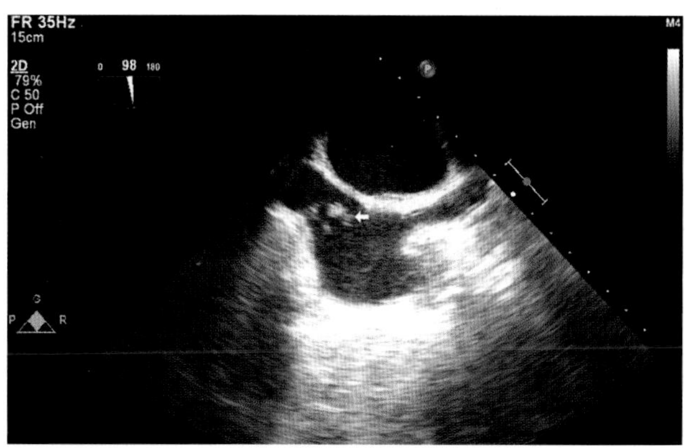

Figure 43.1. ME bicaval view.

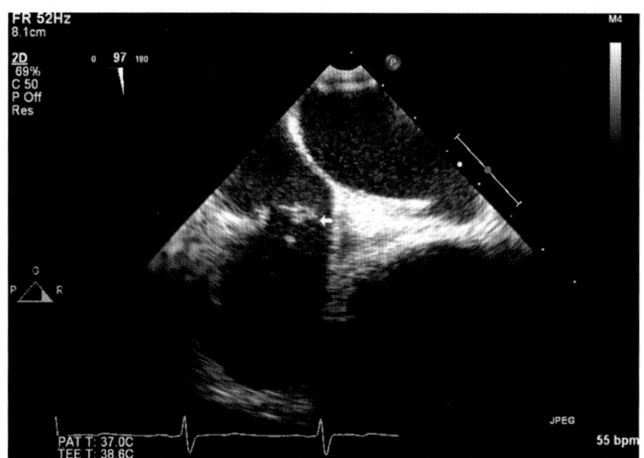

Figure 43.2. Modified ME bicaval view.

QUESTION 43.1. Two ME bicaval views were obtained as part of a comprehensive CPB exam (Figs. 43.1 and 43.2, Videos 43.1 and 43.2). What anatomic structure is the mass noted by the arrow most likely associated with?

A. Crista terminalis
B. Eustachian valve (EV)
C. Chiari network
D. Both B and C

QUESTION 43.2. The most likely diagnosis for the mass noted by the arrow is

A. Vegetation
B. Thrombus
C. Normal finding
D. Thebesian valve

QUESTION 43.3. What is the best approach to further manage the mass noted in the RA?

A. Conservative: postoperative anticoagulation
B. Conservative: follow-up transthoracic echo
C. Surgical evaluation of the mass
D. Antibiotics

ANSWERS AND DISCUSSION

QUESTION 43.1: The correct answer is D.

An important indication for placement of TEE in an otherwise uncomplicated CABG is the diagnosis of unknown pathology that can be treated during the procedure. The identification of an unknown intracardiac mass is an important example of this indication.

The RA is separated into two parts by a muscular ridge called the crista terminalis. It is most prominent near the SVC ostium and extends anteriorly fading out to the right of the IVC ostium. The crista terminalis divides the trabeculated portion of the RA from the smooth-walled venous component. It is a normal anatomic structure in the RA typically seen in the ME bicaval view near the entrance of the SVC into the RA. This mass in the case above is noted near the IVC.

The anterior border of the IVC has a fold of tissue, the EV, which is an embryological remnant of the right valve of the sinus venosus. In utero, the EV diverted blood flow from the IVC across the fossa ovalis into the LA. Although absent in some patients, the EV varies greatly in size, possibly extending all the way to the fossa ovalis. The EV is best seen in the ME bicaval view near the entrance of the IVC into the RA. The EV can be differentiated from other pathologic structures based on its characteristic location near the IVC. The structure seen could be associated with the EV given its location.

A Chiari network is a meshwork of fibers originating at or near the EV and IVC. It is derived from the sinus venosus, like the EV, and often described as an EV that is very large having a thin delicate lace-like structure. It is seen in approximately 2% of patients having TEE performed. Distinction of this structure from a pathologic intracardiac mass is made by its typical echocardiographic appearance and location in the RA. The structure noted by the arrow could also be associated with a Chiari network.

QUESTION 43.2: The correct answer is C.

Vegetations in the RA vary in appearance typically originating on the atrial side of atrioventricular valves, such as the TV. They are mobile, irregularly shaped, heterogeneous structures. Intravenous drugs users and indwelling intravenous catheters or wires associated with pacemakers or defibrillators increase the risk of right-sided endocarditis. History of fever, elevated white blood cell count, and/or positive blood cultures raise the suspicion of endocarditis in a patient with a newly detected intracardiac mass. This patient didn't have a history of fever or infection prior to their surgery, which makes the diagnosis of endocarditis less likely.

Thrombus is the most common intracardiac mass in the vena cava and RA. Thrombus in the deep venous system can embolize to the RA and become entrapped there. RA thrombus can form in situ, especially in patients with right-sided catheters and/or wires. RA low-flow states such as patients with AFib, cardiomyopathy, or tricupid valve stenosis predispose to the formation of RA thrombus. RA thrombi appear as mobile irregular masses of any size. A thrombus that is embolic from the deep venous system may not have a point of attachment in the RA. Thrombi that are formed in the RA can be attached to any of its walls, RA appendage (especially in low-flow states), IVC, SVC, EV, Chirai network, or any catheter or wire. This mass does have a point of attachment in the RA, but the patient does not have history consistent with thrombus formation (low-flow state, catheters in the RA, hypercoagulable state), which makes the diagnosis of thrombus less likely.

Thebesian valves are associated with the CS ostium.

QUESTION 43.3: The correct answer is C.

The unusual appearance of this structure adds to the complexity of decision-making. Converting from off-pump to on-pump revascularization is potentially more problematic than resection versus not. Although the patient's medical history and echocardiographic evaluation make endocarditic vegetation or thrombus unlikely, surgical inspection is likely warranted to rule out both diagnoses. Intraoperative inspection of the RA revealed a tangled Chiari network that was excised. Evidence of obstruction to flow by CFD would lend toward exploration of the mass.

TAKE-HOME LESSON:

Knowledge of pathologic masses in the heart and understanding of the normal structures, anatomic variants, and possible artifacts assist in surgical evaluation and medical therapy for these structures.

SUGGESTED READING

Coddens J. Cardiac masses. In: Mathew JP, Ayoub CM, eds. *Clinical Manual and Review of Transesophageal Echocardiography*. New York: McGraw-Hill; 2005.

Heller LB, Aronson S. Imaging artifacts and pitfalls. In: Savage R, Aronson S, eds. *Comprehensive Textbook of Intraoperative Transesophageal Echocardiography*. Philadelphia: Lippincott Williams & Wilkins, 2005.

Miller JP, Perrino AC, Hillel Z. Common artifacts and pitfalls of clinical echocardiography. In: Perrino AC, Reeves ST, eds. *A Practical Approach to Transesophageal Echocardiography*. 2nd ed. Philadelphia: Lippincott Williams & Wilkins, 2008.

Spencer K. Assessment of cardiac masses. In: Savage R, Aronson S, eds. *Comprehensive Textbook of Intraoperative Transesophageal Echocardiography*. Philadelphia: Lippincott Williams & Wilkins, 2005.

Moderate

CASE 44

A 45-year-old male is undergoing AVR for severe AS. The surgeon is asking for your help in positioning the CPB cannulas

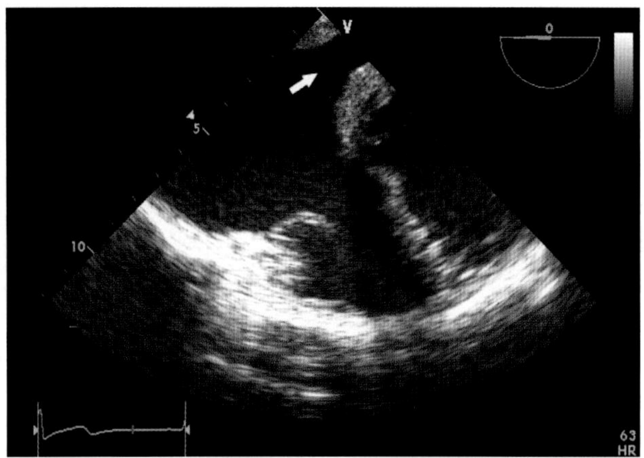

Figure 44.1.

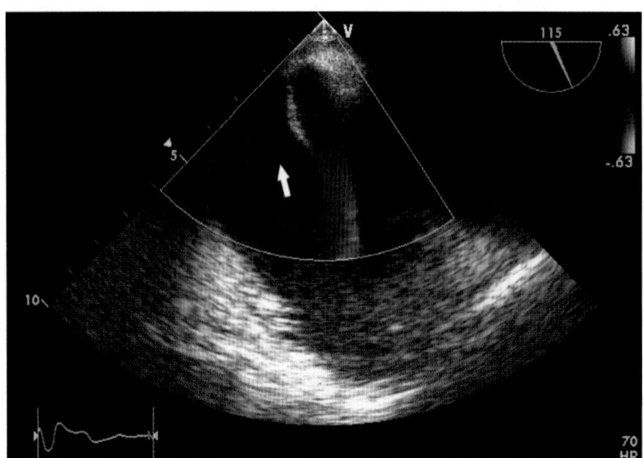

Figure 44.2.

QUESTION 44.1. Which structure is demonstrated by the arrows in Figure 44.1, Video 44.1 (lower esophageal four-chamber) and Figure 44.2, Video 44.2 (modified ME bicaval)?

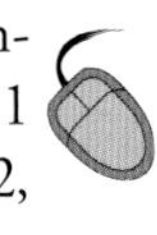

A. SVC

B. ASD

C. CS

D. IVC

QUESTION 44.2. Despite TEE guidance, the surgeon is having difficulty introducing the retrograde cardioplegia cannula into the CS (arrow, Fig. 44.3 and Video 44.3). A modified bicaval view reveals the presence of which structure (Fig. 44.4 and Video 44.4)?

A. Atrial wall

B. Thebesian valve

C. Eustachian valve

D. Chiari network

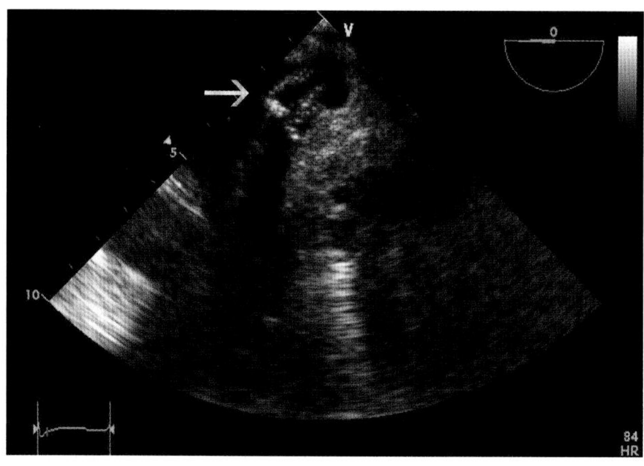

Figure 44.3.

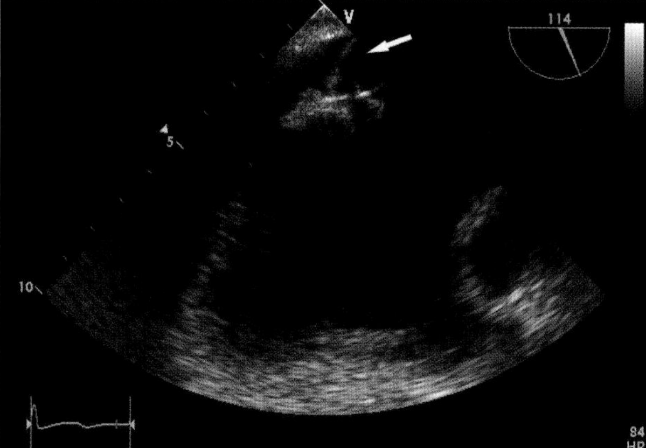

Figure 44.4.

QUESTION 44.3. If the surgeon is unable to insert the retrograde cardioplegia cannula, what other options are at his disposal?

A. Use a smaller cannula

B. Cancel surgery

C. Proceed with a beating/fibrillating heart

D. Directly infuse the cardioplegia into the coronary ostia

QUESTION 44.4. After some struggling, the surgeon is successful inserting the CS catheter (Fig. 44.5, CS catheter in proper position [arrow]). CPB is initiated but adequate cardioplegia cannot be maintained. According to Figure 44.6 (lower esophageal bicaval view with arrow demonstrating tip of CS catheter, Video 44.6), what do you think has occurred?

A. Delivery system malfunction

B. CS catheter was displaced after initial correct positioning

C. CS catheter was inserted into the IVC initially

D. CS catheter was inserted into the SVC initially

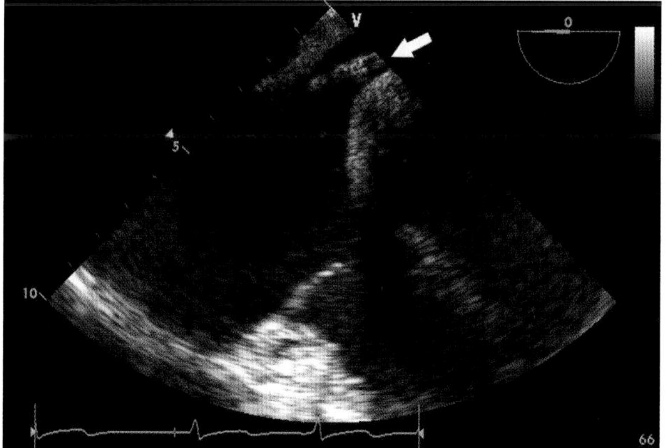

Figure 44.5.

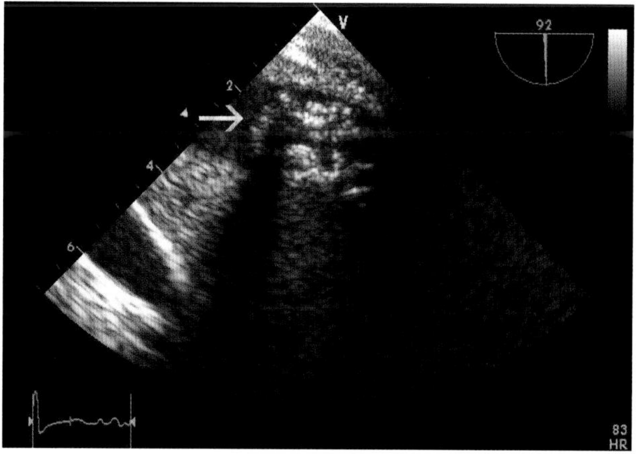

Figure 44.6.

ANSWERS AND DISCUSSION

QUESTION 44.1: The correct answer is C. The CS can usually be visualized from a lower ME 4CH view as the TEE probe is advanced toward the TG level (Fig. 44.1). It appears as a longitudinal structure on the right side of the TEE screen entering the RA. The CS can also be visualized from a modified bicaval view at around 110 degree by rotating the TEE probe slightly to the patient's right (Fig. 44.2). In Figure 44.2, the IVC is then seen just to the right of the CS. The modified bicaval view is particularly helpful to guide CS cannulation with the retrograde cardioplegia catheter. The IVC and CS are anatomically near each other as they enter the RA and are seen on the left side of the TEE screen in the bicaval views. On the other hand, the SVC is visualized on the right side of the TEE screen in the ME bicaval view. ASDs are abnormal connections between the left and the RA that can be seen in the ME bicaval views. CFD and injection of agitated saline will demonstrate a shunt between the right and the left atrium and confirm the diagnosis of an ASD. A dilated CS (>1 cm) is suggestive of elevated right atrial pressures and may be associated with the presence of a persistent left SVC, which can be confirmed by injecting agitated saline into a peripheral IV in the left arm.

QUESTION 44.2: The correct answer is B. The Thebesian valve is a small fold of the endocardium located at the entry to the CS. It can be of various lengths and may impede or obstruct the insertion of a retrograde cannula. Although the CS catheter may well bump against the atrial wall as the surgeon attempts to insert it into the CS, the image shown clearly depicts a membrane in front of the CS (Fig. 44.4). The Eustachian valve, also known as the valve of the IVC, serves to channel oxygenated blood from the lower extremities toward the foramen ovale in the fetus. It normally regresses after birth but remnants of variable lengths are often seen. The Chiari network is a remnant of the right venous valve that normally regresses during embryogenesis. It usually presents as a long web-like, fenestrated filament originating from the IVC and extending into the RA. Both Eustachian and Thebesian valves are usually much shorter than a Chiari network, although differentiation of the three structures on 2D TEE can prove difficult. In the Figures 44.3 and 44.4 and Videos 44.3 and 44.4 shown, the strict location of the membrane in front of the CS makes the diagnosis of a Thebesian valve the most likely answer.

QUESTION 44.3: The correct answer is D. The use of retrograde cardioplegia is not mandatory for AV surgery. However, cardioplegia of a heart with a hypertrophied LV myocardium as seen in AS is often difficult without both ante- and retrograde routes. Nevertheless, for short-duration CPB procedures, a single cycle of antegrade cardioplegia in the aortic root can be given to stop the heart prior to aortotomy. AVR on an empty but beating or fibrillating heart has also been described but is not a common practice. Surgeons could try to use a CS catheter of a different size and shape or attempt to insert it under direct vision via a small incision in the RA. For prolonged CPB, cardioplegia can be selectively infused into the coronary ostia via specially designed cannulas. This approach comes with a risk of causing iatrogenic coronary ostial stenosis in the months following surgery. In any case, many alternative strategies for cardioplegia are available and surgery should not be cancelled.

QUESTION 44.4: The correct answer is B. It is not unusual for a CS catheter to get dislodged during CPB. In this case, the CS catheter was properly placed in the CS, and then expelled from the CS when cardioplegia infusion was initiated or dislodged with surgical manipulation of the heart. One of the clues of correct CS catheter placement, besides effective cardioplegia, is the pressure measured in the CS upon infusion. Normal values are in the 28 to 35 mm Hg range. Lower values suggest CS catheter dislodgement or incomplete occlusion of the CS. In this case, the CS catheter was placed in the CS (Fig. 44.5 and Video 44.5), then found in the IVC (Fig. 44.6 and Video 44.6). Cardioplegia was then directly infused into the coronary ostia as previously described.

TAKE-HOME LESSON:

Correct placement of the CS catheter can be confirmed using lower esophageal four-chamber and bicaval views. The lower esophageal four-chamber view is a modification of the ME view, obtained by advancing the probe from the standard view until the CS is seen posterior to the MV.

SUGGESTED READING

Miller JP, Perrino AC, Hillel Z. Common artifcats and pitfalls of clinical echocardiography. In: Perrino AC, Reeves ST, ed. *A Practical Approach to Transesophageal Echocardiography.* Philadelphia: Lippincott Williams & Wilkins, 2008: 417.

Weiss SJ, Augoustides JG. Transesophogeal echocardiography for coronary revascularization. In: Perrino AC, Reeves ST, ed. *A Practical Approach to TEE.* 2nd ed. 310-311.

CASE 45

A 65-year-old male is scheduled for three-vessel CABG for severe coronary artery disease. He was admitted with unstable angina (Canadian classification score of 4) and shortness of breath NYHA class III. His medical history is significant for hypertension and chronic renal insufficiency.

The intraoperative CPB TEE exam reveals the images shown in Videos 45.1 to 45.3 and Figures 45.1 and 45.2. 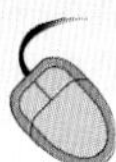

QUESTION 45.1. The images are consistent with

A. Normal AV
B. Bicuspid stenotic AV
C. Sclerosis of the AV but no stenosis
D. Calcific AV stenosis

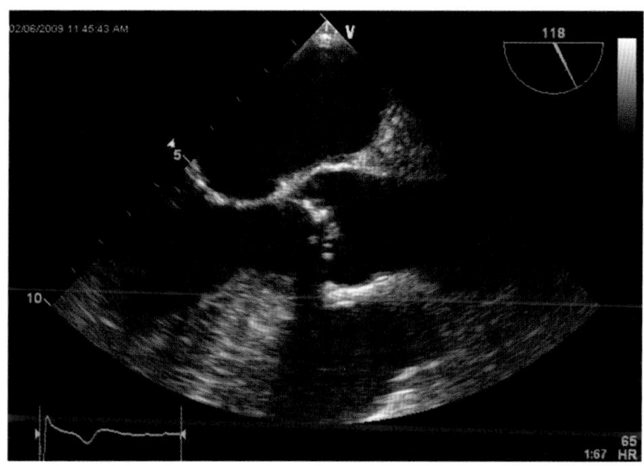

Figure 45.1.

QUESTION 45.2. The surgeon inquires about the severity of AV stenosis. What echocardiographic parameters would you measure to assess the severity of AV stenosis?

A. 2D planimetry
B. Peak and mean pressure gradients
C. LVOT/AV TVI ratio
D. All of the above

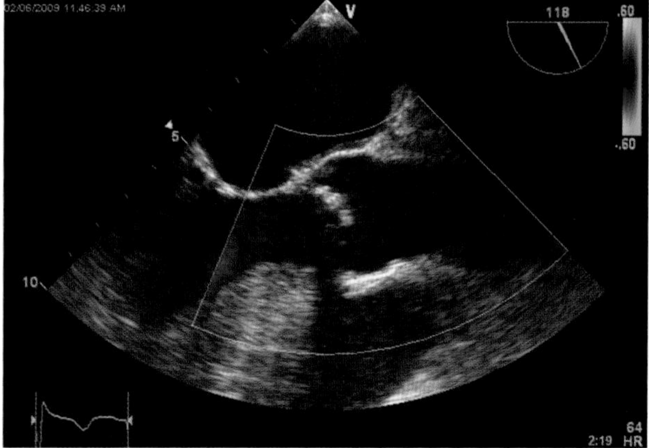

Figure 45.2.

QUESTION 45.3. Which measure of stenosis severity is BEST for making a clinical decision in a patient with an LVEF <20%?

A. Catheterization "peak to peak" (LV to aorta) pressure gradient
B. Gorlin valve area
C. Aortic Doppler maximum jet velocity
D. Dimensionless index

QUESTION 45.4. CW interrogation of the AV from the Deep TG LAX view is commonly used to define the severity of AV stenosis. Which one of the following conditions is not obtainable in this view?

A. Subaortic membrane
B. MR
C. Pulmonic stenosis
D. LVOT obstruction

QUESTION 45.5. After a complete comprehensive TEE exam, the summaries of significant echo findings are as follows:

LVEF 56%

AVA by planimetry 1.11 cm^2

AVA by continuity equation is 1.02 cm^2

Peak gradient 47 mm Hg

Mean gradient 28 mm Hg

What would be the next appropriate step in intraoperative surgical management?

A. Proceed with a coronary bypass
B. Proceed with coronary bypass and AVR
C. Obtain a stat cardiology consult
D. Abort the surgical procedure and wake up the patient
E. It is out of my area of expertise to make any recommendations

ANSWERS AND DISCUSSION

QUESTION 45.1: The correct answer is D: Calcific AV stenosis.

Age-related degenerative calcific AV stenosis is the most common cause of AS in adults. The prevalence of AV abnormalities detected by echocardiography increases with age, with 2% of population older than 65 years having isolated AV stenosis, whereas one third of the population has sclerosis without stenosis.

The images in Figures 45.1 and 45.2 are significant for a tricuspid AV that appears grossly abnormal with significant thickening of the AV cusps and restricted opening. Observe the hyperechogenicity created by calcium deposits on the free edges of the leaflets and the corresponding shadows that obscure the far field structures. Calcific changes usually start in the central part of leaflets, resulting in a three-pointed (peace sign) shaped orifice.

Cusp on a normal AV would appear thin, supple, and mobile. The tricuspid AV might have a bicuspid appearance if two of the cusps are fused; however, the hinge points of insertion differ between bicuspid and TV.

A sclerotic valve is a common finding in elderly population and its echocardiographic signature would be thickening of the cusps without narrowing of the AV opening.

QUESTION 45.2: The correct answer is D: All of the above.

There is no single value that defines severity of AV stenosis; however, a set of corroborated hemodynamic and natural history data can provide an accurate assessment of the stenosis.

The AHA/ACC guidelines for valvular heart diseases recommend the following criteria in defining severity of AV stenosis:

Indicator	Mild	Moderate	Severe
Jet velocity (m/s)	Less than 3	3.0–4.0	Greater than 4.0
Mean gradient (mm Hg)	Less than 25	25–40	Greater than 40
Valve area (cm^2)	Greater than 1.5	1.0–1.5	Less than 1.0
Valve area index (cm^2/m^2)			Less than 0.6

The incidental finding of AV stenosis in a patient scheduled for CABG surgery limits the valve assessment to TEE examination (additional clinical picture inquiries, MRI or cardiac catheterization data are not available). The AVA can be estimated echocardiographically by two methods: planimetry and via the continuity equation.

The planimetric measurement of the AV in the ME AV SAX view is prone to inaccuracies due to severe echogenic material (calcification) on the free edges of the AV and resulting shadows that obscure the opening of the valve anteriorly (Fig. 45.3).

In addition, the plane of interrogation could be "off" leading to overestimation of the AVA. One must attempt to find the smallest orifice view in which to perform the planimetry measurements. Hence, planimetry of the AVA is difficult and less accurate than the continuity equation for assessing the severity of AS. The continuity equation valve area can be calculated using the following equation:

$$AVA = 3.14(r_{LVOT})^2 \times LVOT_{TVI}/AV_{TVI}$$

where AVA = aortic valve area

r_{LOVT} = radius of LVOT

LOVT = left ventricle outflow tract

TVI = time velocity integral

AV = aortic valve

TVI of the AV can be obtained by tracing the AV CW Doppler velocity envelope in the deep TG view (Fig. 45.4). The TVI of the LVOT could be generated from PW Doppler velocity envelope in LVOT (deep TG or TG LAX views) or as demonstrated in Figure 45.4 from the inner envelop of the CW velocity. The diameter of LVOT can be measured in ME AV LAX view (Fig. 45.5). Inaccurate measurement of LVOT diameter and poor alignment between Doppler signals with blood flow are the major factors contributing to errors in calculating AVA via the continuity equation.

The mean and peak (instantaneous) gradients are derived from tracing AV CW Doppler velocity envelope. It is important to appreciate that these gradients can be low when the patient has significantly depressed LV function.

Although the valve gradients are flow dependent (low SV generates low gradient and vice versa), the ratio of $LVOT_{TVI}/AV_{TVI}$ is independent of any change in SV (flow) because the LVOT and AV velocities change proportionately. A $LVOT_{TVI}/AV_{TVI}$ ratio ≤ 0.25 is a very useful flow-independent indicator for severe AS.

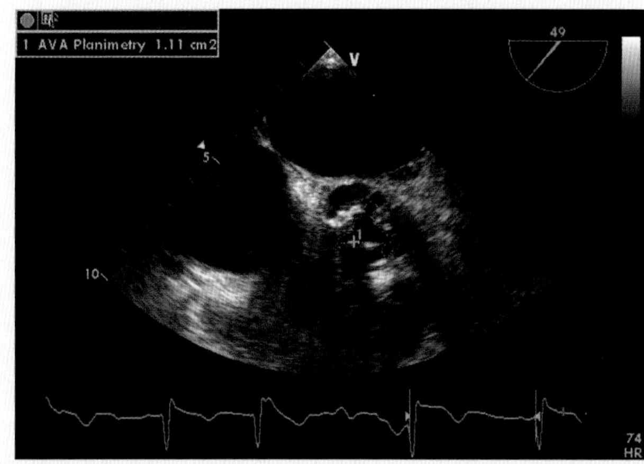

Figure 45.3.

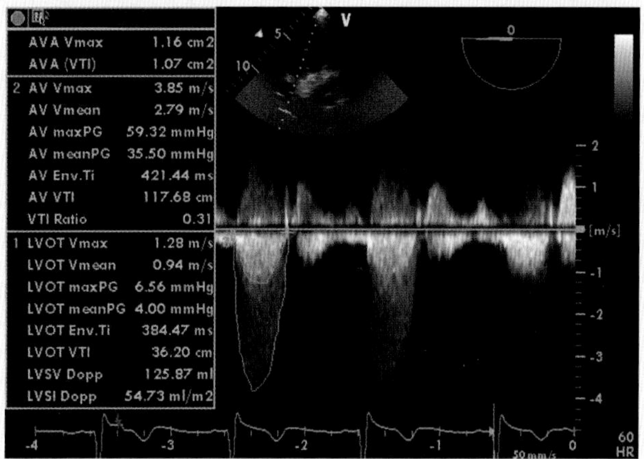

Figure 45.4.

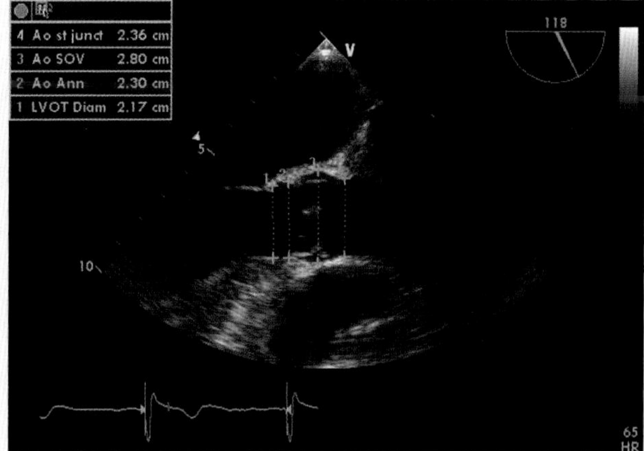

Figure 45.5.

QUESTION 45.3: The correct answer is D: Dimensionless index.

There are several parameters describing the severity of AV stenosis: peak and mean transaortic gradients, peak Doppler jet velocity, Gorlin valve area, continuity equation valve area, AV resistance, LV stroke work loss. Each proposed parameter for evaluating AV stenosis, when examined closely, varies with the flow rate through AV. There is one exception: dimensionless index or the $LVOT_{TVI}/AV_{TVI}$ ratio.

Frequently, this can be derived from a single image of deep TG CW Doppler aortic exam when a "double envelope" is generated: the cursor of CW Doppler is aligned with the transaortic blood flow and two envelopes are identified; the lower velocity envelope belongs to LVOT and the higher velocity is from the AV as demonstrated in Figure 45.4. There are advantages to using the double envelope technique: the beat-to-beat variability of measurements is eliminated since both the LVOT and AV VTI measurements can be obtained from the same SV. A dimensionless index ≤ 0.25 is equivalent to severe AV stenosis. There are no correlation data between the dimensionless index and less severe AV stenosis.

QUESTION 45.4: The correct answer is C: pulmonary stenosis.

The CW Doppler obtained from deep TG LAX view appears as a dense signal with negative velocities (flow directed away from the TEE probe) during LV systole. There are several lesions that generate a negative CW Doppler envelope and must be differentiated from AV stenosis on the basis of peak velocity, accompanying diastolic flow, pixel Doppler flow appearance, flow duration or ejection time, and location of the interrogation view.

All of the above-mentioned lesions generate clinically a systolic murmur. The deep TG view CW Doppler beam passes through ascending aorta, AV, LVOT, and LV cavity. Any narrowing of the systolic blood flow along this path would create a gradient of pressures pictured as a negative envelope. For instance, LV septal hypertrophy could generate a gradient of pressures that needs to be differentiated from that of an AV stenosis gradient. The flow velocity of dynamic LVOT obstruction produces a late-peaking dagger-shaped velocity envelope that increases in magnitude during a Valsalva maneuver.

At times, the deep TG interrogation window could be difficult to obtain or the image quality is poor especially when the LV is enlarged. In consequence, the CW Doppler beam could erroneously encounter the MV or even the TV regurgitant blood flows, which are in close vicinity with the AV flow. Both tricuspid and MV insufficiency generate a systolic murmur and a systolic negative CW envelope that needs to be differentiated from an AV stenosis origin. The TV velocity has the typical variation with respiration and the Doppler envelope "density" would appear less homogenous than that of the AV. The MR jet is normally 4 to 5 m/s and always higher than that of the AV jet of the same patient. In addition, the MV jet duration is longer than that of AS because the regurgitant mitral jet occurs not only in systole but also during isovolemic relaxation and contraction.

The pulmonary valve is anatomically oriented perpendicular to the AV. Pulmonary valve stenosis will generate a Doppler spectrum almost identical to that of AV stenosis. Since the pulmonic valve is perpendicular to the AV, it is not possible to obtain a Doppler flow velocity pattern in the deep TG LAX view. The angle of Doppler interrogation will be 90 degrees; therefore, the Doppler equation will equal zero—(cos 90 = 0).

QUESTION 45.5: The correct answer is B: Proceed with coronary bypass and AVR.

The AHA recommends in "patients with severe AS, with or without symptoms, who are undergoing CABG should undergo AVR at the time of the revascularization procedure." Based on the more accurate continuity equation AVA of ~1.0 the patient should undergo valve replacement surgery following a conversation with their referring physician.

TAKE-HOME LESSON:

An unexpected intraoperative finding of AS is a patient planned for isolated CABG surgery poses significant intraoperative TEE decision making challenges. The age of the patient, expected survival with or without AVR, the estimated rate of progression, and the risks of the combined surgical procedure should be balanced when AVR is contemplated.

SUGGESTED READING

Bonow RO, Carabello BA, Chatterjee K. ACC/AHA 2006 Guidelines for the management of patients with valvular heart disease. *JACC.* 2006;48:e1–e148.

Moderate

CASE 46

A 66-year-old woman presents for CABG, tricuspid ring, and possible MV repair. The outpatient echo report notes "severe MR." The images shown in Figures 46.1 to 46.4 were captured in the prebypass period (see also Videos 46.1, 46.2, 46.3, and 46.4).

QUESTION 46.1. True or False? The prebypass exam confirms the preoperative diagnosis of severe MR.

A. True

B. False

QUESTION 46.2. The Carpentier classification of the MR is

A. Type 1

B. Type 2

C. Type 3a

D. Type 3b

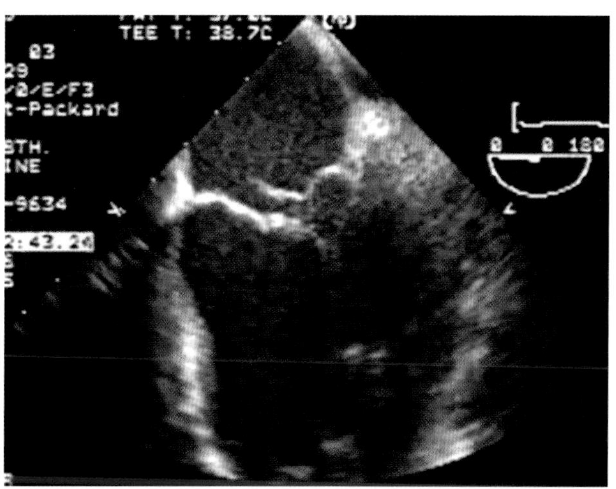

Figure 46.1. ME 4CH view, 2D (see also Video 46.1).

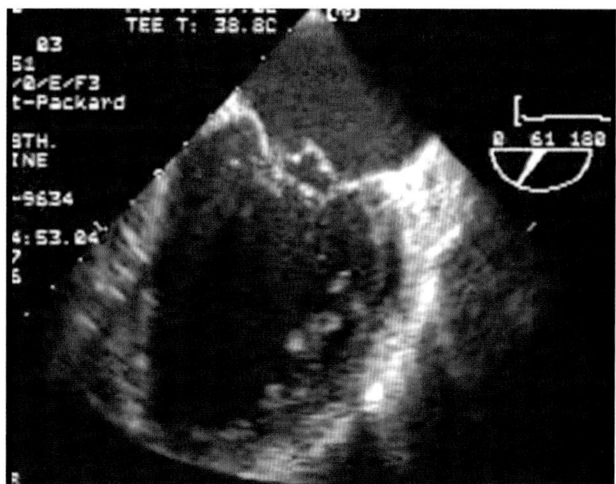

Figure 46.2. ME bicommissural view, 2D (see also Video 46.2).

QUESTION 46.3. What is the pathophysiology of the MR?

A. Endocarditis
B. Prolapse of the posterior leaflet
C. Prolapse of the anterior leaflet
D. Prolapse of the posterior and anterior leaflets

The images shown in Figures 46.5 and 46.6 are obtained following separation from CPB.

QUESTION 46.4. What surgical procedure was performed?

A. Posterior leaflet repair
B. Posterior leaflet repair and ring annuloplasty
C. Insertion of bileaflet mechanical prosthesis
D. Insertion of bioprosthetic valve

QUESTION 46.5. The most likely mechanism of the MR is

A. Residual prolapse of the posterior leaflet
B. Perivalvular leak
C. Intravalvular coaptation failure
D. Annular dilatation

The MV repair was revised and the patient was transported to the ICU. The following morning the patient is dyspneic and an echo exam is performed.

QUESTION 46.6. Figure 46.7A,B shows the major cause of MR to be

A. Leaflet coaptation failure
B. Dehisced mitral ring
C. Endocarditis
D. New onset SAM of the anterior leaflet of the MV

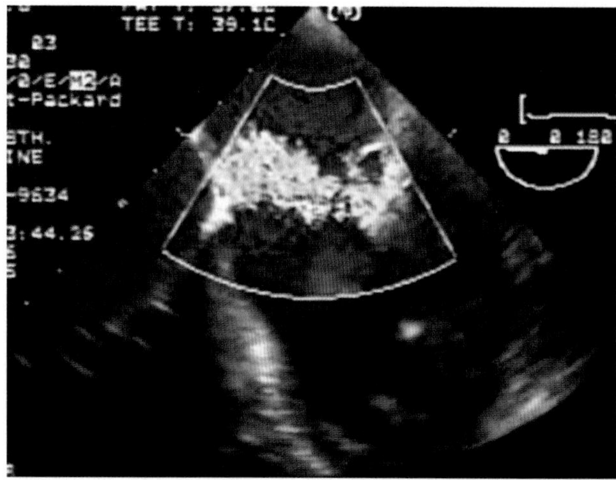

Figure 46.3. ME 4CH view, with CFD (see also Video 46.3).

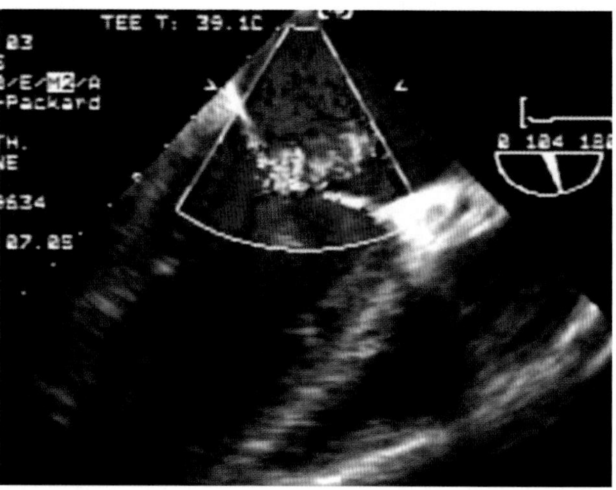

Figure 46.4. ME 2CH view, with CFD (see also Video 46.4).

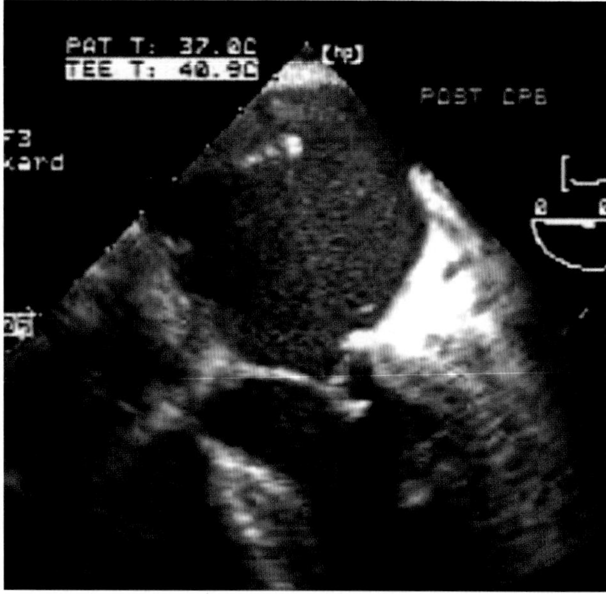

Figure 46.5. ME 4CH view (see also Video 46.5).

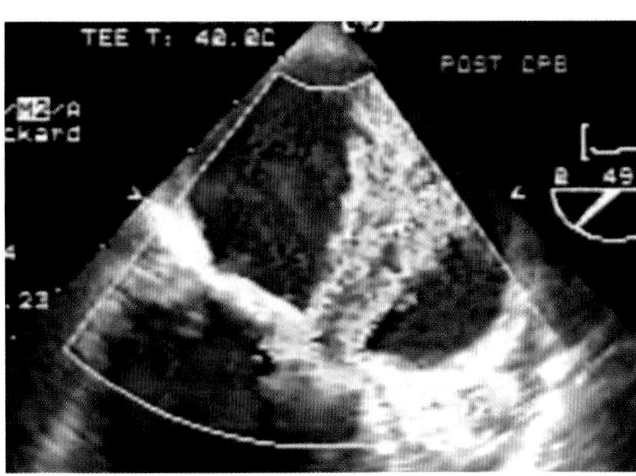

Figure 46.6. ME commissural view, with color Doppler, immediately post bypass (see also Video 46.6).

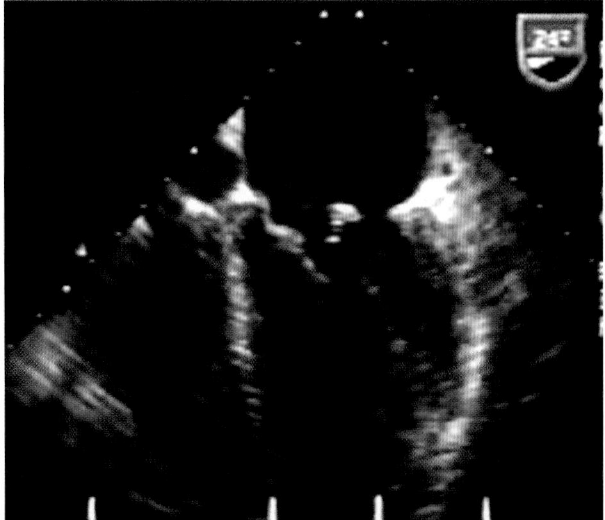

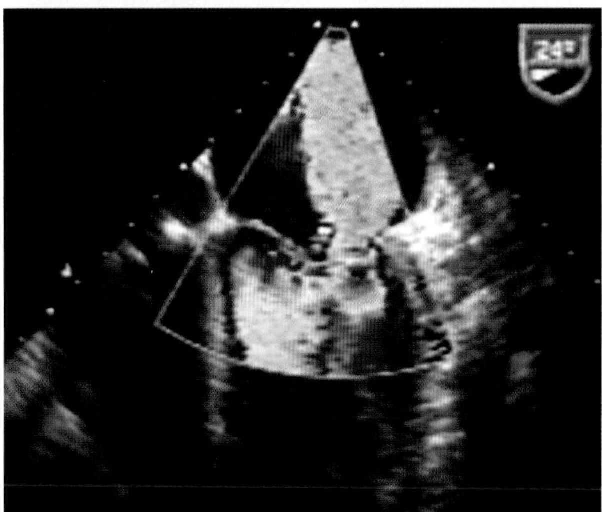

Figure 46.7. ME 4CH view in 2D (**A**) and CFD (**B**) (see also Video 46.7).

ANSWERS AND DISCUSSION

QUESTION 46.1: The correct answer is A: True. The exam is consistent with severe MR. Several features of the prebypass exam confirm the preoperative diagnosis of severe MR. These include an eccentric jet with a large vena contracta. Note that the length of the jet in this case exceeds the margins of the selected color Doppler box. In addition, as the jet impacts on the interatrial septum, the jet size will underestimate MR severity due to the Coanda effect.[1] For a more detailed discussion of the TEE signs of severe MR, please see Cases 50 and 67.

QUESTION 46.2: The correct answer is B: Type 2. There is structural abnormality of the MV leaflets and excessive motion as demonstrated on the 2D images. Type 1 would present with normal leaflet motion and is associated with conditions such as annular dilatation or perforated mitral leaflet. Type 3 would demonstrate restricted leaflet motion that is usually the result of rheumatic disease (3a), or an enlarged LV and tethering on the chordate (3b). For a more detailed description of the various types of MR, see Case 16.

QUESTION 46.3: The correct answer is B: Prolapse of the posterior leaflet. The ME 4ch image shows a flail P2 segment of the posterior leaflet extending into the left atrium (Fig. 46.1). The ME commissural view also shows a prolapsed segment that could represent the A2 scallop of the anterior leaflet as this segment is typically visualized in this imaging plane. However, the known flail posterior leaflet seen in the ME 4ch view and the anteriorly directed color jet suggests that the observed prolapsed segment in both ME views is the P2 segment of the posterior leaflet, not the anterior leaflet. While P2 is not normally visible in the ME commissural cross section, its presence is consistent with the redundant, prolapsed leaflet extending anteriorly, and "invading" the scanning plane. Answer A (*endocarditis*) is incorrect: Endocarditis can cause destruction or perforation of a leaflet, but it rarely causes chordal rupture. Answers C (*anterior prolapse*) and D (*bileaflet prolapse*) are also incorrect: Figure 46.1 does not show prolapse of the anterior leaflet. Identification of the correct pathology is critically important to selecting the correct surgical plan for repair or replacement. Again, for more detail, the reader is referred to Cases 16, 50, and 67.

QUESTION 46.4: The correct answer is B: Posterior leaflet repair and ring annuloplasty. Compared to the prebypass images the posterior leaflet has been shortened and an annuloplasty ring is seen in cross section. Leaflet repair is advisable whenever it is feasible and, in experienced surgical hands, it has a high success rate. Answer A (*posterior leaflet repair without ring*) is incorrect. Leaflet repair is rarely performed without a ring to support the repair. Answers C and D (*mechanical and bioprosthetic repairs*) are also incorrect: Figure 46.5 and Video 46.5 show no hallmarks typical of a mechanical or bioprosthetic valve. Note also that the amount of acoustic shadowing is much less in a valve repair, compared to a valve replacement. Finally, the color Doppler exam shows significant residual MR that warranted additional surgical intervention.

QUESTION 46.5: The correct answer is C: Intravalvular coaptation failure. Figure 46.6 and Video 46.6 show a large, central residual MR jet. Answer A (*residual prolapse of the posterior leaflet*) is incorrect: The posterior leaflet segment has been resected and Figure 46.5 and Video 46.5 reveal a shortened posterior leaflet with no evidence of prolapse. Answer B (*perivalvular leak*) is incorrect: Strictly speaking, a perivalvular leak (which denotes a leak *around* the valve) can only occur in a prosthetic valve or in a procedure where the annulus has been detached and reattached to the heart. But the term is commonly applied to leaks around an annuloplasty ring as well. Figure 46.6 and Video 46.6 clearly show the MR jet traveling *within* the valve, thus a perivalvular leak is excluded. Answer D (*annular dilatation*) is also incorrect: The annulus, supported by the ring implant, is not dilated.

QUESTION 46.6: The correct answer is B: Dehisced mitral ring. In Figure 46.7 and Video 46.7, the supporting ring has lost its posterior anchor to the annulus and can be seen within the atrium with 2D imaging. CFD reveals severe regurgitation with flow now occurring *between* the ring and the annulus. Compare this flow pattern to that seen immediately post bypass where the regurgitation occurred *within* the valve itself. Answer D (*new onset of SAM*) is incorrect: There is no evidence of SAM of the anterior mitral leaflet. Answer C is also incorrect, as endocarditis is extremely unlikely only hours after the surgery. Finally, answer A (leaflet coaptation failure) is not correct as only a small amount of the regurgitation *originates between* the mitral leaflets with the majority traversing a path between the annulus and the dehisced mitral ring. Immediately following this echocardiogram the patient was returned to the OR for life-saving MV replacement surgery.

TAKE-HOME LESSON:

MR has many mechanisms. Echocardiographic imaging is valuable to determine the specific etiology and proper treatment.

REFERENCE

1. Cheung AT. Prosthetic valves. In: Perrino AC, Reeves ST, eds. *A Practical Approach to Transesophageal Echocardiography*. Philadelphia: Lippincott Williams & Wilkins; 2008.

SUGGESTED READING

Lambert AS. Mitral regurgitation. In: Perrino AC, Reeves ST, eds. *A Practical Approach to Transesophageal Echocardiography*. Philadelphia: Lippincott Williams & Wilkins; 2008.

Moderate

CASE 47

A 63-year-old male is undergoing cardiac surgery. TEE examination of the descending aorta reveals the images shown in Video 47.1 and Fig. 47.1.

QUESTION 47.1. What is your diagnosis?

A. Grade 5 aortic atheroma
B. Artifact
C. Aortic aneurysm
D. Aortic dissection

QUESTION 47.2. In Figure 47.1 and Video 47.1, what is represented by the numbers 1 and 2?

A. 1 true lumen, 2 false lumen
B. 1 false lumen, 2 true lumen
C. 1 true lumen, 2 artifact
D. 1 artifact, 2 true lumen

QUESTION 47.3. According to Figure 47.2 and Video 47.2, what type of aortic dissection is the patient suffering from?

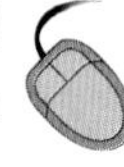

A. Type A
B. Type B
C. Type II
D. Type IIIb

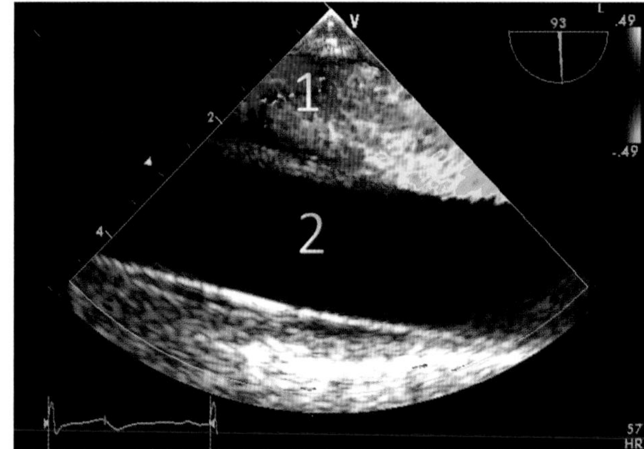

Figure 47.1. Desc Ao LAX view, color Doppler. See also Video 47.1.

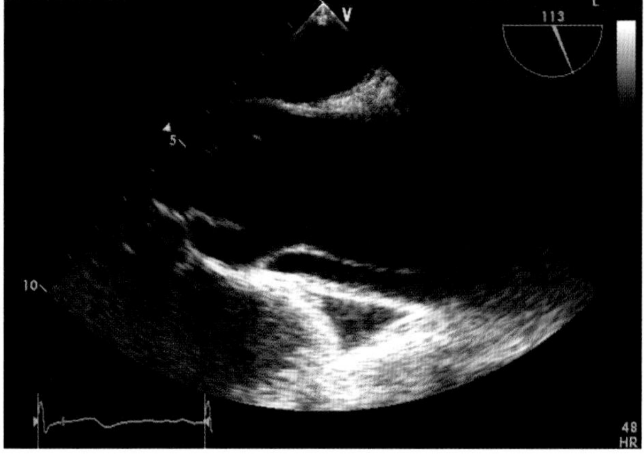

Figure 47.2. Modified ME view, ascending aorta. See also Video 47.2.

QUESTION 47.4. What is shown in Figures 47.3 and 47.4 and seen in Videos 47.3 and 47.4?

A. Aortic cannula

B. Re-entry point

C. Aortic debris

D. Aortic rupture

QUESTION 47.5. According to Figures 47.5 and 47.6 and Video 47.5, what worrisome complication may occur as a result of the extension of this dissection?

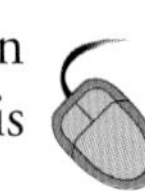

A. Obstruction of forward flow by the dissection flap

B. Pericardial tamponade

C. Myocardial infarction

D. AI

QUESTION 47.6. What vessel is the arrow pointing to in Figure 47.7 and seen in Video 47.7?

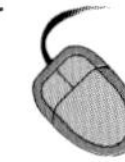

A. Aortic rupture

B. CS

C. PDA

D. Left subclavian artery

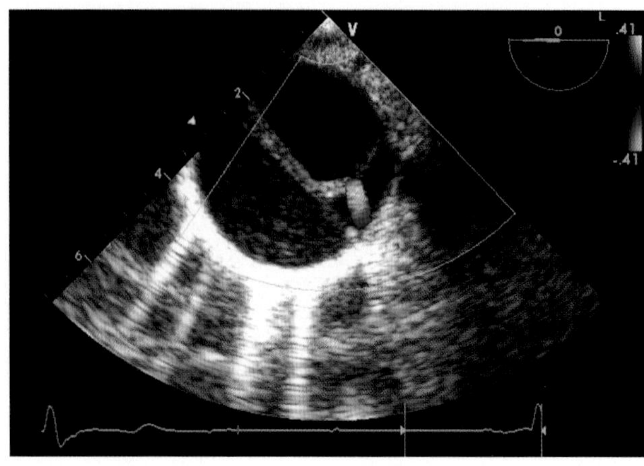

Figure 47.3. Desc Ao SAX view, color Doppler. See also Video 47.3.

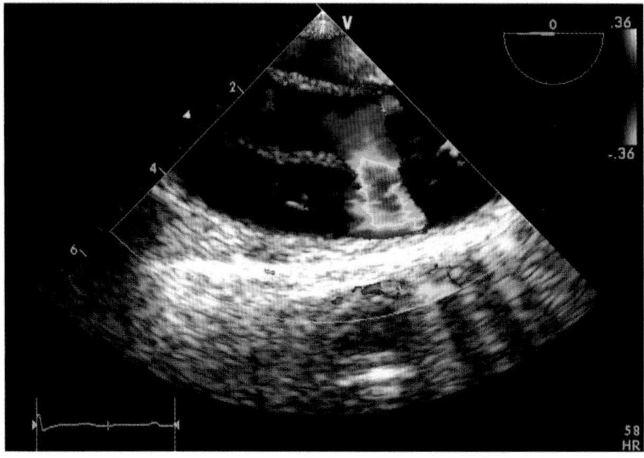

Figure 47.4. UE Aortic Arch LAX view, color Doppler. See also Video 47.4.

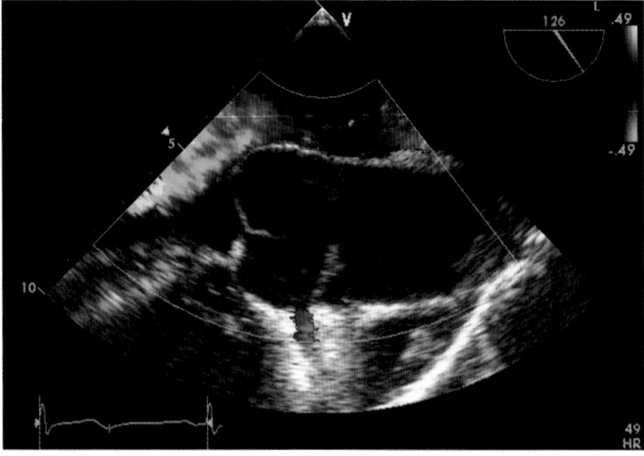

Figure 47.5. ME AV LAX, color Doppler. See also Video 47.5.

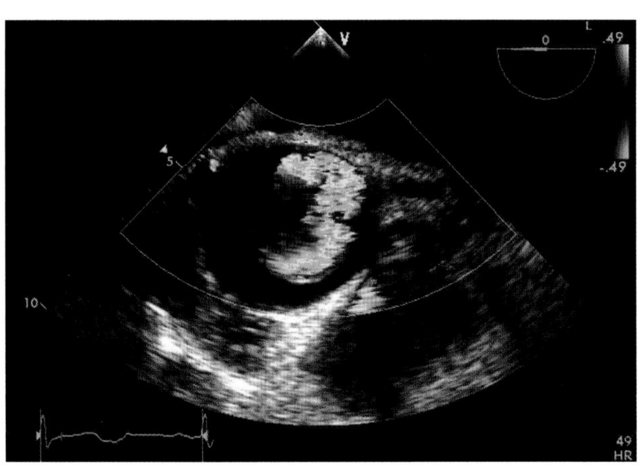

Figure 47.6. Modified ME AV LAX, color Doppler. See also Video 47.6.

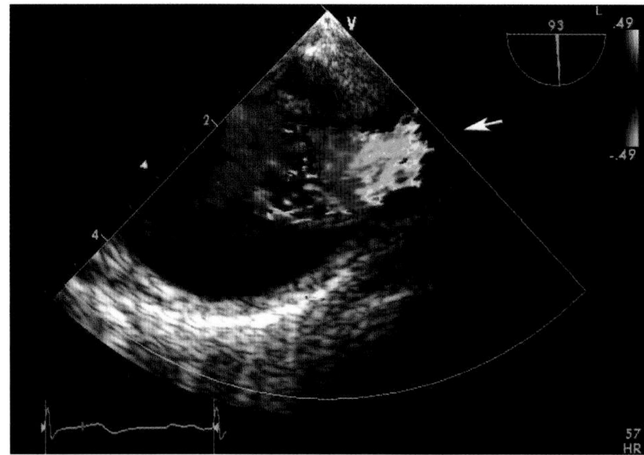

Figure 47.7. UE Aortic Arch SAX view, color Doppler, close-up. See also Video 47.7.

ANSWERS AND DISCUSSION

QUESTION 47.1: The correct answer is D: Aortic dissection.

Aortic dissection, a surgical emergency of the aorta, is caused by a single or multiple tears in the intimal wall. Blood under pressure can then dissect the layers from the media to produce a false lumen and an intimal flap. An example of such a flap is shown in Figure 47.6 and Video 47.6. Grade 5 atheromas are defined as protruding plaques >5 mm with mobile components. They are seen extending into the aorta from the vessel wall and would not have a linear aspect. One must be vigilant when making the diagnosis of aortic dissection as reverberations and side-lobe artifacts can mimic its appearance. Aortic aneurysm is defined as an abnormal dilation of the aortic diameter, which is not the case here.

QUESTION 47.2: The correct answer is A: 1 true lumen, 2 false lumen.

In Figure 47.2, the true lumen is identified as number 1 and the false lumen as number 2. Typically, in the ME LAX, the intimal flap will move such that it expands in systole. Furthermore, flow velocity will be higher in the true lumen and color Doppler interrogation will show blood flow moving slightly earlier. The false lumen is typically larger than the true lumen's diameter, involving half to two thirds of the circumference, and expands in diastole. Sometimes, clots or venous stasis (spontaneous echo contrast) can be seen inside this channel. The false lumen can rupture into the pericardium, the pleural space, or the abdomen. TEE is therefore helpful in differentiating the true lumen from the false lumen—which is crucial, especially during procedures such as endovascular aortic stenting. If the image were a normal aorta and an artifact, the lower image would mirror the upper and there would not be a difference in the direction of flow during the cardiac cycle.

QUESTION 47.3: The correct answer is A: Type A.

In the Stanford classification of aortic dissections, type A refers to dissection involving the ascending part of the aorta (with or without AI) and any extension into other aortic sections, whereas type B aortic dissection refers to involvement of the descending aorta, distal to the left subclavian artery. Type A dissections are surgical emergencies while type B dissections may be medically treated. The DeBakey classification defines type I as involvement of the ascending aorta extending into the descending aorta; type II as a dissection limited to the ascending section of the aorta; and type III as a dissection limited to the descending aorta (IIIa thoracic aorta, IIIb extension into the abdominal aorta). Numerous imaging modalities provide for the diagnosis of aortic dissection, all of which have benefits and detractors. TEE is highly effective in the diagnosis of aortic dissection of the proximal ascending aorta and descending thoracic segment, with reported sensitivity and specificity close to 100%. However, visualization of the aortic arch, distal thoracic aorta, and abdominal segment can be variable with TEE. CT, angiography, MRI, and TEE can all provide the diagnosis, and the modality of choice at your institution will depend on factors such as hemodynamic status and availability of various modalities.

QUESTION 47.4: The correct answer is B: Re-entry point.

The intimal tear creates one or several entry and re-entry points through which blood may enter and exit the false lumen. The intimal tear frequently occurs in the thoracic aorta. Blood can be seen entering the false lumen in systole. The aortic cannula has a completely different appearance on TEE and is usually seen in the ascending aorta. Aortic debris, another term for mobile or complex atheromas, does not have the linear appearance shown in the examples. Aortic rupture would involve extraluminal blood collection. The structure (flap) demonstrated is intraluminal.

QUESTION 47.5: The correct answer is C: Myocardial infarction.

In the images shown, the dissection stopped just short of the left main and right coronary ostia. Should it have dissected further, myocardial infarction could have occurred. When aortic dissection extends beyond the sinotubular junction, enlargement of the aortic root can result in AI, not seen in this case. Extension into the pericardium can result in tamponade; there was no evidence in the case presented. Finally, the flap seen in Figure 47.4 and Video 47.4 can appear to be obstructing forward flow. However, remember that the aorta is a tridimensional structure that should be examined in orthogonal views. Complete obstruction of forward flow is rare and fatal.

QUESTION 47.6: The correct answer is D: Left subclavian artery.

The vessel demonstrated by the arrow in Figure 47.6 is most likely the left subclavian artery; it is seen at 90 degrees in this close-up of the UE Aortic Arch SAX view. Tears or entry points in type III dissection begin distal to this point. Retrograde dissection extending into the left carotid may cause complications ranging from transient neurological symptoms to a stroke. A PDA is a congenital anomaly seen most often in children but sometimes in adults. It is a communication between the descending aorta and the left PA. When present, a PDA would be seen at around 40 degrees in the ME ascending aortic short-axis view with rotation to the left. The CS is a vessel draining into the RA at the level of the atrioventricular junction. Although seen on the right side of the TEE screen at zero degrees, it is clearly not an aortic structure. Aortic rupture leads to rapid lethal hemorrhage. When present, disruption of the aortic wall is seen as a thick intraluminal medial flap moving with each contraction. This medial flap is typically thicker than the intimal flap of aortic dissection as it is composed of both intimal and medial layers of the aortic wall.

TAKE-HOME LESSON:

TEE is a powerful diagnostic tool when aortic dissection is suspected. A complete TEE examination of the aorta should be done in order to assess and identify the intimal tear, the aortic true lumen, the extension of dissection, and potential complications as they all will have an impact on management.

SUGGESTED READING

Acute Aortic Dissection. *Kirklin/Barratt-Boyes Cardiac Surgery*. 3rd ed. Philadelphia: Churchill Livingston Publishers; 2003:1820–1849.

Aorta. In: Denault AY, Couture P, Tardif JC, et al., eds. *Transesophageal Echocardiography Multimedia Manual: A Perioperative Transdisciplinary Approach*. Marcel Dekker; 2005:261–283.

Shiga T, Wajima Z, Apfel CC, et al. Diagnostic accuracy of transesophageal echocardiography, helical computed tomography, and magnetic resonance imaging for suspected thoracic aortic dissection: systematic review and meta-analysis. *Arch Intern Med.* 2006;166(13):1350–1356.

Moderate

CASE 48

A 68-year-old male with a history of MV prolapse with worsening fatigue and dyspnea presents for MV repair.

QUESTION 48.1. The MV is repaired and the aortic cannula is removed after termination of CPB. A hematoma is noted at the cannulation site. What is the next most appropriate step in the care of this patient?

A. Monitor the hematoma and reassess if it grows in size
B. Do nothing since the patient is hemodynamically stable
C. Give protamine to prevent the hematoma from expanding
D. Echocardiographically assess the aorta for possible dissection

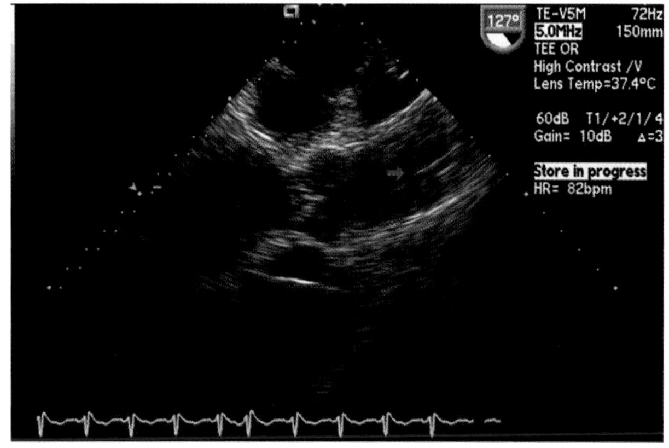

Figure 48.1. ME AV LAX.

QUESTION 48.2. What is the linear echo density (arrow in Fig. 48.1 and Video 48.1) seen in the ascending aorta in this patient?

A. Calcified plaque
B. Aortic intramural hematoma
C. Aortic dissection
D. Artifact

QUESTION 48.3. Examination of the descending aorta reveals (Fig. 48.2 and Video 48.2)

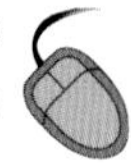

A. Aortic intimal flap
B. Aortic intramural hematoma
C. Pleural effusion
D. Aortic luminal artifact

QUESTION 48.4. The hematoma seen on the aorta is unchanged. What view of the aorta is seen in Figure 48.3 and Video 48.3?

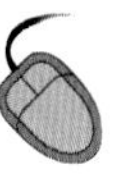

A. Descending aortic short axis
B. ME ascending aortic short axis
C. UE Aortic Arch SAX
D. Epiaortic view of the ascending aorta
E. ME ascending aortic long axis

QUESTION 48.5. TEE is limited in the examination of which of the following areas of the aorta?

A. Mid ascending aorta
B. Proximal aortic arch
C. Proximal descending aorta
D. Distal descending aorta

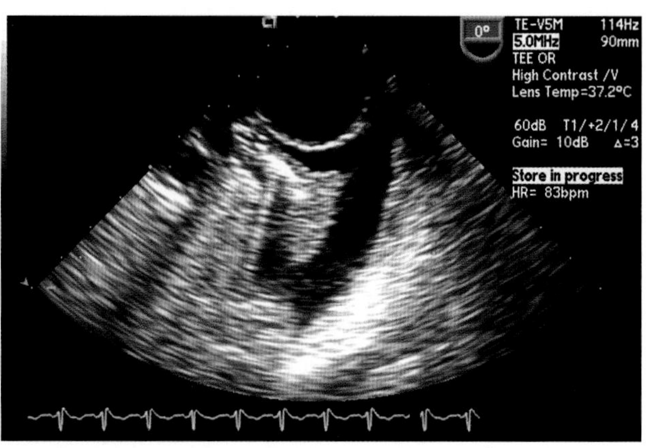

Figure 48.2. Descending aortic short axis.

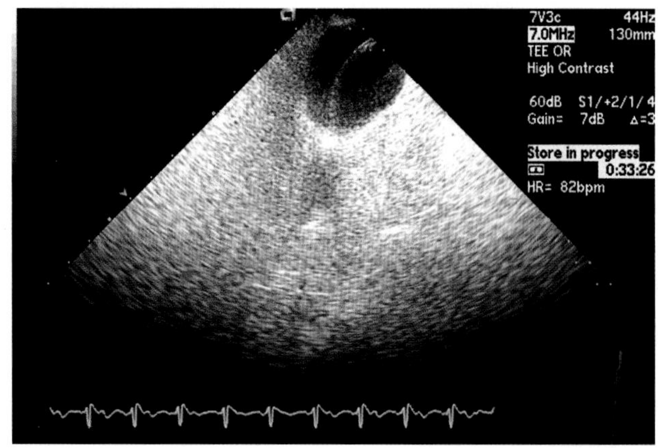

Figure 48.3. Aortic dissection flap.

ANSWERS AND DISCUSSION

QUESTION 48.1: The correct answer is D. Although the patient has a stable hematoma around the cannulation site, it is a sign of possible aortic injury. A complete examination of the aorta should be performed to rule out intimal dissection or intramural hematoma. An unrecognized aortic injury has both increased short-term and long-term morbidity and mortality.

QUESTION 48.2: The correct answer is D. The linear echo density in the ascending aorta is an artifact. Reverberation and side-lobe artifacts are the most common types of artifacts that mimic intimal flaps in the ascending aorta. An intramural hematoma would appear as a greater than 7-mm thick, crescent-shaped density in the wall of the aorta. It usually extends greater than 1 cm along the long axis of the aorta. It is important to differentiate an intramural hematoma from the mural thrombus within the lumen of the aorta. Intramural hematomas do not have a dissection flap. No dissection flap is seen in the image ruling out an aortic dissection in the proximal to mid ascending aorta. A calcified plaque can produce both reverberation and side-lobe artifacts in the ascending aorta, typically originating from a plaque at the sinotubular junction.

QUESTION 48.3: The correct answer is C. A moderate-sized left pleural effusion is seen in descending aortic short-axis view. The other possible answers are incorrect (see the answer for question 48.2).

QUESTION 48.4: The correct answer is D. Epiaortic echocardiographic views do not have a multiplane indicator on the viewing screen since epiaortic or transthoracic probes do not have that capability. All of the other views are obtained with a TEE probe.

QUESTION 48.5: The correct answer is B. Visualization of the distal ascending aorta and proximal aortic arch is limited on TEE because of the location of the air-filled trachea and left main bronchus between the probe and the aorta. In this patient, the dissection was localized to the distal ascending aorta, which could not be visualized with TEE. The addition of the epiaortic exam revealed a dissection flap in the TEE "blind-spot." The patient went back on CPB to repair the ascending aortic dissection.

TAKE-HOME LESSON:

Intramural hematoma, cannula hematoma, and aortic dissection are similar pathologies in the spectrum of aortic injury. Identification of a new aortic pathology necessitates evaluation for remote extension of the disease. Artifacts are common with ultrasound assessment of the aorta; multiple imaging planes are recommended to confirm the diagnosis.

SUGGESTED READING

Glas KE, Swaminathan M, Reeves ST, et al. Guidelines for the performance of a comprehensive intraoperative epiaortic ultrasonographic examination: recommendations of the American society of echocardiography and the society of cardiovascular anesthesiologist; endorsed by the society of thoracic surgeons. *J Am Soc Echocardiogr*. 2007;20:1127–1135.

Nienaber CA, Kodolitch Y, Petresen B, et al. Intramural hemorrhage of the thoracic aorta: diagnostic and therapeutic implications. *Circulation*. 1995;92:1465–1472.

Pantin EJ, Cheung AT. Transesophageal echocardiographic evaluation of the aorta and pulmonary artery. In: Konstadt SN, Shernan SK, Oka Y, eds. *Clinical Transesophageal Echocardiography*. Philadelphia: Lippincott Williams & Wilkins; 2003:215–244.

Moderate

CASE 49

A 45-year-old female presents to the cardiac OR for MV repair after a 10-year history of MV prolapse. Following induction of anesthesia you insert a TEE probe as part of your routine intraoperative management (Videos 49.1 and 49.2).

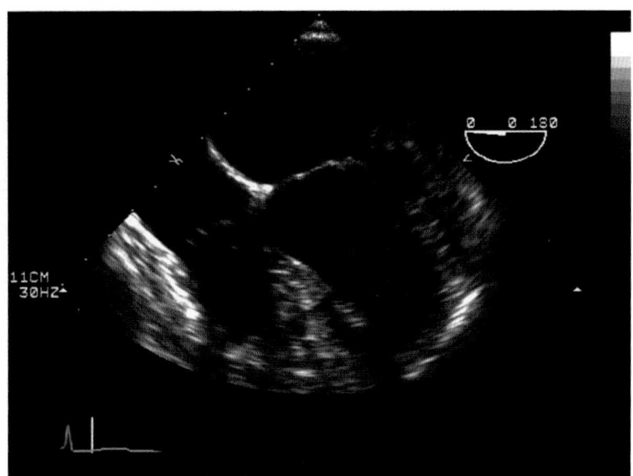

Figure 49.1. ME 4CH view, 2D. See also Video 49.1.

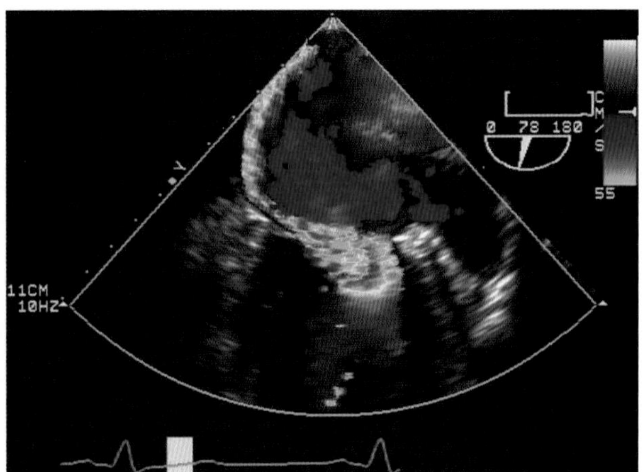

Figure 49.2. ME 2CH view (modified), CFD. See also Video 49.2.

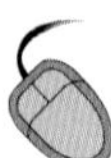

QUESTION 49.1. The 2D examination of the MV (Fig. 49.1) can provide direct information on all of the following except

A. RV
B. Structural abnormality
C. Location of leaflet defects
D. Hemodynamic effects of MR on the rest of the heart

QUESTION 49.2. Which of the following statements is *false*, regarding the CFD appearance of wall hugging MR jets (Fig. 49.2)?

A. The aliasing surface area of a wall hugging jet correlates poorly with its severity
B. The appearance of CFD of an eccentric jet is affected by gain settings but not by the aliasing velocity
C. A wall hugging jet should be considered severe until proven otherwise
D. A wall hugging jet almost always points to a structural leaflet problem

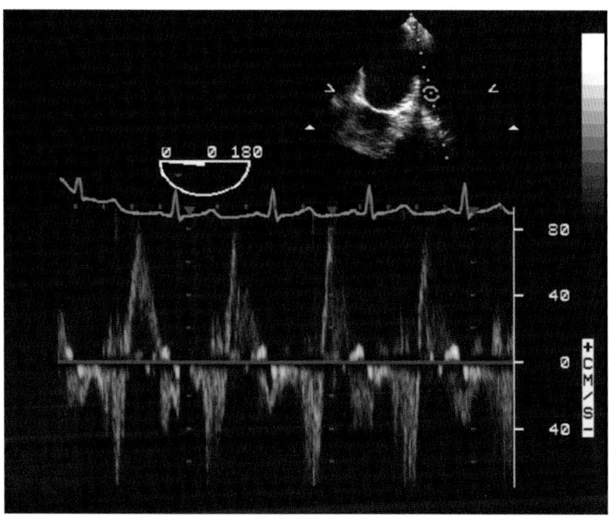

Figure 49.3. PW Doppler of the LUPV.

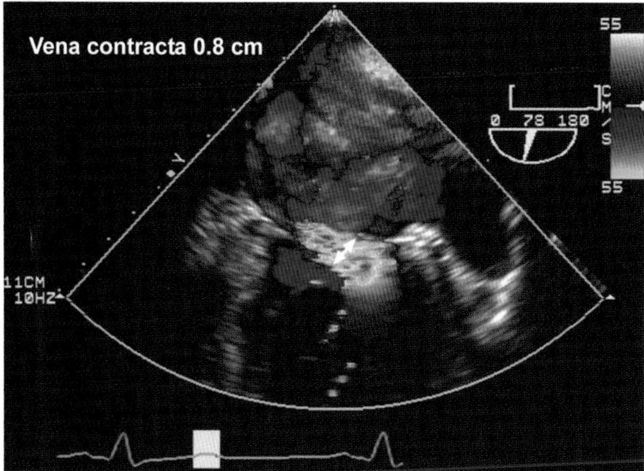

Figure 49.4. ME 2CH view (modified), with CFD, to illustrate the *vena contracta (white arrow).*

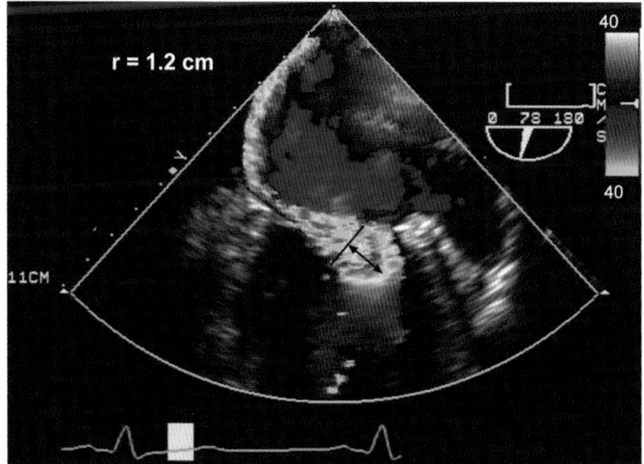

Figure 49.5. ME 2CH view (modified), with CFD, illustrating the proximal flow convergence area, used in the PISA method.

QUESTION 49.3. The PVF pattern in Figure 49.3 is most consistent with what severity of MR?

A. Trace MR
B. Mild MR
C. Moderate MR
D. Severe MR

QUESTION 49.4. In Figure 49.4, a *vena contracta* of 0.8 cm is most consistent with which of the following?

A. Trace MR
B. Mild MR
C. Moderate MR
D. Severe MR

QUESTION 49.5. Which of the following is true regarding the PISA method?

A. PISA can be used to determine RV
B. PISA is especially useful in the assessment of wall hugging jets
C. PISA has the advantage of not being dependent on gain and Nyquist limit adjustments
D. An EROA >0.2 cm^2 correlates with severe MR

QUESTION 49.6. Based on Figure 49.5, if the patient's arterial blood pressure is 115 mm Hg and the PCWP is 15 mm Hg, what is the EROA?

A. 0.72 cm^2, consistent with severe MR
B. 1.44 cm^2, consistent with severe MR
C. 1.2 cm^2, consistent with severe MR
D. The EROA cannot be calculated without knowing the peak mitral velocity

ANSWERS AND DISCUSSION

QUESTION 49.1: The correct answer is A: RV. The 2D examination of the MV is arguably the most important part of the assessment of MR, as it provides significant information on the structure of the valve, the pathophysiologic mechanism of MR, and often the etiology. Leaflet thickness and mobility, coaptation defects, annular dilatation and calcification, as well as subvalvular pathology (chordae tendinae, papillary muscles, and supporting LV walls), are all important elements of the diagnosis of MR. A systematic 2D MV analysis also allows one to pinpoint lesions to specific segments of the MV. Finally, the 2D examination may provide indirect indicators of the severity and chronicity of the MR: for example, LA enlargement, LV volume overload and/or signs of pulmonary hypertension, all suggest more severe, hemodynamically significant MR. The RV is estimated using calculations obtained from Doppler assessment. It cannot be calculated from 2D measurements alone.

QUESTION 49.2: The correct answer is B: The appearance of CFD of an eccentric jet is affected by gain settings but not by the aliasing velocity. CFD is the best tool to screen for the presence of MR. It also provides a semiquantitative assessment of its severity. The surface area of the aliasing jet correlates with its severity, provided that the gain *and* the aliasing velocity are adjusted properly (this is a potential major pitfall of CFD). Studies have shown that if the surface area of the jet is greater than 40% of the surface area of the left atrium, the MR is likely to be severe. Unfortunately, this technique is *not reliable in wall hugging jets*, due to the Coanda effect and the distortion of the jet by the atrial wall. Wall hugging jets are *almost always caused by a structural abnormality* of the mitral leaflets. As such, they should be investigated closely and should always be *considered severe until proven otherwise*.

QUESTION 49.3: The correct answer is D: Severe MR. Normal PVF is biphasic, occurring during ventricular systole (the S wave) and early diastole following MV opening (the D wave). There is also a small amount of flow reversal after atrial contraction (the A wave). The normal flow pattern is forward (toward the left atrium) in both systole and diastole, meaning that both the S and D waves are upright. In the presence of increasing MR, the S wave becomes progressively blunted, until it eventually becomes reversed. This means that the MR causes transient retrograde systolic flow in the pulmonary veins. When present, this sign is very specific for severe MR, but it is not necessarily sensitive, especially if the MR is chronic and the left atrium is very dilated and compliant. In this example, there is frank systolic flow reversal, consistent with severe MR.

QUESTION 49.4: The correct answer is D: Severe MR. The vena contracta is defined as the narrowest point of the color Doppler jet as it passes through the mitral regurgitant orifice. This measurement has been shown to correlate with quantitative measurements of MR severity, made at the time of cardiac catheterization. A vena contracta of 3 mm or less correlates with mild MR, while a vena contracta greater than 7 mm is associated with severe MR.[1] This technique is most accurate when the mitral regurgitant orifice is round and has significant limitations when the orifice is eccentrically shaped. Indeed, significant underestimation or overestimation can occur depending on which axis is measured.

QUESTION 49.5: The correct answer is A: PISA can be used to determine RV. The PISA method allows a quantitative EROA and RV. It is based on the physics of flow acceleration and the continuity equation. In short, blood flowing toward the mitral regurgitant orifice accelerates along a series of concentric hemispheres of isovelocity. By measuring the radius of the hemisphere where the blood reaches the aliasing velocity, and measuring the peak velocity and VTI of the regurgitant flow, one can calculate the EROA. Since it is a color Doppler-based technique, it is very dependent on gain and Nyquist limit settings, and changing the Nyquist limit can significantly affect the shape of the isovelocity hemispheres. PISA can be of limited benefit in situations of oddly shaped regurgitant orifices, multiple orifices, and wall hugging jets that are difficult to align with the Doppler beam.

An introduction to the PISA method in evaluating MR is available in Ref. 2 and a more detailed review in Ref. 3.

QUESTION 49.6: The correct answer is A: 0.72 cm^2, consistent with severe MR.

The PISA calculation is as follows:

EROA $= (2\pi r^2)\, V_{aliasing}/V_{max}$, where r is the radius of the PISA hemisphere, measured between the regurgitant orifice and the point at which the color changes from red to blue; $V_{aliasing}$ is the Nyquist limit and V_{max} is the peak mitral velocity measured by CW Doppler. When certain conditions are met, that is when $V_{max} = 5$ m/s and $V_{aliasing} = 40$ cm/s the PISA formula simplifies to EROA $= r^2/2$. These conditions are met when the difference between the arterial blood pressure and the PCWP is about 100 mm Hg and when the Nyquist limit is set at about 40 cm/s.

So, in this example, EROA $= (1.2)^2/2 = 0.72$ cm^2. An EROA < 0.2 cm^2 is consistent with mild MR, while an EROA > 0.4 cm^2 is associated with severe MR.[1]

TAKE-HOME LESSON:

Eccentric MR jets (as opposed to central jets) usually suggest a *structural* mitral leaflet problem and should always be carefully evaluated. The severity of wall hugging jets can easily be underestimated and they should be considered severe until proven otherwise.

REFERENCES

1. Lambert S. Mitral Regurgitation. In: Perrino AC, Reeves ST, eds. *A Practical Approach to Transesophageal Echocardiography.* 2nd ed. Philadelphia: Lippincott Williams & Wilkins, 2008.
2. Lambert AS. Proximal isovelocity surface area should be routinely measured in evaluating mitral regurgitation: a core review. *Anesth Analg.* 2007;105(4):940–943.
3. Zoghbi WA, Enriquez-Sarano M. Recommendations for evaluation of the severity of native valvular regurgitation with two-dimensional and Doppler echocardiography. *J Am Soc Echocardiogr.* 2003;16(7):777–802.

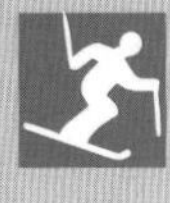

Moderate

CASE 50

A 76-year-old diabetic woman presents to the hospital with heart failure, fever, and a systolic murmur. Her blood cultures grow *Staphylococcus aureus*. After her TTE demonstrates MR, a TEE is performed for diagnostic purposes.

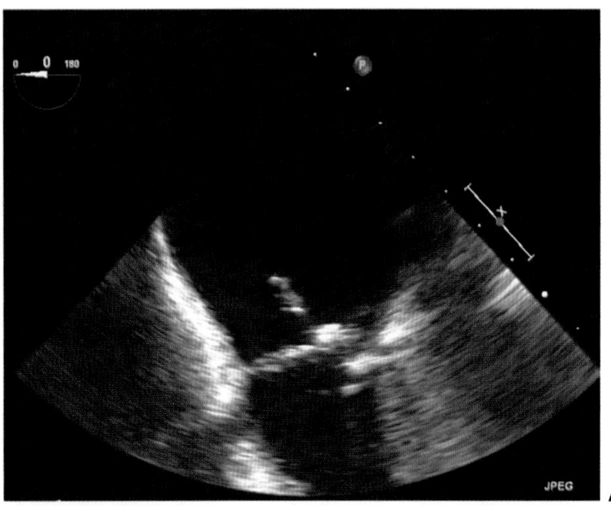

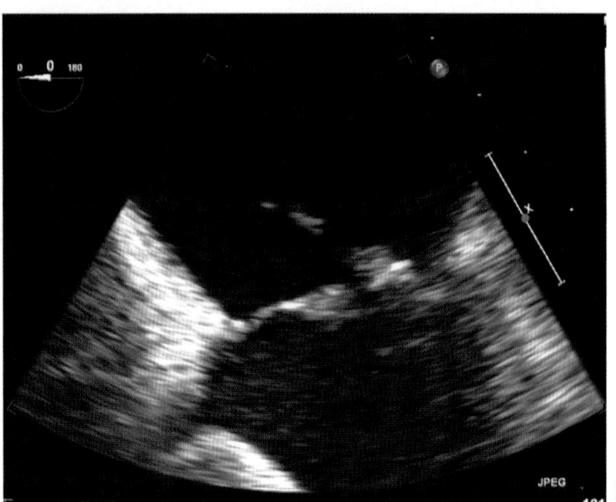

Figure 50.1. ME 4CH views of the MV.

QUESTION 50.1. The echocardiography on Figure 50.1A,B (and in Video 50.1) is most consistent with:

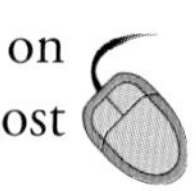

A. Vegetation on the MV
B. Long thrombus on MV
C. Posterior leaflet (P2) prolapse
D. MV stenosis
E. MV billowing

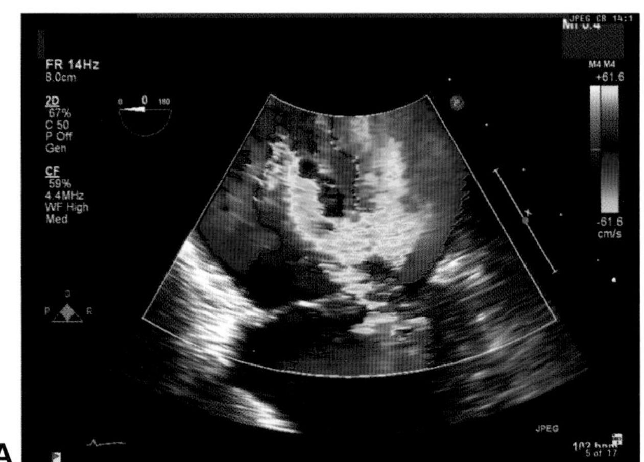

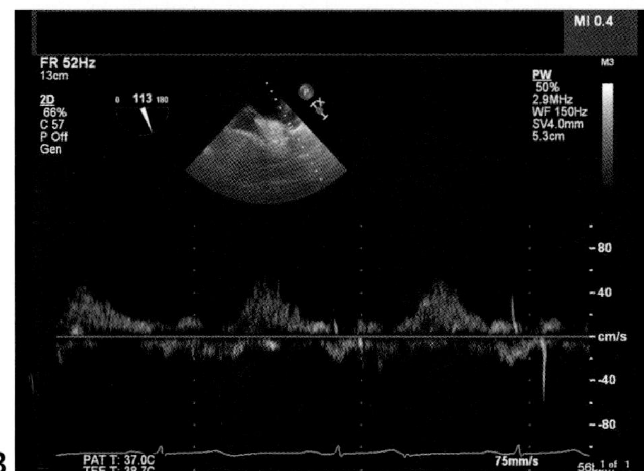

Figure 50.2. **A**: Color Doppler image of the MV, ME 4CH view. **B**: PW Doppler of the right upper PVF.

QUESTION 50.2. How severe is the MR (Fig. 50.2A,B and Video 50.2A,B)?

A. Trace

B. Mild

C. Moderate

D. Severe

The patient is treated with intravenous antibiotics and diuretics, but over the next week she continues to have intractable heart failure, with pulmonary edema, rising creatinine, increasing peripheral edema and liver congestion with an elevated international normalized ratio (INR). The decision is made to send her to the OR for MV replacement. You are called to perform the intraoperative TEE.

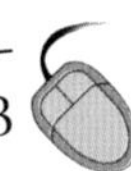

QUESTION 50.3. What complication of endocarditis is depicted on this echo (Fig. 50.3A,B and Video 50.3A,B)?

A. Perforation of the posterior leaflet

B. Abscess formation

C. Paravalvular leak of the MV

D. Fistula to the RA

E. MAC

QUESTION 50.4. The patient undergoes patching of the abscess and MV replacement with a bioprosthesis. She is transferred to the ICU. What important investigation is strongly indicated in this patient postoperatively, given the intraoperative TEE findings?

A. Fractional excretion of sodium

B. Chest x-ray

C. CT scan of the head and abdomen

D. V/Q scan

E. Myocardial perfusion scan

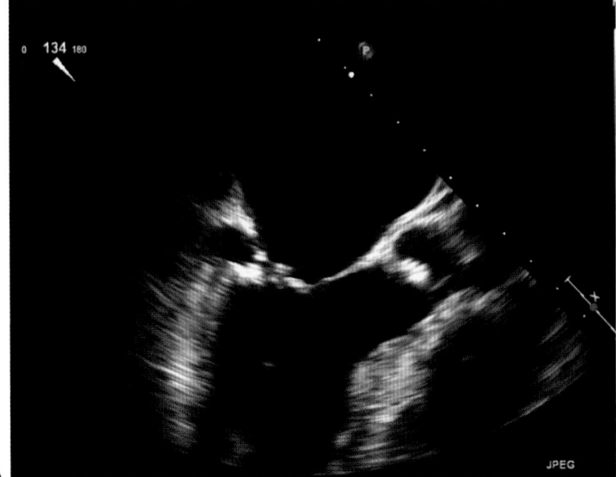

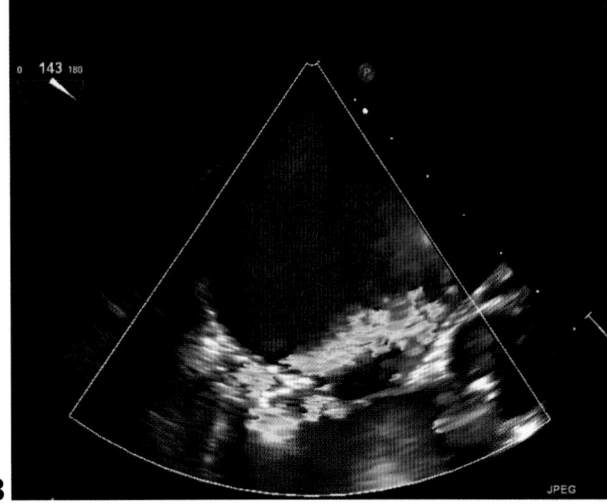

Figure 50.3. 2D echocardiogram and color Doppler image of the MV, ME LAX.

ANSWERS AND DISCUSSION

QUESTION 50.1: The correct answer is A: Vegetation on the MV. Although TEE cannot define tissue pathology, the clinical presentation and imaging are consistent with vegetation and endocarditis. Two masses can be seen on the middle scallop of the posterior leaflet of the MV (P2): a large bright vegetation, firmly attached to the posterior leaflet, and a long mobile vegetation extending from the first one. Despite the fact that it is severely disrupted, the posterior leaflet is not prolapsed. A thrombus could conceivably appear long and filamentous, especially when attached to an indwelling catheter.

QUESTION 50.2: The correct answer is D: Severe. The MR jet fills most of the left atrium; it is broad-based, eccentric, with a visible area of flow convergence PISA and is associated with blunting of the systolic PVF. Although the PVF pattern does not show systolic flow reversal, when the complete exam is evaluated collectively, the findings are consistent with severe MR.

QUESTION 50.3: : The correct answer is B: Abscess formation. A large abscess, measuring 1.7 cm × 0.9 cm can be seen in the posterior mitral annulus. It extends behind P2 medially toward P3. The mitral leaflet is disrupted, resulting in intravalvular MR, but it is not perforated. On the color Doppler loop, flow can be seen entering from the LV into the abscess cavity, then out into the LA. Although this constitutes a fistula formation, it communicates with the left atrium, not the right. Paravalvular leaks, strictly speaking, only exist in prosthetic valves (although the mechanism here is somewhat similar in that blood flows *around* the valve rather than *through* it). Finally, MAC is present in this patient, but it is not a short-term complication of endocarditis.

Figure 50.4 uses 3-D echocardiography to view the MV from the atrium and shows the large vegetation adherent to the P2 scallop and the abscess just above and posterior to P2–P3 scallops.

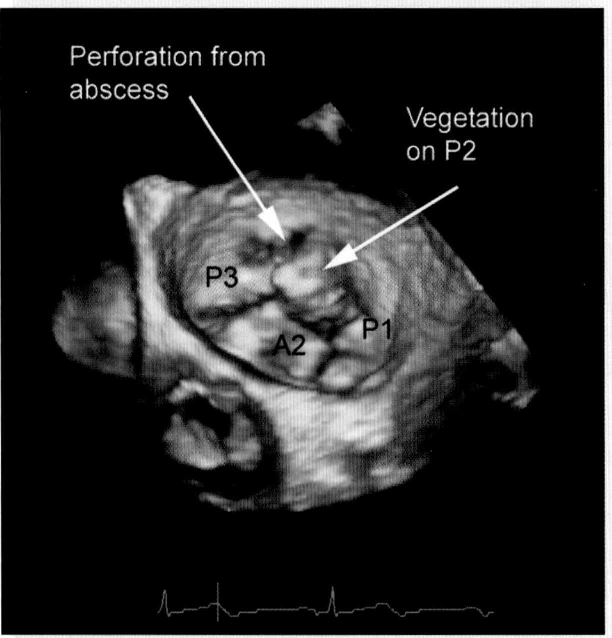

Figure 50.4. 3D echocardiogram of the MV.

QUESTION 50.4: The correct answer is C: CT scan of the head and abdomen.

The long filamentous vegetation is conspicuously *absent* from the second study. One hopes that antibiotic therapy has caused it to be reabsorbed, but given the short time interval of therapy, embolization to the brain or another organ is a concern. Diagnostic imaging, especially of the brain, is strongly indicated.

TAKE-HOME LESSON:

Perivalvular abscess formation is a serious complication of MV endocarditis and it may result in fistula formation. Although less common than in prosthetic valves, periannular spread of infection also occurs in native MV. TEE is central to the diagnosis and management of patients with endocarditis.

SUGGESTED READING

Baddour LM, Wilson WR, Bayer AS, et al. Infective endocarditis: diagnosis, antimicrobial therapy, and management of complications: a statement for healthcare professionals from the Committee on Rheumatic Fever, Endocarditis, and Kawasaki Disease, Council on Cardiovascular Disease in the Young, and the Councils on Clinical Cardiology, Stroke, and Cardiovascular Surgery and Anesthesia, American Heart Association: Endorsed by the Infectious Diseases Society of America. *Circulation*. 2005;111:e394–e434.

Moderate

CASE 51

A 60-year-old male underwent fluoroscopically guided placement of an endovascular stent. The surgical team is ready to remove the femoral artery sheath if the TEE is acceptable. The images shown in Figures 51.1 and 51.2 were obtained.

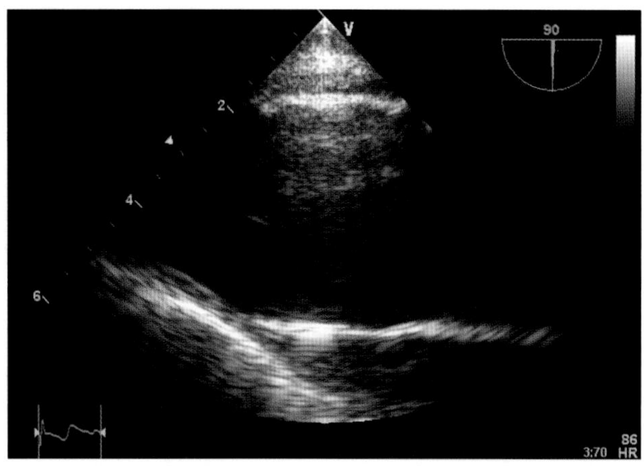

Figure 51.1. LAX of descending aorta.

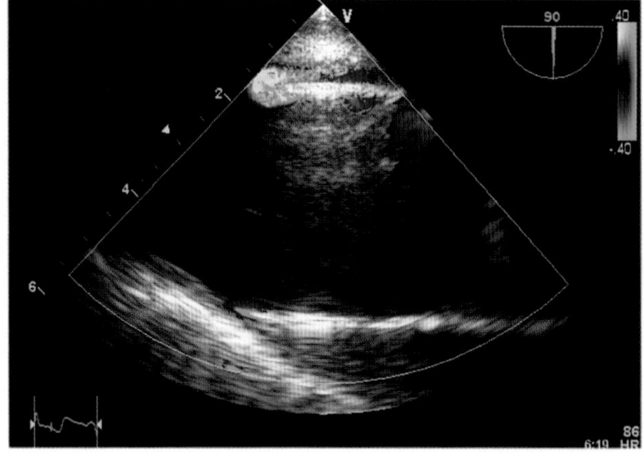

Figure 51.2. LAX of descending aorta with CFD. See also Video 51.1.

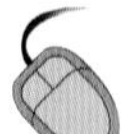

QUESTION 51.1. The most likely etiology of the echo still image shown Figure 51.2–51.5 is:

A. Traumatic aortic injury
B. Aortic dissection
C. Aortic graft in good position
D. Unsatisfactory aortic graft position

QUESTION 51.2. To further evaluate the aorta you would:

A. Examine the aorta in short axis
B. Examine the aorta with pulse wave Doppler
C. Examine the aorta with color Doppler
D. Examine the aorta with CW Doppler

QUESTION 51.3. The surgical management (Fig 51.2) is:

A. None, this is a normal echo finding for endovascular aortic reconstruction (EVAR)
B. Adjust/repeat EVAR
C. Proceed to emergent open repair
D. Follow-up imaging after discharge

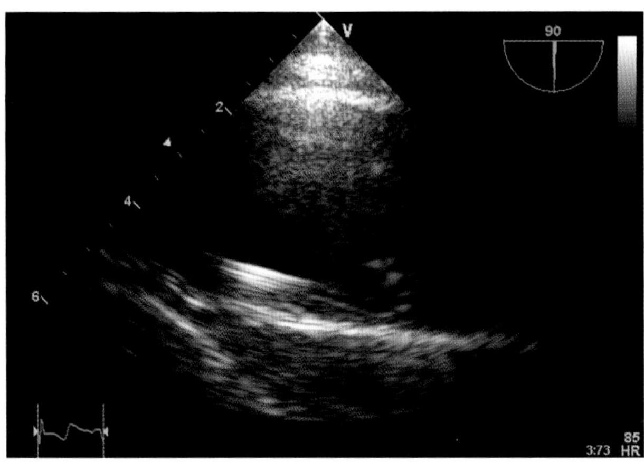

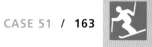

Figure 51.3. LAX of descending aorta. See also Video 51.2.

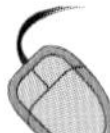

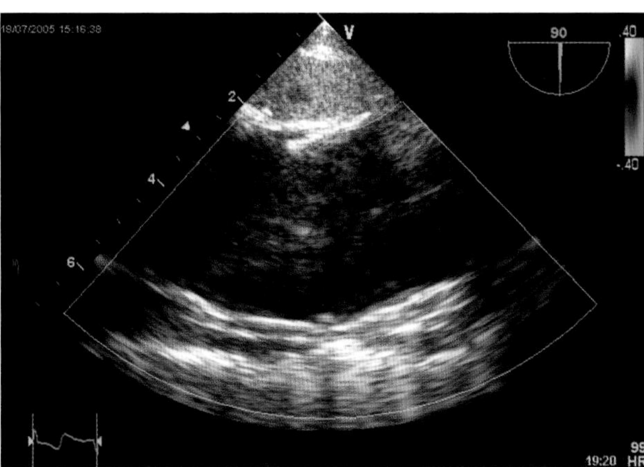

Figure 51.4. LAX of descending aorta.

QUESTION 51.4. The echocardiographic finding in Figure 51.3:

A. Guide wire in true lumen
B. Guide wire in false lumen
C. Acute dissection
D. Side-lobe artifact

QUESTION 51.5. What has occurred in Figure 51.4?

A. Deployment of an additional stent
B. Balloon modification of existing stent
C. No change
D. Aortic disruption

ANSWERS AND DISCUSSION

QUESTION 51.1: The correct answer is D: Unsatisfactory aortic graft position. Making this diagnosis with a still frame is challenging, and while it can be done it is recommended you review a video image to confirm the diagnosis. The graft does not exclude the entire aneurysmal portion of the aorta. By convention the markers along the left lateral border of the image are in 1-cm increments, so this aorta is 5 cm below the level of the graft. The aortic graft is identifiable within the aorta and the distal edge is demonstrated by the blue arrows (Fig. 51.5).

ANSWER A: Answer A can be excluded as an option due to the uniform enlargement of the aorta. A trau-

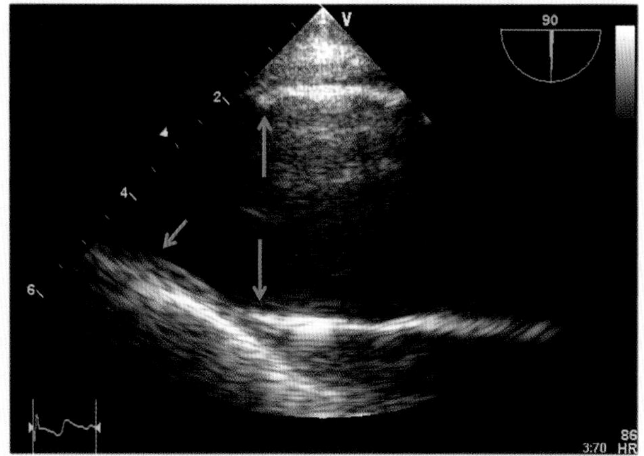

Figure 51.5. LAX of descending aorta.

matic rupture would show an intimal flap and a localized area of dilatation, or a corresponding effusion if there was an associated rupture.

ANSWER B: Answer B is excluded by the appearance of the aorta, and dissection is not the most likely etiology in this clinical scenario. A dissection is possible during EVAR, but not as common as unsatisfactory graft deployment. The graft and aortic cavity may give the appearance of a dissection flap and false lumen, but close inspection reveals the aortic wall is graft material and not normal aortic wall.

ANSWER C: Answer C is incorrect. The graft does not extend distally enough to reach the normal aorta (red arrow) distal to the aneurysmal aorta. Without firm purchase, endoleak is probable and the distal graft may be unstable and migrate.

QUESTION 51.2: The correct answer is C: Examine the aorta with color Doppler. The diseased aorta should be surveyed along its length in long and short axis with color Doppler searching for an endoleak. The analogous exam would be that of Type A or B aortic dissection in search of re-entry points (Fig. 51.2).

ANSWER A: Answer A is incorrect. Examining the aorta in short axis allows measurement of the landing zone but does not exclude a leak.

ANSWERS B and D: Answers B and D are incorrect. Endoleak rarely causes enough flow to be noted in pulse wave or CW Doppler of the aorta. However, PW examination of an endoleak, initially noted by color Doppler, may identify the direction and relative amount of flow.

QUESTION 51.3: The correct answer is B: Adjust/repeat endovascular repair. The distal end of the graft must reach normal aorta by bridging with a second graft.

ANSWER A: Answer A is incorrect. The graft is not well positioned in an appropriate landing zone. Endoleak with CFD near the probe is evident.

ANSWER C: Answer C is not unreasonable in the setting of hemodynamic instability after graft deployment.

ANSWER D: Answer D is incorrect. The complication should be repaired during this examination.

QUESTION 51.4: The correct answer is A: Guide wire in the lumen. The "J" form of the wire can be seen transiting from distal to proximal aorta (yellow arrow).

ANSWER B: Answer B is incorrect. The aorta is aneurysmal in this case. There is no "false lumen." The possibility of the guide wire entering the aneurysmal aorta *outside* the graft, however, does exist.

ANSWER C: Answer C is incorrect. Linear artifacts can frequently be confused with dissections. In this case, the linear structure is not an artifact, and the structure can be confirmed as a guide wire by asking the surgeon to move the wire.

ANSWER D: Answer D can be excluded by same method as in answer C. In addition, side-lobe artifacts typically cross anatomic structures and this wire is clearly intraluminal.

QUESTION 51.5: The correct answer is A: Deployment of an additional stent. A second stent has been advanced into the initial stent. The doubled outline of the overlapping stents can be seen in Figure 51.6 (yellow arrows).

ANSWER B: Answer B is incorrect. It is possible in some settings of an endoleak to modify the end of the graft with balloon reinflation at the leak site. In this case, however, the leak is due to a diameter mismatch of aneurysmal aorta and the graft.

ANSWER C: Answer C is incorrect. The overlapping grafts indicate repeat stenting.

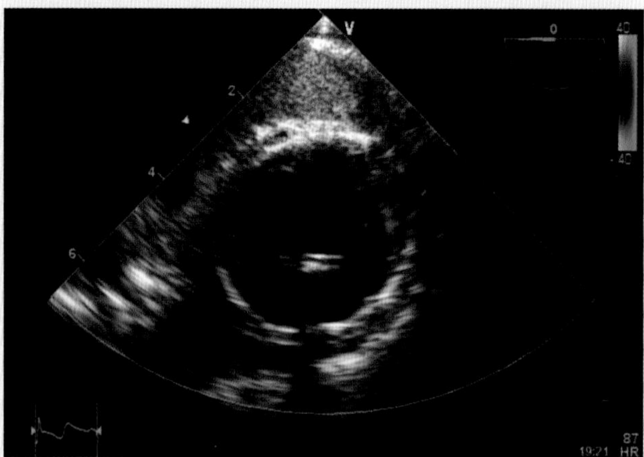

Figure 51.6. Short-axis view of descending aortic grafts.

TAKE-HOME LESSON:

Intraoperative TEE allows confirmation of adequate stent deployment and presence or absence of an endoleak. TEE evaluation of the aorta should be performed if there are acute hemodynamic changes during or after stent deployment.

SUGGESTED READING

Koschyk DH, Nienaber CA, Knap M, et al. How to guide stent-graft implantation in type B aortic dissection? Comparison of angiography, transesophageal echocardiography, and intravascular ultrasound. *Circulation.* 2005;112(9 suppl):I260–I264.

Rapezzi C, Rocchi G, Fattori R, et al. Usefulness of transesophageal echocardiographic monitoring to improve the outcome of stent-graft treatment of thoracic aortic aneurysms. *Am J Cardiol.* 2001; 87(3):315–319.

Rocchi G, Lofiego C, Biagini E, et al. Transesophageal echocardiography-guided algorithm for stent-graft implantation in aortic dissection. *J Vasc Surg.* 2004; 40(5):880–885.

Schütz W, Gauss A, Meierhenrich R, et al. Transesophageal echocardiographic guidance of thoracic aortic stent-graft implantation. *J Endovasc Ther.* 2002;9(suppl): II14–II19.

Moderate

CASE 52

A 34-year-old woman presented to the cardiac catheterization suite for a correction of a congenital heart problem. Views from her baseline TEE exam are presented in Video 52.1.

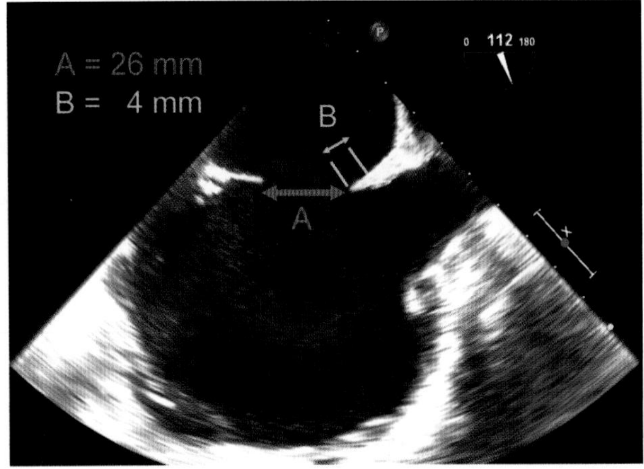

Figure 52.1.

QUESTION 52.1. What is the patient's congenital heart lesion?

A. A sinus venosus ASD
B. A secundum ASD
C. A primum ASD
D. A persistent left superior vena cava

A ME bicaval view is shown in Figure 52.1, with relevant measurements. An Amplatzer septal occluder device is chosen to repair this patient's congenital heart lesion.

QUESTION 52.2. Is the chosen device appropriate for this patient?

A. No, there is not adequate tissue to deploy the device
B. No, the defect is too large
C. No, it is not indicated for this patient's lesion
D. Yes, this is an appropriate choice

Several minutes following deployment of the device, the patient becomes short of breath. Postprocedural TEE views are shown in Video 52.2.

QUESTION 52.3. What is the cause of the patient's shortness of breath?

A. The device has migrated into the PA
B. The device migrated into the aorta
C. The patient has developed an acute thrombus in the PA
D. The patient's shortness of breath is not likely related to the device

QUESTION 52.4. What should be the next step in patient management?

A. Perform cardiac angiography to rule out coronary artery disease
B. Obtain a stat cardiac MRI
C. Administer thrombolytics
D. Transport emergently to the OR

ANSWERS AND DISCUSSION

QUESTION 52.1: The correct answer is B: A secundum ASD. A secundum ASD is the most common type of ASD and is confined to the fossa ovalis. A tissue defect is present in the interatrial septum that allows communication between the right and the left atria. It is usually seen best in either the ME 4CH or bicaval view. A primum ASD is part of a category of findings known as endocardial cushion defects. Unlike a secundum ASD, a primum ASD is adjacent to the mitral and TV and may also be associated with a cleft MV or VSD. A sinus venosus ASD would most commonly occur at the junction of the RA and SVC. An enlarged CS would suggest a persistent left superior vena cava, which is not present in this patient.

QUESTION 52.2: The correct answer is A: No, there is not adequate tissue to deploy the device. The septal occluder device consists of two flat discs that plug the defect by overlapping surrounding atrial tissue. There is some disagreement about the requisite amount of tissue, or "rim," needed for proper device seating. However, there are reports of migrating devices when the device has less than 5 mm of tissue to "grab onto." The maximum size of ASDs that can be occluded with the device is changing, but currently there are devices that can occlude defects as large as 40 mm. Since the patient has a secundum ASD, this would be an appropriate choice if the patient had a larger rim of tissue.

QUESTION 52.3: The correct answer is A: The device has migrated into the PA. The video presents an upper aortic arch short-axis view and the device can be seen in the main PA, just above the pulmonic valve. The arrow in Figure 52.2 points to the device. It is not in the aorta. There is no thrombus shown in the video.

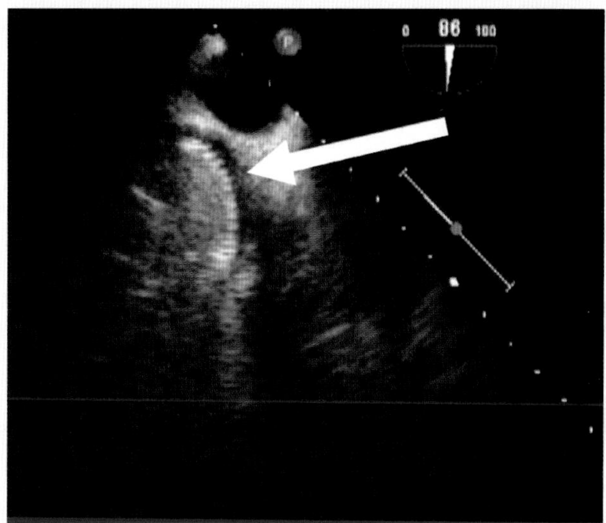

Figure 52.2.

QUESTION 52.4: The correct answer is D: Transport emergently to the OR. Although misplaced devices can sometimes be retrieved in the catheterization suite, this device has migrated outside of the heart and retrieving it without significant damage to the pulmonary and TV is unlikely. Time is also of the essence, as it will become harder to surgically remove the device the more distal it migrates. Other diagnostic tests, such as coronary angiography and MRI, are unnecessary. Administering thrombolytics would do nothing to resolve the problem and likely make surgical removal more dangerous.

TAKE-HOME LESSON:

Amplatzer Septal Occluders can be used to close secundum ASDs, but the ASD cannot be too large and there must be an adequate rim of tissue to seat the device.

SUGGESTED READING

Cooke JC, Gelman JS, Harper RW. Echocardiologists' role in the deployment of the Amplatzer Septal Occluder device in adults. *J Am Soc Echocardiogr.* 2001;14:588–594.

Tuong QA, Gupta V, Bezarra HG, et al. The traveling Amplatzer: rare complication of percutaneous atrial septal occluder device embolism. *Circulation.* 2008;118:e93–e96.

Moderate

CASE 53

A 60-year-old woman undergoes MV repair for a flail anterior leaflet segment. After separation from CPB, the patient is hemodynamically unstable, despite multiple inotropes and IABP. You obtain the TEE images shown in Figure 53.1 and Video 53.1.

QUESTION 53.1. The echocardiographic image in Figure 53.1 and Video 53.1 is most consistent with

A. Moderate ischemic MR
B. Severe MR suggesting inadequate repair
C. Severe paravalvular leak
D. Mild MR of no clinical significance

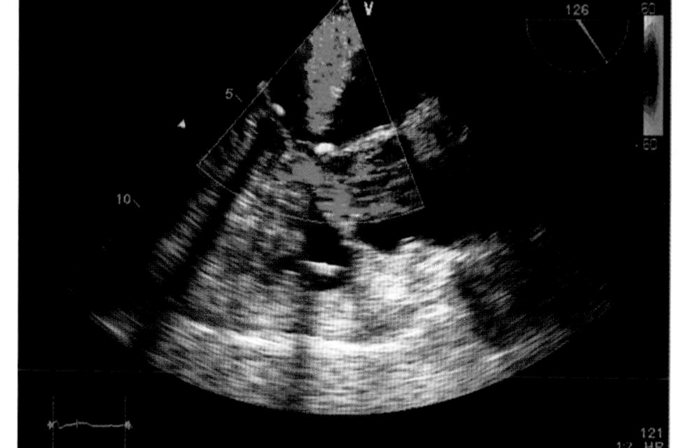

Figure 53.1. ME AV LAX with CFD. See also Video 53.1.

QUESTION 53.2. Based on what you see in Figure 53.1 and Video 53.1, what is the *most likely* cause of the MR?

A. Residual prolapse of the anterior mitral leaflet
B. Overriding of the posterior mitral leaflet
C. SAM of the MV with LVOT obstruction
D. Paravalvular leak

QUESTION 53.3. To help you better understand the *mechanism* of the MR, which of the following spectral Doppler examinations would be most helpful?

A. CW Doppler through the MV
B. PW Doppler through the MV
C. PW Doppler of the pulmonary veins
D. CW Doppler through the LVOT and AV

QUESTION 53.4. The spectral Doppler waveform on Figure 53.2 is most consistent with which of the following pathology:

A. AI

B. MR

C. AS

D. LV outflow obstruction

QUESTION 53.5. Careful examination of the 2D images in Figure 53.3 and Video 53.2 helps to confirm the diagnosis of SAM of the MV with dynamic LVOT obstruction. Which of the following treatments would be useful?

A. Fluid administration

B. Vasoconstrictors

C. Stopping the intra-aortic balloon

D. All of the above

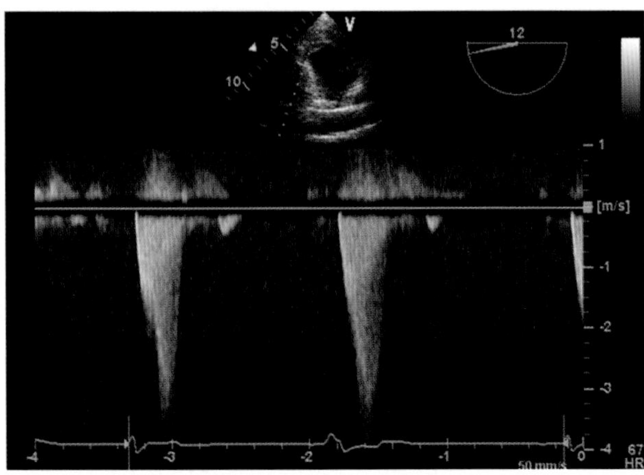

Figure 53.2. CW Doppler profile obtained from the deep TG LAX view.

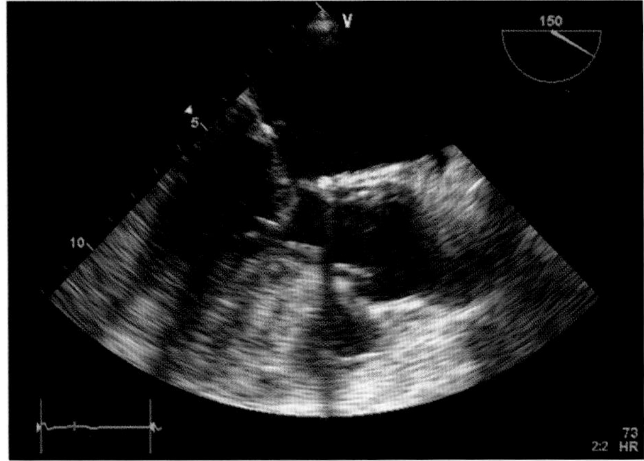

Figure 53.3. ME LAX of the AV. See also Video 53.2.

ANSWERS AND DISCUSSION

QUESTION 53.1: The correct answer is B: Severe MR suggesting inadequate repair. In Figure 53.1, the MR jet is large and it fills a large portion of the dilated left atrium. This is consistent with at least moderate-to-severe MR. The central origin and direction of the jet could be consistent with either structural *or* ischemic MR, but in the context of a MV repair, one must immediately suspect that the repair is at fault. The exact mechanism of the regurgitation requires further investigation with a detailed 2D examination. Answer A is incorrect: LV ischemia can lead to chamber dilation and tethering of the mitral leaflets, causing MR. This patient, however, appears to have good overall contractility, which is unlikely in severe ischemia. Answer C is incorrect: strictly speaking, the term paravalvular leak (literally a leak *beside* the valve) tends to be reserved for cases when the MV is removed and another one (a prosthesis) is reattached in its place. If a leak occurs between that valve and the rest of the heart, one has a paravalvular leak. In certain cases of mitral repair where part of the valve is detached and reattached to the annulus (such as a sliding annuloplasty), some experts believe that you could also have a paravalvular leak (controversy exists as to whether this represents a paravalvular defect or a defect *within* the leaflet itself, but such a discussion is beyond the scope of this case). In any case, such leaks originate near the annulus and can travel inside or outside the annuloplasty ring, if it is dehisced. In this case, the jet originates in the center of the valve and the ring is well seated. Moreover, the repair of an anterior leaflet flail typically does not involve a sliding annuloplasty and it is highly unlikely to cause a paravalvular leak. Finally, answer D is incorrect: this is not a mild jet.

QUESTION 53.2: The correct answer is C: SAM of the MV with LVOT obstruction. SAM is an *intrinsic* MV problem where the coaptation occurs abnormally high on the leaflets, producing redundant mitral tissue that can then be displaced anteriorly in systole. This creates two hemodynamic problems: LVOT obstruction and MR. Various anatomic factors have been described, which predispose a patient to develop SAM after MV repair. These anatomic factors, like a long posterior leaflet, short anterior leaflet, and small LV cavity, tend to bring the mitral coaptation point closer to the LVOT. After an anterior leaflet repair, the anterior leaflet is often shortened compared to the posterior leaflet. This results in the coaptation point being brought closer to the interventricular septum, greatly increasing the risk of SAM. An undersized annuloplasty ring will only worsen the problem. Answer A is incorrect: anterior leaflet prolapse tends to cause *eccentric* MR directed posterolaterally over the posterior leaflet. For the same reason, answer B is incorrect: an overriding posterior leaflet would likely give rise to an *eccentric* jet directed anteromedially over the anterior leaflet. This patient has a *central* regurgitant jet. Finally, see the discussion of Question 53.1 for why answer D is incorrect.

QUESTION 53.3: The correct answer is D: CW Doppler through the LVOT and AV. Figure 53.1 and Video 53.1 show a lot of MR but they also show high velocity (aliasing) flow in the LVOT. The high velocities in the LVOT are not typical with MR and warrant further interrogation of the LVOT with CW Doppler to better identify the causal factor (see answer to Question 53.4 for more detail). Answer A is incorrect: while CW through the MV can help characterize the *severity* of MR by the spectral Doppler density, it offers no clue as to the mechanism of the MR. Likewise pulmonary vein flow is important in quantifying the severity of MR, but it provides little information on the mechanism. Thus, answer C is incorrect. Finally, answer B is incorrect: due to its physical properties, PW Doppler can only measure relatively slow velocities and it is of limited use in assessing stenotic or regurgitant high velocity jets.

QUESTION 53.4: The correct answer is D: LV outflow obstruction.

The ECG shows that the timing of this jet is clearly systolic. This, along with the direction of the jet, rules out AI (answer A). Answer B is incorrect for several reasons: On the 2D image at the top, the cursor is positioned along the LVOT, not the MV. Second, the shape of the spectral Doppler signal is *asymmetrical* and it peaks in *late* systole. MR flow is typically *pansystolic, symmetrical*, and it peaks in *mid*-systole. Third, the peak gradient of this jet is about 3.5 m/s, which is typically too slow for MR (using the formula $\Delta P = 4V^2$, it would translate into a systemic blood pressure of 60–70 mm Hg, possible in this scenario but not likely). Typical MR velocity is in the range of 5 to 6 m/s. This leaves two possibilities: LVOT obstruction or valvular AS. The *shape* of the spectral Doppler signal provides the best clue to the diagnosis. Indeed, *fixed* orifices (such as those seen in MR or valvular AS) usually lead to parabolic, symmetrical spectral Doppler signals and the velocity peaks in *mid*-systole. By contrast, in a case of *dynamic* outflow obstruction, the gradient will increase as the chamber size decreases and the peak velocity will occur in *late* systole. The characteristic *dagger-shaped* or *saber-shaped* spectral Doppler appearance in Figure 53.2 is in fact pathognomonic of a dynamic LVOT obstruction.

QUESTION 53.5: The correct answer is D: All of the above. This patient has SAM of the MV as a result of the repair. The 2D echocardiogram demonstrates that the coaptation of the MV occurs high up on the valve leaflets, resulting in a lot of *redundant* tissue. In addition, the anterior leaflet and subvalvular apparatus are seen pulled anteriorly toward the LVOT in systole. This disrupts the valve geometry and results in severe MR. One of the important contributing factors in this condition is the fact that the LV is small. Any medical treatment that increases the size of the ventricle will reduce the amount of obstruction and improve the cardiac output. Fluid administration, increasing the afterload with vasoconstrictors, reduction in inotropic and balloon counterpulsation support, and administration of β-blockers have all been advocated as possible means of reducing or eliminating SAM.

If the SAM and severe MR persist despite all these treatments, return to CPB for further repair may be necessary. However, it is worth noting that retrospective series have shown that postmitral repair SAM tends to *improve and eventually disappear* in the vast majority of patients.

TAKE-HOME LESSON:

Careful evaluation allows one to *anticipate* complications such as postrepair SAM. Severe LVOT obstruction is an example of heart failure where conventional treatments, such as inotropes, vasodilators, and IABP, often worsen the condition. TEE allowed for the proper diagnosis and management.

SUGGESTED READING

Brown ML, Abel MD, Click RL, et al. Systolic anterior motion after mitral valve repair: is surgical intervention necessary? *J Thorac CV Surg.* 2007;133:136–143.

Maslow A, Regan MM, Haering JM, et al. Echocardiographic predictors of left ventricular outflow tract obstruction and systolic anterior motion of the mitral valve after mitral valve reconstruction for myxomatous valve disease. *J Am Coll Cardiol.* 1999;34(7):2096–2104.

CASE 54

A 68-year-old male is scheduled to undergo redo-sternotomy for ascending aorta and arch aneurysm repair. The surgeon has decided to obtain femoral access prior to redo sternotomy for possible femoral artery—femoral vein bypass. He is having trouble accessing the femoral vein. He has asked for your assistance with ultrasound.

QUESTION 54.1. From the image in Figure 54.1, what can you tell your surgeon?

A. The femoral artery is anterior to the femoral vein
B. The femoral artery is posterior to the femoral vein
C. Cannulation should be attempted in the other groin
D. Both A and C

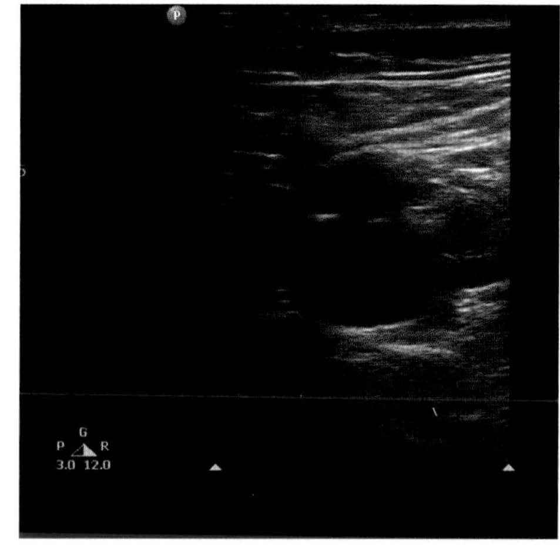

Figure 54.1.

QUESTION 54.2. Which image (Fig. 54.2A or 54.2B) shows the left femoral artery and vein?

A. Figure 54.2A
B. Figure 54.2B
C. Both 54.2A and 54.2B
D. Neither 54.2A nor 54.2B
E. Cannot tell

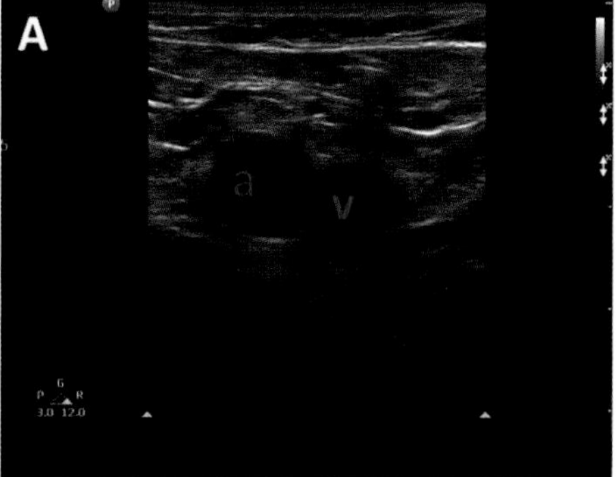

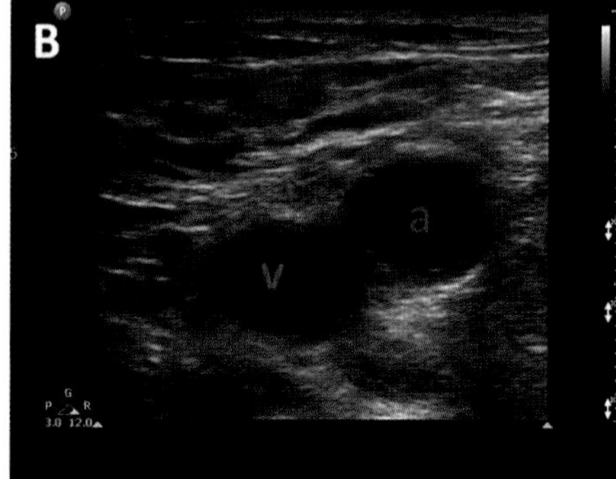

Figure 54.2.

QUESTION 54.3. True or False?

After successful cannulation and insertion of a wire in the femoral vein, TEE will show the guidewire in the RA (Fig 54.3).

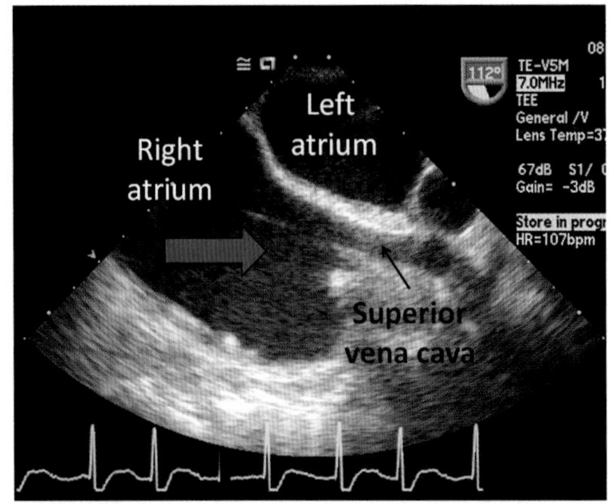

Figure 54.3.

ANSWERS AND DISCUSSION

QUESTION 54.1: The correct answer is D.

The femoral artery (a) is usually the smaller, more round, less compressible, pulsatile structure with a thicker intimal lining. CFD can also be an asset in differentiating vascular structures by examining the direction and velocity of flow. In this case, the femoral artery is anterior to the femoral vein (v) (Fig. 54.4), rather than the usual position of being lateral to the femoral vein. If possible, the surgeon should obtain access in the other groin.

QUESTION 54.2: The correct answer is E.

Always check the orientation of the ultrasound probe. Without knowing which side is medial versus lateral, it is not possible to tell if one is looking at the left groin or the right groin in either picture.

QUESTION 54.3: The correct answer is False

If there are multiple catheters and wires in the RA (central venous catheters and pacemakers), it may be difficult to confirm that this wire is coming from the IVC. Figure 54.3 shows a wire in the RA, that is entering the SVC (red arrow). If the surgeon used a long wire (similar to the one used for insertion of an intra-aortic balloon), the guidewire should be imaged entering the RA from the IVC (Fig. 54.5, red arrow). The echocardiographer should attempt to image the IVC in the liver as it enters the RA to confirm that the wire is coming from the femoral vein.

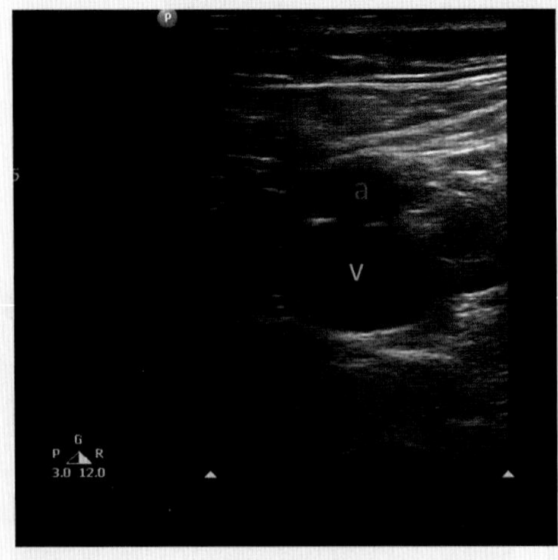

Figure 54.4.

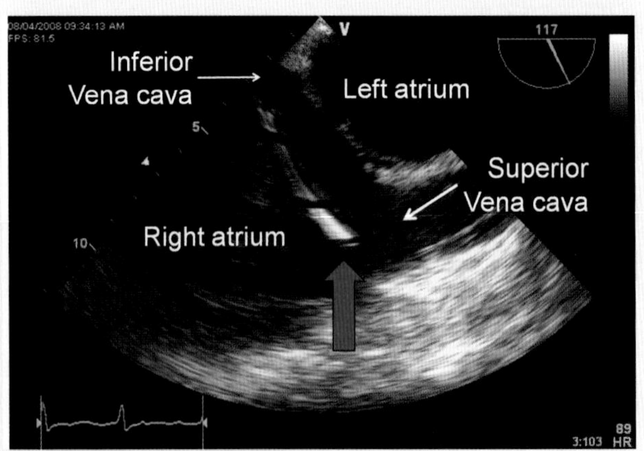

Figure 54.5.

TAKE-HOME LESSON:

- **Orientation of the ultrasound probe is important in determining the anatomy of the vascular structures in the groin.**
- **Compression, color and PW Doppler, and femoral vessel anatomy help differentiate the veins from arteries.**
- **Confirming a femoral wire is coming from the IVC into the RA is essential.**

SUGGESTED READING

Sharma RM, Mohan CVR, Setlus R, et al. Ultrasound guided central venous cannulation. *Methods Med.* 2006;62:371–372.

Moderate

CASE 55

A 55-year-old female with HOCM presents for septal myectomy via aortotomy. An intraoperative TEE was performed.

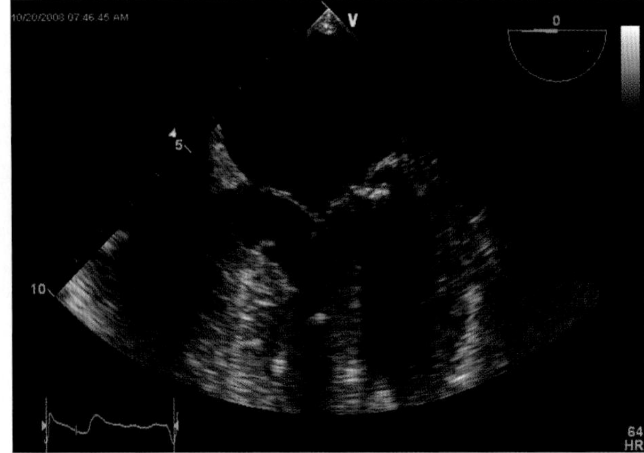

Figure 55.1.

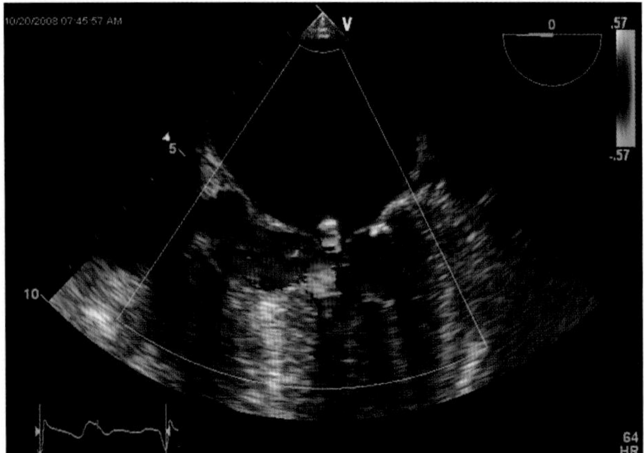

Figure 55.2.

QUESTION 55.1. The TEE images in Figures 55.1 and 55.2, and Videos 55.1 and 55.2 are suggestive of which of the following *except*:

A. HOCM

B. SAM of the MV

C. Subaortic membrane

D. MR

QUESTION 55.2. Which TEE imaging techniques are needed to confirm and quantify the presenting diagnoses?

A. 2D echocardiography

B. M-mode

C. CFD

D. PW Doppler/CW Doppler

E. All of the above

QUESTION 55.3. Which features define HOCM?

A. LVH > 11.0 mm
B. LV septal to LV free wall thickness ratio > 1.5:1.0
C. LVOT obstruction
D. All of the above

QUESTION 55.4. Which of the following are common echocardiographic findings associated with HOCM?

A. LV diastolic dysfunction
B. Mitral stenosis
C. Dilated cardiomyopathy
D. Aortic regurgitation

QUESTION 55.5. Which features commonly contribute to SAM and are associated LVOT obstruction?

A. Posterior positioning of the MV coaptation point
B. Shortened mitral leaflets
C. Posterior MAC
D. Basal septal hypertrophy

QUESTION 55.6. Which echocardiographic measurements are most helpful in directing the surgical management of HOCM?

A. Septal hypertrophy position and dimensions
B. Length of anterior mitral leaflets at end-diastole
C. CSept distance
D. AL:PL ratio
E. All of the above

QUESTION 55.7. The following are potential surgical complications following surgery for HOCM *except*

A. VSD
B. Posterior leaflet of MV injury
C. Right coronary cusp of AV injury
D. Conduction abnormalities
E. LAD injury

ANSWERS AND DISCUSSION

QUESTION 55.1: The correct answer is C. The TEE images provided demonstrate features of HOCM and SAM. These features will be described in subsequent answers to questions. A subaortic membrane is not appreciated in the images provided.

QUESTION 55.2: The correct answer is E. 2D and M-mode TEE allow for assessment of myocardial thickness, chamber dimensions, identification and localization of LVOT dynamics, and valvular dysfunction. CFD facilitates assessment of valvular function. PW Doppler and CW Doppler permit the measurement of velocities and associated gradients for quantification of functional dynamics.

QUESTION 55.3: The correct answer is D. The diagnostic criteria for HOCM are

1. LVH (>11 mm) in the absence of LV dilation and predisposing hypertrophic conditions, such as AS and systemic hypertension.
2. LV septal to LV free wall thickness ratio > 1.3:1.0.

The diagnosis of HOCM includes the above criteria plus evidence of LVOT obstruction.

QUESTION 55.4: The correct answer is A. LV diastolic dysfunction occurs in nearly all patients with HOCM due to the decreased compliance associated with increased wall thickness and mass. MR due to SAM of the anterior mitral leaflet is a common pathology created by the structural and functional abnormalities of HOCM. LVOT obstruction is by definition part of HOCM. The mechanisms of LVOT obstruction are complex with LV hypertrophy and abnormalities of the MV apparatus being the major contributing factors. Conditions likely to generate LVOT obstruction are asymmetrical prominence of the basal septum, narrowed LVOT (<25 mm), and MV apparatus abnormalities.

QUESTION 55.5: The correct answer is C. Anterior positioning of the MV coaptation can result from multiple factors that include redundant or elongated

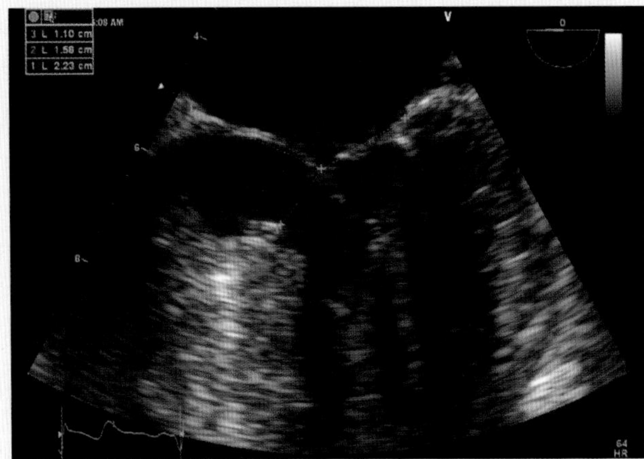

Figure 55.3.

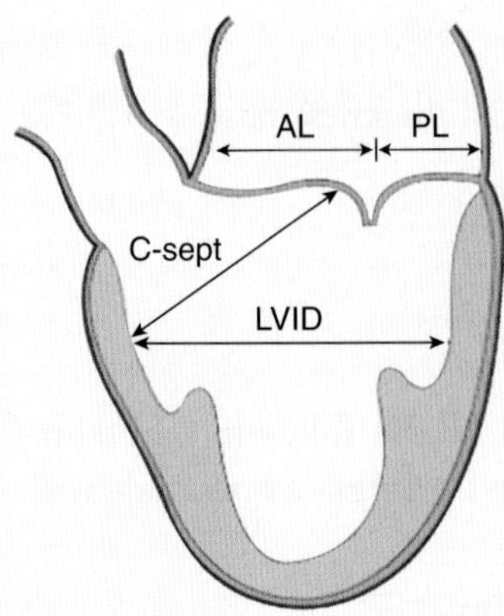

Figure 55.4.

mitral leaflets, chordal laxity, and anteriorly positioned papillary muscles. A C-Sept distance <2.5 cm (Fig. 55.3, measurements #3) and an AL:PL ratio <1.3:1.0 in the five-chamber view increase the risk of SAM (Fig. 55.3, measurements #1/#2, and Fig. 55.4). MV annulus abnormalities (i.e., posterior annular calcification) distort the normal systolic posterior mitral annular motion that results in a narrowing of the LVOT. Mid-septal hypertrophy causes redirection of the intraventricular flow such that it originates from a more posterior and lateral direction. This altered flow pattern creates mitral paravalvular flow dynamics in which the anterior mitral leaflet is "pushed" anteriorly into the LVOT. This mechanism is supported by Doppler evidence that SAM begins at low LVOT velocities. Thus, SAM is created not only by Venturi effects of high velocity LVOT flow but also by altered LV inflow and outflow patterns. Each of these conditions increases the susceptibility to SAM-associated LVOT obstruction.

QUESTION 55.6: The correct answer is E. There is little consensus as to which specific echocardiographic parameters best guide presurgical and postsurgical decisions for HOCM. However, all measurements that define the dynamic interactions of intraventricular structures are key to directing the surgical interventions. Thus, all measurements that delineate the position and extent of septal hypertrophy relative to common surgical and echocardiographic identifiable landmarks (i.e., AV annulus) are crucial. Such measurements would include

1. Distance from the AV annulus to the upper point of the septal hypertrophy
2. Distance from the AV annulus to the point of maximal septal hypertrophy
3. Distance from the AV annulus to the point of septal contact with the MV
4. Thickness of intraventricular septum at the tips of the mitral leaflets at end-diastole

The ME AV LAX view is usually a good imaging plane in which to achieve the above measurements (Video 55.3).

Some authors suggest that the distance from the AV annulus to the tip of the anterior mitral leaflets at end-diastole should be the minimal apical extent of the myectomy. Surgical intervention is generally considered adequate if the postinterventional TEE indicates a resting LVOT peak gradient <30 mm Hg or a pharmacologically provoked LVOT gradient <50 mm Hg and MR of moderate or less severity. Identification of anteriorly positioned papillary muscles is helpful if papillary myotomy is a consideration. Parameters that assess risk factors for SAM such as C-Sept distance and AL:PL ratio are useful in guiding MV interventions.

QUESTION 55.7: The correct answer is B. The potential complications associated with surgical septal myectomy are directly related to the resection of septal tissues that include VSD, interruption of conduction pathways, and laceration of septal perforator branches of the LAD artery. In addition, both right coronary cusp of AV and anterior leaflet of the MV injuries can occur due to the limited surgical exposure afforded by the aortotomy.

TAKE-HOME LESSON:

LV diastolic dysfunction occurs in nearly all patients with HOCM due to the decreased compliance associated with increased wall thickness and mass. MR due to SAM of the anterior mitral leaflet is a common pathology created by the structural and functional abnormalities of HOCM.

SUGGESTED READING

Grigg LE, Wigle ED, Williams WG, et al. Transesophageal Doppler echocardiography in obstructive hypertrophic cardiomyopathy: clarification of pathophysiology and importance in intraoperative decision making. *J Am Coll Cardiol.* 1992;20(1):42–52.

Marwick TH, Stewart WJ, Lever HM, et al. Benefits of intraoperative echocardiography in the surgical management of hypertrophic cardiomyopathy. *J Am Coll Cardiol.* 1992;20(5):1066–1072.

Sherrid MV, Chaudhry FA, Swistel DG. Obstructive hypertrophic cardiomyopathy: echocardiography, pathophysiology, and the continuing evolution of surgery for obstruction, *Ann Thorac Surg.* 2003; 75(2):620–632. Review [Erratum in: *Ann Thorac Surg.* 2003;75(5):1684].

Moderate

CASE 56

A 69-year-old previously healthy male presents with acute onset unilateral upper extremity weakness. A CT scan revealed a small cerebral infarct. Carotid ultrasonography, tests for hypercoagulable states, and MRI failed to elicit an etiology for the infarct. The patient was referred for a TEE to complete the stroke workup.

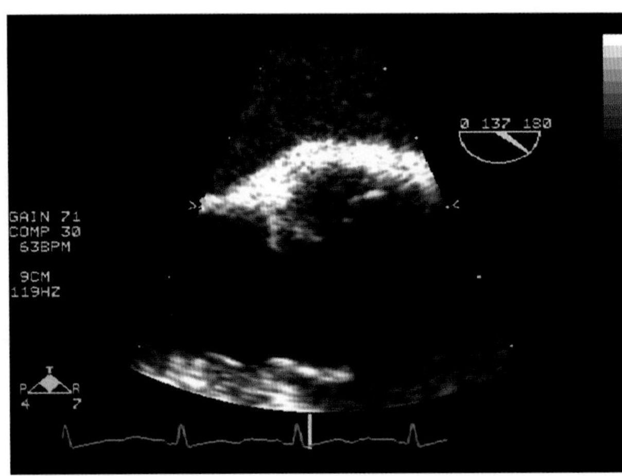

Figure 56.1. ME AV LAX (zoom).

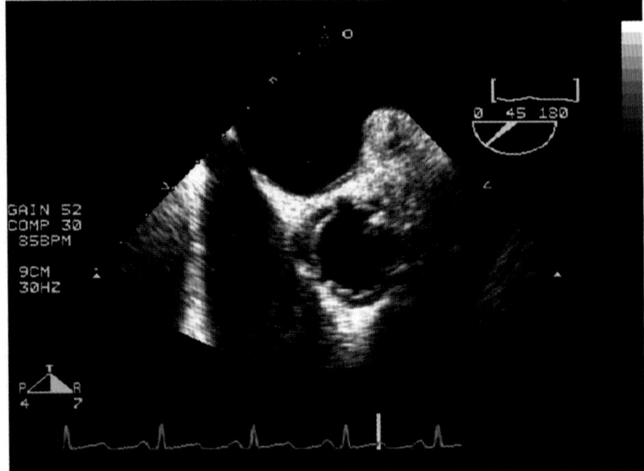

Figure 56.2. ME AV SAX.

QUESTION 56.1. During TEE examination a mass is seen on the AV in a zoomed ME AV LAX (Fig. 56.1 and Video 56.1). What is the most likely diagnosis of the mass?

A. Nodule of arantii
B. Papillary fibroelastoma
C. Vegetation from infective endocarditis
D. Lambl's excrescence

QUESTION 56.2. What would be the most appropriate next step in the management of this patient?

A. Patient requires no further management as this is a normal variant
B. Patient requires anticoagulation to prevent further strokes
C. Patient requires excision of the AV mass
D. Patient requires replacement of the AV

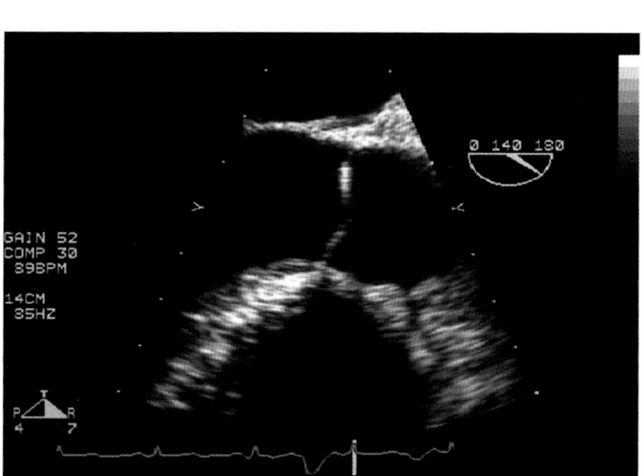

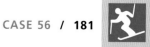

Figure 56.3. ME AV LAX.

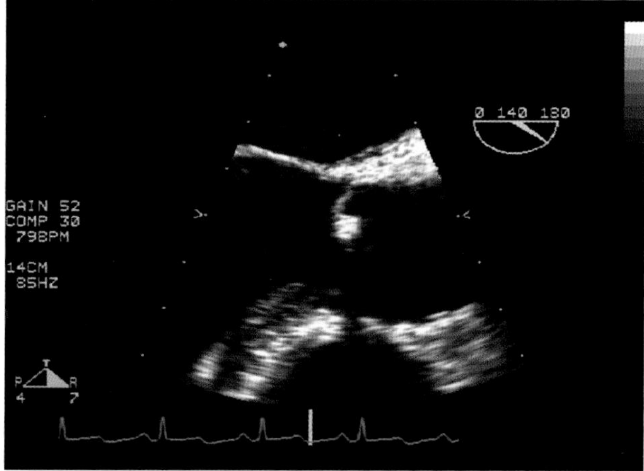

Figure 56.4. ME AV LAX.

QUESTION 56.3. Six years later the patient presents with new ST segment elevation myocardial infarction on ECG. TTE demonstrated reduced LV function. Coronary angiography demonstrated 90% stenosis of LAD not amenable to percutaneous intervention. The patient is scheduled to have a CABG. An intraoperative TEE is performed. The AV mass seen in short axis appears on the left coronary cusp (Fig. 56.2 and Video 56.2). In order to identify the mass in long axis, an adjustment was made to the ME LAX of the AV (Fig. 56.3 and Video 56.3 to Fig. 56.4 and Video 56.4). What adjustment was made?

A. The TEE probe was withdrawn
B. The TEE probe was advanced
C. The TEE probe was turned to the patient's right
D. The TEE probe was turned to the patient's left

QUESTION 56.4. What is the most appropriate management option for this patient?

A. Perform CABG to the LAD
B. Perform CABG and start postoperative anticoagulation
C. Perform CABG and AVR
D. Perform CABG and excise the lesion noted on the AV
E. Perform an aortotomy and remove the lesion noted on the AV

ANSWERS AND DISCUSSION

QUESTION 56.1: The correct answer is D: Lambl's excrescence.

Lambl's excrescences are thin, mobile, filiform structures that occur at contact margins of a valve. They most commonly occur on the aortic and MV although involvement of pulmonic and TV has been reported. They may occur as a single strand, in rows or in clusters. They are less than 1 mm in thickness and between 1 and 5 mm in length. The pathogenesis is believed to be related to endothelial trauma in areas of high stress (valve contact margins). Fibrin deposits develop over the injured area with subsequent overgrowth of the endothelium. On histopathological examination Lambl's excrescences contain a central core of elastic connective tissue and a single layer of endothelial cells. They are found in increasing frequency with increasing age. *Nodules of arantii* are small fibrous nodules that can be seen at the center of the free edge of each cusp of the AV. Cardiac papillary fibroelastomas are the third most common benign tumors of the heart, after myxomas and lipomas. Papillary fibroelastomas are small, avascular masses. Frequently, they are mobile with a thin stalk and have a mean diameter of 3 × 10 mm. They may have multiple papillary fronds. Histologically, papillary fibroelastomas consist of a central core of dense connective tissue, surrounded by a layer of loose connective tissue and covered by hyperplastic endothelial cells. Surgical resection is recommended because even small lesions (3 to 4 mm) can cause cerebral or coronary infarction.

The patient's medical history is not typical of infective endocarditis and the valve appears structurally normal.

QUESTION 56.2: Answer B is correct. Patient requires anticoagulation to prevent further strokes. Transesophageal should be considered as part of the complete workup of patients who have had a stroke. Asymptomatic patients who are found to have evidence of Lambl's excrescences should be monitored closely. If there is evidence of a single stroke in a patient with Lambl's excrescences, anticoagulation is advised. Any suggestion of a subsequent stroke should prompt consideration of removal of the excrescences. Although debridement of the Lambl's excrescences will be therapeutic, it needs to be weighed against associated perioperative risks of excision. In the presence of a second stroke or transient ischemic attack excision may be indicated. Valve replacement is not warranted in an otherwise normal valve.

QUESTION 56.3: Answer D is correct. The TEE probe was turned to the patient's left. Video 56.3 shows the AV in ME LAX. The right coronary cusp is visible as the lower leaflet of the AV and the noncoronary and left coronary cusps (with the giant Lambl's excrescence) move in and out of plane. By turning the TEE probe to the patient's left, the left coronary cusp is maintained in the viewing plane throughout the cardiac cycle.

Advancing or withdrawing the probe would move the entire valve out of view. Turning the TEE probe to the patient's right would bring the noncoronary cusp into plane.

QUESTION 56.4: Answer D is correct. Perform CABG to the LAD and excise the lesion noted on the AV. Angiographic evidence of coronary disease necessitates intervention with CABG. The mass noted on the left coronary cusp has increased in size. It is in the same location at the Lambl's excrescence seen 6 years prior. The larger mass could be a Lambl's excrescence that has grown in size due to multiple excrescences adhering to one another, otherwise known as a giant Lambl's excrescence. Giant Lambl's excrescences have been associated with embolization and coronary ostial obstruction resulting in myocardial infarction. The mass could also be a fibroelastoma of the AV, but since the patient had a previous history of Lambl's excrescences, a giant Lambl's is more likely. There is disagreement whether giant Lambl's excrescences and fibroelastomas are actually different pathologies. Both giant Lambl's and fibroelastomas can look very similar on echocardiographic exam. The final diagnosis is made by histopathologic examination. Given the size of the mass on the left coronary cusp and increase in associated complications, excision is recommended. CABG alone does not address the mass; valve replacement is not indicated when the valve is otherwise normal.

TAKE-HOME LESSON:

Lambl's excrescences are thin, mobile, filiform structures that occur at contact margins of a valve. Presence of symptoms determines medical (anticoagulation) versus surgical (excision) management.

Lambl's excrescence can typically be excised without the need for AVR.

SUGGESTED READING

Aggarwal A, Leavitt BJ. Images in clinical medicine: giant Lambl's excrescences. *N Engl J Med.* 2003; 349(25):e24.

Aziz F, Baciewicz FA. Lambl's excrescences: review and recommendations. *Tex Heart Inst J.* 2007;34(3): 366–368.

Jaffe W, Figueredo VM. An example of Lambl's excrescences by transesophageal echocardiogram: a common misinterpreted lesion. *Echocardiography.* 2007;24(10): 1086–1089.

Wolf RC, Spiess J, Vasic N, et al. Valvular strand and ischemic stroke. *Eur Neurol.* 2007;57(4):227–231.

CASE 57

A 55-year-old man presents with a history of exertional dyspnea and fatigue. A TTE demonstrates moderate-to-severe MV regurgitation. The patient is taken to the OR for mitral repair. You perform an intraoperative TEE and obtain the images shown in Figure 57.1 and Video 57.1.

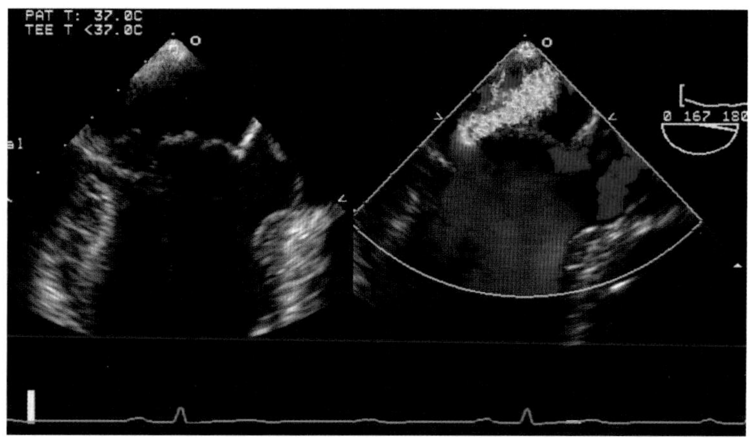

Figure 57.1. ME LAX of the MV, 2D and CFD. See also Video 57.1.

QUESTION 57.1. Based on the image, the echocardiographic appearance of the valve is most consistent with which of the following?

A. Normal MV leaflets with dilated mitral annulus
B. Myxomatous MV with bileaflet prolapse
C. Myxomatous MV with posterior leaflet prolapse
D. Parachute MV

The surgeon performs a complex MV repair, including a quadrangular resection with sliding plasty of the posterior leaflet, chordal transfer to the anterior leaflet using both native (hybrid flip-over technique) and artificial (Gore-Tex) cords, and a band annuloplasty.

Following separation from CPB, the patient is in sinus rhythm at 90 with a cardiac index of 2.0 L/min/m^2. You obtain the images shown in Figures 57.2 and 57.3 and in Videos 57.2 and 57.3.

You measure the mean diastolic gradient across the MV and perform planimetry. The mean diastolic gradient is 6.78 mm Hg and the estimated MV area by planimetry is 2.5 cm^2. There is trace MR.

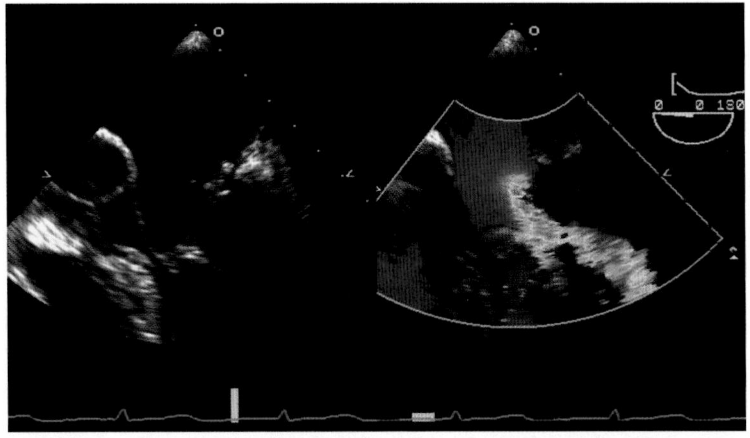

Figure 57.2. ME 4CH view of the MV in 2D and CFD. See also Video 57.2.

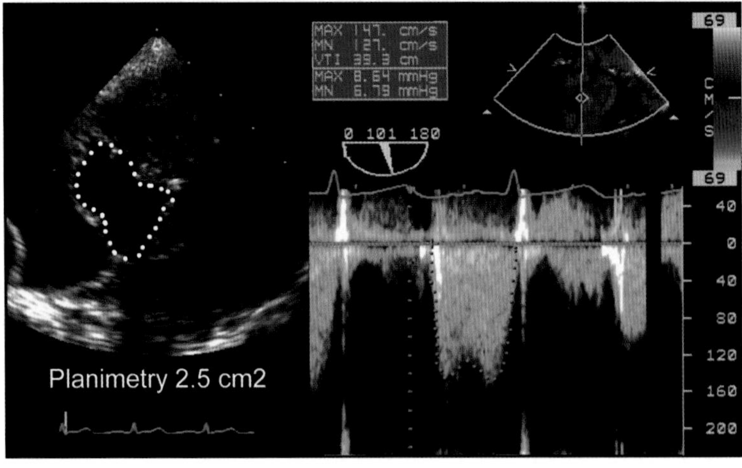

Figure 57.3. TG SAX view of the MV in systole. CW Doppler of the MV. See also Video 57.3.

QUESTION 57.2. If you want to rule out mitral stenosis after MV repair, which of the following MV assessments is *least* preload dependent?

A. Mean diastolic gradient
B. PHT
C. Peak diastolic gradient
D. Planimetry in the TG SAX view

QUESTION 57.3. In Figures 57.2 and 57.3 and in Videos 57.2 and 57.3 images are most consistent with:

A. SAM of the MV
B. Severe mitral stenosis
C. Moderate mitral stenosis
D. An adequate MV repair

QUESTION 57.4. What should you do?

A. Give protamine; this is a good repair
B. Measure the MV area using the continuity equation
C. Advise the surgeon to go back on CPB for further repair
D. Administer volume and a β-blocker

The surgeon agrees that the repair is suboptimal. He re-repairs the valve by removal of cords from the restricted anterior leaflet. The second aortic cross-clamp time is only 15 minutes. The hemodynamics are similar after the second separation from CPB.

QUESTION 57.5. After the second repair, the images in Figures 57.4 and 57.5 are consistent with

A. A successful operation
B. Significant MR
C. The need for a MV replacement
D. SAM of the MV

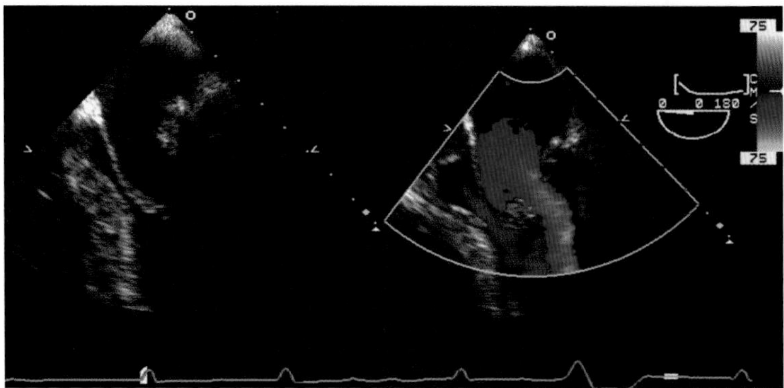

Figure 57.4. ME five-chamber view of the MV, 2D and CFD. See also Figure 57.5.

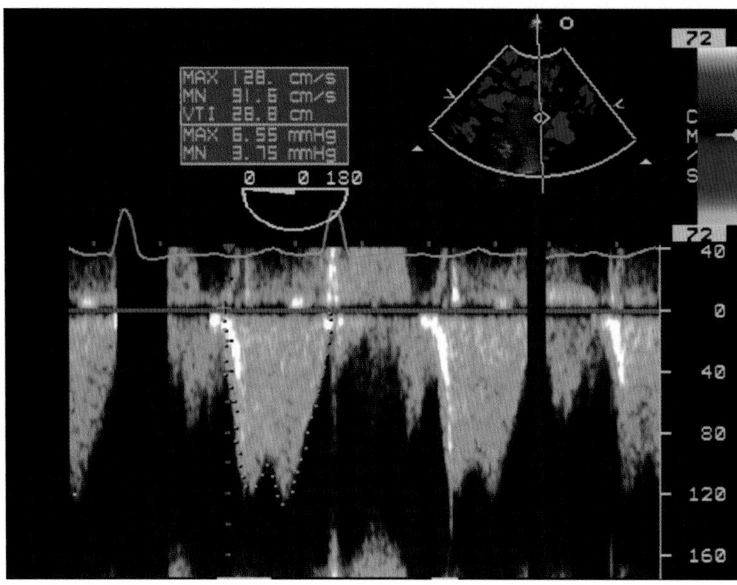

Figure 57.5. CW Doppler of the MV after second repair.

ANSWERS AND DISCUSSION

QUESTION 57.1: The correct answer is B: Myxomatous MV with bileaflet prolapse. The MV leaflets appear thickened and redundant, consistent with myxomatous degeneration. *Both* leaflets are seen to cross the annular plane in systole, so answer C is incorrect. The posterior leaflet does prolapse more than the anterior leaflet, resulting in an anteriorly directed jet. The annulus is not dilated, so answer A is incorrect. Finally, answer D is incorrect: a parachute MV is a form of congenital disease in which all chordae tendinae insert into a single papillary muscle resulting in mitral stenosis. Figure 57.6 shows an example of a parachute MV in a different patient.

QUESTION 57.2: The correct answer is D: Planimetry in the TG SAX view. The assessment of mitral stenosis post MV repair is difficult and it shouldn't rely on a single technique. Unfortunately, none of these methods is completely preload independent, but planimetry of the MV is believed to be the *least* dependent on loading conditions. Answers A and C are incorrect: Pressure gradients, regardless of the view in which they are obtained, are very dependent on loading conditions, and these change frequently and quickly after separation from bypass. Mean pressures are said to be less sensitive to preload than peak pressures, but not completely independent. Note that while they are dependent on loading conditions, gradients *should still be obtained* for a more complete picture of the MV function. But they *should be interpreted with the understanding that they are dependent on loading conditions*. Finally, answer B is incorrect: PHT is affected by left ventricular compliance as much as by MV function

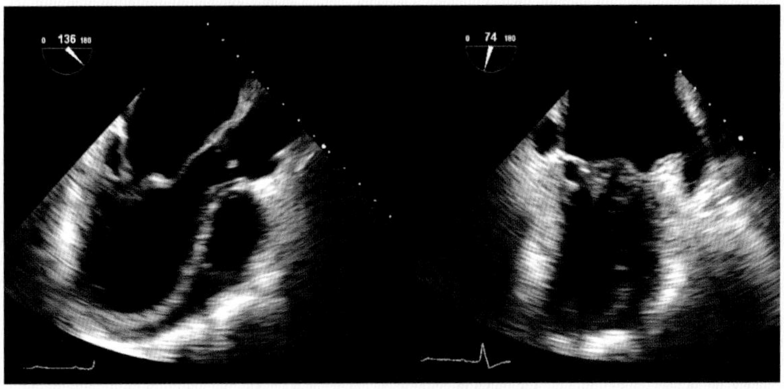

Figure 57.6. Parachute MV, seen in the ME LAX (left) and ME commissural view (right). See also Video 57.4.

and it too can change frequently and unpredictably in the immediate postbypass period, making this technique unreliable.

QUESTION 57.3: The correct answer is C: Moderate mitral stenosis. The 2D appearance of the MV demonstrates mobility of the base and mid-portion of the anterior leaflet with restricted motion of the tip. Although this appearance of the anterior leaflet can be seen after chordal transfer or insertion of artificial cords, it is quite pronounced in this case. And while the MV planimetry, performed *at the level of the base of the leaflets*, showed a reassuring valve area of 2.5 cm^2, the stenosis in this case is at the *tip* of the leaflets. CFD confirms aliased flow consistent with moderate mitral stenosis. Finally, while not diagnostic in itself, a mean diastolic gradient of 6.79 mm Hg in the face of a cardiac index of 2.0 $L/min/m^2$ is also worrisome. This in no way contradicts the answer to Question 57.2, but emphasizes the fact that mitral stenosis assessment post repair should be multimodal and no single sign or technique can be used in isolation.

QUESTION 57.4: The correct answer is C: Advise the surgeon to go back on CPB for further repair.

This repair is suboptimal. The elevated mean diastolic gradient confirms the 2D and CFD impression of moderate mitral stenosis. As stated above, the cardiac index is only 2.0 $L/min/m^2$, HR 90, and therefore the elevated gradient cannot be explained by a high flow state and/or marked tachycardia. The MV area can be calculated using the continuity equation, but it takes time and precision and is not necessary given the information you already have. Answer A is incorrect, as all the features of a good mitral repair are not present. These include mild or less MR, no SAM of the MV and no mitral stenosis. The first two criteria are met, but not the third. Answer D would be the correct medical approach to reduce LVOT obstruction caused by SAM, but this is not an issue in this case.

QUESTION 57.5: The correct answer is A: A successful operation. The 2D appearance of the valve demonstrates increased anterior leaflet mobility. CFD shows laminar flow across the valve, in sharp contrast to Figure 57.2. The mean diastolic transvalvular gradient is in the expected range of 2 to 4 mm Hg. There is trace MR and no SAM of the valve.

TAKE-HOME LESSON:

Reliance on a single estimate of valve performance can lead to the diagnostic miss of significant stenosis.

SUGGESTED READING

Savage RM, Shiota T, Stewart WJ, et al. Assessment in mitral valve surgery. In: Savage R, Aronson S, et al., eds. *Comprehensive Textbook of Intraoperative Transesophageal Echocardiography*. Philadelphia: Lippincott Williams & Wilkins; 2005:443–533.

Verma S, Mesana TG. Mitral-valve repair for mitral-valve prolapse. *N Engl J Med.* 2009;361(23):40–48.

Moderate

CASE 58

A 56-year-old woman is being prepared for CABG and MV replacement. Preoperatively, a PA catheter is placed using the RIJ vein approach. Placement was uneventful with a PA pressure of approximately 53/30 mm Hg.

TEE was performed after uneventful induction and intubation of the patient. Initial exam of the ascending aorta is displayed in Figures 58.1 to 58.3.

Further investigation from a slightly different depth and angle revealed this abnormal exam of the ascending aorta (Fig. 58.4 and Video 58.1).

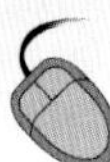

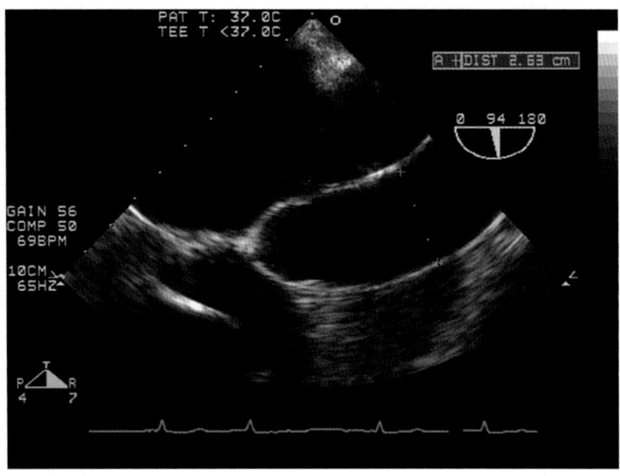

Figure 58.1. ME LAX of the ascending aorta.

QUESTION 58.1. What is the etiology of the reflective mass in the ascending aorta?

A. The PA catheter was inadvertently floated down the right carotid artery into the aortic arch
B. Aortic dissection has occurred
C. This is a common artifact
D. The TEE probe is malfunctioning

In the same patient, the ME LAX (ME LAX) of the AV was notable for the structure seen in Figure 58.5 and Video 58.2. The ME LAX view with CFD is presented for comparison (Fig. 58.6 and Video 58.3).

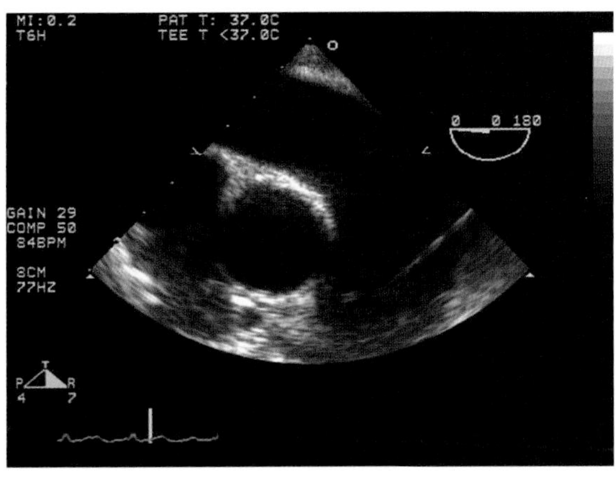

Figure 58.2. ME SAX of the ascending aorta.

QUESTION 58.2. What is the source of this structure at the AV?

A. Congenital sinus of Valsalva anuerysm of the AV

B. Normal anatomy of AV

C. Prolapse of the right coronary cusp due to a localized dissection in aortic root

D. Vegetation on the left coronary cusp of the AV

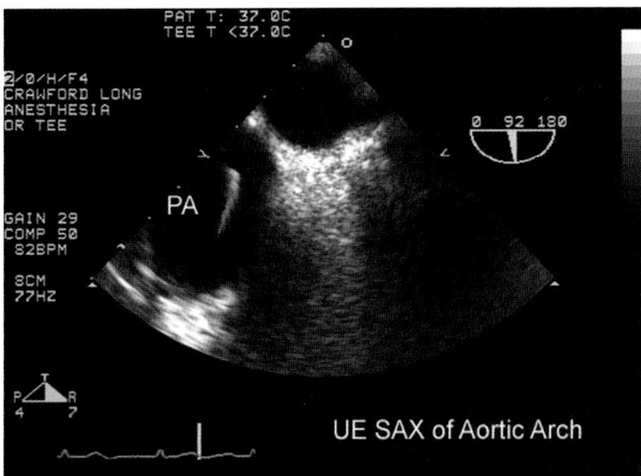

Figure 58.3 UE SAX of the aortic arch.

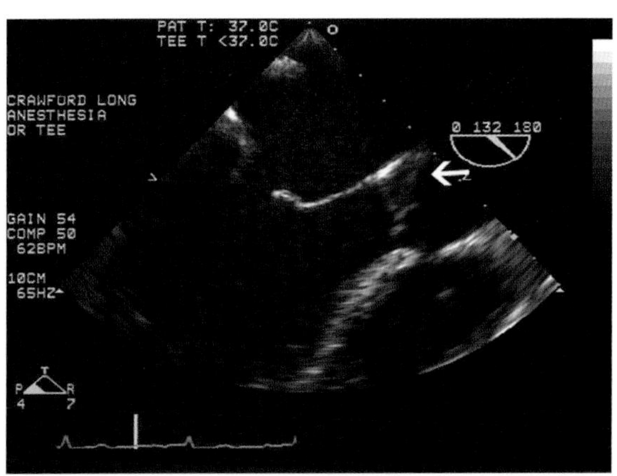

Figure 58.5. ME LAX of the AV. See also Video 58.2.

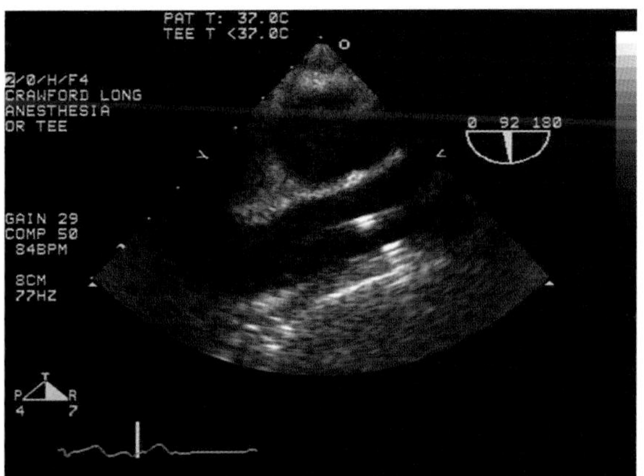

Figure 58.4. ME LAX of the ascending aorta. See also Video 58.1.

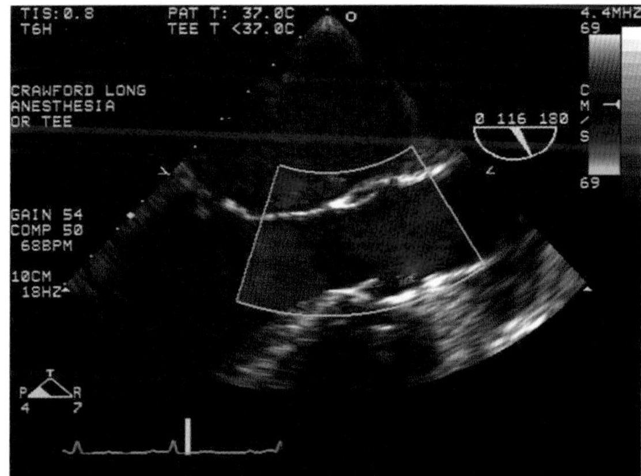

Figure 58.6. ME LAX of the AV with CFD. See also Video 58.3.

ANSWERS AND DISCUSSION

QUESTION 58.1: The correct answer is C: This is a common artifact.

Linear masses and indistinct artifacts in the aorta are remarkably common and paticularly troubling. It is important to realize that 25% to 40% of all exams of the aorta may be notable for some type of image degradation and artifactual mass that can confound the rare but criticial diagnosis of intimal disruption of the aorta.

Three types of artifacts are frequently seen in the aorta. The most common are side-lobe artifacts and reverberation (multipath) artifacts. Both are dependent on a strong reflection of the ultrasound energy. Side-lobe artifacts cause degradation of the lateral resolution and typically are seen at a consistent depth from the probe across lateral anatomic boders. Reverberation artifacts degrade the longitudinal resolution and will be seen to cross normal anatomic borders at repetitive distances, in a parallel line from the direction of the probe.

A third possible confounder is called "beam-width" artifact. Realize that the 2D image we see is actually formed by 3D ultrasound signals. As the width of the ultrasound beam increases with increasing depth, it becomes possible that the ultrasound system may incorrectly locate a structure such as a PA catheter into the 2D image of the adjacent aorta (Figs. 58.7 and 58.8).

ANSWER A: The PA catheter was inadvertently floated from the right carotid artery to the aorta is incorrect.

Figures 58.2 and 58.3 clearly demonstrate the PA catheter in the PA and not in the proximal ascending aorta. It is critical to understand the anatomy of these views for a complete exam of the ascending aorta!

ANSWER B: Aortic dissection has occurred is incorrect.

Aortic dissection can occur at any point in the aorta and track retrograde to the heart or antegrade to the abdomen. A thorough exam of the ascending aorta, the

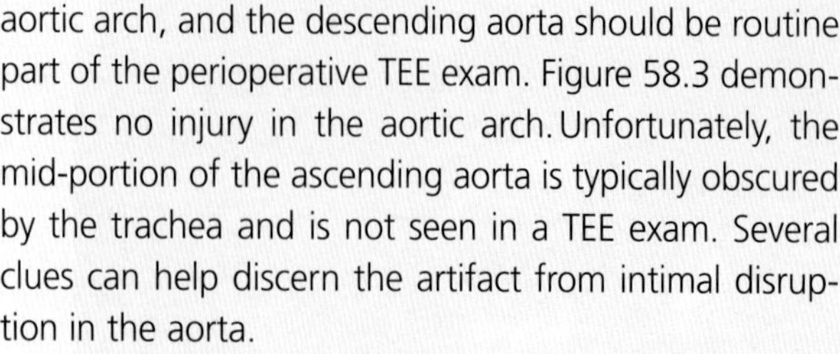

aortic arch, and the descending aorta should be routine part of the perioperative TEE exam. Figure 58.3 demonstrates no injury in the aortic arch. Unfortunately, the mid-portion of the ascending aorta is typically obscured by the trachea and is not seen in a TEE exam. Several clues can help discern the artifact from intimal disruption in the aorta.

1. Artifacts often have fuzzy, indistinct borders within the aorta.
2. Linear artifacts do not rapidly oscillate in systole.
3. Linear artifacts commonly extend across anatomic borders as straight line.
4. Reverberation artifacts will commonly extend directly to the probe.
5. CFD across an artifact will show homogenous CFD without a communicating jet.

ANSWER D: The TEE probe is malfunctioning is incorrect.

A potentially dangerous assumption! If a thorough exam is not definite then pull the PA catheter out and reassess.

QUESTION 58.2: The correct answer is B: Normal anatomy of AV.

This mass represents normal coaptation of the noncoronary cusp and left coronary cusp of the AV. This coaptation can often be demonstrated with probe rotation in the ME LAX view of the AV. Other than the more distal right coronary cusp, it can be difficult to name which specific cusp is seen in this view shown in Figures 58.9 and 58.10.

ANSWER A: Congenital, noncoronary sinus of Valsalva aneurysm is incorrect.

A congenital sinus of Valsalva aneurysm causes significant dilatation of the aortic root and typically impinges on surrounding structures outside, such as the RV. It typically does not present as an intra-aortic mass.

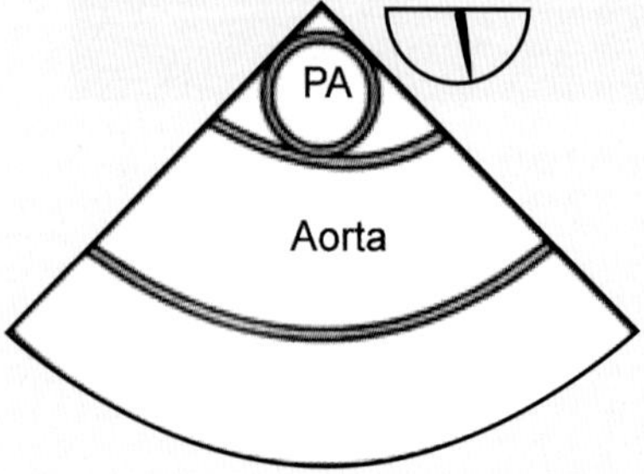

ME LAX of the Ascending Aorta

Figure 58.7.

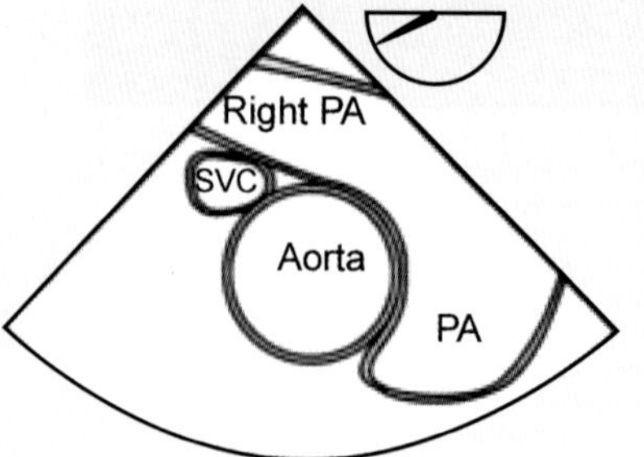

ME Ascending Aorta SAX

Figure 58.8.

ANSWER C: Prolapse of the right coronary cusp due to a localized dissection in aortic root is incorrect.

Figures 58.5 and 58.6 represent normal appearing anatomy. Videos 58.2 and 58.3 confirm normal motion and normal systolic flow without any AI from AV disruption.

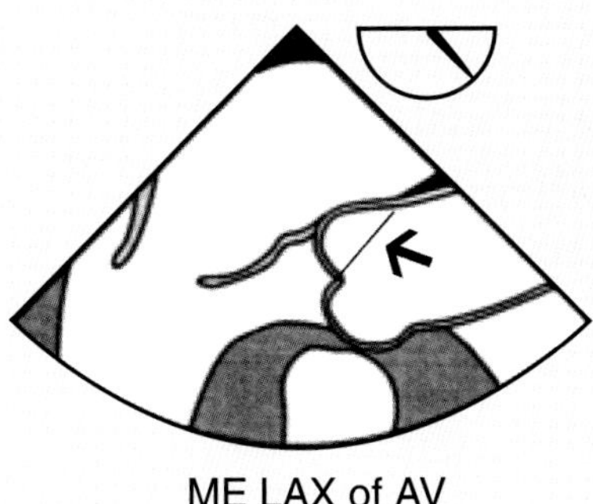

Figure 58.9.

ANSWER D: Vegetation on the left coronary cusp of the AV is incorrect.

AV vegetations are typically irregular and oscillate rapidly throughout the systolic ejection. They are highly associated with valvular stenosis or regurgitation. Laminar flow and normal leaflet motion are evident in the presented image.

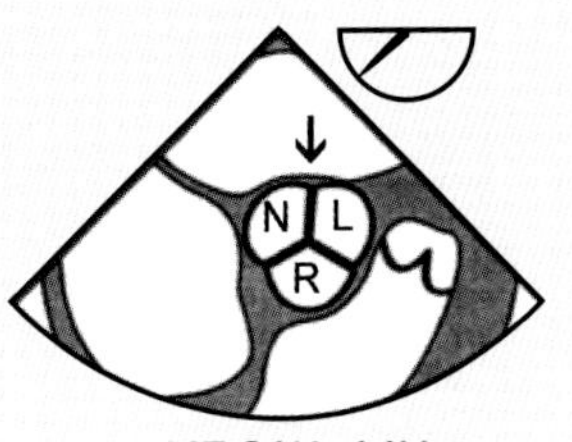

Figure 58.10.

TAKE-HOME LESSON:

Aortic artifacts are common and potentially misleading. A logical and thorough exam of the AV, aorta, and aortic arch is critical to successfully rule out false positive pathology.

SUGGESTED READING

Applebe AF, Walker PG, Yeoh JK, et al. Clinical significance of origin of artifacts in transesophageal echocardiography of the thoracic aorta. *J Am Coll Cardiol.* 1993;21:754–760.

Payne KJ, Ikonomidis JS, Reeves ST. Transesophageal echocardiography of the thoracic aorta. In: Perrino AC, Reeves ST, eds. *A Practical Approach to Transesophageal Echocardiography*. 2nd ed. Philadelphia: Lippincott Williams & Wilkins; 2007:321–343.

Vignon P, Spencer KT, Rambaud G, et al. Differential transesophageal echocardiographic diagnosis between linear artifacts and intraluminal flap of aortic dissection or disruption. *Chest.* 2001;119:1778–1790.

Moderate

CASE 59

An 83-year-old man is undergoing coronary arterial revascularization. A TEE exam is performed prior to surgical incision and the TG mid-SAX view of the LV is shown in Video 59.1. An M-mode cursor is placed across the middle of inferolateral and anteroseptal segments of the LV as shown in Figure 59.1.

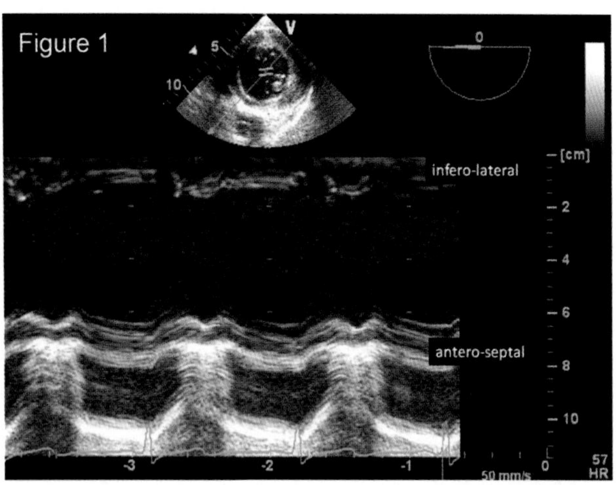

Figure 59.1.

QUESTION 59.1. Which of the following statements regarding the segmental motion is correct?

A. The inferolateral and anteroseptal walls are contracting synchronously
B. The inferolateral and anteroseptal walls are contracting asynchronously
C. The two segments are akinetic
D. None of the above statements are correct

Following an uneventful revascularization, the patient is weaned off CPB. The TG mid-SAX view of the LV is shown in Video 59.2. An M-mode cursor is placed across the middle of infero-lateral and antero-septal segments of the LV as shown in Figure 59.2.

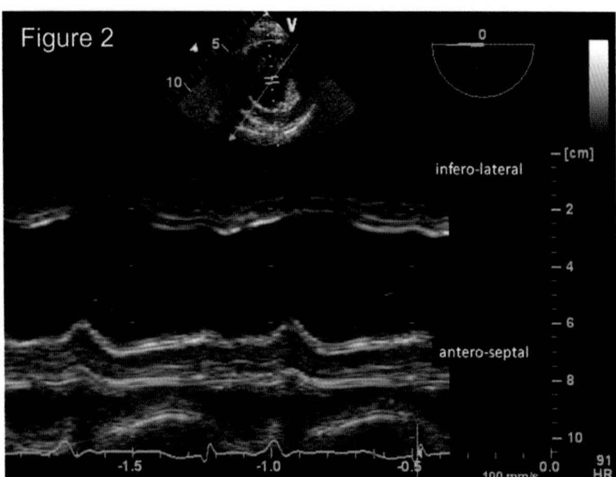

Figure 59.2.

QUESTION 59.2. Which of the following statements regarding the segmental motion is correct?

A. The inferolateral and anteroseptal walls are contracting synchronously
B. The inferolateral and anteroseptal walls are contracting asynchronously
C. The two segments are akinetic
D. None of the above statements are correct

ANSWERS AND DISCUSSION

QUESTION 59.1: The correct answer is A: The infero-lateral and antero-septal walls are contracting synchronously. M-mode allows the highest temporal resolution of all echocardiographic modes. Here, the cursor has been placed across the middle of diametrically opposite segments. The endocardium clearly moves toward the center of the cavity of the LV almost at the same time. Both infero-lateral and antero-septal segments have synchronous motion, as shown in Figure 59.3. Asynchronous contraction would result in a much larger time delay from when one wall moves inward to when the other wall moves inward. It is clearly shown in both the M-mode figure (Figs. 59.1 and 59.2) and the 2D video clip (Video 59.2) that these walls are moving inward, and therefore not akinetic.

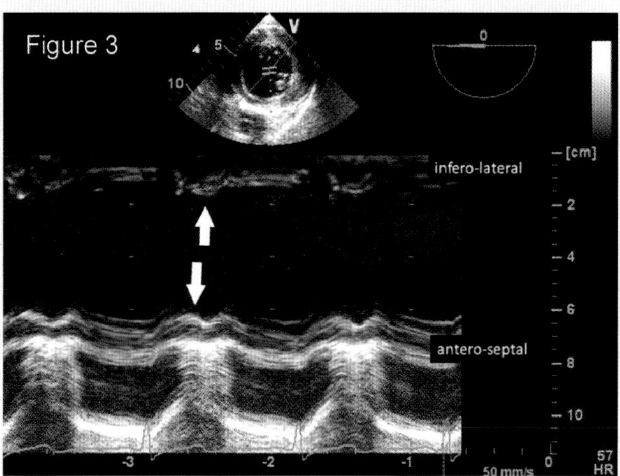

Figure 59.3.

QUESTION 59.2: The correct answer is B: The inferolateral and anteroseptal walls are contracting asynchronously. Temporary pacing is frequently required in patients following cardiac surgery. In the early postoperative period, patients may suffer from hemodynamically significant arrhythmias and temporary pacing may be required to optimize cardiac function. Epicardial pacing wires, which tend to be the most common method of lead placement in cardiac surgery patients are usually placed on the epicardium of the RA and RV. Because of the lead location, the external electrical impulse is not conducted along the intrinsic pacing pathway, but instead travels first to the right and then to the left cardiac chambers. As a result, there exists a left bundle branch block, and the interventricular septum will be activated and contract earlier than the rest of the LV segments. Consequently, the anteroseptal segment will manifest inward endocardial excursion much earlier than the diametrically opposite infero-lateral segment. Compare the time between the inward movements of the two walls in Figure 59.4 to that of Figure 59.3. There is a much greater degree of separation in Figure 59.4.

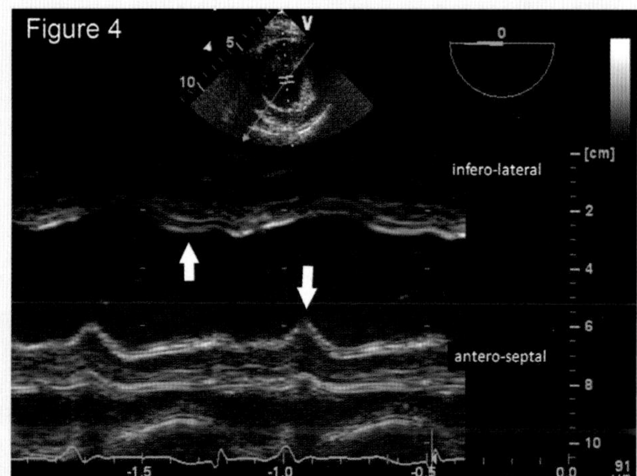

Figure 59.4.

TAKE-HOME LESSON:

Ventricular septal motion abnormalities are common post cardiac surgery if external pacing wires are utilized.

SUGGESTED READING

Elmi F, Tullo NG, Khalighi K. Natural history and predictors of temporary epicardial pacemaker wire function in patients after open heart surgery. *Cardiology*. 2002;98:175–180.

Hurlé A, Gómez-Plana J, Sánchez J, et al. Optimal location for temporary epicardial pacing leads following open heart surgery. *Pacing Clin Electrophysiol.* 2002;25:1049–1052.

Moderate

CASE 60

A 68-year-old woman with end-stage pulmonary fibrosis presents to the hospital with a systolic murmur. After investigation, she is taken to the OR for surgery. Following induction of anesthesia, the TEE images shown in Figure 60.1 and Video 60.1 are obtained.

QUESTION 60.1. Based on Figure 60.1 and Video 60.1, the most likely diagnosis is

A. AS

B. Aortic root aneurysm

C. Aortic dissection

D. Normal AV

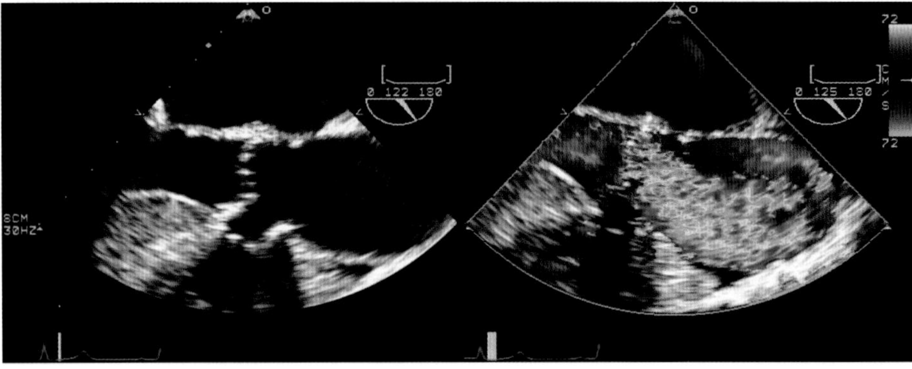

Figure 60.1. ME long axis of the AV in 2D (left) and CFD (right). See also Video 60.1.

An AV intervention is performed, after which the TEE images shown in Figures 60.2 to 60.4 and Videos 60.2 to 60.4 are obtained:

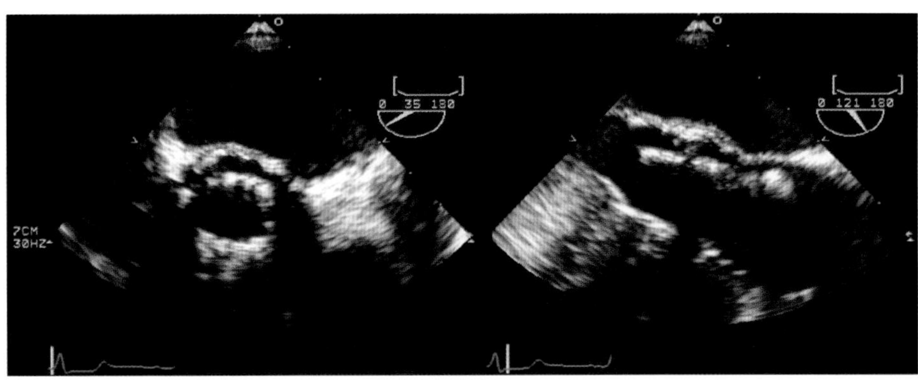

Figure 60.2. Post-procedure ME short-axis (left) and long-axis (right) view of the AV, in 2D. See also Video 60.2.

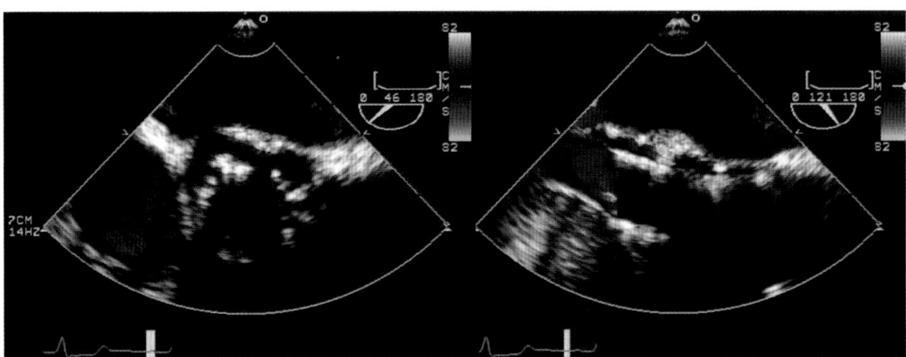

Figure 60.3. Post-procedure ME short-axis (left) and long-axis (right) view of the AV, with CFD. See also Videos 60.3 and 60.4.

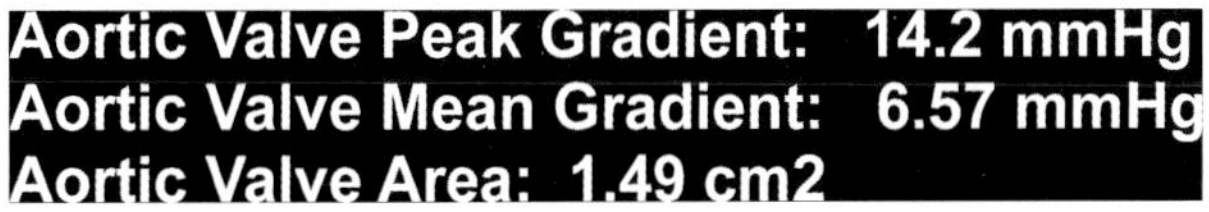

Aortic Valve Peak Gradient: 14.2 mmHg
Aortic Valve Mean Gradient: 6.57 mmHg
Aortic Valve Area: 1.49 cm2

Figure 60.4. Hemodynamic measurements on the AV, post procedure.

QUESTION 60.2. The procedure performed was

A. A conventional surgical AVR
B. An endovascular repair of an aortic root aneurysm
C. A percutaneous AVR
D. A percutaneous closure of a membranous VSD

QUESTION 60.3. The postprocedural images and hemodynamics show that the procedure resulted in

A. Severe stenosis and severe regurgitation
B. Severe stenosis and mild regurgitation
C. No AS and severe transvalvular aortic regurgitation
D. No AS and mild periprostheic regurgitation

As part of a complete postprocedure TEE examination, the images shown in Figures 60.5 and 60.6 and in Video 60.5 are obtained. The patient is hemodynamically stable without support from inotropes or vasopressors.

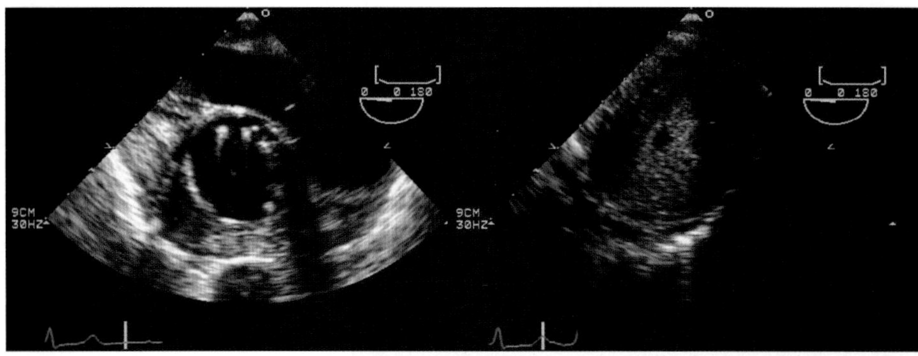

Figure 60.5. Upper esophageal short-axis view of the aorta (left). TG mid-papillary view of the LV at end-systole (right).

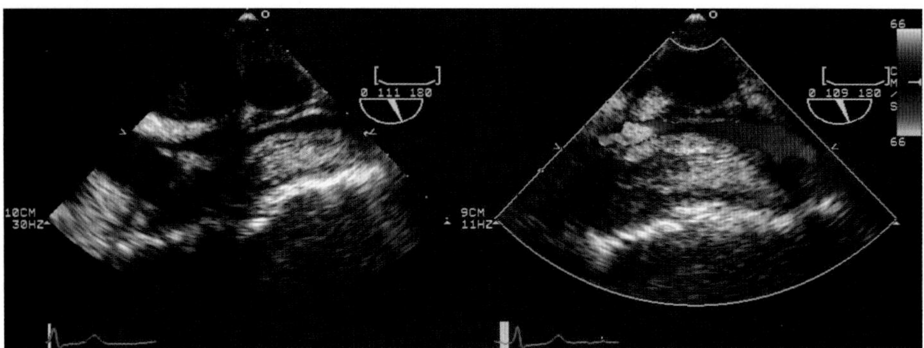

Figure 60.6. ME bicaval view, modified by withdrawing the probe slightly, in order to demonstrate the SVC in long axis, in 2D on the left and with CFD on the right. See also Video 60.5.

QUESTION 60.4. The TEE images displayed in Figure 60.5 and 60.6 and in Video 60.5 are most consistent with which of the following?

A. Periaortic hematoma
B. Type A aortic dissection
C. Intrapericardial fluid
D. Intraluminal aortic thrombus
E. A and C are correct

QUESTION 60.5. In light of the TEE findings, what is (are) the most concerning issue(s)?

A. Impending cardiac tamponade
B. Acute prosthetic dysfunction
C. Potential injury to the ascending aorta
D. A and C are correct
E. All of the above are correct

ANSWERS AND DISCUSSION

QUESTION 60.1: The correct answer is A: AS. Figure 60.1 and Video 60.1 show a heavily calcified and restricted AV and Figure 60.1 also shows aliasing systolic flow across the AV, all consistent with significant AS. This also explains the patient's systolic murmur. Answer B (*aortic root aneurysm*) is incorrect: while there is mild poststenotic dilatation of the ascending aorta, it is not an aortic root aneurysm. Answer C (*aortic dissection*) is incorrect: There is no evidence of an aortic flap. Finally, answer D is incorrect: this is not a normally functioning AV.

QUESTION 60.2: The correct answer is C: A percutaneous AVR.

The postprocedural images (Figs. 60.2 and 60.3 and Videos 60.2 to 60.4) show a structure across the AV extending both above and below the aortic annulus. Within this structure, thin and mobile leaflets can be seen opening in systole and closing in diastole (Video 60.2). The leaflets sit within the aorta a little distal to the native aortic annulus. This structure is a Medtronic CoreValve prosthesis, which was inserted percutaneously using a retrograde femoral arterial approach. Answer A (*conventional AVR*) is incorrect: this structure is not a conventional bioprosthetic or mechanical valve. Answer B (*endovascular repair of an aortic root aneurysm*) is incorrect: Endovascular repair of aortic aneurysms and dissections is being increasingly used to treat thoracic aortic disease. These procedures were initially limited to the descending aorta but now, in association with arch debranching operations, are more frequently relied on to treat aortic arch pathology. However, endovascular repair is at this time not used to treat aortic *root* disease. Furthermore, the preprocedural images do not show an aortic root aneurysm. Answer D is also incorrect. There is no VSD. Even if there had been, the foreign structure crosses the AV and is clearly not a septal occlusion device; those are round or oval discs, which straddle the ventricular septum.

The Medtronic CoreValve prosthesis produced by Medtronic CV (Luxembourg) (Fig. 60.7) was developed as an alternative to surgical AVR in patients who were felt to be at unacceptable risk for a cardiac surgical procedure requiring a sternotomy and CPB. It consists of a porcine pericardial prosthesis mounted within a nitinol frame, which expands into place when deployed from the specialized catheter delivery system. These studies reveal the prosthesis results in a significant reduction in the mean gradient to 3.2 ± 5.2 mm Hg and 87% of cases had mild or no aortic periprosthetic regurgitation. The remainder had moderate periprosthetic regurgitation only. The complication rates are remarkably low considering that these implantations were performed in patients felt to be too sick to be candidates for conventional AV surgery.

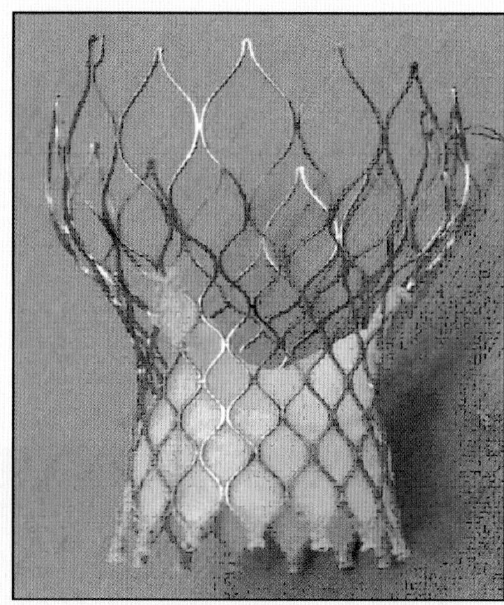

Figure 60.7. A CoreValve Revalving Prosthesis (Medtronic CV, Luxembourg) consisting of a bioprosthetic valve mounted on a self-expanding nitinol frame. (Courtesy of Dr. Marino Labinaz.)

QUESTION 60.3: The correct answer is D: No AS and mild periprostheic regurgitation. The postprocedural images show the percutaneous AV in place. The leaflets are moving normally. The transvalvular gradients are 14.2 mm Hg (peak) and 6.5 mm Hg (mean), with an EOA of 1.49 cm^2. Since these values do not indicate severe prosthetic AS, both answers A and B are incorrect. The CFD images show trivial transvalvular aortic regurgitation only. Hence answer C is also incorrect. The images do show that there is mild posterior periprosthetic regurgitation, where calcification of the annulus has prevented a close fit of the prosthesis with the native wall. There is also systolic flow through this small defect. Since these devices are self-expanding and not sewn into the aortic annulus, periprosthetic leaks are common, but usually mild. Twenty-one percent of patients require balloon inflation of the annulus of the frame to alleviate significant periprosthetic leaks,[1] with highly successful results.

QUESTION 60.4: The correct answer is E: Periaortic hematoma and intrapericardial fluid. Figure 60.5 shows a large hematoma anterior to the right of the ascending aorta, extending around (and compressing) the SVC (Fig. 60.6 and Video 60.5). It is marked by arrows in Figures 60.8 and 60.9. There is also a small echo-free space anterior to the severely hypertrophied LV. This raises serious concerns about an aortic injury and leakage of blood into the pericardium. Answer B (*aortic dissection*) is incorrect: there is no intimal flap to suggest a dissection. Finally, answer D (*intraluminal thrombus*) is incorrect: the mass appears to be *outside* the aortic wall, therefore not an intramural hematoma, nor is it an intraluminal thrombus on the prosthesis.

QUESTION 60.5: The correct answer is D: Impending cardiac tamponade and potential injury to the ascending aorta. Aortic root dissection or perforation and cardiac tamponade are recognized complications of a percutaneous AV implantation[1,2,3] and can be life threatening. The patient may ultimately require surgery via a sternotomy to correct these problems. In this case, because of the patient's general medical condition, there was great reluctance to perform a sternotomy. She was observed for several hours with TEE. She remained hemodynamically stable and there was no expansion of the hematoma or pericardial effusion. Accordingly, the patient was extubated and managed conservatively. Serial echocardiograms over the next few days showed no significant changes and the patient was discharged home in good condition. Answers B and E are incorrect, since there is no evidence of prosthetic malfunction.

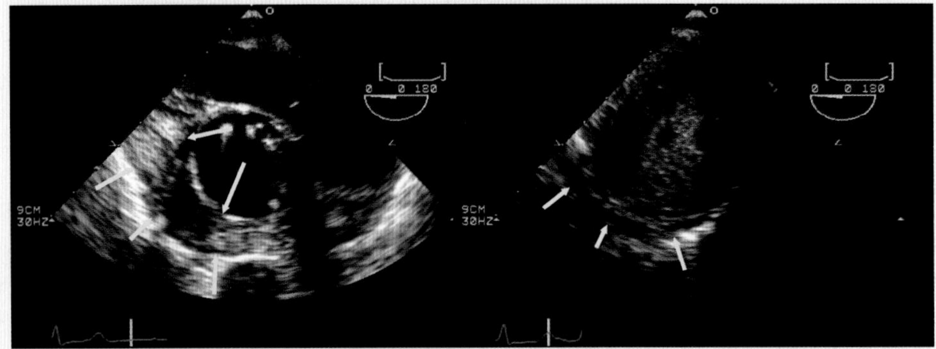

Figure 60.8. Same as Figure 60.5, with *arrows* demonstrating the periaortic hematoma and the small pericardial fluid.

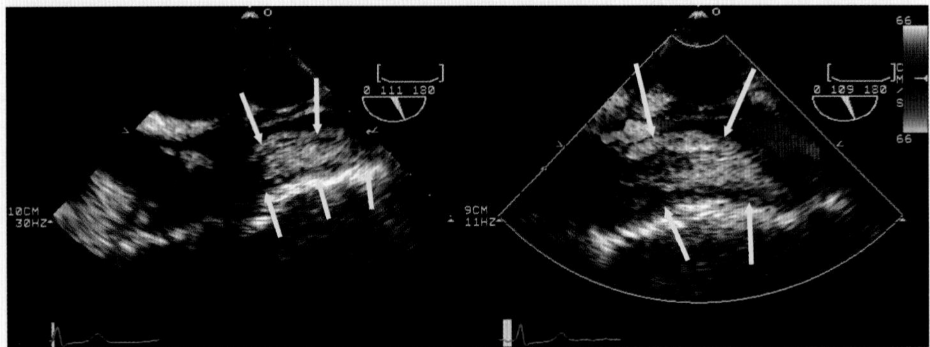

Figure 60.9. Same as Figure 60.6, with *arrows* demonstrating the periaortic hematoma compressing the SVC.

REFERENCES

1. Grube E, Laborde JC, Gerckens U, et al. Percutaneous implantation of the CoreValve self-expanding valve prosthesis in high-risk patients with aortic valve disease. The Sieburg first-in-man study. *Circulation.* 2006;114:1616–1624.
2. Piazza N, Grube E, Gerckens U, et al. Procedural and 30-day outcomes following transcatheter aortic valve implantation using the third generation (18Fr) CoreValve Revalving system: results from the multicentre, expanded evaluation registry 1 year following CE mark approval. *EuroIntervention.* 2008;4:242–249.
3. Tamburino C, Capodanno D, Mulè M, et al. Procedural success and 30 day clinical outcomes after percutaneous aortic valve replacement using current third generation self-expanding CoreValve prosthesis. *J Invasive Cardiol.* 2009;21:93–98.

SUGGESTED READING

Berry C, Oukerraj L, Asgar A, et al. Role of trans-esophageal echocardiography in percutaneous aortic valve replacement with the CoreValve Revalving system. *Echocardiography.* 2008;25(8):840–848.

Grube E, Laborde JC, Zickmann B, et al. First report on a human percutaneous transluminal implantation of a self expanding valve prosthesis for interventional treatment of aortic valve stenosis. *Catheter Cardiovasc Interv.* 2005;66:465–469.

Moderate

CASE 61

A 64-year-old man underwent an uncomplicated four-vessel CABG earlier today. Approximately 6 hours after he arrives in the ICU, you are called to perform an emergent TEE for hemodynamic instability. The patient has received multiple blood products over the past few hours, is intubated, and is being mechanically ventilated.

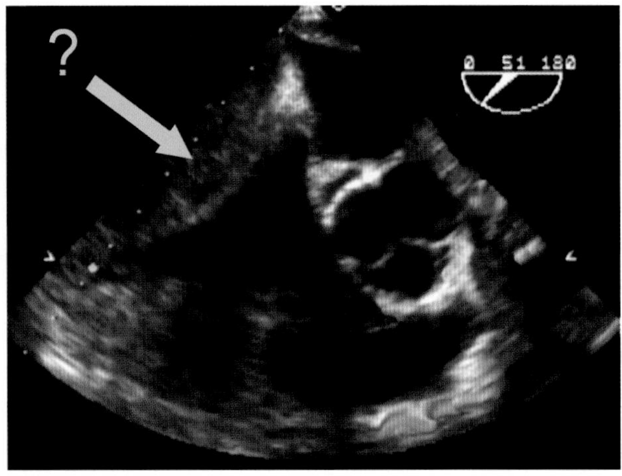

Figure 61.1.

QUESTION 61.1. A TEE probe is placed, yielding the ME images obtained in Video 61.1. The most significant finding is:

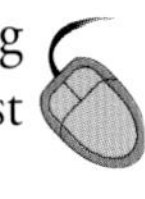

A. Severe TR
B. A large ASD
C. A large VSD
D. Compression of the RA
E. A large pleural effusion

QUESTION 61.2. What is the arrow most likely pointing to in Figure 61.1?

A. Liver
B. Clotted blood
C. Lung tissue
D. A myxoma
E. A normal intracardiac structure

QUESTION 61.3. Video 61.2 is a TG mid-SAX view obtained from this patient. What is your final diagnosis?

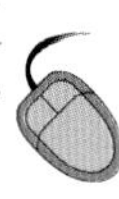

A. Tension pneumothorax
B. Hepatic carcinoma
C. Constrictive pericarditis
D. Pericardial tamponade
E. None of the above

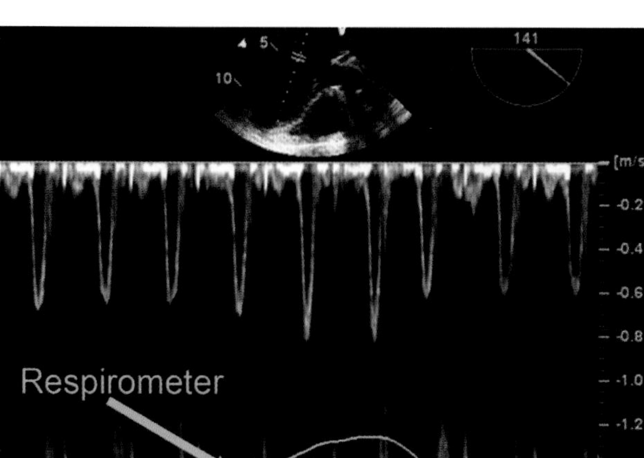

Figure 61.2.

QUESTION 61.4. Is the mitral inflow pattern seen in Figure 61.2 consistent with this patient's diagnosis?

A. Yes, because there is an increase in the early transmitral pressure gradient
B. Yes, because there is a decrease in the early transmitral pressure gradient
C. No, because there is an increase in the early transmitral pressure gradient
D. No, because there is a decrease in the early transmitral pressure gradient
E. Figure 61.2 is not a transmitral inflow tracing

QUESTION 61.5. The most appropriate management of this patient would be to

A. Administer β-blockers to prevent myocardial ischemia
B. Administer a loading dose of milrinone to increase contractility
C. Order a ventilation-perfusion (VQ) scan to rule out pulmonary embolism
D. Perform cardiac catheterization to ensure all grafts are patent
E. Return to the operating room (OR) for mediastinal exploration

ANSWERS AND DISCUSSION

QUESTION 61.1: The correct answer is D. The most significant finding in Video 61.1 is compression of the RA. Figure 61.3 is a frame from the second half of Video 61.1 showing 2D and CFD right ventricle (RV) inflow-outflow views. There is clearly a mass causing invagination of the RA. Note that the CFD demonstrates reduced cavity size of the RA. The first half of the video, a ME 4CH view, shows the presence of a pericardial effusion, suggesting that may be where the compressing mass is located. TR would be seen as a high velocity jet into the RA during systole. There is no evidence of either a VSD or an ASD in Video 61.1. Pleural effusions are not typically seen in the views presented.

QUESTION 61.2: The correct answer is B. The arrow is most likely pointing to clotted blood. As discussed above, there is clearly compression of the RA. The borders of the RA are seen, indicating the mass is external to the heart. Therefore it would not be a myxoma, nor a normal intracardiac structure. The mass does not have the aerated appearance of lung tissue, which would be unlikely to cause right atrial compression anyway. Given the clinical situation, it is more likely that the mass is clot formed from postcardiac surgical bleeding rather than an extremely enlarged liver.

QUESTION 61.3: The correct answer is D. The diagnosis for this patient is pericardial tamponade. Video 61.2 demonstrates a large amount of what appears to be clotted blood in the pericardial space (see Fig. 61.4, a still frame from Video 61.2). Note that the separation between the splanchnic pericardium (i.e. epicardium) and the parietal pericardium is greater than 2 cm, indicating a large effusion—filled with some clotted blood in this case. Separation of less than 0.5 cm would be considered small, and medium size would be between 0.5 and 2 cm. Given the clinical scenario, the large effusion, and the demonstrated right atrial compression, the diagnosis of cardiac tamponade can easily be made. Note that in the postcardiac surgical patient, other signs of tamponade, such as RV collapse during diastole or LA collapse, may not be seen because clot formation may be localized causing a regional tamponade. Constrictive pericarditis would not be expected immediately following cardiac surgery, and

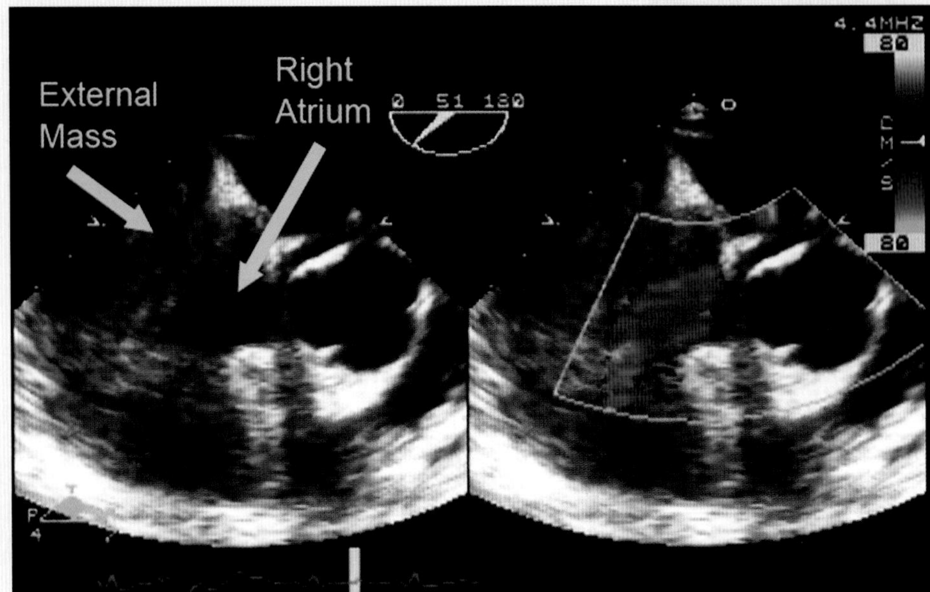

Figure 61.3.

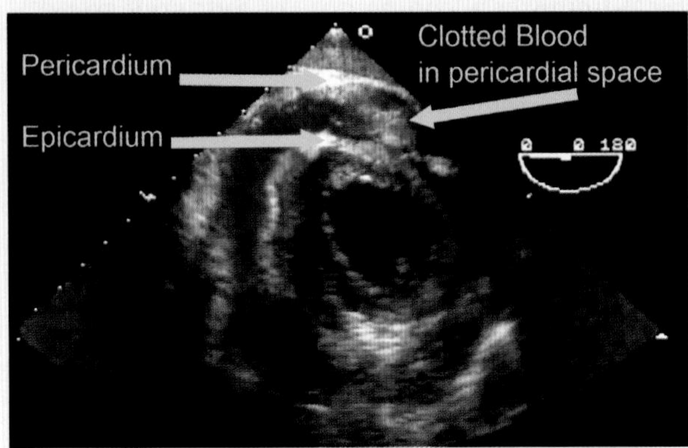

Figure 61.4.

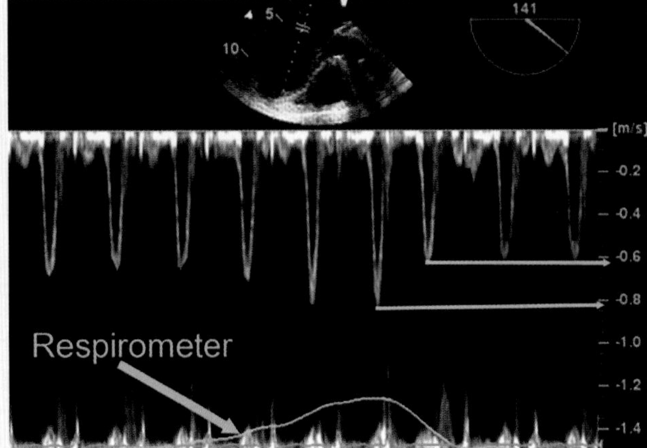

Figure 61.5.

there would be tight adhesion of the pericardium to the epicardium.

QUESTION 61.4: The correct answer is A: Yes, because there is an increase in the early transmitral pressure gradient. As shown in Figure 61.5, the E wave height on transmitral inflow increases about 33% (from ~60 to 80 cm/s) during the positive pressure inspiration, indicated by the hump in the respirometer waveform. Normally in a mechanically ventilated patient, inspiration will not cause a significant increase in E wave velocity. However, tamponade causes increased filling of the LV at the expense of the RV (exaggerated ventricular interdependence) and the early transmitral gradient increases during positive pressure inspiration. Note that this is exactly the opposite of what would happen in a *spontaneously* breathing patient, where inspiration would decrease the left-sided filling pressures and cause a decreased mitral E wave velocity.

QUESTION 61.5: The correct answer is E. The most appropriate management of this patient would be to return to the OR for mediastinal exploration. The presence of cardiac tamponade is a life-threatening condition that mandates a reopening of the chest in order to relieve the compression of the heart. Medical management before the chest is opened would include ensuring adequate preload, keeping a faster heart rate, and maintaining high systemic vascular resistance ("*keep 'em fast, full, and tight*"). Administering either a β-blocker that could decrease heart rate or loading milrinone that could cause vasodilatation would be detrimental to the patient. Going to the radiology suite or catheterization lab would also be inadvisable since both would delay treatment with unnecessary tests.

TAKE-HOME LESSON:

Hemodynamic instability following cardiac surgery should raise the suspicion of cardiac tamponade. Bleeding and clot formation can cause localized compression of cardiac chambers, impairing filling, and decreasing cardiac output. The diagnosis of tamponade can be made with TEE, which should prompt a return to the OR.

SUGGESTED READING

Tsang TSM, Oh JK, Seward JM. Diagnosis and management of cardiac tamponade in the era of echocardiography. *Clin Cardiol.* 1999;22:446–452.

Wann S, Passen E. Echocardiography in pericardial disease. *J Am Soc Echocardiogr.* 2008;21:7–13.

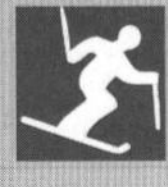

Moderate

CASE 62

A 2-year-old child presents to his pediatrician. A murmur is detected and the child is referred for the following TEE. A few selected images and videos are shown (Figs. 62.1 and 62.2, and Videos 62.1 to 62.3).

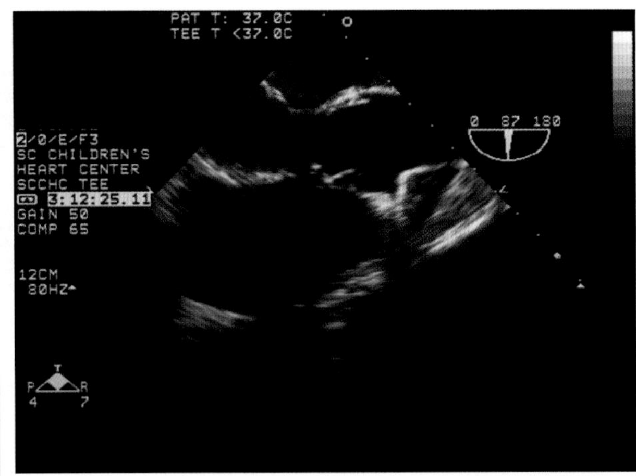

Figure 62.1.

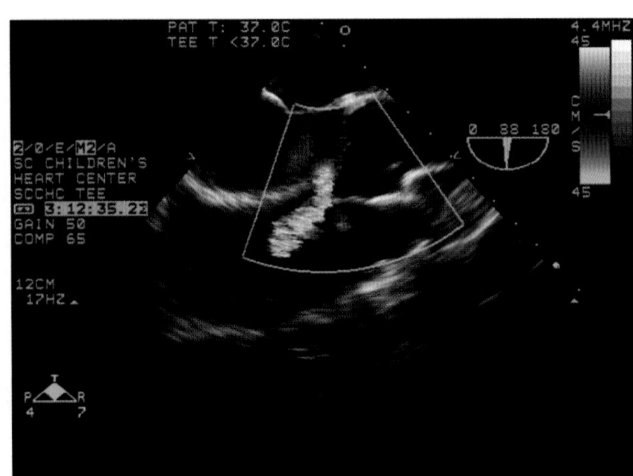

Figure 62.2.

QUESTION 62.1. What is the diagnosis?

A. Inlet VSD
B. Perimembranous VSD
C. Doubly committed outlet (subarterial VSD)
D. Muscular VSD

QUESTION 62.2. What associated pathology is commonly found with a perimembranous VSD?

A. Ventricular septal aneurysm
B. Aortic regurgitation
C. Primum ASD
D. Cleft MV

QUESTION 62.3. Spectral Doppler evaluation of what abnormality(ies) can allow estimation of PA systolic pressure?

A. MR
B. AI
C. Tricuspid insufficiency
D. VSD flow

ANSWERS AND DISCUSSION

QUESTION 62.1: Answer B—Perimembranous VSD—is correct.

VSDs are classified by location into four major groups: perimembranous, muscular, doubly committed outlet (subarterial), and inlet defects (Fig. 62.3).

A perimembranous defect accounts for approximately 70% of VSDs and occupies most of the membranous septum.

ANSWER A: Inlet VSDs account for approximately 5% of all VSDs and are located in close proximity to the atrioventricular valves in the posterior or inlet portion of the ventricular septum. Hence answer A is incorrect.

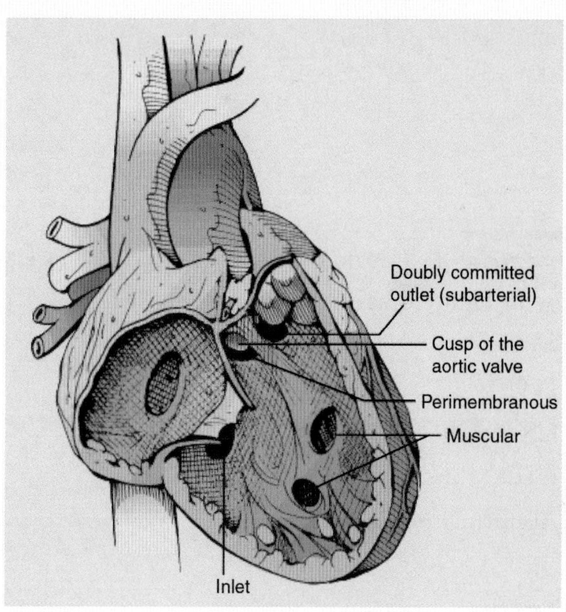

Figure 62.3.

ANSWER C: Doubly committed outlet (subarterial) VSDs are located in the infundibular septum immediately below the pulmonic valve. Hence answer C is incorrect.

ANSWER D: Muscular VSDs account for 20% of all VSDs and are located in the muscular portion of the ventricular septum. They can be isolated but are frequently multiple. Hence answer D is incorrect.

QUESTION 62.2: Answers A and B—Ventricular septal aneurysm and aortic regurgitation—are correct.

Perimembranous defects are associated with ventricular septal aneurysms that appear as a tissue pouch composed of TV tissue. A ventricular septal aneurysm can frequently limit the flow of blood across a perimembranous VSD. AV cusp herniation through the perimembranous defect can result in aortic regurgitation. Answer C is incorrect since a primum ASD is most commonly associated with an inlet VSD. Answer D is incorrect since cleft MV is most commonly associated with an AV canal defect.

QUESTION 62.3: Answers C and D—Tricuspid insufficiency and VSD flow—are correct.

In the absence of outflow tract obstruction, estimation of PA systolic pressure can be performed by either of the following calculations:

ANSWER C:

TR jet velocity

PA systolic pressure = RV systolic pressure

PA pressure = $4(V_{TR})^2$ + RA pressure

or

ANSWER D:

RV systolic pressure = Systolic blood pressure – $4(V_{VSD})^2$

TAKE-HOME LESSON:

A perimembranous defect is the most common type of VSD (approximately 70% of VSDs) and occupies most of the membranous septum.

SUGGESTED READING

Rouine-Rapp K, Miller-Hance WC. Transesophageal echocardiography for congenital heart disease in the adult. In: Perrino A, Reeves ST, eds. *A Practical Approach to Transesophageal Echocardiography,* 2nd ed. Philadelphia: Lippincott Williams & Wilkins; 2008: 366–400.

Perrino A, Reeves ST, eds. *A Practical Approach to Transesophageal Echocardiography.* 2nd ed. [Chapter 18]. Philadelphia: Lippincott Williams & Wilkins; 2008.

CASE 63

A 53-year-old man with known bicuspid AV and moderate-to-severe aortic regurgitation presents for AVR. A CT of the thorax showed a supracardiac partial anomalous pulmonary venous drainage to the left subclavian vein.

A transesophageal examination is performed after induction of general anesthesia and before institution of CPB.

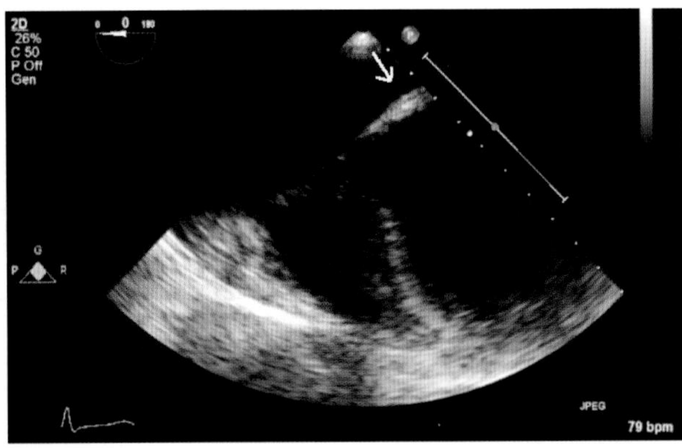

Figure 63.1. Modified ME 4CH view.

QUESTION 63.1. What is the structure marked by arrow in Figure 63.1?

A. SVC
B. IVC
C. CS
D. ASD
E. Abnormal pulmonary vein

QUESTION 63.2. How is the diagnosis of persistent left vena cava usually confirmed?

A. Examination with CFD
B. Injection with agitated saline through a right arm peripheral intravenous line
C. Injection with agitated saline through a left arm peripheral intravenous line
D. Examination with PW Doppler

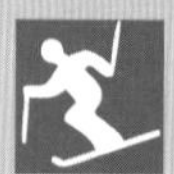

QUESTION 63.3. How does this finding change the management of the case?

A. There will be no change
B. The case will be cancelled
C. There will be a change in the venous cannulation technique
D. There will be a change in the mode of cardioplegia administration

QUESTION 63.4. What are the overall implications of this finding?

A. None
B. There is a left to right shunt with the potential of right heart overload
C. There is a right to left shunt with no consequences
D. Precautions should be taken during central venous cannulation

ANSWERS AND DISCUSSION

QUESTION 63.1: The correct answer is C. The structure marked by the arrow shown in Figure 63.1 is a dilated CS. A dilated CS can be found in many clinical situations including RV dysfunction, severe TR, elevated right atrial pressure, coronary arteriovenous fistula, anomalous pulmonary or hepatic venous return in the CS, and persistent left superior vena cava (PLSVC).[1,2] PLSVC is the most common variation in the thoracic venous system. PLSVC is present in 0.5% of the general population and can be associated with other cardiac anomalies such as bicuspid AV, ASD, and coarctation of aorta. PLSVC can also be concomitant with the absence of the right SVC in which case the RIJ vein and the right subclavian vein empty through an innominate vein in the PLSVC.

Our patient had bicuspid AV and a partial anomalous pulmonary venous return. He presented with the most common subtype of PLSVC in which both right and left SVC are present as demonstrated by the normal course of the PA catheter floated after induction through the RIJ vein cordis.

QUESTION 63.2: The correct answer is C. The presence of a PLSVC is diagnosed by a dilated CS (more than 1 cm) (Fig. 63.2), the opacification of the CS before the RA after injection of agitated saline in a peripheral intravenous line in the left upper extremity, as identified by the arrow in Figure 63.3. Also, agitated saline can be observed in the PLSVC as it travels laterally to the aortic arch (Fig. 63.4), crosses the posterior wall of the left atrium (Fig. 63.5), and passes between the left atrium appendage and left upper pulmonary vein (Figs. 63.6 and 63.7). With injection of agitated saline in a peripheral intravenous line in the right upper extremity, if the

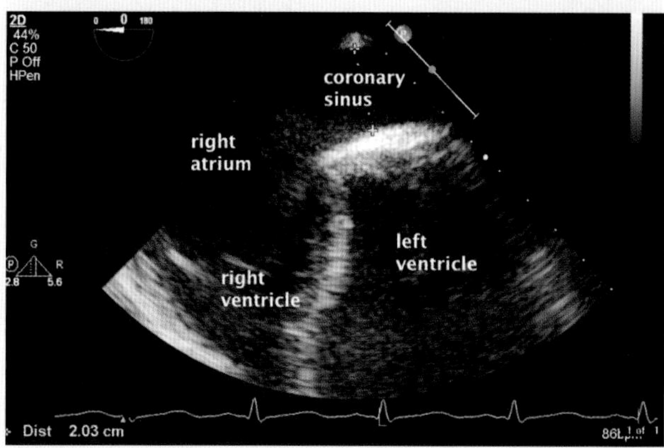

Figure 63.2. Modified ME 4CH view. The CS has been measured at 2.03 cm.

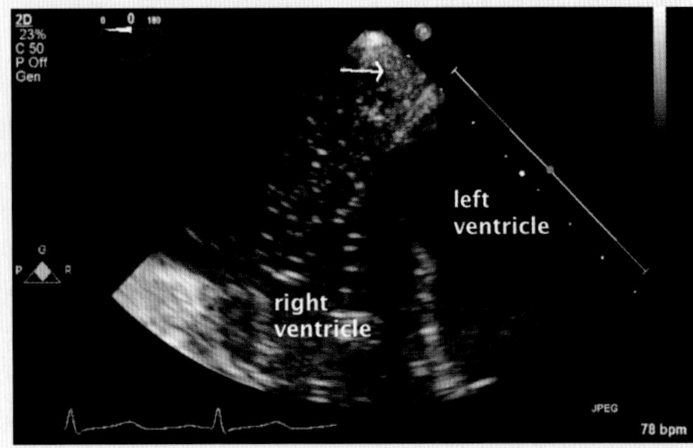

Figure 63.3. Modified ME 4CH view. Agitated saline is noted entering the RA through the CS marked by arrow.

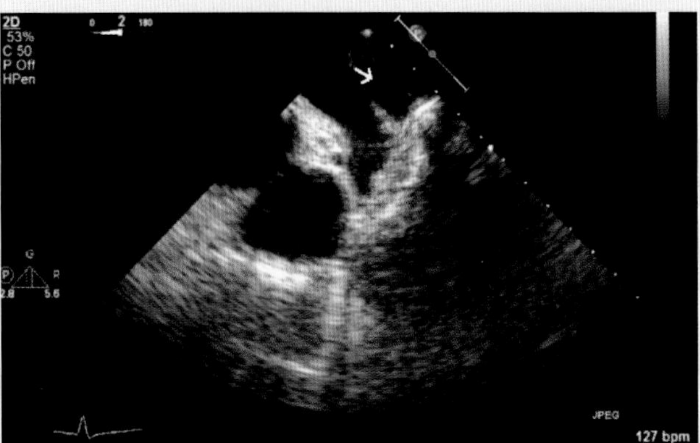

Figure 63.6. The arrow identifies the PLSVC between the left atrium appendage and the LUPV.

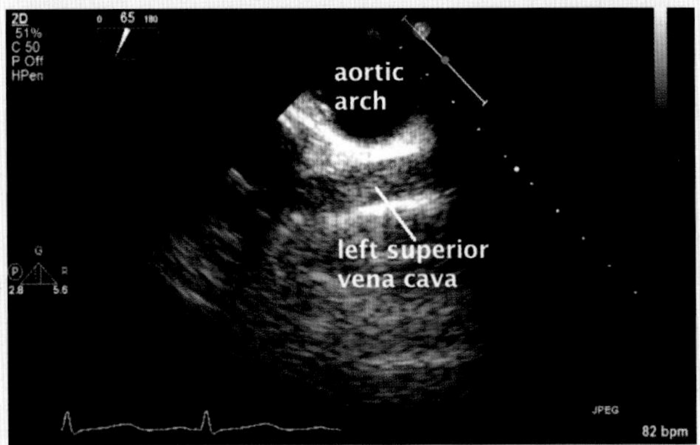

Figure 63.4. UE aortic arch SAX view.

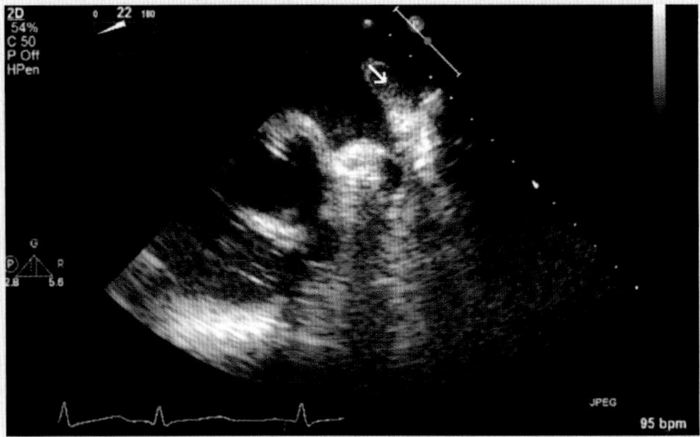

Figure 63.7. The arrow identifies the PLSVC after injection of agitated saline.

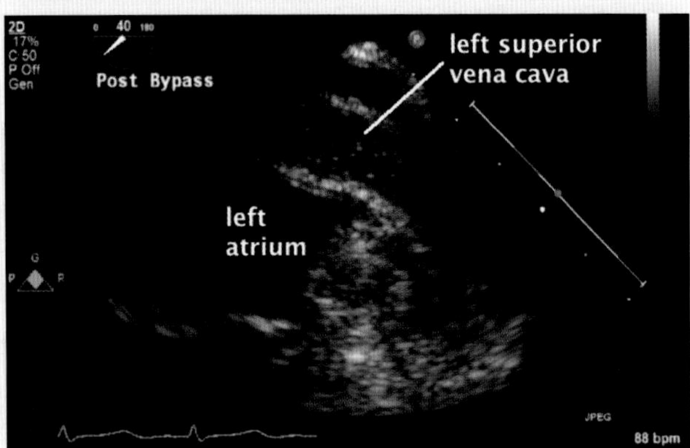

Figure 63.5. Modified ME 4CH view zoomed-in on the left atrium.

opacification of the CS occurs before opacification of the RA, the PLSVC is concomitant with an absent right SVC.

QUESTION 63.3: The correct answer is D. In patients with a significant degree of aortic regurgitation undergoing AVR, until the opening of the aortic root when the cardioplegic solution can be administered selectively through the coronary arteries, the administration of cardioplegia should be done in a retrograde fashion through a catheter placed in the CS. In the presence of a PLSVC, however, the administration of retrograde cardioplegia would be ineffective in providing myocardial protection and could result in infusing the cardioplegic solution in the cerebral circulation. In this patient the largest size catheter was placed in the CS. The PLSVC was identified as a vascular structure between the LAA and the LUPV and a vascular clamp was used to occlude it.

QUESTION 63.4: The correct answer is D. In most cases, PLSVC empties through the CS in the RA; however, in about 10% of the cases it empties in the left atrium resulting in a small right-to-left shunt. In patients with PLSVC, care should be taken when placing central venous catheters, PA catheters, or pacing wires through the left venous system as these procedures can be technically challenging or can result in damage to the CS.

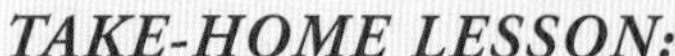

TAKE-HOME LESSON:

A dilated CS can be found in many clinical situations, including RV dysfunction, severe TR, elevated right atrial pressure, coronary arteriovenous fistula, anomalous pulmonary or hepatic venous return in the CS, and persistent left superior vena cava.

REFERENCES

1. Goyal SK, Punnam SR, Verma G, et al. Persistent left superior vena cava: a case report and review of literature. *Cardiovasc Ultrasound.* 2008;6:50.
2. Hasel R, Barash PG. Dilated coronary sinus on prebypass transesophageal echocardiography. *J Cardiothorac Vasc Anesth.* 1996;10:432–435.

Moderate

CASE 64

A 64-year-old male is presenting to the OR for AVR and CABG surgery. Past medical history is positive for hypertension, cerebrovascular accident, and diabetes mellitus. You are performing the intraoperative TEE when the surgeon asked if the patient has a PFO.

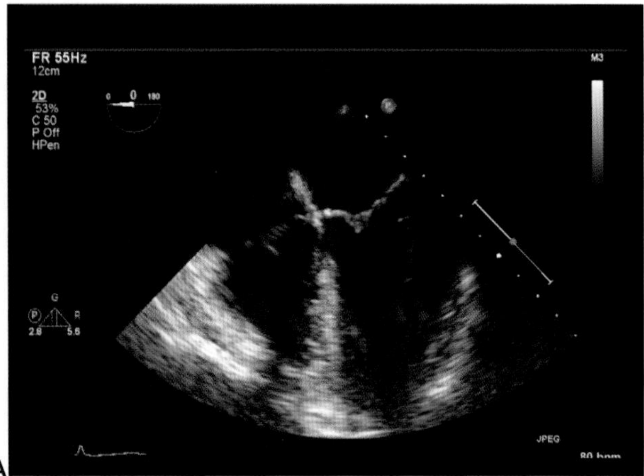

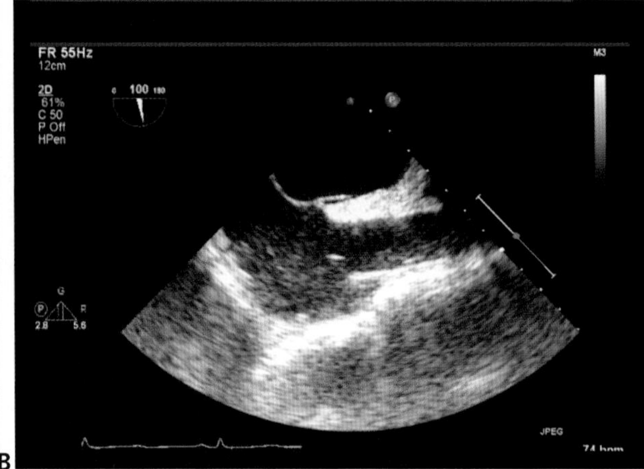

Figure 64.1. **A:** ME 4CH view. **B:** ME bicaval view. See also Videos 64.1 and 64.2.

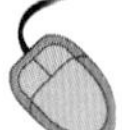

QUESTION 64.1. Which view provides the highest fidelity images of the interatrial septum?

A. ME 4CH view
B. ME bicaval view
C. Deep TG view
D. ME five-chamber view

QUESTION 64.2. In Figure 64.1 A and B, the Examination of the interatrial septum suggests

A. ASD secundum type
B. ASD primum type
C. PFO
D. Sinus venosus

You choose to perform CFD imaging to further evaluate the interatrial septum (Fig. 64.2).

QUESTION 64.3. Which Doppler setting is optimal for interrogation of suspected ASD or PFO?

A. High Nyquist limit map
B. Low Nyquist limit map
C. Speckle tracking
D. Tissue Doppler

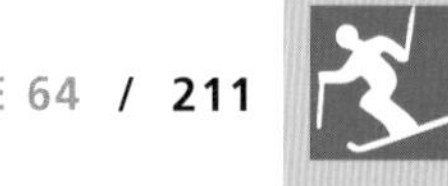

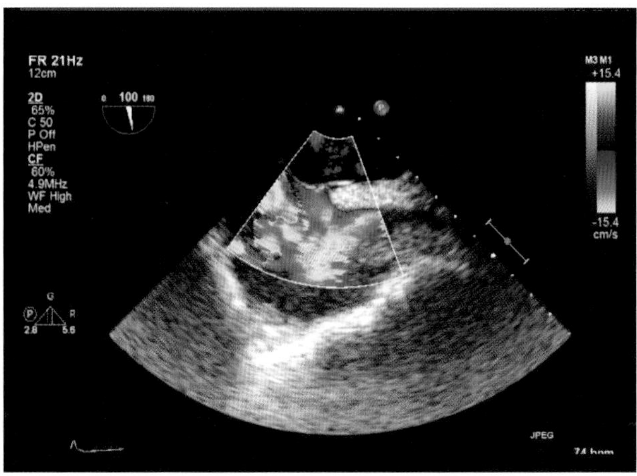

Figure 64.2. ME bicaval view with CFD. See also Video 64.3.

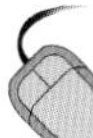

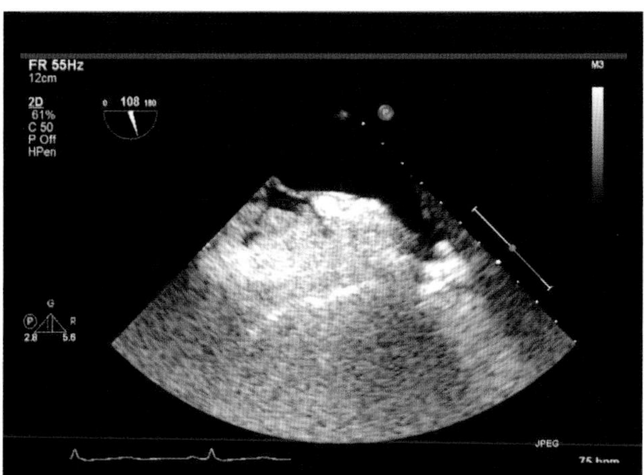

Figure 64.3. 2D ME bicaval view with contrast saline agitation. See also Video 64.4.

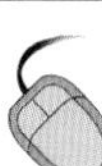

QUESTION 64.4. At that point, you inform the surgeon:

A. Yes, there is PFO

B. No, there is no PFO

C. An ASD primum is present

D. I am not sure

You decide to perform a contrast study by injecting agitated saline through the RIJ vein catheter (Figs. 64.3 and 64.4).

QUESTION 64.5. What determines a successful saline agitation test?

A. If 1, 2, and 3 are correct

B. If 1 and 3 are correct

C. If 2 and 4 are correct

D. If 4 is correct

E. If all are correct

1. Full opacification of the RA with air bubbles
2. Bowing of the interatrial septum toward the left atrium
3. The speed of the injection
4. Bowing of the interatrial septum toward the RA

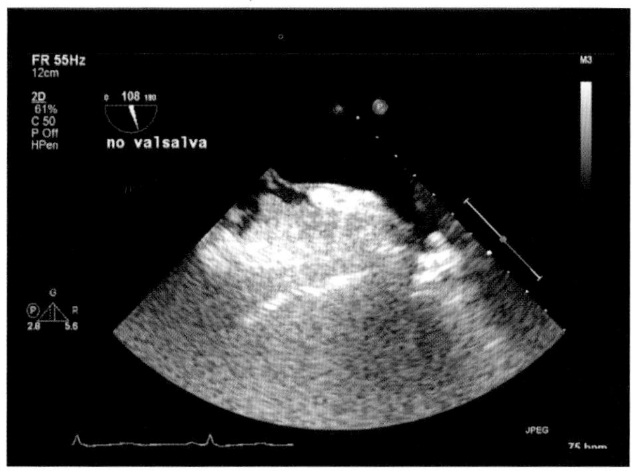

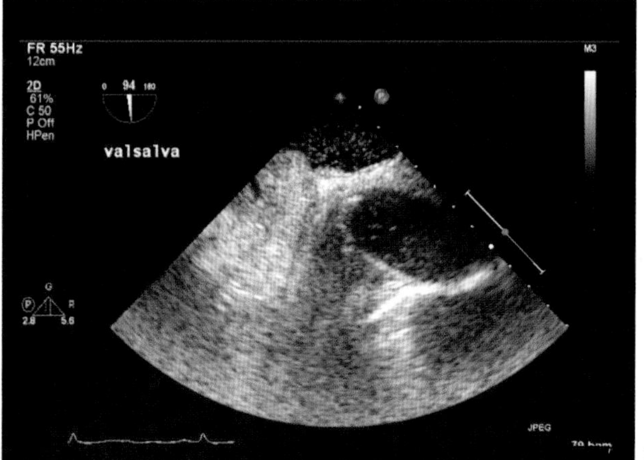

Figure 64.4. 2D ME bicaval view with saline contrast agitation. **A:** Without Valsalva. **B:** With Valsalva. See also Videos 64.5 and 64.6.

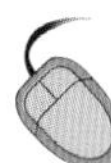

QUESTION 64.6. When applying Valsalva maneuver in conjunction with contrast injection to diagnose PFO, bubbles appear in the left atrium:

A. At the beginning of Valsalva
B. At the release of Valsalva
C. At the middle of Valsalva
D. At anytime during the Valsalva

QUESTION 64.7. Based on the above findings what information would you relay to the surgeon? The surgeon repaired the PFO, Post repair finding is illustrated in Figure 64.5.

A. Positive PFO
B. Negative PFO
C. Indeterminate
D. Persistent left superior vena cava

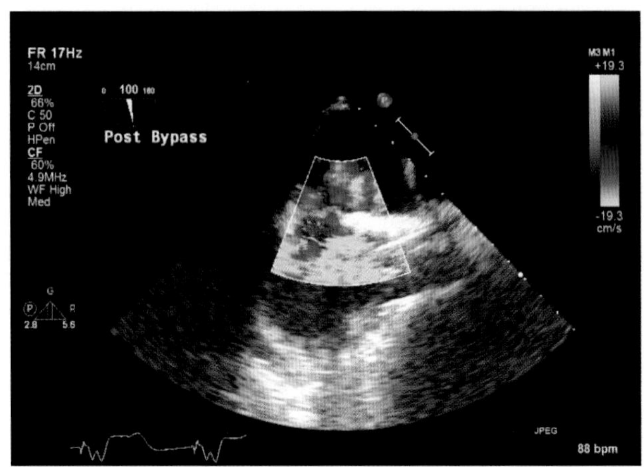

Figure 64.5. ME bicaval view with CFD post repair of PFO. See also Video 64.7.

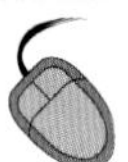

ANSWERS AND DISCUSSION

QUESTION 64.1: The correct answer is B: ME bicaval view.

The interatrial septum has a thin region centrally called the foramen ovale and thicker regions anteriorly and posteriorly called the "Limbus." Pathology can be associated with each of these regions requiring a full evaluation of the septum in its entirety. This is achieved by using multiple imaging planes. The ME bicaval view has the advantage of providing a high-quality imaging of the interatrial septum as the ultrasound beam is aligned perpendicular to the septum producing strong specular reflections. In views such as the ME 4CH, deep TG or the ME five chamber, the ultrasound beam travels parallel to the septum. This has the disadvantages of low-intensity reflections. In addition, the interatrial septum is located in the far field in the deep TG view that further compromises image quality.

QUESTION 64.2: The correct answer is C: PFO.

During the early embryologic development of the heart, the interatrial septum is formed of septum primum with a foramen secundum present at its upper part and septum secundum that develops later on the right side of the septum primum. In effect, the septum secundum extends like a curtain over the foramen secundum forming the foramen ovale. The septum primum acts like a one-way flap valve allowing oxygenated blood to flow from the RA toward the left atrium. The high pulmonary resistance and consequent high right atrial pressure during the intrauterine life ensures the patency of this foramen ovale. At birth, blood flows through the lungs and the pulmonary resistance markedly drops and hence the right atrial pressure. This results in fusion of the septum primum and septum secundum and closure of the foramen ovale. This fusion may not be permanent but rather functional in some patients resulting in a patent foramen ovale. In disease states associated with increase in RA pressures such as RV infarction, pulmonary embolism, or the use of high levels of positive end expiratory pressure (PEEP), this potential probe-patent PFO may open and cause right-to-left shunt of deoxygenated blood exacerbating the hypoxemia with a potential for paradoxical emboli. Such flow can be detected using CFD (Fig. 64.6).

ASDs are actual defects in the septum in which discontinuity of the septum is visible. Different types of ASD occur that can be characterized by the location of this defect: with answer A, ASD secundum, a complete defect is observed at the midportion of the interatrial septum at the location of the foramen ovale. With answer B, primum ASD, a defect at the base of the septum is observed at the level of the endocardial cushion. This defect is often associated with cleft anterior mitral leaflet. With answer D, sinus venosus, the defect is usually observed at the superior region of the septum in proximity to the orifice of the SVC.

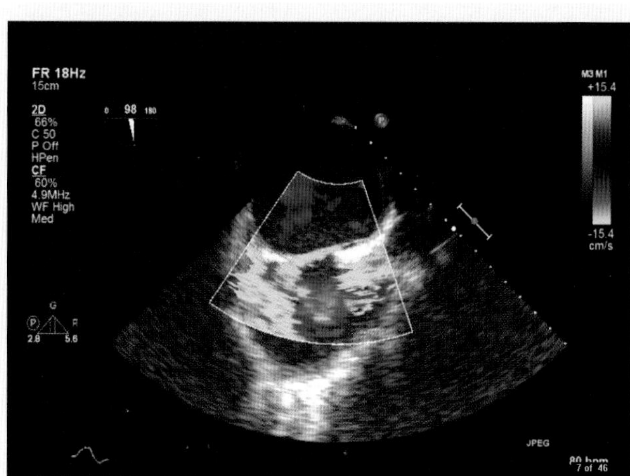

Figure 64.6. ME bicaval view with CFD showing right to left flow through a PFO. See also Video 64.8.

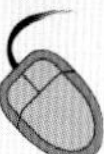

It is often associated with anomalous drainage of the pulmonary veins.

QUESTION 64.3: The correct answer is B: Low Nyquist limit map.

Blood flow velocity through the PFO is dependent on the pressure gradient between the right and the left atria. Since the pressures in both atria are relatively low, a low Nyquist limit map (<30 cm/s) is chosen to best detect the low velocity flow. With answer A, using a high Nyquist limit (>30 cm/s) map, the echocardiographer may not detect the low velocity flow. Speckle tracking and tissue Doppler are modalities used to track soft tissue motion, not blood flow.

QUESTION 64.4: The correct answer is D: I am not sure.

Answer A—Yes, there is a PFO—is incorrect as the CFD did not demonstrate a PFO. Answer B, No, there is no PFO, is also incorrect despite the lack of flow through the PFO by CFD. A lack of positive CFD is not definitive because flow may not be present due to a lack of positive pressure gradient between the right and the left atria or the imaging plane itself may not interrogate the blood flow. Given the highly suspicious 2D findings on this patient, further evaluation such as contrast injection is warranted.

QUESTION 64.5: The correct answer is A. Full opacification of the RA with air bubbles, bowing of the interatrial septum toward the left atrium, and the speed of the injection.

Blood appears black in conventional 2D ultrasound because of the extensive scattering that happens to the ultrasound beam by the RBCs and hence the returning signals are very weak. Contrast ultrasound results from the scattering of incident ultrasound at a gas/liquid interface, increasing the strength of the returning signal. This technique is used commonly to detect PFO in conjunction with 2D imaging and color Doppler flow. The technique can be performed with the use of two 10-mL syringes placed on adjacent stopcocks. Each syringe is filled with 5 mL saline (or alternatively blood) and 0.2 mL of air. Saline is agitated between the two syringes by alternately depressing the syringe plungers with the stopcocks positioned such that the saline is transferred back and forth from one syringe to the next. The agitated saline is then injected rapidly through the wide bore intravenous catheter (20 G or greater), preferably close to the RA to achieve full opacification of the RA happens. A PFO is diagnosed if three or more microbubbles are seen in the left atrium within three cardiac cycles of atrial opacification. Late appearance of bubbles in the left atrium may be secondary to transpulmonary flow. A crude quantification of the PFO is possible with small shunt defined as 3 to 10 bubbles, medium shunt as 10 to 20 bubbles, and large shunt as >20 bubbles. Contrast study can diagnose PFO at normal respiration pattern, but in patients with high suspicion for PFO with negative color Doppler flow and negative contrast study, provocative tests might be needed to transiently increase the pressure in the RA over the left atrium. These provocative tests include coughing, straining, or most effectively the Valsalva maneuver. If Valsalva maneuver is performed successfully, the interatrial septum should bow transiently toward the left atrium.

QUESTION 64.6: The correct answer is B: At the release of Valsalva.

Valsalva maneuver is defined as forced expiration against a closed glottis. This increase in intrathoracic pressure during the maneuver decreases the venous return and consequently the right atrial pressure. At the release of the Valsalva the intrathoracic pressure suddenly drops and the pressure gradient produces a marked increase in the venous return and a transient increase in the right atrial pressure. This is manifested on TEE as bowing of the interatrial septum toward the left atrium. Because of the physiology described, answers A, C, and D are incorrect as they are not reliably associated with a positive right atrial to LA pressure gradients.

QUESTION 64.7: The correct answer is A: Positive PFO.

The saline agitation test with a provocative test (Valsalva maneuver) is positive for PFO. In addition, the 2D and the color Doppler images were suspicious though not diagnostic in themselves. The incidence of PFO has been reported in an autopsy study to be around 27%, while the intraoperative incidentally discovered PFO has been reported to be 17%. The decision to repair an incidentally discovered PFO during cardiac surgery is complex and depends on the patient's medical history and the surgical operation. Surgeons are more tempted to correct PFO in younger patients, patients with history of cerebrovascular accidents, transient ischemic attacks, or during mitral or TV surgery. Surgical correction of PFO requires change of venous cannulation from two-stage venous cannula to bicaval cannulation; it may prolong the duration of CPB and may increase the risk of transient postoperative AFib.

Persistent left superior vena cava is a rare congenital anomaly with an incidence of 0.3% of general population. It results from failure of regression of left anterior and common cardinal veins and left sinus horn. It connects to the RA through the CS in 90% of the cases. It is diagnosed by echocardiography by having a dilated CS (>2 cm in diameter) and appearance of air bubbles in the CS during a saline agitation test in any of the left upper extremity veins. In the case presented here, the saline agitation was injected through the RIJ vein.

TAKE-HOME LESSON:

Intraoperative diagnosis of PFO requires understanding several echocardiographic modalities including 2D, color Doppler flow and the use of contrast ultrasound with provocative tests.

SUGGESTED READING

Hagen PT, Scholz DG, Edwards WD. Incidence and size of patent foramen ovale during the first 10 decades of life: an autopsy study of 965 normal hearts. *Mayo Clin Proc.* 1984;59(1):17–20.

Konstadt SN, Louie EK, Black S, et al. Intraoperative detection of patent foramen ovale by transesophageal echocardiography. *Anesthesiology.* 1991;74(2):212–216.

Krasuski RA, Hart SA, Allen D, et al. Prevalence and repair of intraoperatively diagnosed patent foramen ovale and association with perioperative outcomes and long-term survival. *JAMA.* 2009;302(3):290–297.

Maslow A, Perrino AC. Principles and technology of two-dimensional echocardiography. In: Perrino AC, Reeves ST, eds. *A Practical Approach to Transesophageal Echocardiography.* 2nd ed. Philadelphia: Lippincott Williams & Wilkins; 2007.

Stewart MJ. Contrast echocardiography. *Heart.* 2003; 89(3):342–348.

CASE 65

A 65-year-old male with hypertension presented 4 days ago with anterior lateral ST segment elevation on his ECG. He now has acute onset pulmonary edema and a new heart murmur. A TEE is performed (Fig. 65.1, Video 65.1).

QUESTION 65.1. What is the diagnosis?

A. Acute TR
B. Acute MR
C. Acute ASD
D. Acute VSD

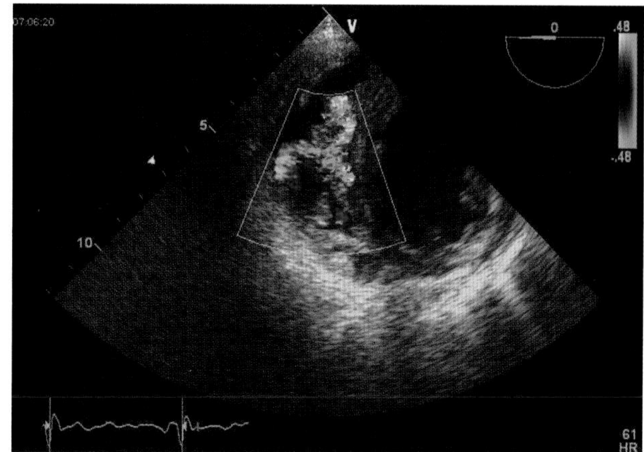

Figure 65.1.

QUESTION 65.2. The total extent of the VSD was unable to be evaluated with TEE. What other options are available intraoperatively?

A. Epiaortic scanning
B. Epicardial scanning
C. MRI
D. CT

QUESTION 65.3. The patient undergoes epicardial scanning. The VSD is visualized in Figure 65.2 and Videos 65.2 and 65.3.

This image plane is called

A. Epicardial LV LAX
B. Epicardial two-chamber
C. Epicardial LV basal SAX
D. Epicardial LV mid SAX

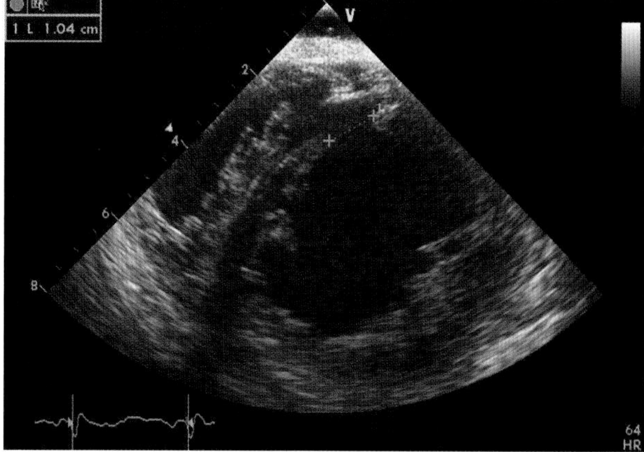

Figure 65.2.

ANSWERS AND DISCUSSION

QUESTION 65.1: The correct answer is D: Acute VSD.

Maillier et al. described the usefulness of TEE in evaluating patients suspected of having a post-infarction VSD. In a prospective study of 15 consecutive patients, TEE was able to identify septal ruptures in 14 out of 15 patients.[1] The VSD was directly visualized in the TG SAX view in all patients and the transesophageal imaging planes in only seven patients. TEE was concordant with intraoperative finding with regards to the number, size, type, location, and associated lesions. This TG view does not demonstrate the TV, MV, or atrial septum, thus making these answers incorrect.

QUESTION 65.2: The correct answer is B: Epicardial scanning.

Intraoperative TEE is the most commonly used technology but maybe unable to adequately evaluate an anterior muscular VSD due to poor visualization in the far field. Epicardial echocardiography is an excellent choice and allows high-resolution imaging in this location. In order to aid in visualization of the postinfarction VSD, a technical pearl is to ask the surgeon to palpate the thrill associated with the VSD and to place the probe on this area of the heart. Epiaortic imaging is totally confined to the aorta, but the epiaortic probe maybe useful for epicardial imaging. The other technologies, MRI and CT, are impractical in the OR.

QUESTION 65.3: The correct answer is D: Epicardial LV mid SAX. In 2007, The American Society of Echocardiography and the Society of Cardiovascular Anesthesiologists published guidelines for performing a comprehensive epicardial echocardiography examination.[2] Seven standard views were described with corresponding transthoracic nomenclature.

TAKE-HOME LESSON:

Epicardial imaging is an excellent technique to master when looking at anterior cardiac structures or when TEE is contraindicated.

REFERENCES

1. Maillier B, Metz D, Nazeyrollas P, et al. Value of transesophageal echocardiography in post-infarction septal ruptures. *Arch Mal Coeur Vaiss.* 1996;89:695–702.
2. Reeves ST, Glas KE, Eltzschig H, et al. Guidelines for performing a comprehensive epicardial echocardiography examination: recommendations of the American Society of Echocardiography and the Society of Cardiovascular Anesthesiologists. *Anesth Analg.* 2007;105:22–28.

CASE 66

A 63-year-old man with essential hypertension and severe MR treated with an angiotensin converting enzyme (ACE) inhibitor presents to the OR for a repair of his MV. After induction of anesthesia, the TEE images shown in Figures 66.1 to 66.3 are obtained.

QUESTION 66.1. The images are most consistent with

A. Mild MR
B. Moderate MR
C. Severe MR
D. There is no problem with the valve, you should wake him up and go to the golf course

QUESTION 66.2. Based upon these images, your diagnosis of the MV pathology is

A. Leaflet restriction
B. Leaflet prolapse
C. Annular dilatation
D. Functional regurgitation

QUESTION 66.3. To confirm your diagnosis and localize the pathology, which additional cross sections of the MV should you obtain?

A. ME mid-commissural view (60 degrees)
B. ME 2CH view (90 degrees)
C. ME LAX (120 degrees)
D. TG basal short axis (0 degree)
E. All of the above

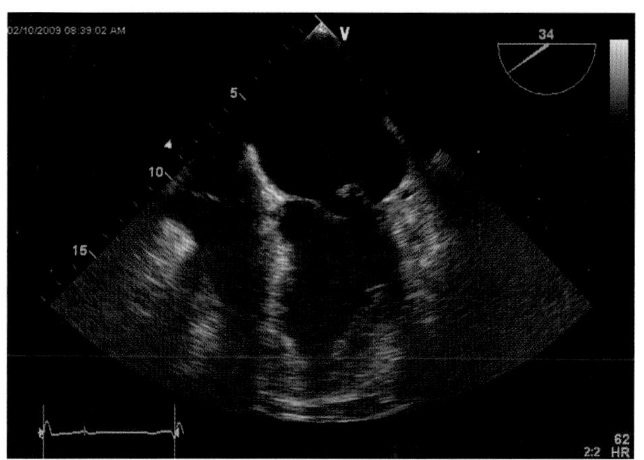

Figure 66.1. ME 4CH view, 2D. See also Video 66.1.

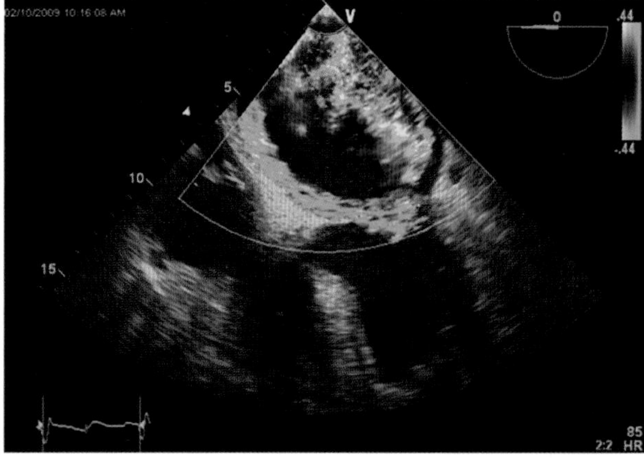

Figure 66.2. ME 4CH view with CFD. See also Video 66.2.

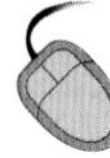

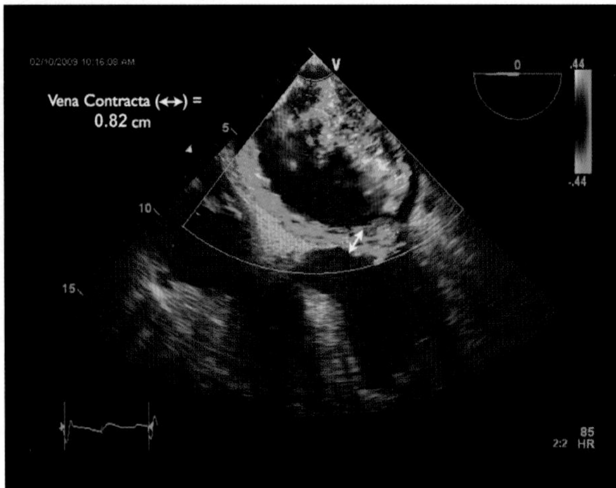

Figure 66.3. ME 4CH view with CFD and measurement of vena contracta.

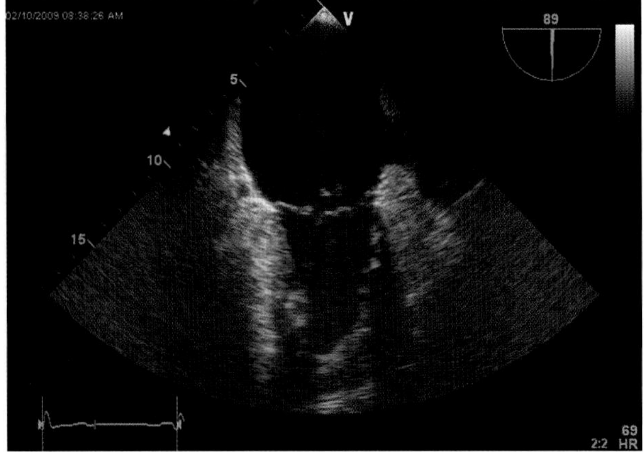

Figure 66.4. ME mid-commissural view, 2D. See also Video 66.3.

QUESTION 66.4. Using Figures 66.1 and 66.4 and Videos 66.1 and 66.3, *which segment* of the MV is most likely affected?

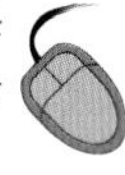

A. P1

B. P2

C. P3

D. A2

QUESTION 66.5. What is the most appropriate way for the surgeon to correct this patient's problem?

A. Replace the valve

B. Repair the valve by resecting the diseased segment and placing an annular ring

C. Place an annular ring without any leaflet repair

D. Place a cardiac support device

ANSWERS AND DISCUSSION

QUESTION 66.1: The correct answer is C: Severe MR. CFD interrogation with an aliasing velocity of 0.44 m/s, combined with a vena contracta of 0.82 cm, indicates severe MR. The length of the anteriorly directed jet shown in Figures 66.2 and 66.3, which travels up the anterior leaflet of the MV extending to the top of the left atrium, also indicates severe MR. The characteristic wall-hugging jet is created by the *Coanda effect.* This is a physical principle by which jets directed toward a wall will track tightly along the wall's surface rather than spread into the cavity and they will appear smaller than regurgitant jets directed centrally. A wall-hugging jet should always be considered *severe until proven otherwise.* Figure 66.3 demonstrates the measurement of the *vena contracta*. This is the narrowest point of the regurgitant jet at its base, and it is frequently used to grade the severity of MR. A vena contracta width of 0.3 cm is associated with mild, 0.3 to 0.69 cm moderate, and ≥0.7 cm severe MR.

QUESTION 66.2: The correct answer is B: Leaflet prolapse.

Carpentier classified MR based on leaflet motion (Fig. 66.6). Leaflets whose tips project above the mitral annulus, as in this case, are said to be *prolapsing*. In Figure 66.5, the arrow points to the prolapsing posterior leaflet. Answers A (*leaflet restriction*) and C (*annular dilatation*) are incorrect: in MR caused by leaflet restriction and annular dilatation, the leaflet tips remain at or below the annulus. Note that mitral annular dilatation may develop as a result of LV volume overload in chronic MR of *any etiology*, but it is not the main reason for MR in this particular patient. Finally, answer D (*functional*

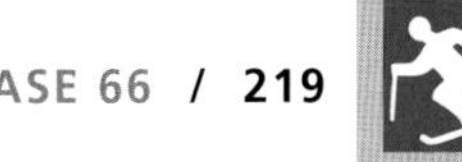

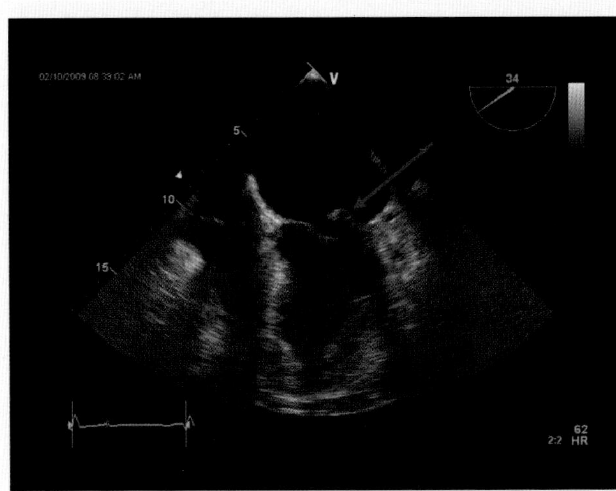

Figure 66.5. ME 4CH view, 2D, with arrow.

regurgitation) is incorrect: In functional MR, the mitral leaflets are usually structurally normal, but because of LV dysfunction, there is posterior and apical displacement of the papillary muscle, resulting in *tethering* of the mitral leaflets and central MR (see Cases 89 and 105 for a detailed discussion of this topic).

QUESTION 66.3: The correct answer is E: All of the above. Creating a mental 3D representation of the MV from 2D images requires obtaining images in multiple imaging planes.

QUESTION 66.4: The correct answer is B: P2. By viewing the ME 4CH and mid-commissural views, it becomes clear that this lesion is isolated to P2, the middle scallop of the posterior leaflet. In the four-chamber view, the posterior leaflet is displayed on the right side of the screen. In that view, one most often sees the A2 and P2 segments, but anteflection of the probe will reveal the A1/P1 segments while retroflection will move the scanning plane toward the A3/P3 segments (Fig. 66.7A). In the ME commissural view, one typically sees the P3, A2, and P1 segments, but when P2 is prolapsed, it will appear above A2 in the same cross section.

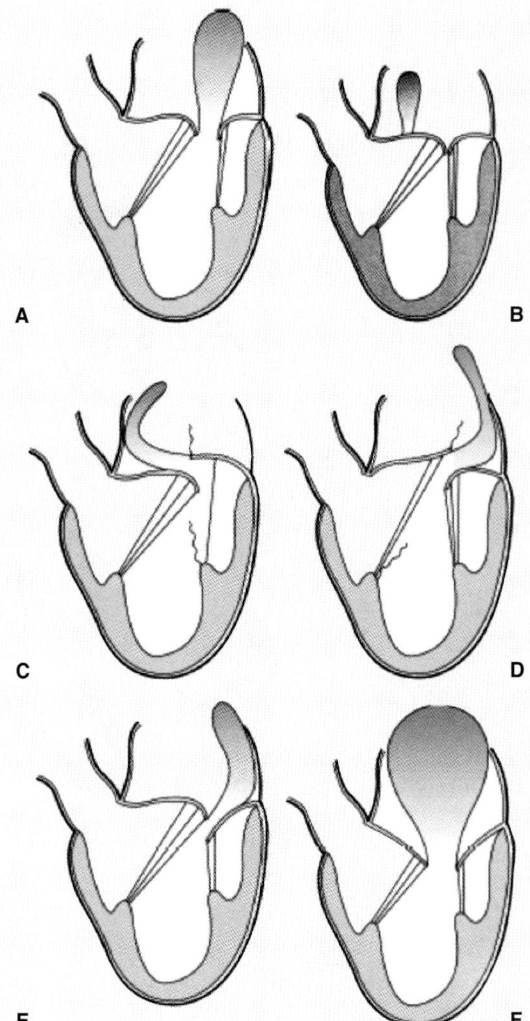

Figure 66.6. Carpentier's classification of MR based on leaflet motion. In type 1, the leaflet motion is normal and the MR jet tends to be central. In type 2, there is excessive leaflet motion and the MR jet is typically directed away from the diseased leaflet. In type 3 lesion, the leaflet motion is restricted and is further subdivided into type 3a (structural) and 3b (functional). In type 3 lesions, the regurgitant jet maybe directed away from the diseased leaflet if only one leaflet is affected, or it may be central if both mitral leaflets are equally affected. (From Perrino AC, Reeves ST, eds. *A Practical Approach to Transesophageal Echocardiography.* 2nd ed. 2008, with permission.)

QUESTION 66.5: The correct answer is B: Repair the valve by resecting the diseased segment and placing an annular ring. The patient with isolated posterior leaflet prolapse is best served by having a MV repair. Valve repair, when possible, is preferable to MV replacement. Isolated P2 prolapse is one of the easiest MV lesions to repair and, in the hands of an experienced surgeon, it has a very high success rate. Answer A (*valve replacement*) is incorrect: MV replacement is rarely required for this type of lesion. The most common repair technique is a *triangular* or *quadrangular* resection of the diseased segment, with or without a *sliding annuloplasty,* followed by a placement of an *annuloplasty ring* (Fig. 66.8). Answer C (*placement of a ring alone*) is incorrect: placement of an annuloplasty ring alone is often used in MR caused by a dilated mitral annulus, or in functional MR, but it would not be appropriate in this case. Finally, answer D is incorrect: *a cardiac support device* is an experimental device that is placed over the epicardial surface of the heart much like a sock. It is designed to constrict the heart and is used in the setting of a dilated cardiomyopathy. Again, it would not be enough in this case.

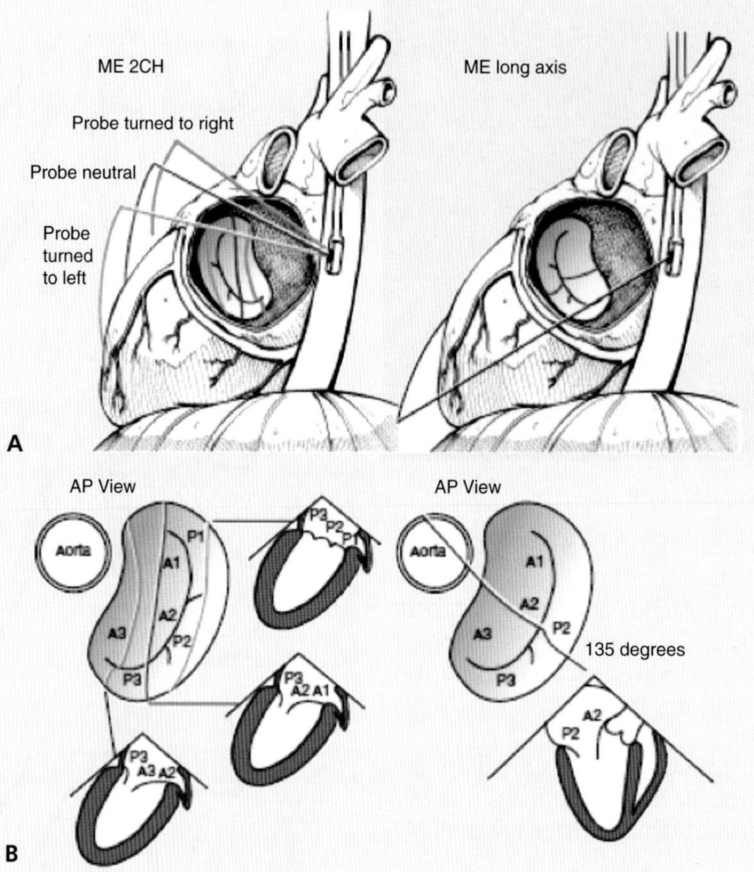

Figure 66.7. How the MV is sliced at multiple scan angles. (From Perrino AC, Reeves ST, eds. *A Practical Approach to Transesophageal Echocardiography*. 2nd ed. 2008, with permission.)

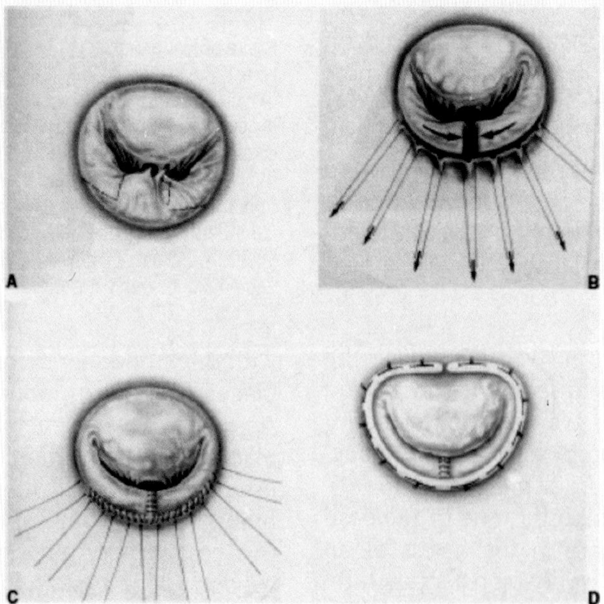

Figure 66.8. Illustrated MV repair with resection of the diseased segment (P2), a sliding annuloplasty, and placement of an annular ring. (From Jebara VA, Mihaileanu S, Acar C, et al. Left ventricular outflow tract obstruction after MV repair: results of the sliding leaflet technique. *Circulation*. 1992;88:30–34, with permission.)

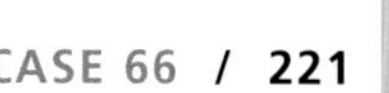

TAKE-HOME LESSON:

The MV examination requires multiple imaging planes in order to convey critical functional and structural anatomy to the surgeon. Prolapse of the P2 scallop of the MV is the most common structural causes of MR and it has a very high rate of successful repair.

SUGGESTED READING

Jebara VA, Mihaileanu S, Acar C, et al. Left ventricular outflow tract obstruction after mitral valve repair: results of the sliding leaflet technique. *Circulation.* 1992;88:30–34.

Lambert AS. Mitral regurgitation. In: Perrino AC, Reeves ST, eds. *A Practical Approach to Transesophageal Echocardiography.* Philadelphia: Lippincott Williams & Wilkins; 2008:171–188.

Starling, RC, Jessup M, Oh JK, et al. Sustained benefits of the CorCap cardiac support device on left ventricular remodeling: three year follow-up results from the Acorn clinical trial. *Ann Thorac Surg.* 2007;84(4): 1236–1242.

Moderate

CASE 67

A 78-year-old woman presented with symptomatic bradycardia, upper abdominal pain, nausea, and vomiting. ECG findings were consistent with inferior wall Q waves and ST elevation. She was intubated because of persistent hypotension and required vasoactive medications to maintain a systolic arterial pressure in the nineties. An emergent TEE was performed.

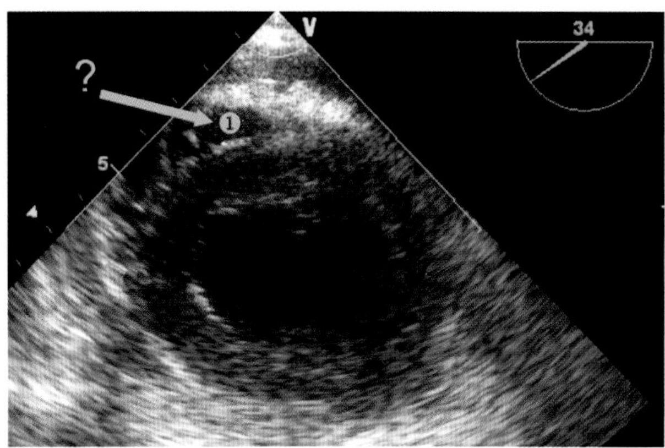

Figure 67.1.

QUESTION 67.1. Figure 67.1 shows a TG view of the LV. Where is the number "1" located?

A. In a pericardial effusion
B. In the CS
C. In the RV
D. In the right pulmonary vein

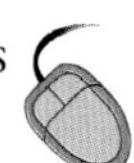

QUESTION 67.2. Additional information is given in Video 67.1. What is the diagnosis?

A. Normal blood flow within the LV
B. An VSD
C. HOCM
D. Pseudoaneurysm of the LV

QUESTION 67.3. The patient's arterial blood pressure is 90/50. From the data in Figure 67.2 (maximum velocity indicated is 2.5 m/s), what is the RV systolic pressure?

A. 115 mm Hg
B. 75 mm Hg
C. 65 mm Hg
D. 25 mm Hg

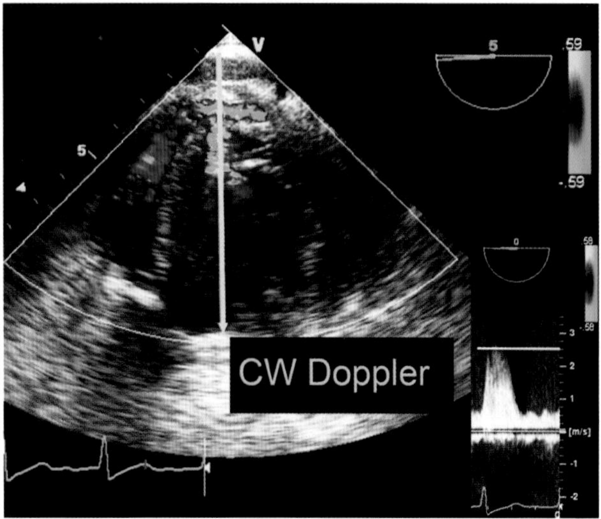

Figure 67.2.

Moderate

ANSWERS AND DISCUSSION

QUESTION 67.1: The correct answer is C. The number "1" is located in the RV.

ANSWER A: It is helpful to identify the epicardium (the bright, echogenic line at the top of the sector image) and follow it as it transitions from the left to the RV. This proves that the cavity space denoted with the number "1" is intracardiac. Since it is located within the heart, it can therefore not be in the pericardial space, so answer A—pericardial effusion—is incorrect.

ANSWER B: The usual tomographic planes to visualize the CS are a modified ME 4CH view or the bicaval view (the CS is seen in long axis) or at the top of the basal inferior segment in the ME 2CH view (the CS is imaged in cross section). Therefore, answer B)—CS—is also incorrect.

ANSWER D: The pulmonary veins are imaged at the level of the AV in the ME views. Therefore, answer D—right pulmonary vein—is also incorrect.

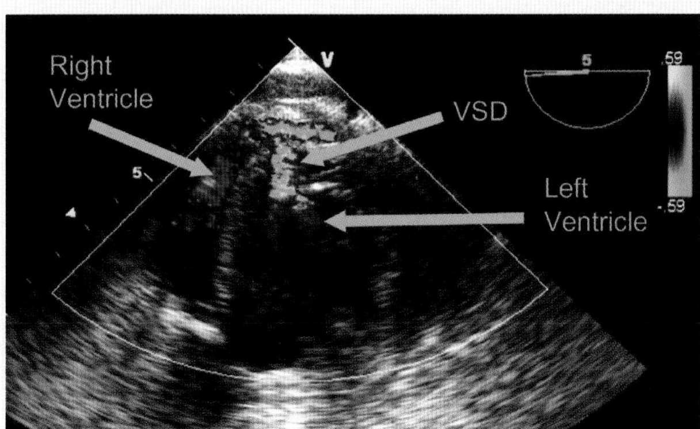

Figure 67.3.

QUESTION 67.2: The correct diagnosis is B: An inter-VSD.

ANSWER A: In the deep TG view shown in Video 67.1, there is clearly blood flowing from the LV to the RV (Fig. 67.3), which is not a part of normal LV blood flow. Therefore, answer A is incorrect.

ANSWER C: TEE is usually superior to transthoracic echo in identifying postinfarct disruptions of the ventricular septum. The TG views tend to image breaks in the inferior and inferolateral (posterior) septum better than ME views. Anterior septal ruptures are usually best seen in the ME views. In either case, it is important to place CFD over the region of interest, as small breaks may be difficult to find. Answer C—HOCM—is incorrect because although the myocardium appears to be thickened, the typical features of dynamic obstruction of the LVOT are not present.

ANSWER D: Answer D—A pseudoaneurysm—has a saclike appearance and is a discontinuity of the ventricular wall, but is not a complete rupture. There, answer D is also incorrect.

QUESTION 67.3: The correct answer is C: 65 mm Hg. The simplified Bernoulli equation ($\Delta P = 4V^2$) can be used to find the pressure difference between two cardiac chambers. In this particular case, Figure 67.2 indicates that CW Doppler was placed through the VSD, yielding a maximum velocity of 2.5 m/s. The difference between the right and LV is then $[4 \times (2.5 \text{ m/s})^2] = 25$ mm Hg. Since the CW Doppler signal is above the baseline, indicating flow toward the transducer, the higher pressure is in the LV, which was stated to be 90 mm Hg during systole. The RV pressure is therefore 25 mm Hg, or $90 - 25 = 65$ mm Hg.

TAKE-HOME LESSON:

Ventricular septal rupture is a rare complication of myocardial infarction, best imaged in TG views utilizing CFD echocardiography. The direction of blood flow is usually from the LV to the RV.

SUGGESTED READING

Burke AP, Virmani R. Pathophysiology of acute myocardial infarction. *Med Clin N Am.* 2007;91: 553–572.

Obarski TR, Rogers PJ, Dcbaets DL, et al. Assessment of postinfarction ventricular septal ruptures by transesophageal Doppler echocardiography. *J Am Soc Echocardiogr.* 1998;8:728–734.

Moderate

CASE 68

A 61-year-old morbidly obese woman undergoes a MV replacement for rheumatic mitral stenosis. Her comorbidities include obstructive sleep apnea, chronic renal insufficiency, and AFib. A 31 mm mechanical bileaflet prosthesis is inserted uneventfully and the postoperative course is uneventful. The patient is anticoagulated with warfarin and discharged home. Three weeks postoperatively, she returns to the hospital with severe CHF. Following readmission to the ICU, the TEE images shown in Figures 68.1 to 68.3 are obtained:

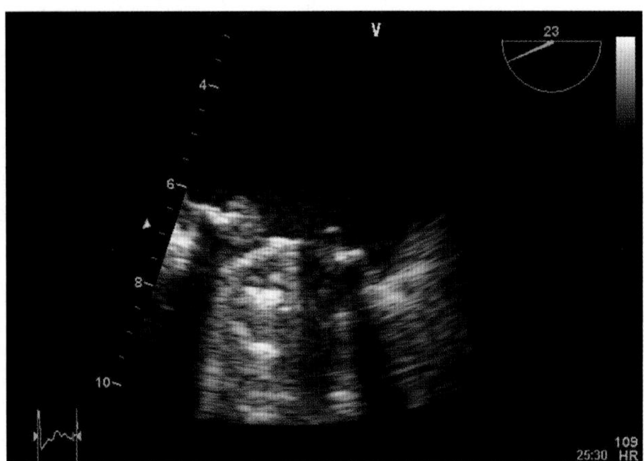

Figure 68.1. ME 4CH view (modified) of the MV prosthesis in *diastole*. See also Video 68.1.

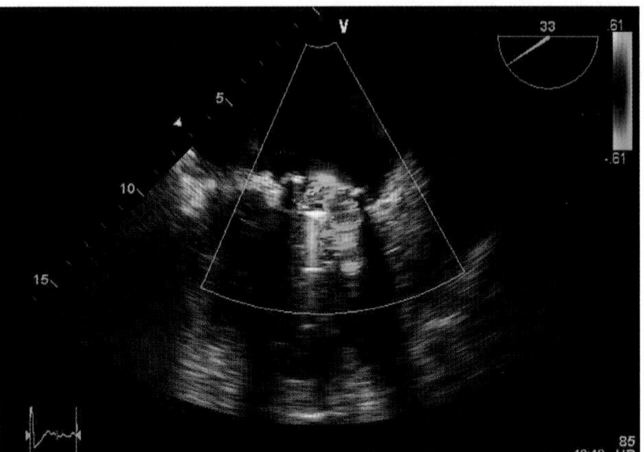

Figure 68.2. ME 4CH view (modified) of the MV prosthesis *in diastole*, with CFD. See also Video 68.2.

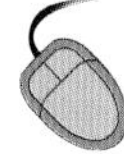

QUESTION 68.1. Based on Figures 68.1 to 68.3, what abnormality of the mitral prosthesis is likely to explain the patient's clinical deterioration?

A. There is no abnormality of the mitral prosthesis
B. Dehiscence of the mitral prosthesis
C. Obstruction of the mitral prosthesis
D. Acute perforation of the mitral prosthesis

QUESTION 68.2. Which of the following conditions *could be consistent* with Figures 68.1 to 68.3?

A. Pannus formation
B. Thrombosis
C. Endocarditis
D. All of the above

QUESTION 68.3. Which of the following statements is *true* regarding the differentiation of thrombus from pannus formation in obstructed mechanical valve prostheses?

A. Thrombosis is much more common than pannus formation
B. A history of inadequate anticoagulation suggests thrombus rather than pannus

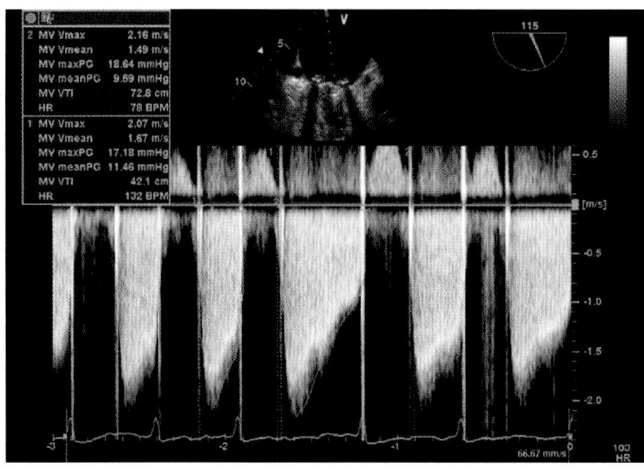

Figure 68.3. CW Doppler of the MV prosthesis.

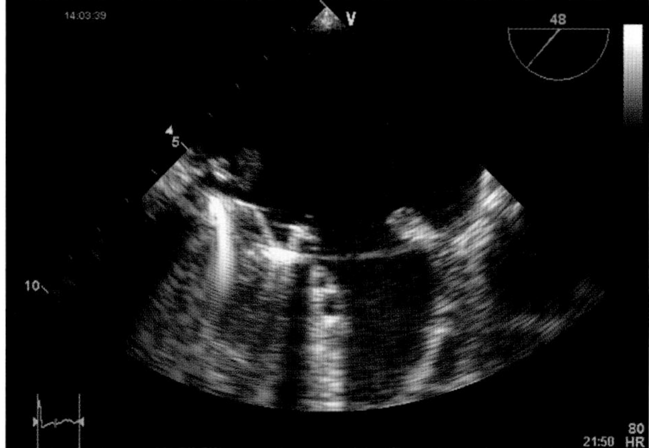

Figure 68.4. ME 4CH view (modified) of the mitral prosthesis 30 minutes after administration of tPA. See also Video 68.3.

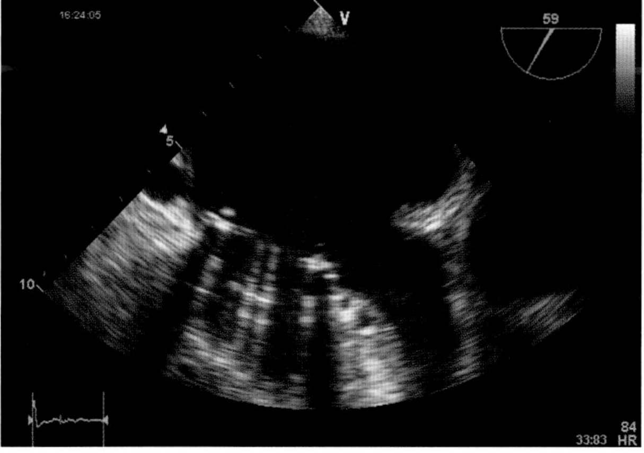

Figure 68.5. ME view (modified) of the mitral prosthesis, approximately 3 hours after administration of tPA. See also Video 68.4.

C. Thrombosis is associated with a shorter duration of time from valve insertion to malfunction

D. All of the above statements are true

The patient's condition deteriorates rapidly, requiring intubation and large doses of inotropic and vasopressor support. She becomes anuric, hypoxemic, and severely acidotic, with a serum lactate of 15 mmol/L. Her International Normalized Ratio (INR) rises to 6.4. Initial workup rules out heparin-induced thrombocytopenia (HIT).

QUESTION 68.4. Given the clinical scenario, what is the recommended management of this patient?

A. Immediate return to the OR for redo-MV replacement

B. Systemic thrombolysis

C. Correct the coagulopathy with fresh frozen plasma

D. Nothing can be done to reverse this condition

Given the extreme hemodynamic instability and profound acidosis and coagulopathy, it is felt that the patient is at too high risk for surgery and thrombolysis is attempted. Figure 68.4 and Video 68.3 show the mitral prosthesis 30 minutes following administration of systemic tissue plasminogen activator (tPA). Figure 68.5 and Video 68.3 show the same mitral prosthesis approximately 3 hours following administration of tPA.

QUESTION 68.5. Given the images in Figures 68.5 and 68.6, and Video 68.4, what would you do now?

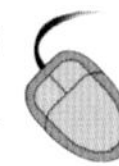

A. Immediately send the patient to the OR for emergency MV replacement

B. Schedule the patient for a semi-elective redo-MV surgery in 2 weeks

C. Conservative management—there appears to be complete resolution of the situation

D. Repeat the thrombolysis after 24 hours

The patient's condition improved markedly over the next 48 hours; she was extubated 3 days after thrombolysis and she was discharged from the ICU.

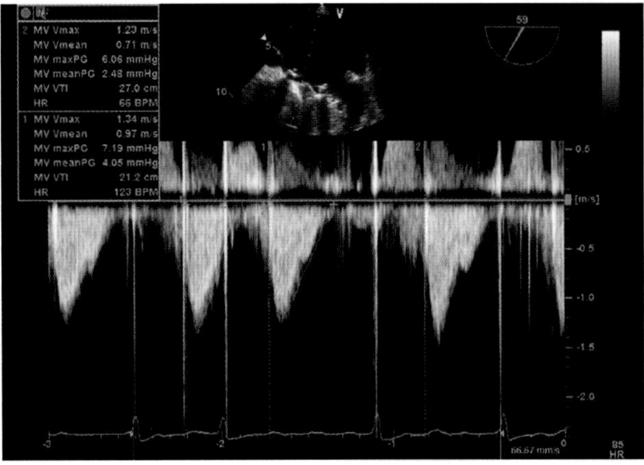

Figure 68.6. CW Doppler of the MV after administration of tPA.

ANSWERS AND DISCUSSION

QUESTION 68.1: The correct answer is C: Obstruction of the mitral prosthesis. On Figure 68.1 and Video 68.1, one can see a mass obstructing the left orifice of the mitral prosthesis. One of the two leaflets is clearly immobile, resulting in aliasing CFD through the other orifice in Figure 68.2 and Video 68.2. The mass can be described as *soft tissue density*, with a diameter of about 2 cm. It seems attached to the prosthetic leaflet and the sewing ring. Hemodynamically, the clinical picture is that of mitral stenosis, and the degree is at least moderate to severe, based on a mean diastolic gradient of 9.6 to 11.4 mm Hg (Fig. 68.3). Answer B is incorrect: prosthetic dehiscence presents as a MR (usually severe) and abnormal movement of the mitral sewing ring, often described as "rocking" of the valve. This valve is well seated. Answer D is also incorrect: perforation can occur in bioprosthetic valves but does not apply to mechanical valves.

QUESTION 68.2: The correct answer is D: All of the above. The differential diagnosis of a prosthetic obstruction includes thrombosis, pannus formation, and endocarditis. Any of these conditions could theoretically produce the echocardiographic images presented here. In this case, the clinical scenario is most consistent with acute thrombosis of the mitral prosthesis. Pannus formation, a fibrous tissue ingrowth that can develop on prosthetic valves, tends to take many months to develop and it is unlikely within 3 weeks of surgery. Acute endocarditis could present as a valve obstruction, but more commonly it affects the sewing ring and results in dehiscence of the prosthesis. This patient is most likely suffering from acute thrombosis of MV. Of all types of valves, mechanical valves in the mitral position have the highest risk of thrombosis, a catastrophic complication that carries a high mortality rate. For that reason, constant and carefully monitored anticoagulation of all mechanical mitral prostheses is paramount. The AHA/ACC guidelines recommend maintaining an INR of 2.5 to 3.5 for all mechanical prostheses in the mitral position. Patients with a coagulation abnormality, such as HIT, are at particularly high risk for valve thrombosis.

QUESTION 68.3: The correct answer is D: All of the above statements are TRUE.

The distinction of thrombus from pannus on obstructed prosthetic valves is important, especially since thrombolysis has emerged in recent years as an alternative to surgery. Although no single criterion by *itself* is enough to make a diagnosis, several factors can help the clinician differentiate between the two. One review of 24 obstructed prosthetic valves that were inspected surgically[1] revealed that the time from initial valve replacement to valve obstruction was almost three times longer in pannus formation than thrombosis (178 vs. 62 months). A history of inadequate anticoagulation was also four times more common in thrombosis than pannus formation. However, the functional status of the patients was similar (and generally poor) in both the cases. Hemodynamically, the valve gradients and effective valve areas were similar, although thrombosis seemed to be more common in the mitral position, while pannus formation occurred more frequently in aortic prostheses. Echocardiographically, the leaflet motion was abnormal in all patients with thrombosis, but only in 60% of patients with pannus. And although the *size* and *mobility* of the mass seen by TEE were similar in both the diseases, the *echo density* tended to be higher in pannus than thrombus: 92% of thrombi had the same tissue density as myocardium, while only 29%

of pannus formations were described as "soft tissue" density. Along with the timing of onset and the anticoagulation status, the echo density of the mass was the most reliable indicator of thrombus versus pannus formation.

QUESTION 68.4: The correct answer is B: systemic thrombolysis. Given the high likelihood that this lesion is a thrombus and given the severe cardiogenic shock, an immediate return to surgery would likely carry a high mortality. A review of 39 reoperations for mitral prosthetic thrombosis reported a 64% mortality.[2] Thrombolysis has emerged as a reasonably low risk and effective alternative to surgery, and it is recommended as first-line treatment for prosthetic valve thrombosis, especially in critically ill patients. In a series of 68 thrombosed prosthetic valves,[3] thrombolysis provided complete resolution in 85% of patients, partial resolution in 6%, and failure of treatment in 9%. Major hemorrhage was reported in two patients and rethrombosis occurred in 11 patients (all of whom, except one, were successfully rethrombolysed). An older but similar study found identical results: 83% of 12 patients with prosthetic valve thrombosis were successfully treated with thrombolytic therapy.[4]

QUESTION 68.5: The correct answer is C: Conservative management, there appears to be complete resolution of the situation. Figure 68.4 and Video 68.3 show that the clot has partially dissolved 30 minutes after administration of tPA. At 3 hours post-tPA (Fig. 68.5 and Video 68.4), one can see that the mass has completely disappeared and both leaflets of the mitral prosthesis are moving well (although one cannot completely rule out embolization of some fragments, hopefully they have dissolved as well with systemic tPA). Figure 68.6 shows an acceptable mean gradient of 2.48 mm Hg across the valve, suggesting that the obstruction has been eliminated. Appropriate management at this stage would be to maintain proper anticoagulation and closely watch for hemorrhagic complications. Answers A and B are incorrect: There appears to be complete resolution of the obstruction, so there is no need for repeat surgery, now or in 2 weeks. Furthermore, surgery immediately after thrombolysis would carry a high risk of massive bleeding, but it may be the only option left in infrequent cases where thrombolysis is unsuccessful. Finally, answer D is incorrect: repeat thrombolysis would only be indicated if the thrombosis recurs after a successful initial treatment.

TAKE-HOME LESSON:

Prosthetic valve obstruction is a serious complication, which can present as heart failure. TEE is important in identifying the obstruction, but the differential diagnosis depends on the timing and clinical presentation, and a careful history is crucial in diagnosing the cause. The treatment is most often surgical, although thrombolysis can be considered in selected cases.

REFERENCES

1. Barbetseas J, Nagueh SF, Pitsavos C, et al. Differentiating thrombus from pannus formation in obstructed mechanical prosthetic valves: an evaluation of clinical, transthoracic and transesophageal echocardiographic parameters. *J Am Coll Cardiol.* 1998;32:1410–1417.
2. Caceres-Loriga FM, Pérez-López H, Morlans-Hernández K, et al. Thrombolysis as first choice therapy in prosthetic heart valve thrombosis. A study of 68 patients. *J Thromb Thrombolysis.* 2006;21(2):185–190.
3. Podesta A, Carmagnini E, Parodi E, et al. Thrombosis of mechanical valve prosthesis: thrombolysis vs surgical treatment. Report of two cases, personal experience and review of the literature. *Minerva Cardioangiol.* 2000;48(10):309–315.
4. Silber H, Khan SS, Matloff JM, et al. The St. Jude valve. Thrombolysis as the first line of therapy for cardiac valve thrombosis. *Circulation.* 1993;87: 30–37.

Moderate

CASE 69

A 49-year-old male with a history of myocardial infarction (Q waves in V3–V6 and I and aVL) was scheduled to undergo elective coronary revascularization. After tracheal intubation, a TEE probe was inserted and a comprehensive TEE examination was performed. The ME 4CH view is shown in Video 69.1.

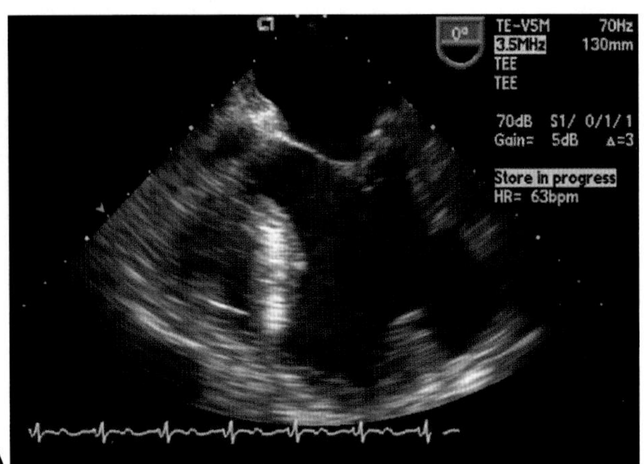

A

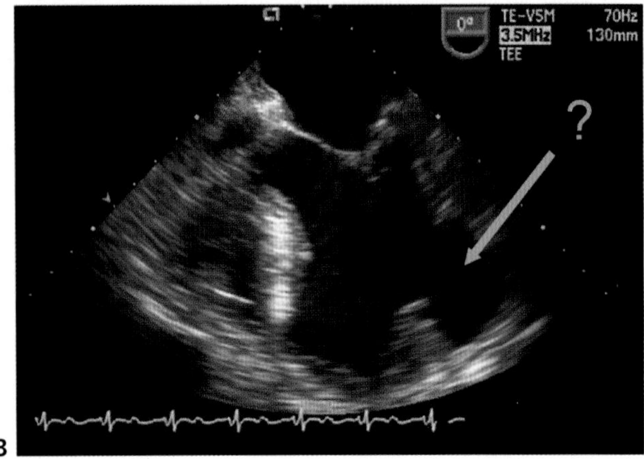

B

Figure 69.1.

QUESTION 69.1. What is the pathology highlighted by the arrow (Fig. 69.1)?

A. A pericardial effusion
B. A ventricular thrombus
C. A ventricular pseudoaneurysm
D. A ventricular diverticulum

QUESTION 69.2. All of the following distinguish a pseudoaneurysm from a true aneurysm *except*

A. A pseudoaneurysm does not contain all myocardial layers
B. The "neck" to maximal "sac" diameter ratio is smaller in a pseudoaneurysm
C. A pseudoaneurysm has an abrupt transition between normal and abnormal myocardium
D. All of the above statements are true

QUESTION 69.3. What is the proper treatment for this patient?

A. Percutaneous drainage of the collection
B. Conservative management, with β-blockers and afterload reduction
C. Coronary stent placement
D. Coronary revascularization and excision of the affected area

ANSWERS AND DISCUSSION

QUESTION 69.1: The correct answer is C. The arrow in Figure 69.1 is pointing to a ventricular pseudoaneurysm. Postmyocardial infarction rupture of the left ventricule is rare and is associated with sudden death. When there is a discontinuity of the ventricular wall that is contained by the surrounding tissues (epicardium or pericardium) a ventricular pseudoaneurysm is created. A LV pseudoaneurysm has the appearance of a sac, with an opening ("neck") communicating with the LV cavity. The aneurysmal cavity may demonstrate pulsation (shown in Video 69.1), with the pseudoaneurysm size increasing in systole, contrary to the ventricular cavity that decreases. Sometimes the application of DTI may be of assistance in making the diagnosis, by colorizing the myocardial motion, not blood flow. Video 69.2 shows DTI of the pseudoaneurysm. In this case, the cavity can be seen surrounded by a thin layer of myocardium.

Pericardial effusion is an incorrect answer because the echolucent space communicates directly with the ventricular cavity. In a pericardial effusion there is clear separation between the epicardium and the pericardium by the pericardial collection. A LV thrombus is not specifically seen in Figure 69.1, although the presence of thrombus should be actively sought after in patients with a ventricular pseudoaneurysm. A ventricular diverticulum is a congenital anomaly not associated with coronary artery disease. A ventricular diverticulum has a narrow neck like a pseudoaneurysm, but also has contractile function and is characterized by systolic ejection of blood into the LV cavity, rather than systolic expansion as seen in a pseudoaneurysm.

QUESTION 69.2: The correct answer is D: All of the above statements are true.

There are several distinguishing characteristics between a "true" and a "pseudo" ventricular aneurysm. A pseudoaneurysm is a rupture of the ventricular wall that is contained by either epicardium or pericardium. A true ventricular aneurysm, on the other hand, contains all layers of the myocardium. Pseudoaneurysms are characterized by a narrow neck. The neck to maximal sac diameter is <0.5, as shown in Figure 69.2. True aneurysms usually have broad necks, with a neck to maximal sac diameter of >0.9. Because a pseudoaneurysm is a rupture of the ventricular wall, pseudoaneurysms have an abrupt transition between the aneurysmal sac and the normal myocardium. This transition tends to be much smoother in a true aneurysm.

QUESTION 69.3: The correct answer is D. This patient should undergo coronary revascularization and excision of the affected area. LV aneurysms and pseudoaneurysms are complications of myocardial infarction. They typically develop within 3 months of the event. LV pseudoaneurysms require surgical treatment, because the lack of myocardial fibers in the wall of the sac predisposes them to rupture. Leaving the weakened area alone, by using either medical treatment or revascularization, predisposes the patient to a catastrophic rupture. Drainage of the fluid collection would be used for a pericardial effusion.

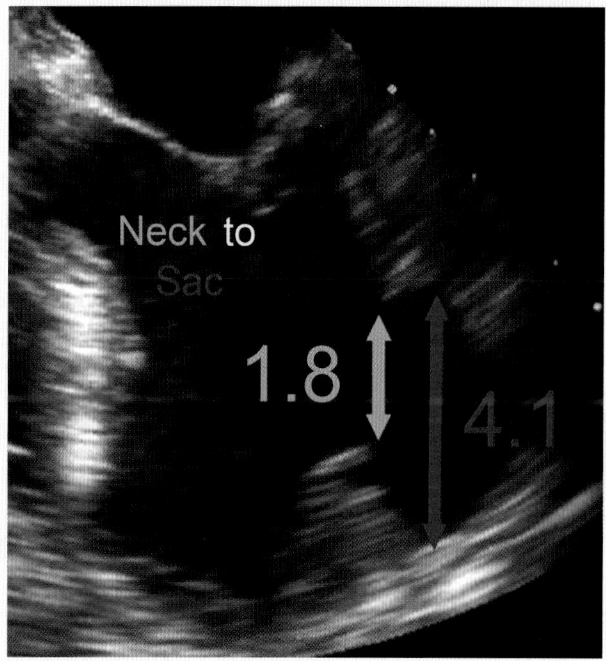

Figure 69.2.

TAKE-HOME LESSON:

A pseudoaneurysm can develop following a myocardial infarction and should be differentiated from a true aneurysm. They are prone to rupture and surgical resection of the aneurysmal sac is advisable.

SUGGESTED READING

Brown SL, Gropler RJ, Harris KM. Distinguishing left ventricular aneurysm from pseudoaneurysm. A review of the literature. *Chest.* 1997;111:1403–1409.

Cay S, Tufekcioglu O, Ozturk S, et al. Left ventricular diverticulum with contractile function in an unusual site. *J Am Soc Echocardiogr.* 2006;19:1293.33–1296.e6.

May BV, Reeves ST. Contained rupture of a left ventricular pseudoaneurysm. *Anesth Analg.* 2007;105:38–39.

Roelandt JRTC, Sutherland GR, Yoshida K, et al. Improved diagnosis and characterization of left ventricular pseudoaneurysm by Doppler color flow imaging. *J Am Coll Cardiol.* 1988;12:807–811.

Moderate

CASE 70

The following TEE was performed to evaluate a 69-year-old, 80-kg patient who became hemodynamically unstable during an exploratory laparotomy for unexplained ascites. The patient is otherwise healthy and total blood loss is estimated at 1500 cc. The anesthesiologist attempted to place a PA catheter but was unsuccessful. The CVP is noted to be elevated.

You place the TEE probe without difficulty. The first views obtained are shown in Figures 70.1 to 70.4.

QUESTION 70.1. What should be done next?

A. Abandon insertion of RIJ vein catheter
B. Proceed with insertion of RIJ vein catheter
C. Insert a central venous line via a femoral vein
D. Insert a central venous line via subclavian vein

QUESTION 70.2. The object identified by the * in image Figure 70.2 most likely represents

A. Thrombus
B. Atrial myxoma
C. Renal cell carcinoma (RCC)
D. Lipomatous infiltration of the interatrial septum

QUESTION 70.3. The most common cardiac tumor is

A. Atrial myxoma
B. Secondary (metastatic) malignant disease
C. Lipoma
D. Sarcom

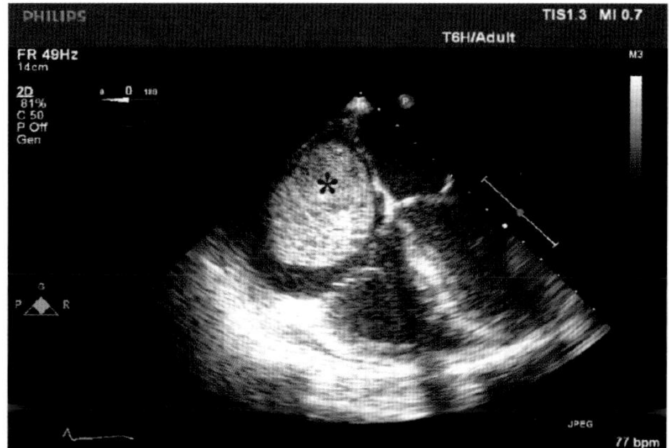

Figure 70.1.

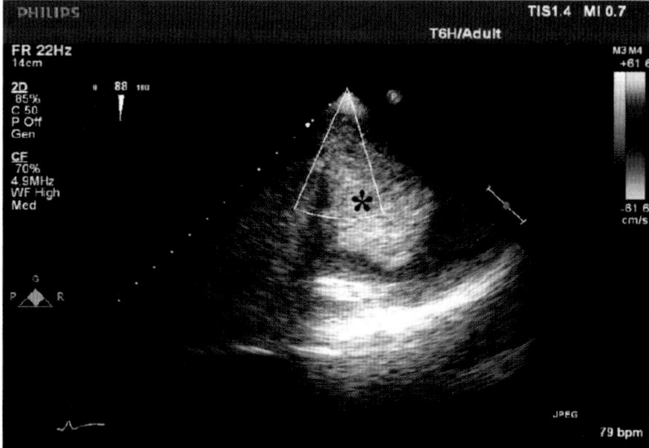

Figure 70.2.

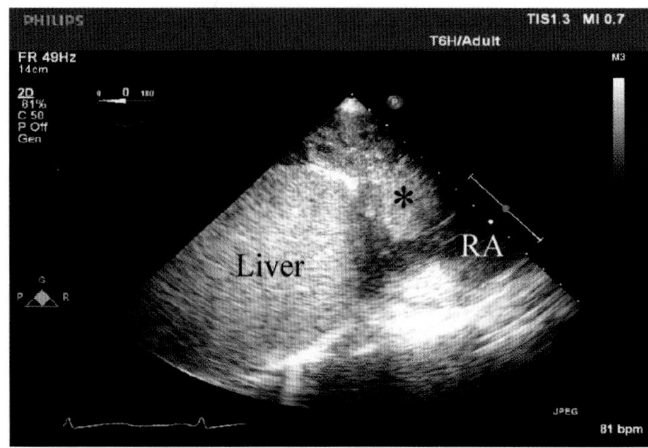

Figure 70.3.

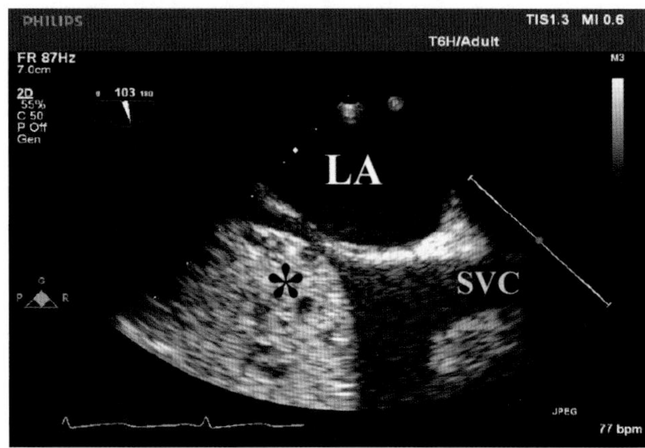

Figure 70.4.

ANSWERS AND DISCUSSION

QUESTION 70.1: The correct answer is B: Proceed with insertion of RIJ vein catheter.

As seen below, the most frequent cardiac tumors are myxomas (appearing with a frequency 3:1 in the left and RA, respectively) and extension/metastasis of tumors via the IVC (with the most frequent being a hypernephroma, or RCC). The patient needs to undergo resection of the tumor, and a central line is necessary for managing the potentially large fluid shifts that may occur during surgical resection. Insertion of a central venous line via a femoral vein will not be helpful, as frequently the IVC needs to be temporarily excluded during manual retraction of the tumor.

QUESTION 70.2: The correct answer is C: RCC.

One unique feature of RCC is its predilection for involvement of the venous system, which is found in 10% of RCCs, more often than in any other tumor type. Other tumors that frequently extend along the IVC into the RA include leiomyosarcoma, hepatoma, and Wilms tumor. While the patient in the above scenario did not carry a diagnosis of cancer, it is important to remember that these tumors are frequently discovered incidentally and should always be considered when evaluating cardiac masses.

In the ME 4CH view, several important observations can be made. Although the size of the mass is its most striking feature initially, other important characteristics to note include its mobility, lack of attachment to any of the walls of the RA, being encapsulated, and not passing through the TV or the fossa ovalis.

In the modified ME bicaval view the tumor is seen within the lumen of the intrahepatic IVC extending into the RA. While not always possible, one should attempt to determine if the mass is adherent to the IVC or simply lying within it. In the video, the tumor appears to be nonadherent. This is important to note as some tumors characteristically have several points of attachment to the IVC (leiomyosarcoma), while others typically are nonadherent (RCC, hepatoma).

In addition to fully characterizing the mass, it is important to perform a thorough examination of all cardiac structures to look for other cardiac anomalies, metastases, and so on. During resection, intraoperative TEE allows monitoring for embolization and positioning of cannula and occlusion balloons. Once resection is complete, intraoperative TEE is essential to look for residual tumor and IVC patency.

ANSWER A: Answer A—thrombus—is incorrect.

While thrombus is the most common etiology of an intracardiac mass in the vena cava and RA, several characteristics help differentiate thrombus from the tumor seen in these images. First, one must divide thrombi into two major categories: embolized thrombi from the deep venous system and thrombi that form in situ in the RA. Embolized thrombi from the deep veins appear as mobile serpiginous irregular masses that often resemble a "cast" of a deep vein. They do not appear well circumscribed or encapsulated. Thrombi that form in situ typically appear homogeneous on echo and appear to have a broad base of attachment to the right atrial wall. Further, they have mobile irregularities extending from their surface and do not appear to be encapsulated.

ANSWER B: Answer B—atrial myxoma—is incorrect.

Myxomas share many characteristics with the tumor seen in these images. They are well-circumscribed, heterogeneous, mobile masses that can sometimes obstruct the atrioventricular valve. Myxomas, however, arise from and are adherent to the atrium, most commonly at the interatrial septum. Myxomas have also been reported to be adherent to the posterior atrial wall, the anterior atrial wall, and the atrial appendage. The mass in the images above is not adherent to the atrium. While right atrial myxomas do occur, they represent only 15%–20% of myxomas with 80% to 85% occurring in the left atrium.

Answer D—lipomatous infiltration of the interatrial septum—is incorrect.

Lipomatous infiltration of the interatrial septum is seen echocardiographically as an echodense thickening of the septum that spares the fossa ovalis. This normal anatomic variant is frequently described as a dumbbell because of its characteristic shape.

QUESTION 70.3: The correct answer is B: Secondary (metastatic) malignant disease.

Secondary malignant disease involving the heart and pericardium is up to 1000 times more common than primary cardiac tumors. The cancers that most commonly metastasize to the heart include lung, breast, esophagus, stomach, kidney, melanoma, lymphoma, and leukemia. These tumors reach the heart by direct extension, hematogenous spread, lymphatic spread, and intraluminal venous extension. Within the group of primary cardiac tumors, myxomas are by far the most common tumor representing over one third of all primary tumors. Myxomas are benign cardiac tumors and are described above.

TAKE-HOME LESSON:

In renal cell carcinoma examine possible tumor extension into cardiac chambers.

SUGGESTED READING

Jadbabaie F. Cardiac masses and embolic sources. In: Perrino A, Reeves ST, eds. *A Practical Approach to Transesophageal Echocardiography.* 2nd ed. Philadelphia: Lippincott Williams & Wilkins; 2008:401–413.

Komanapalli CB, Tripathy U, Sokoloff M, et al. Intraoperative renal cell carcinoma tumor embolization to the right atrium: incidental diagnosis by transesophageal echocardiography. *Anesth Analg.* 2006;102: 378–379.

Martinelli SM, Mitchell JD, McCann RL, et al. Intraoperative transesophageal echocardiography diagnosis of residual tumor fragment after surgical removal of renal cell carcinoma. *Anesth Analg.* 2008;106:1633–1635.

Otto CM. *Practice of Clinical Echocardiography.* 3rd ed. Philadelphia: Saunders; 2007:1108–1128.

Moderate

CASE 71

A 65 year-old male underwent three-vessel CABG 6 hours ago. He is now in the ICU with the following vital signs: blood pressure 80/40 mm Hg, heart rate 71 beats per minute, CVP 24 mm Hg. His mediastinal output decreased from 50 mL/hour to 0 for the last hour. A TEE is performed, and video 71.1 is obtained.

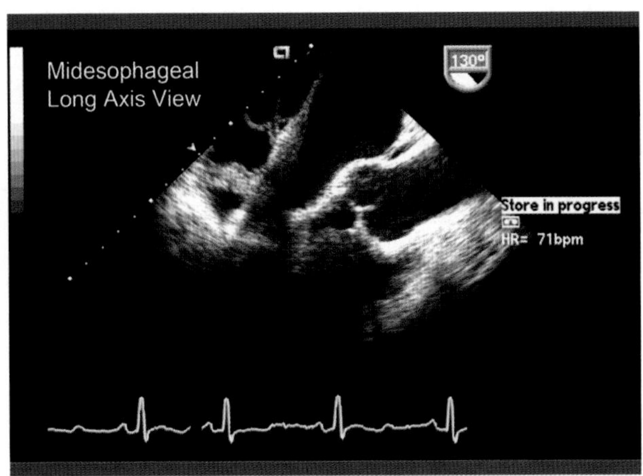

Figure 71.1.

QUESTION 71.1. The images in Video 71.1 and Figure 71.1 show a(n):

A. Left pleural effusion
B. Right pleural effusion
C. Posterior pericardial effusion
D. Anterior pericardial effusion
E. Pulmonary embolism in transit

QUESTION 71.2. The best treatment for this condition is a:

A. Left-sided thoracostomy tube
B. Right-sided thoracostomy tube
C. Pericardial drain
D. Return to the OR for exploration and washout
E. Return to the OR for pulmonary thromboembolectomy

Eighteen hours after resolution of the previous problem, the patient is noted to have ST segment elevation in leads V_3 to V_6. A second TEE exam yields the images found in Video 71.2 and Figure 71.2.

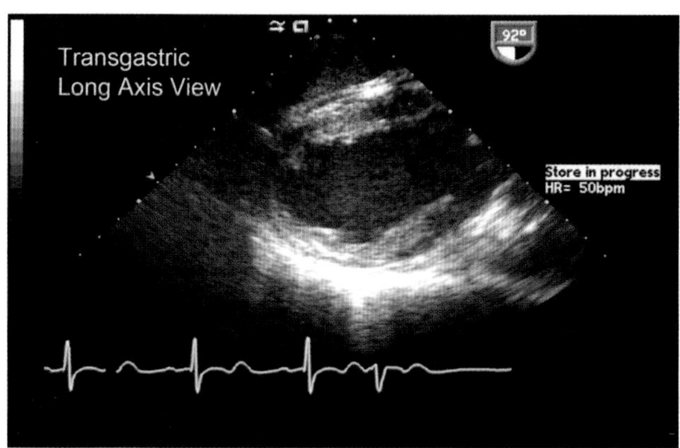

Figure 71.2.

QUESTION 71.3. Which of the following is the most likely diagnosis?

A. Takotsubo cardiomyopathy
B. Hypovolemia
C. Pericarditis
D. RV failure
E. Ventricular pseudoaneurysm

QUESTION 71.4. Which of the following is the most appropriate next step in management?

A. Perform cardiac catheterization
B. Administer 1-L fluid bolus
C. Administer indomethacin
D. Administer nitric oxide
E. Perform emergent surgical re-exploration

ANSWERS AND DISCUSSION

QUESTION 71.1: The correct answer is C. This image shows a posterior pericardial effusion. A number of clues to the diagnosis are apparent from the clinical picture. The patient is hypotensive and his mediastinal drain output has fallen precipitously. Additionally, his CVP is elevated. All of these findings are consistent with postoperative pericardial tamponade. The posterior walls of the LA and LV are compressed by accumulation of echo-free blood in the posterior pericardium, as shown in Figure 71.3. The echodensities in that space are the beginnings of thrombus formation. The pleural spaces are not included in this image. The small portion of the RV that is visible in this image does not show a pulmonary embolism in transit. This patient has a regional, specifically posterior, cardiac tamponade.

QUESTION 71.2: The correct answer is D. The most appropriate management for this patient involves a return to the OR for exploration and washout. It is important to recognize that just because the mediastinal drainage is minimal does not mean that there is not ongoing bleeding. A return to the OR will give the surgical team and the intensive care team an opportunity to determine the source of bleeding, control it, and

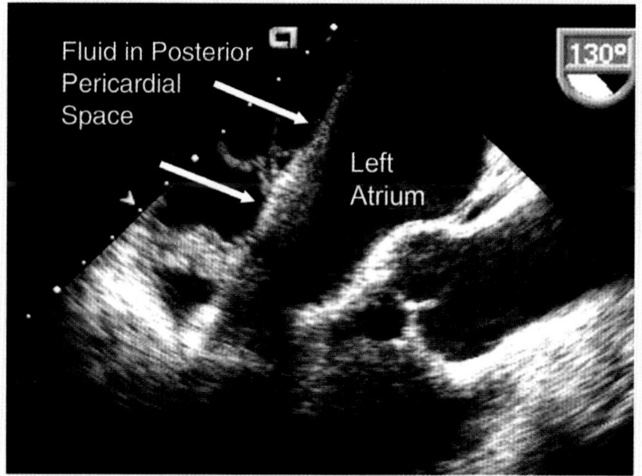

Figure 71.3.

prevent a life-threatening problem. It will also allow the opportunity to remove any clot that has formed resulting in the regional tamponade. Maintaining a high index of suspicion for postoperative bleeding and tamponade is the key to early recognition. Placement of a pericardial drain may or may not be helpful in draining the effusion in this posterior location. While it may address the symptoms of the tamponade, new drain placement does not address the cause of bleeding. A left- or right-sided thoracostomy tube is not indicated, as there is no evidence of pleural effusion. Pulmonary thromboembolectomy is not indicated, as there is no evidence of intravascular clot burden.

QUESTION 71.3: The correct answer is A. The most likely diagnosis is Takotsubo cardiomyopathy. As Video 71.2 shows, the patient has normal wall movement at the base of the heart and anteroapical akinesis. This pattern of RWMA—a normal/hyperkinetic LV base with a newly akinetic or dyskinetic apex—is pathognomonic. Other associated echocardiographic abnormalities can include SAM of MV, MR, and LV outflow tract obstruction. The dysfunction can be severe enough to require pharmacologic or mechanical support of the circulation. The LV appears to be dilated, so the patient is definitely not hypovolemic. The pericardium, seen at the top of the screen, is not thickened or echodense, making the diagnosis of pericarditis unlikely. The RV is not seen. A pseudoaneurysm is not present.

QUESTION 71.4: The correct answer is A. The most appropriate management would be to perform cardiac catheterization. Although the cardiac catheterization will not likely result in any significant findings, acute coronary occlusion must be ruled out in the setting of a recent CABG. This would be the next logical step although the etiology of Takotsubo is not due to coronary occlusion. In fact, the etiology is unknown and the treatment is mostly supportive. Hemodynamic support, including inotropes if needed, and medical management (usually aspirin, β-blockers, and a statin) are the mainstays of therapy. This cardiomyopathy usually resolves within days to weeks.

TAKE-HOME LESSON:

Bleeding is common following cardiac surgery and must be considered when there is hemodynamic instability, even when there is no chest tube output. Coronary occlusion must also be contemplated, even though wall motion abnormalities can have other etiologies.

SUGGESTED READING

Akashi YJ, Goldstein DS, Barbara G, et al. Takotsubo cardiomyopathy: a new form of acute reversible heart failure [Review]. *Circulation.* 2008;118:2754–2762.

Imren Y, Tasoglu I, Oktar GL, et al. The importance of transesophageal echocardiography in diagnosis of pericardial tamponade after cardiac surgery. *J Card Surg.* 2008;23:450–453.

Pinney SP, Mancini DM. Myocarditis and specific cardiomyopathies. In: Fuster V, O'Rourke RA, Walsh RA, et al., eds. *Hurst's the Heart.* 12th ed. New York: McGraw-Hill Publishers; 2008:878.

Prasad A, Lerman A, Rihal CS. Apical ballooning syndrome (Tako-Tsubo or stress cardiomyopathy): a mimic of acute myocardial infarction [see comment] [Review]. *Am Heart J.* 2008;155:408–417.

CASE 72

A 65-year-old woman with history of peripheral vascular disease and insulin-dependent diabetes mellitus presents for elective coronary revascularization. During the prebypass period, and prior to heparin administration, the TEE image shown in Figure 72.1 was obtained.

QUESTION 72.1. Choose the correct answer.

A. Aortic dissection
B. PA catheter artifact
C. Side-lobe artifact
D. Lambl's excrescences

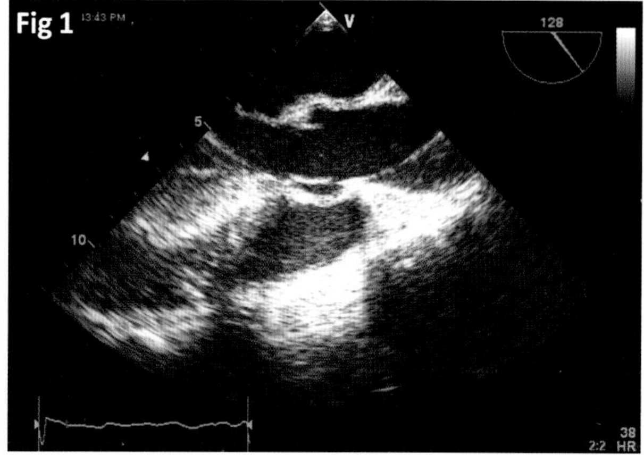

Figure 72.1.

ANSWERS AND DISCUSSION

QUESTION 72.1: The correct answer is C: Side-lobe artifact.

Side-lobe artifact is a linear imaging artifact produced by the side lobes of the ultrasound beam. In addition to the central sound beam, there are always additional ultrasound beams, diverging at an angle from the central beam. Typically, the side lobes do not produce images because their energy is significantly reduced. However, a strong reflector (such as a calcium deposit) can cause the weaker ultrasound signals to reflect to the probe. The ultrasound machine will misinterpret the location of the true reflector because it assumes that all reflections originate from the central beam. As the central beam sweeps from side to side, a lateral artifact of consistent depth is created. In this case, it gave the impression of an aortic dissection flap. The side-lobe artifacts cross anatomic boundaries and are placed within the same radius away from the transducer (Fig. 72.2). They usually disappear with adjustment of the depth or angle of the transducer.

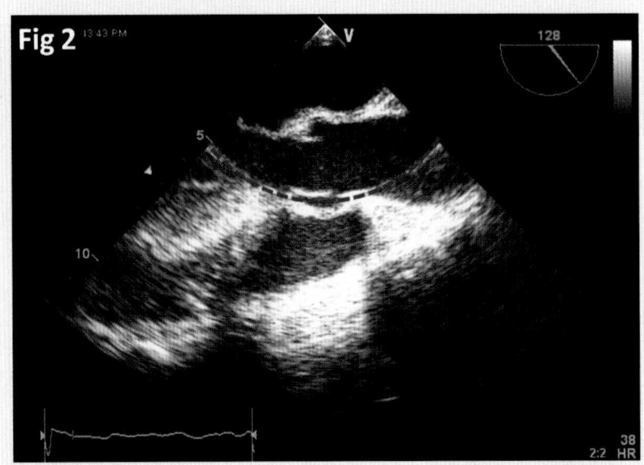

Figure 72.2. **A:** Side-lobe artifact created by calcium deposit at the aorta-sinus of Valsalva junction (ME AV LAX view). **B:** The side-lobe artifact is displayed as a curved line at the level of the true object with the brightest area corresponding to the calcium deposit.

ANSWER A: Answer A—*Aortic dissection*—is incorrect, as the structure crosses the anatomic boundaries (which is shown as a curvilinear line from underneath the anterior mitral leaflet to the ascending aorta).

ANSWER B: Answer B—*PA catheter artifact*—is incorrect. The structure is seen inside the aorta, not the RV, which is located underneath it.

ANSWER D: Answer D—*Lambl's excrescences*—is incorrect. Lambl's excrescences are thin, filament-like attachments seen floating from the tips (not the body) of the AV cusps, protruding into the aortic lumen in systole as well as diastole. The imaged structure is "attached" to the sinotubular junction.

TAKE-HOME LESSON:

Side-lobe artifact is seen as a curvilinear mass that crosses normal anatomic planes. It is necessary to examine the object in multiple angles to distinguish the true reflector from the artifact.

SUGGESTED READING

Vignon P, Spencer KT, Preux PM, et al. Differential transesophageal echocardiographic diagnosis between linear artifacts and intraluminal flap of aortic dissection or disruption. *Chest*. 2001;119:1778–1790.

Moderate

CASE 73

A 54-year-old man with congenital bicuspid AV is undergoing elective surgery. The ME AV and aorta LAX is seen in Videos 73.1 and 73.2 and in Figure 73.1.

QUESTION 73.1. The principal diagnosis is

A. Severe AS

B. Severe AI

C. Aortic dissection

D. None of the above

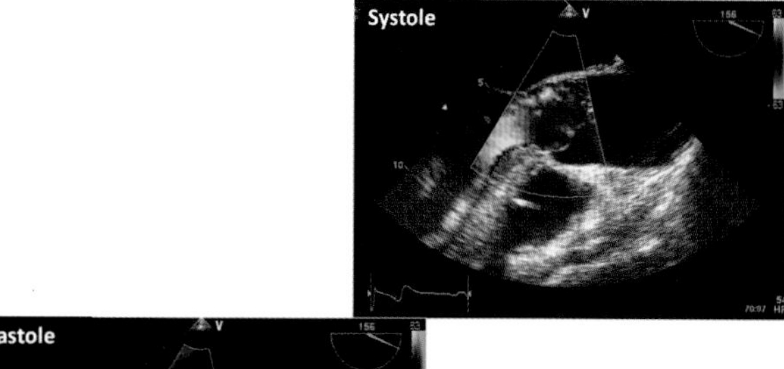

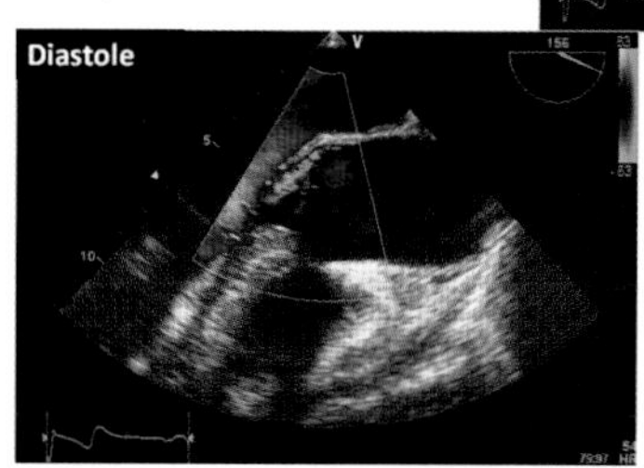

Figure 73.1.

QUESTION 73.2. In Figure 73.2 (from another patient), match the dimensions a, b, c, and d with one of the following:

A. Sinotubular junction

B. Ascending aorta

C. Aortic annulus

D. Sinus of Valsalva

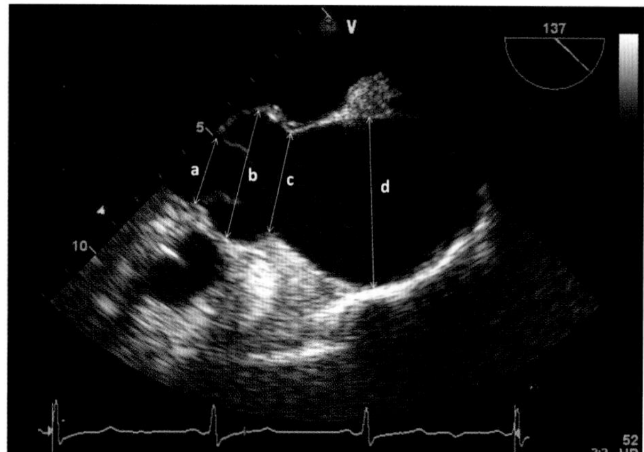

Figure 73.2.

QUESTION 73.3. The most appropriate treatment of this patient based on the dimensions a, b, and c (Fig. 73.3) is

A. Repair of ascending aorta distal to sinotubular junction
B. Replacement of ascending aorta distal to aortic annulus
C. Replacement of AV only
D. Do nothing

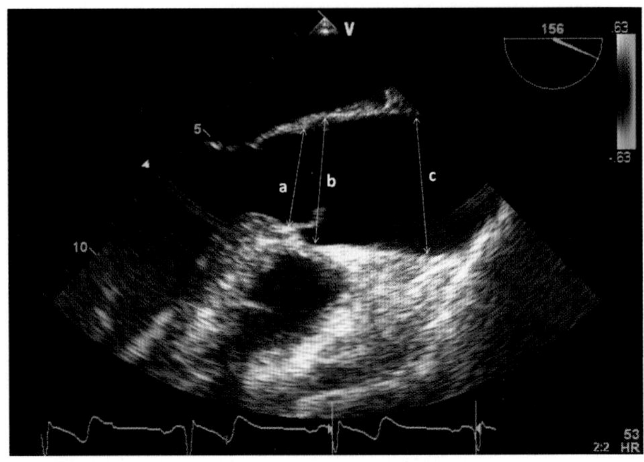

Figure 73.3.

ANSWERS AND DISCUSSION

QUESTION 73.1: The correct answer is D: None of the above.

AV function is normal: there is laminar flow in systole and a small jet of AI in diastole. Both these findings are inconsistent with either severe AS or insufficiency. There is no dissection flap in the proximal ascending aorta.

QUESTION 73.2:
A = c, Aortic annulus
B = d, Sinus of Valsalva
C = a, Sinotubular junction
D = b, Ascending aorta

QUESTION 73.3: The correct answer is B: Replacement of ascending aorta distal to aortic annulus.

This patient with a bicuspid valve has aortic root dilation starting at the level of the aortic annulus, transitioning to the area of the sinuses of Valsalva and beyond in the ascending aorta. Note that the sinuses of Valsalva are almost obliterated and the entire aortic root resembles a tube (compare with the normally appearing aortic root of Fig. 73.2). Irrespective of the condition of the AV, the aorta is dilated and in need of repair/replacement.

The three sinuses of Valsalva correspond to each of the three coronary cusps and are the site of local expansion of the aortic root. Each sinus is defined inferiorly by the attachments of an aortic cusp and superiorly by the sinotubular junction. An aneurysm is a local (saccular) or circumferential (fusiform) dilatation of >1.5 the expected normal diameter. The mean diameter of the sinus of Valsalva is 3.4 cm in men and 3.1 cm in women. In general, the diameter of the sinuses of Valsalva is greater than the diameter of the ascending aorta.

An aneurysm of the sinus of Valsalva is either congenital or acquired as a result of trauma, endocarditis, syphilis, tuberculosis, or Behcet disease. Sinus of Valsalva aneurysm is uncommon (0.14% to 0.23%) and may be associated with bicuspid AV and AI. The aneurysm may rupture into any of the cardiac chambers, the pericardium, or cause compression of neighboring anatomic (chamber or vascular) structures. Aneurysms of the right CS of Valsalva tend to rupture into the RV while those of the noncoronary cusp tend to rupture into the RA.

In this patient with bicuspid AV, the proper approach is to replace the bicuspid valve as well as the ascending aorta distal to the aortic annulus with a composite graft.

TAKE-HOME LESSON:

A sinus of Valsalva aneurysm is a local (saccular) or circumferential (fusiform) dilatation of >1.5 the expected normal diameter.

SUGGESTED READING

Pacini D, Di Marco L, Suarez SM, et al. Aortic valve-sparing operations: early and midterm results. *Heart Surg Forum*. 2006;9:E650–E656.

Rosenberger P, Cohn LH, Fox JA, et al. Sinus of Valsalva aneurysm obstructing the right ventricular outflow tract. *Anesth Analg*. 2006;102:1660–1661.

Vetrugno L, Bassi F, Giordano F, et al. Imaging a large unsuspected sinus of Valsalva aneurysm dissecting into interventricular septum. *Anesth Analg*. 2008;106:1387–1389.

Moderate

CASE 74

A 35-year-old male presents with a history of exertional chest pain. He has a family history of sudden death in two of his paternal uncles. Catheterization shows single-vessel disease of the LAD along with a high pressure gradient across his AV. He presents for CABG and AVR. During the intraoperative TEE examination a CW Doppler across the AV reveals the image shown in Figure 74.1.

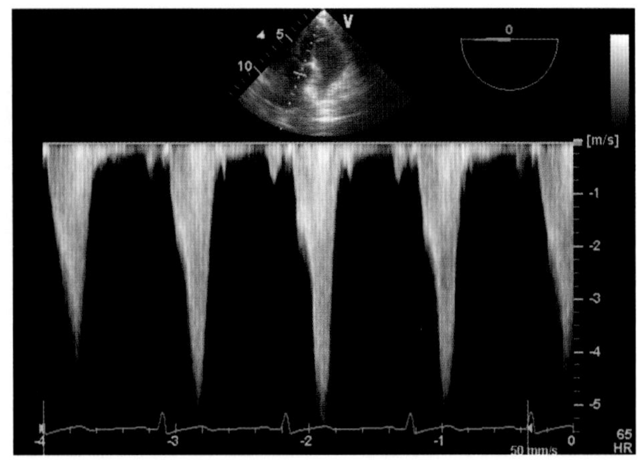

Figure 74.1. Deep TG CW Doppler of aortic outflow.

QUESTION 74.1. What does this pattern suggest?

A. Normal flow velocity profile
B. AS
C. Dynamic obstruction
D. AI

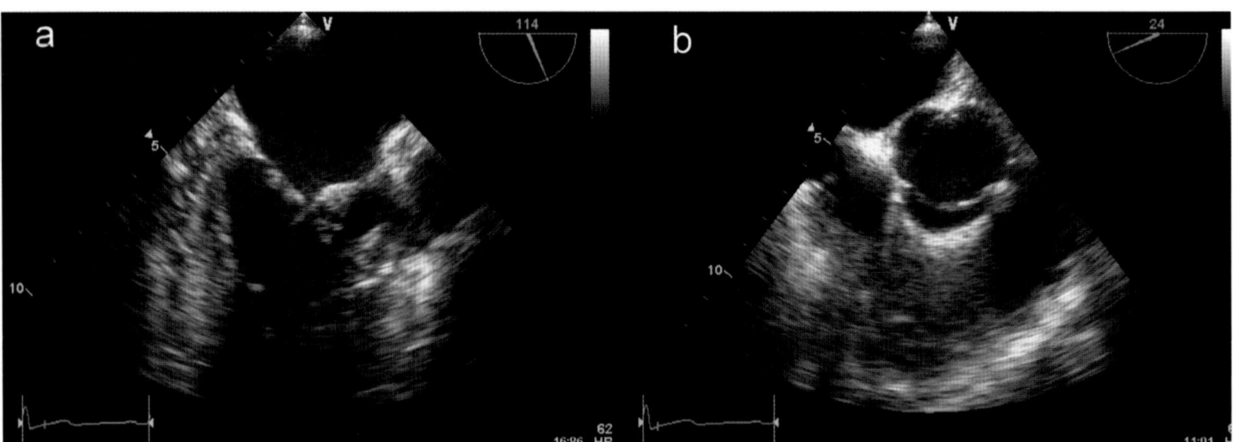

Figure 74.2. **A:** ME AV LAX. **B:** ME AV SAX.

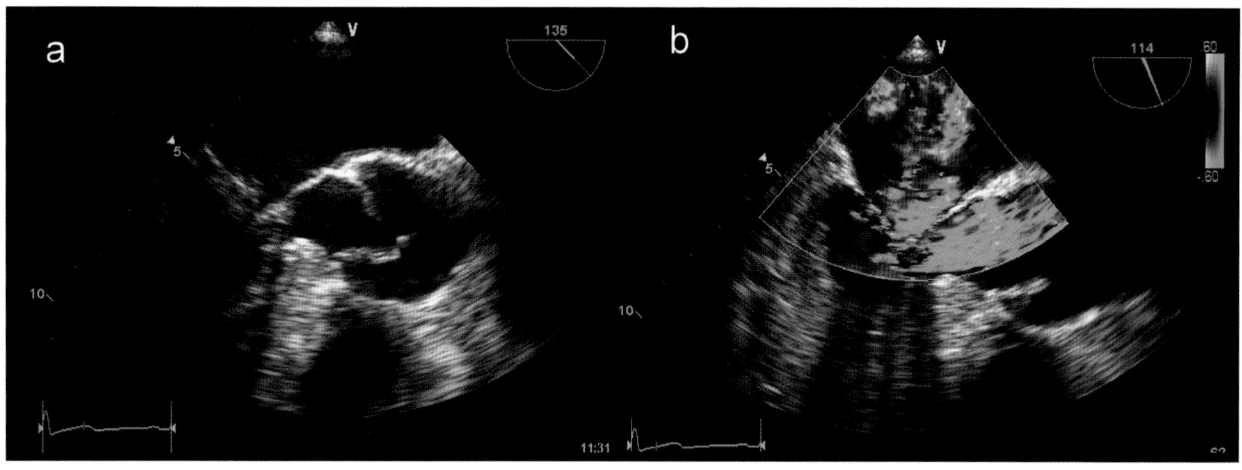

Figure 74.3. **A:** ME aortic outflow in systole. See also Video 74.1. **B:** ME aortic outflow with CFD.

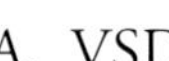

QUESTION 74.2. After reviewing Figures 74.2 and 74.3 how can you account for the velocity gradient detected on Doppler?

A. Commissural fusion

B. Subaortic membrane

C. HOCM

D. Figure 74.2A and 74.2B are normal; Doppler of MR mistaken for Doppler of LVOT

QUESTION 74.3. What associated finding is demonstrated in Figure 74.3 and Video 74.1?

A. VSD

B. MV prolapse

C. SAM of the mitral leaflet

D. Midsystolic aortic leaflet flutter.

ANSWERS AND DISCUSSION

QUESTION 74.1: The correct answer is C: Dynamic obstruction.

A "dagger-shaped" velocity contour, with peak velocity occurring in late systole, is consistent with dynamic outflow obstruction. The Doppler pattern is typically observed with HOCM and is the result of late systolic flow obstruction as contraction of the thick ventricle obstructs flow. The resulting velocity pattern differs from the pan systolic flow obstruction seen with AS. Importantly, CW Doppler, which has range ambiguity, may be misinterpreted as AS as the line of interrogation usually includes the LV, LVOT, and the AV. It is for this reason that a proper 2D echo is performed to examine the precise anatomy associated with the velocity contour and estimated pressure gradient. CFD will demonstrate turbulent flow within the LVOT (or LV in some cardiomyopathies), clearly below the AV, and aids in differentiating valvular from subvalvular obstruction (Fig. 74.3A, Video 74.1).

Answer A, normal flow velocity profile, is incorrect. The profile is not normal and the peak velocities are very high. The contour demonstrates the typical shape of dynamic obstruction with relatively normal early velocity profile followed by a rapid mid- to late systolic rise in velocity.

Answers B, AS, and D, AI, are incorrect. The velocity profile, although demonstrating high velocities, is not typical of AS. There is no evidence of AI on the Doppler trace; the velocity trace is in a direction away from the apically positioned transducer in this TG interrogation.

QUESTION 74.2: The correct answer is C: HOCM.

Figure 74.2A demonstrates a muscular ridge in the LVOT that extends into the septum. The septum is hypertrophied and, in this patient, measures up to 2.8 cm (Fig. 74.4B). Normal septal thickness in men ranges between 0.6 and 1.0 cm.[1] A value above 1.7 cm is considered severely abnormal. There is also evidence of concentric LV hypertrophy (Fig. 74.4A). The posterior wall thickness should not measure more than 1.0 cm in men. A value of 1.4 to 1.6 cm is considered moderately abnormal. Ventricular hypertrophy in the setting of a normal LV cavity size is responsible for the dynamic obstruction. HOCM is usually the result of an overly thick LV septum that may be found in isolation or affecting additional walls of the LV. Diastolic filling will be impaired—a result of the thick, stiff LV walls.

Hypertrophic cardiomyopathy has several presentations.[2] Hypertrophy may be isolated to the anterior septum (as in this case) or the entire septum. Other forms involve the entire myocardium or just the apical segments.

Answer B, subaortic membrane, is incorrect. Subaortic membrane or a fibromuscular tunnel is a less common cause of subvalvular obstruction. Importantly, no membrane is detected in Figure 74.2 and a velocity profile such as that in Figure 74.1 would not be expected as the obstruction would not be dynamic. Answer A, commissural fusion, is incorrect as the AV is captured as widely patent (Fig. 74.2B). Answer D, Figures 74.2A and 74.2B are normal, is incorrect; Figure 74.2A is not normal. Although a CW Doppler of MR can occur by mistake, the velocity profile would not resemble that of Figure 74.1 as it would be more rounded, without late velocity acceleration.

QUESTION 74.3: The correct answer is C: SAM of the mitral leaflet.

SAM of the mitral leaflet is frequently associated with HOCM. It is the result of abnormal geometric relationships within the LV between the MV, the papillary muscles, and chordae in the presence of hyperdynamic ejection. There will be anterior displacement of the anterior MV leaflet toward the septum causing varying degrees of LVOT obstruction and MR (Figs. 74.1 and 74.3).

Answers A and B are incorrect; VSD and MV prolapse are not normally associated with HOCM. Answer D is incorrect; while systolic *aortic* leaflet flutter is associated with HOCM, it is best appreciated on M-mode echocardiography of the AV.

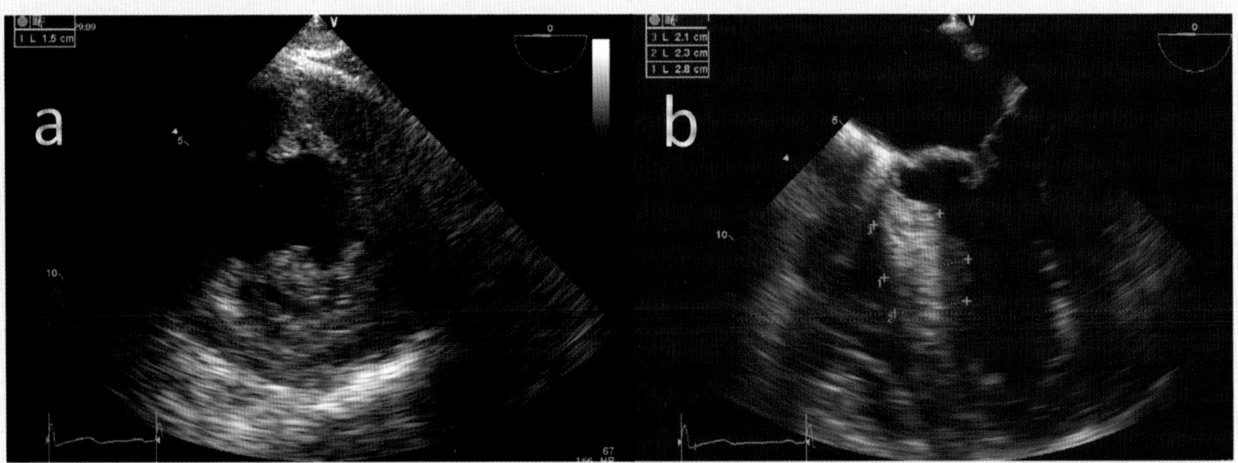

Figure 74.4. **A:** TG midpapillary short-axis view with measurement of the posterior wall of the LV (1.5 cm). **B:** ME 4CH view with septal measurements (largest, 2.8 cm).

TAKE-HOME LESSON:

In case of increased aortic Doppler velocities in the setting of a normal appearing AV, subaortic fixed or dynamic obstructions must be entertained. A dagger-shaped pattern of increased late systolic velocity is diagnostic of a dynamic obstruction. SAM of the mitral leaflet may accompany a dynamic obstruction.

REFERENCES

1. Cohen IS. Aortic stenosis. In: Perrino AC Jr, Reeves ST, eds. *A Practical Approach to Transesophageal Echocardiography*. Philadelphia: Lippincott Williams & Wilkins; 2007.
2. Lang RM, Bierig M, Devereux RB, et al. Recommendations for chamber quantification: a report from the American Society of Echocardiography's Guidelines and Standards Committee and the Chamber Quantification Writing Group, developed in conjunction with the European Association of Echocardiography, a branch of the European Society of Cardiology. *J Am Soc Echocardiogr*. 2005;18:1440–1463.

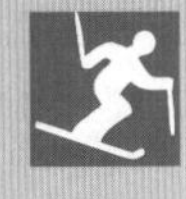

Moderate

CASE 75

A 79-year-old woman presents to the OR for urgent bronchoscopy for removal of foreign body. She is short of breath and has a known systolic ejection murmur. A TEE is performed after induction of anesthesia and removal of the foreign body.

QUESTION 75.1. After reviewing Figure 75.1 and Video 75.1 (ME AV SAX with and without CFD) and Figure 75.2, what is your diagnosis?

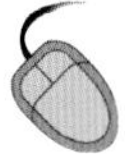

A. AS

B. Pulmonic stenosis (PS)

C. Infective endocarditis

D. PA membrane

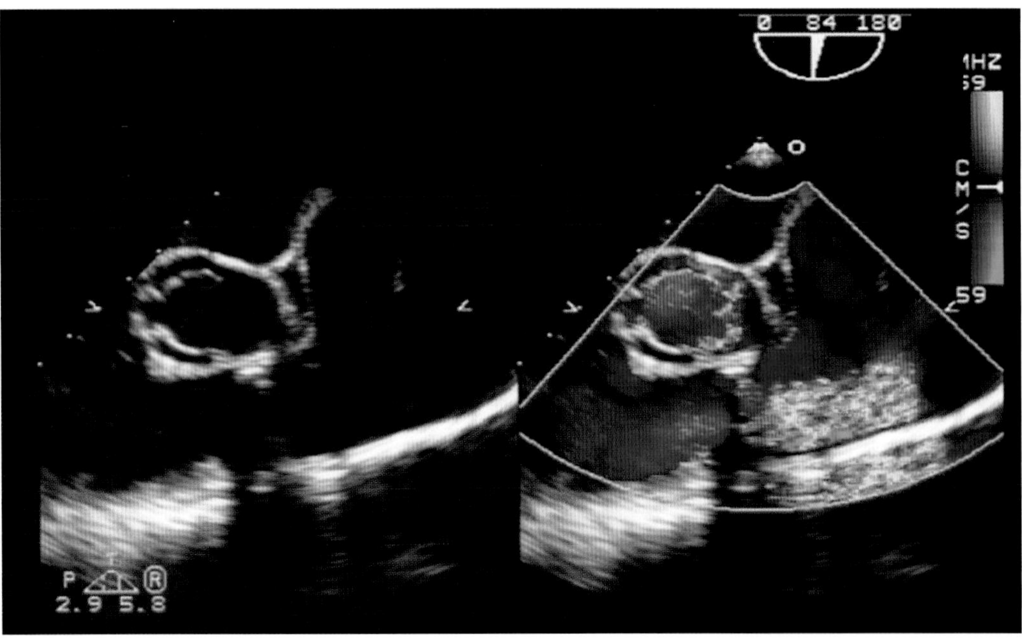

Figure 75.1.

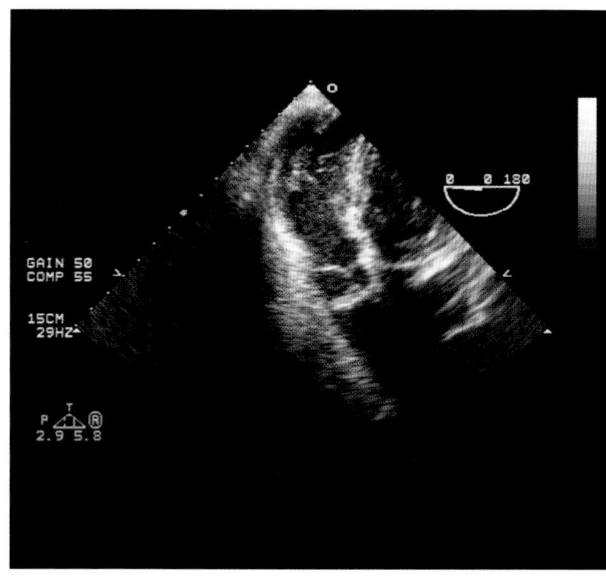

Figure 75.2.

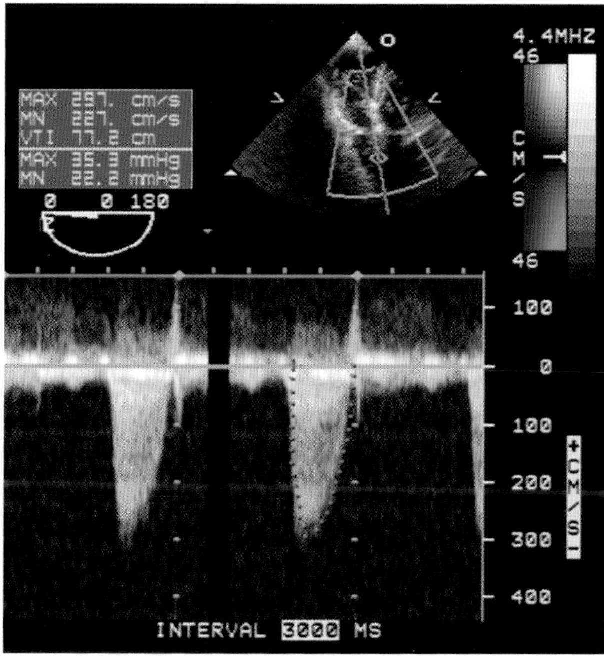

Figure 75.3.

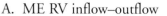

QUESTION 75.2. Which TEE view is represented in Figure 75.2 and Video 75.2?

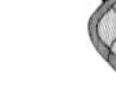

A. ME RV inflow–outflow

B. ME ascending aortic SAX

C. TG RV outflow

D. Basal TG SAX

QUESTION 75.3. Based on the CW spectral Doppler in Figure 75.3, calculate the PA systolic pressure? The CVP is 15 mm Hg.

A. Unable to determine

B. 20 mm Hg

C. 35 mm Hg

D. 50 mm Hg

QUESTION 75.4. What characteristic additional echocardiographic finding should be looked for in this patient?

A. RV dilatation

B. LV hypertrophy

C. RV hypertrophy

D. Small PA

QUESTION 75.5. Which procedure would be best suited to this patient?

A. Leave alone (nothing)

B. Aggressive medical management

C. Balloon dilatation

D. Open cardiac procedure

ANSWERS AND DISCUSSION

QUESTION 75.1: The correct answer is D.

Initial examination of Figure 75.1 and Video 75.1 might suggest calcific pulmonic valve (PV) stenosis (Answer B), but closer examination of Figure 75.2 and Video 75.2 suggests the correct diagnosis of supravalvular pulmonary stenosis (SVPS) from a PA membrane (arrow, Fig. 75.4).

CFD turbulence is seen distal to the membrane with mild pulmonic insufficiency (Fig. 75.1, Video 75.1). A post-stenotic main PA aneurysm, measuring 5.7 cm in diameter, was also detected in this patient (Fig. 75.1).

Answer A is incorrect as Figure 75.1 and Video 75.1 clearly show the AV to be widely patent. Answer C is incorrect as both the pulmonic and AV show no evidence of vegetations (Video 75.1).

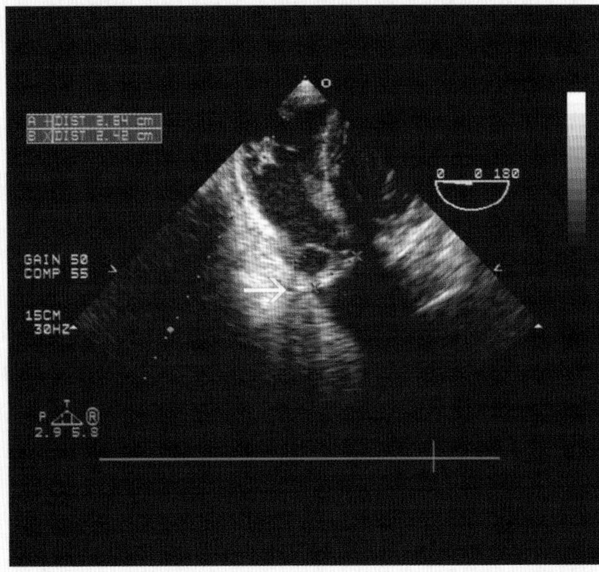

Figure 75.4.

QUESTION 75.2: The correct answer is C.

To obtain this nonstandard TEE view (Video 75.2), the probe is advanced into the basal TG position to acquire a view of the LVOT followed by a rightward (clockwise) turn of the probe and adjustment of the multiplane angle between 0 and 30 degrees in order to optimize the RVOT. This image provides an excellent alternative to the standard upper esophageal (UE) aortic arch short-axis view of the PV and main PA, which was difficult to acquire in this patient due to lung hyperinflation induced by the foreign body and the large PA. The standard UE view is obtained by withdrawing the probe while viewing the descending aorta from the midesophagus until the aortic arch appears (UE aortic arch long axis) and then rotating the multiplane angle to 60 to 90 degrees. Both views provide excellent assessment using 2D imaging of proximal PA pathology and PA dimensions (Fig. 75.4), color Doppler severity of pulmonic insufficiency or stenosis (Fig. 75.5), and allow for parallel CW Doppler alignment (Fig. 75.3, Video 75.3) to aid quantification of stenosis or insufficiency severity. Figure 75.5 is a zoom of the RVOT with and without color Doppler demonstrating the turbulent flow

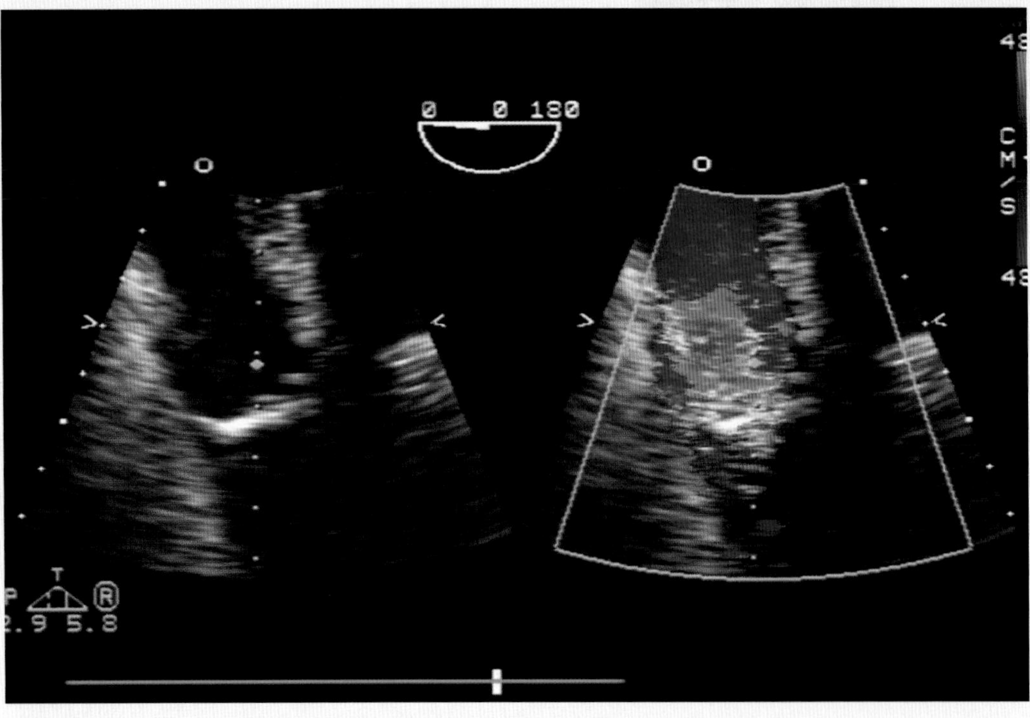

Figure 75.5.

through the narrow PA membrane and flow acceleration above the membrane (Video 75.3).

QUESTION 75.3: The correct answer is A.

There is insufficient information to calculate the PASP. Figure 75.3 is a CW Doppler trace across the PA membrane, which is the pressure difference between the RV and the PA during systole as given by the following equation:

$$4V^2_{\text{PA membrane}} = \text{RVSP} - \text{PASP}$$

or

$$\text{PASP} = \text{RVSP} - 4V^2_{\text{PA membrane}}$$

When obstruction is discrete and confined to one level it is acceptable to use the modified Bernoulli equation. However, if there is a long segment of stenosis and dynamic obstruction as seen, for example, in infundibular hypertrophy, it is difficult to evaluate by CW Doppler and cardiac catheterization may be required.

To calculate the PASP in this patient one must also know the RVSP that is measured from the pressure gradient between the RV and the RA during systole as represented by the peak TR velocity determined from the CW Doppler trace of the TR jet (not given).

$$\text{RVSP} - \text{RAP} = 4V^2_{\text{TR}}$$

or

$$\text{RVSP} = \text{RAP} + 4\text{VTR}^2_{\text{TR}}$$

Combining both equations then:

$$\text{PASP} = (\text{RAP} + 4\text{VTR}^2) - 4V^2_{\text{PA membrane}}$$

Without pulmonic or RVOT obstruction, the PASP is equivalent to the RVSP. However, PS causes pressure loading of the RV resulting in the RVSP being much higher than the PASP.

QUESTION 75.4: The correct answer is C.

PV or PA obstruction typically causes pressure overload of the RV characterized by right ventricular hypertrophy (RVH) rather than volume overload, which leads to RV dilatation (Answer A). RVH is defined by the RV free wall thickness exceeding 5 mm at end-diastole. Chronic pressure loading leads to enhanced trabeculation of the RV and a D-shaped LV cavity in cross section or flat interventricular septum (IVS) with maximal shift toward the LV at end-systole. These features contrast with those of RV volume overload characterized by RV dilatation and maximal displacement of the IVS at end-diastole.

Answer B is incorrect as LVH is not typically associated with RVOT obstruction. Answer D is incorrect as PS can occasionally be associated with post-stenotic dilatation of the main PA trunk giving rise to low pressure PA aneurysms. These may appear as mediastinal masses on chest x-ray but rarely rupture given the high elasticity of the pulmonary vasculature. This contrasts with PA aneurysms associated with pulmonary hypertension that have a higher risk of rupture.

QUESTION 75.5: The correct answer is A.

Management of these patients depends on both patient symptomatology and echo Doppler assessment of the severity of stenosis. Severity of valvular PS is classified as mild when the peak gradient is less than 30 mm Hg, moderate when the gradient is 30 to 50 mm Hg, and severe if the gradient exceeds 50 mm Hg using Doppler echocardiography. Current guidelines now recommend assessment of gradients using Doppler echocardiography that has transitioned from older texts where catheter-based techniques were routinely used to measure peak-to-peak gradients to guide further intervention and follow-up. Recent data has shown a good correlation exists between the peak-to-peak gradient measured by cardiac catheterization and the mean Doppler gradient. The peak instantaneous Doppler gradient consistently overestimates the catheter peak-to-peak gradient by approximately 20 mm Hg.

ANSWER D: Surgical intervention (answer D) is recommended for supravalvular PS if there is severe PS, symptoms (exertional dyspnea, angina, presyncope, syncope) or the presence of other anomalies such as intracardiac shunts or refractory arrhythmia. The long-term results of surgical repair are highly favorable with low risk of recurrence. Clear guidelines are lacking with regard to the management of PA aneurysms. Given that this is a low pressure circuit, the risk of rupture is very low. Thus surgical intervention would be governed by the presence of compressive symptomatology or associated severe pulmonic insufficiency with RV dilatation.

Isolated SVPS is a rare cause of RVOT obstruction with 80% to 90% of cases attributed to valvular PS. SVPS can be secondary to a PA membrane, hour glass deformity of the PV, postsurgical complications of PA banding or stenosis of the main trunk or peripheral branch of the PA. Baseline echocardiography is recommended in all patients and further anatomical delineation should be performed using MRI angiography, CT angiography, or contrast angiography. Periodic follow-up with Doppler assessment of the RVSP at timely intervals as appropriate to the severity should be performed in all patients. Current AHA 2008 guidelines do not recommend routine infective endocarditis (IE) prophylaxis be given as PV endocarditis is very rare.

ANSWER B: Answer B is incorrect. Given this is a mechanically mediated obstructive lesion, medical therapy is largely ineffective except for the use of diuretics to reduced RV loading and dilatation.

ANSWER C: Answer C is incorrect. Percutaneous balloon valvotomy is the treatment of choice in patients with valvular PS (domed morphology) and peripheral branch PA stenosis.

TAKE-HOME LESSON:

Asymptomatic systolic ejection murmurs in the elderly are not always related to the AV.

SUGGESTED READING

ACC/AHA 2008 Guidelines for treatment of adult with congenital heart disease. *Circulation*. 2008;118(23): 2395–2451.

Canadian Cardiovascular Society Consensus Conference 2001 update: Recommendations for the Management of Adults with Congenital Heart Disease (Part II). *Can J Cardiol*. 2001;17(10):1029–1050.

CASE 76

A 25-year-old patient is undergoing septal myectomy for HOCM. A baseline ME LAX during diastole is shown in Figure 76.1.

QUESTION 76.1. What are the margins for the targeted length of resection?

A. From the base of the right coronary cusp of the AV to the point of anterior mitral leaflet septal contact

B. From the base of the right coronary cusp of the AV to 1 cm inferior to the point of anterior mitral leaflet septal contact

C. From the midpoint of the LVOT to the point of anterior mitral leaflet septal contact

D. From the midpoint of the LVOT to 1 cm inferior to the point of the anterior mitral leaflet septal contact

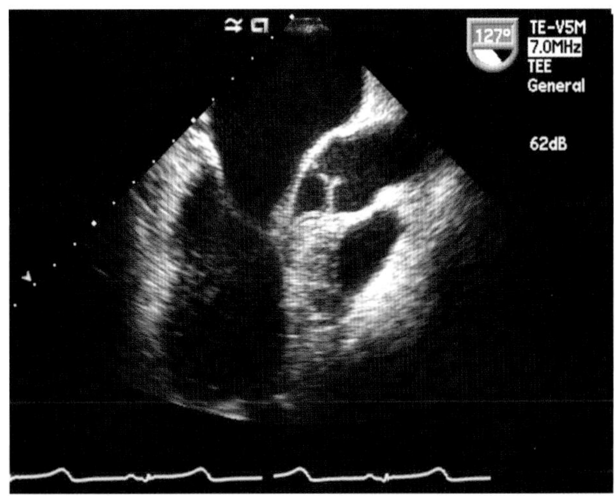

Figure 76.1.

Video 76.1 shows a ME LAX following septal myectomy. Despite an epinephrine infusion, there is difficulty separating from CPB. Figure 76.2 shows the same view during systole with the addition of CFD.

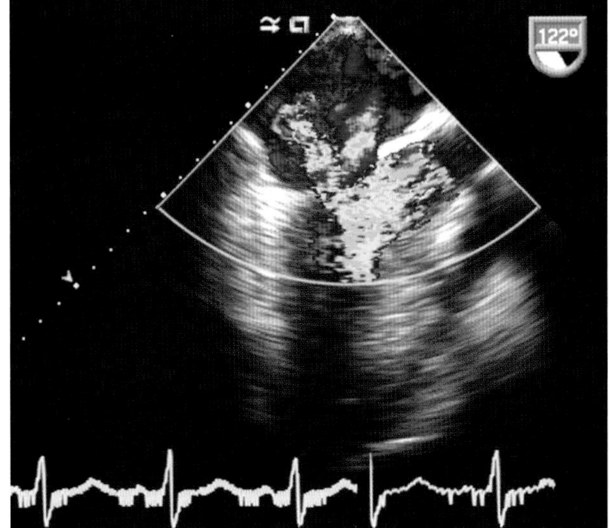

Figure 76.2.

QUESTION 76.2. What is the likely reason for difficulty weaning from CPB?

A. Severe AI

B. Severe MR due to disrupted chordae tendinae

C. Outflow tract obstruction due to SAM

D. Not enough inotropic support

QUESTION 76.3. The surgical team returned to CPB to perform a larger septal myomectomy, what is the most significant finding in video 76.2?

A. Severe AI

B. VSD

C. Severe TR

D. A PFO

QUESTION 76.4. If a large VSD were present, which of the following findings would be expected?

A. Peak systolic velocity of 5 m/s across the VSD using CW Doppler

B. A large Qp:Qs ratio

C. Marked flow turbulence seen in the region of the VSD

D. All of the above

QUESTION 76.5. What is the red arrow pointing to in Video 76.3?

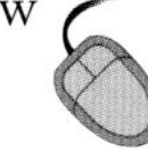

A. A jet of AI

B. A small VSD

C. The RCA

D. A severed septal perforator

ANSWERS AND DISCUSSION

QUESTION 76.1: The correct answer is B. The typical length of a septal myectomy is from the right coronary cusp of the AV to 1 cm inferior to the point of anterior mitral leaflet septal contact. This is illustrated in Figure 76.3, with point "a" being the base of the right coronary cusp and point "b" being 1 cm inferior to the point of anterior mitral leaflet contact. Although some surgeons are performing a more extensive resection, the septal muscle must be resected to at least 1 cm below the point of mitral leaflet contact. Removing less muscle risks failure to relieve the obstruction. The midpoint of the LVOT is not a landmark used for determining where to begin the resection.

QUESTION 76.2: The correct answer is C. The most likely reason for failure to wean from CPB is outflow tract obstruction due to SAM. Video 76.1 demonstrates the characteristic appearance of the interventricular septum following myectomy, although SAM is still present. Figure 76.2, with CFD, shows the classic "Y" sign during systole of turbulent flow in the LVOT and marked MR. Although AI and disrupted chordae tendinae are known complications, they are not demonstrated in this case. Medical treatment for this type of outflow tract obstruction requires less inotropy, rather than more.

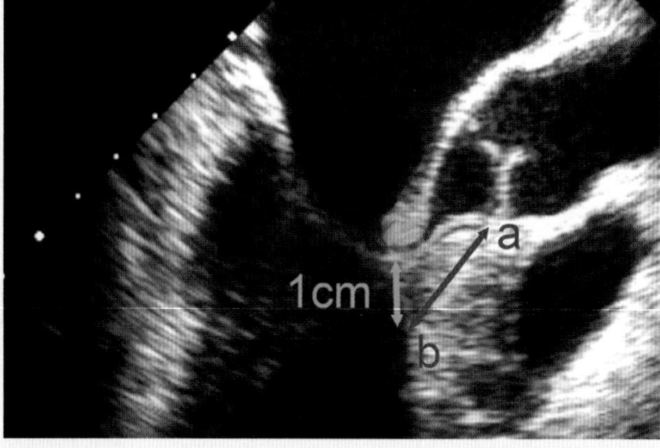

Figure 76.3.

Intraoperative TEE is useful for detecting the most common complications following myectomy, including residual outflow tract obstruction, VSD, MV dysfunction, and AV dysfunction. In some cases, decreased ventricular volumes and other predisposing hemodynamic conditions may reproduce a degree of premyectomy SAM and obstruction. In other cases, reinitiation of bypass for a more extensive myectomy is required.

QUESTION 76.3: The correct answer is B. The most significant finding is a VSD. The video shows turbulent flow around the TV during systole in close association with the LVOT. Upon close inspection, it can be seen that there is flow into the LVOT toward the right heart during diastole. This is indicated in Figure 76.4. Note that blue on CFD indicates flow away from the transducer (located in the middle of the sector field). Severe AI would result in flow moving from the LVOT into the LV, which would be seen as red color, indicating direction of flow toward the transducer. The color seen at the level of the TV is not TR since that would occur during systole, not diastole. This is not the correct location of a PFO.

QUESTION 76.4: The correct answer is B. A large VSD would be expected to have a large Qp:Qs ratio. The Qp:Qs ratio compares the flow of blood through the pulmonary circulation to the flow through the systemic circulation. It can be formally calculated using echocardiography by using the systolic Doppler VTI and corresponding cross-sectional areas to calculate PA and aorta SV. A high Qp:Qs ratio, typically >1.5:1, indicates a larger VSD. The greater the area of communication, the less impediment to flow there is between the two chambers, and these VSDs are termed *nonrestrictive*. A nonrestrictive VSD jet would be expected to have a low peak systolic velocity and less turbulent flow. By contrast, a peak velocity of 5 m/s would indicate a large LV to RV pressure gradient, which is normally present with a restrictive, as well as smaller, VSD.

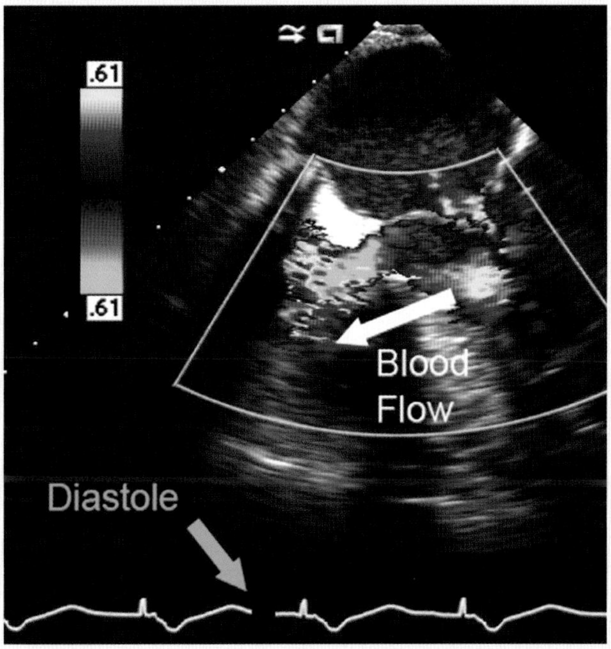

Figure 76.4.

QUESTION 76.5: The correct answer is D. The red arrow in Video 76.3 is pointing toward a severed septal perforator. Many times during the septal myectomy, a branch from the coronary artery perfusing that region can be cut. This causes blood to flow into the LVOT during diastole, as shown in Figure 76.5. There are usually no clinical consequences to this situation. It can, however, often be confused with a VSD or a small jet of AI.

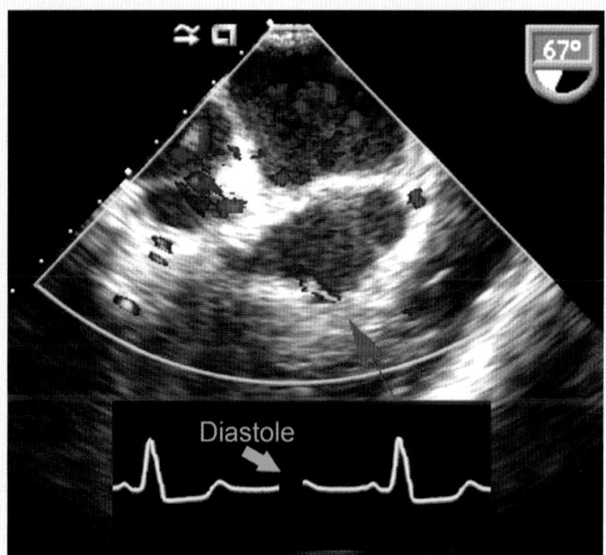

Figure 76.5.

TAKE-HOME LESSON:

The typical resection of a septal myectomy is from the right coronary cusp of the AV to 1 cm inferior to the point of anterior mitral leaflet septal contact. Following septal myectomy, it is important to use TEE to look for complications of the procedure that include iatrogenic VSD, SAM, and valvular damage.

SUGGESTED READING

Sheehan FH. Ventricular shape and function. In: Otto CM, ed. *Textbook of Clinical Echocardiography*. 4th ed. Philadelphia, PA: Saunders; 2009;217–226.

Smedira NG, Lytle BW, Lever HM, et al. Current effectiveness and risks of isolated septal myectomy for hypertrophic obstructive cardiomyopathy. *Ann Thorac Surg*. 2008;85:127–134.

Swaminathan N, DeBruijn NP, Glower DD, et al. Unexpected transesophageal echocardiographic finding after septal myectomy. *J Cardiothorac Vasc Anesth*. 2002;16:384–385.

Woo A, Wigle ED, Rakowski H. Echocardiography in the management of patients with hypertrophic cardiomyopathy. In: Otto CM, ed. *The Practice of Clinical Echocardiography*. 3rd ed. Philadelphia, PA: Saunders; 2007;653–678.

Moderate

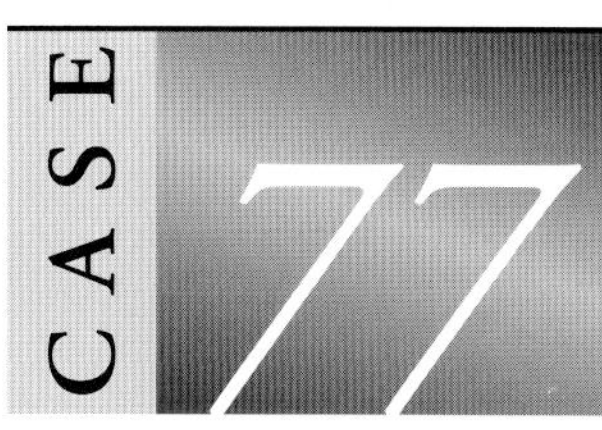

A 67-year-old man is undergoing CABG. The baseline images in Video 77.1 were obtained immediately after induction of anesthesia.

QUESTION 77.1. What segment of the LV contains the highest grade regional wall motion abnormality (RWMA)?

A. Basal anterior
B. Mid anterior
C. Basal septal
D. Apical inferior
E. Basal inferior

QUESTION 77.2. Based on the RWMA in video 77.1, what coronary artery is most likely occluded?

A. LAD
B. Left circumflex artery
C. RCA
D. The posterior descending artery
E. The left main coronary artery

QUESTION 77.3. The LV wall segment indicated by the arrow in Video 77.2 is best described as

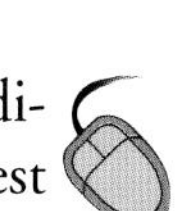

A. Normal
B. Hypokinetic
C. Akinetic
D. Dyskinetic
E. Hyperkinetic

QUESTION 77.4. What coronary artery supplies the LV wall segment indicated by the arrow in Figure 77.1?

A. LAD

B. Left circumflex

C. An obtuse marginal branch

D. The RCA

E. The first diagonal branch

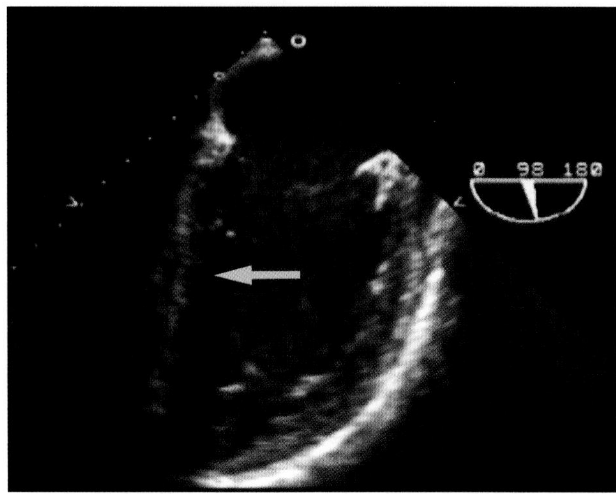

Figure 77.1.

ANSWERS AND DISCUSSION

QUESTION 77.1: The correct answer is B. The highest grade wall motion abnormality is seen in the *mid anterior* segment, which is akinetic. Video shows the ME views of the LV, which can be used to evaluate the standard 17 segments of the LV. These segments are fully described in Ref. 1, and shown in Figures 77.2, 77.3, and 77.4. The septal and inferior walls both display normal wall motion. The anterior basal segment is somewhat hypokinetic, but the mid anterior region is akinetic, making it a higher grade RWMA. The apical anterior segment is also akinetic, but that is not listed as one of the possible answers.

QUESTION 77.2: The correct answer is A. The coronary artery most likely responsible for the RWMA seen is the *LAD*. As discussed in the answer to Question 77.1, the anterior wall appears to be most affected. As shown in Figures 77.2 to 77.4, the LAD is responsible for perfusing the septal, anterior, and anteroseptal walls. The left circumflex artery's perfusion zones are the lateral and posterolateral walls. The right coronary provides perfusion to the inferior wall. If the left main coronary artery were occluded, one would expect RWMA in the territories covered by both the left anterior descending and the left circumflex arteries.

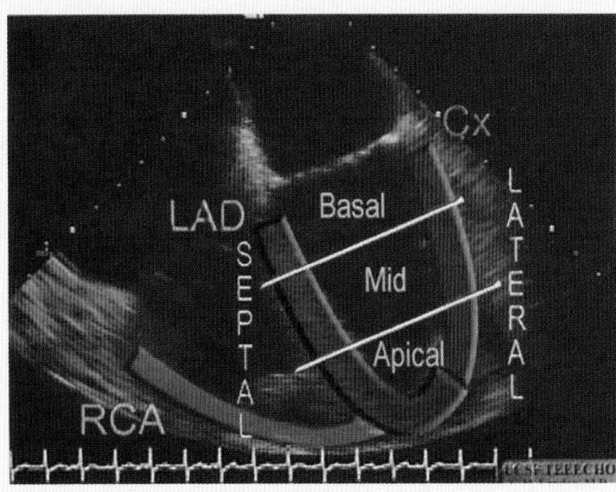

Figure 77.2.

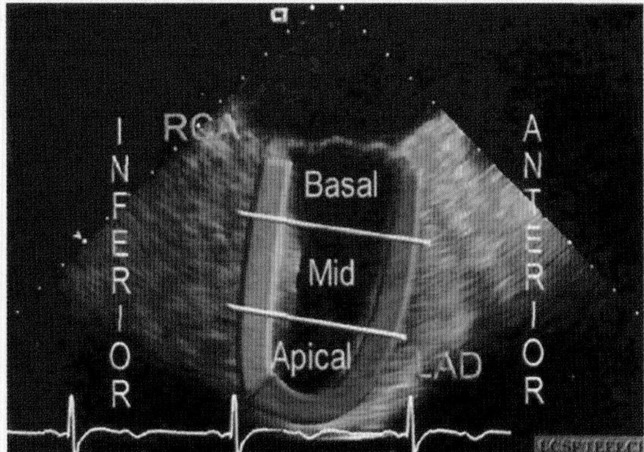

Figure 77.3.

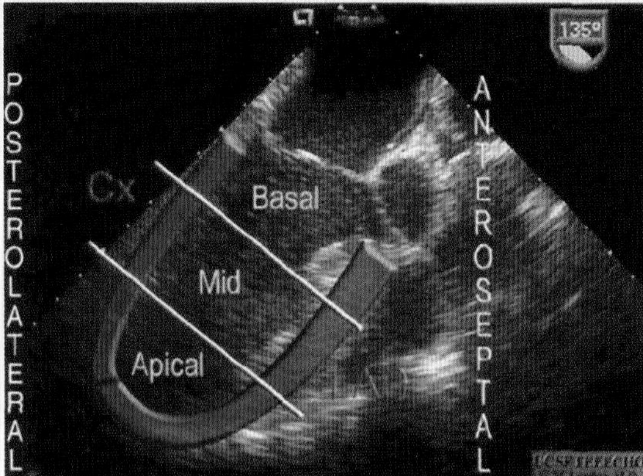

Figure 77.4.

QUESTION 77.3: The correct answer is C. The arrow in Video 77.2 is pointing toward an *akinetic* segment of myocardium. This is the mid anterior wall segment mentioned in Question 77.1. There is little or no wall thickening present and no endocardial excursion in this area. Normal wall motion includes a 30% to 50% thickening of the myocardium. Hypokinetic myocardium will have less thickening than normal and noticeably reduced endocardial excursion. A dyskinetic segment of myocardium will have an outward bulging during systole. Hypercontractile myocardium will have increased wall thickening and endocardial excursion compared to normal myocardium.

QUESTION 77.4: The correct answer is D. The arrow is pointing toward the inferior wall of the LV that is supplied by *the RCA*. As shown in Figures 77.2 to 77.4, neither the LAD nor the left circumflex arteries would be expected to perfuse the inferior wall. Obtuse marginal branches come from the left circumflex artery and diagonal branches come from the LAD.

TAKE-HOME LESSON:

A thorough understanding of the 17 segment model will allow the echocardiographer to assess RWMA and determine associated coronary blood flow abnormalities.

REFERENCE

1. Cerqueira MD, Weissman NJ, Dilsizian V, et al. Standardized myocardial segmentation and nomenclature for tomographic imaging of the heart. *Circulation*. 2002;105:539–542.

SUGGESTED READING

London MJ. Diagnosis of myocardial ischemia. In: Perrino AC Jr, Reeves ST, eds. *A Practical Approach to Transesophageal Echocardiography*. 2nd ed. Philadelphia: Lippincott Williams & Wilkins; 2008:87–104.

Moderate

CASE 78

A 64 year old man is undergoing defibrillator insertion for management of amyloid disease. A comprehensive TEE is performed, and Video 78.1 is obtained to evaluate the mitral leaflets.

QUESTION 78.1. The frame rate of the moving mitral leaflets will be increased the most with:

A. Shallower image sector
B. Deeper image sector
C. Wider image sector
D. Narrower image sector
E. Zoom mode

ANSWER AND DISCUSSION

QUESTION 78.1: Zoom mode or high "regional expansion selection" is selected prior to acquiring the image (it is a preprocessing function) that magnifies the displayed image by increasing the number of pixels within the selected region. Functionally, zoom mode allows selection of a small area of interest within the 2D image. The benefit is augmented spacial resolution, the detractor is smaller field of view.

Another advantage of zoom mode is increased temporal resolution. Rapidly oscillating structures, such as MV leaflets, are more readily evaluated with either zoom mode or M-mode.

The original sector has a frame rate of 50 f/s at a wide angle and 16 cm depth (Video 78.1), the sector with shallower depth (10 cm) or same width has a frame rate of 75 f/s (Video 78.2), and the zoom mode has the greatest frame rate (103 f/s) (Video 78.3). Figure 78.1 is a composite of all the three videos.

Note that the zoom image has a smaller field of view (the depth marks at the left of the sector have a range from 3.5 to 10.5 cm, for a total sector depth of 7 cm).

The correct answer is E: Zoom mode

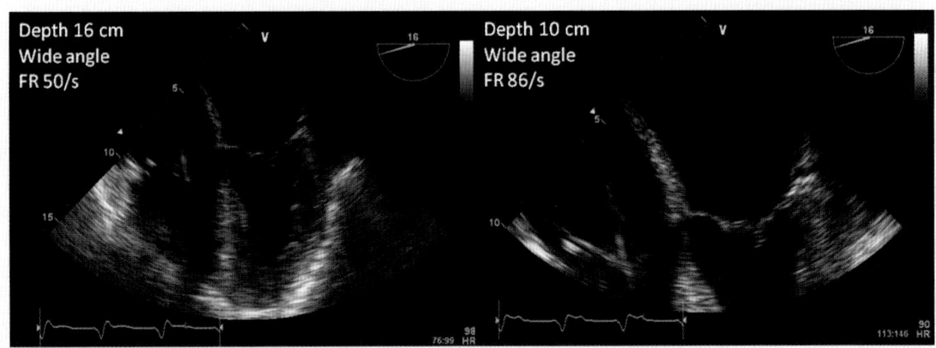

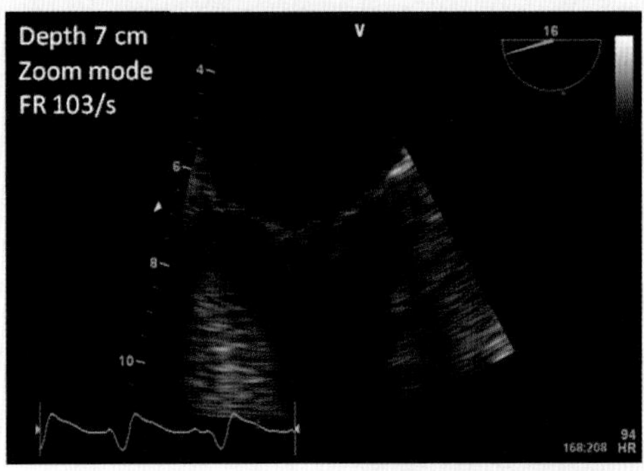

Figure 78.1.

TAKE-HOME LESSON:

Zoom mode increases both spatial and temporal resolution.

SUGGESTED READING

Shernan SK. Optimizing two-dimensional echocardiographic imaging. In: Savage RM, Aronson S, eds. *Comprehensive Textbook of Intraoperative Transesophageal Echocardiography*. 1st ed. Philadelphia: Lippincott Williams & Wilkins; 2005:56–57.

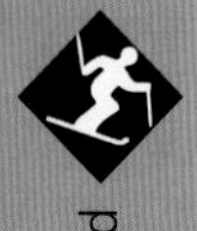

Advanced

CASE 79

A 48 year old male presents with recurrent painful cough, fatigue and persistent pedal edema despite multiple adequate courses of antibiotics for refractory pneumonia. A TEE was performed to assess for etiologies of his pedal edema.

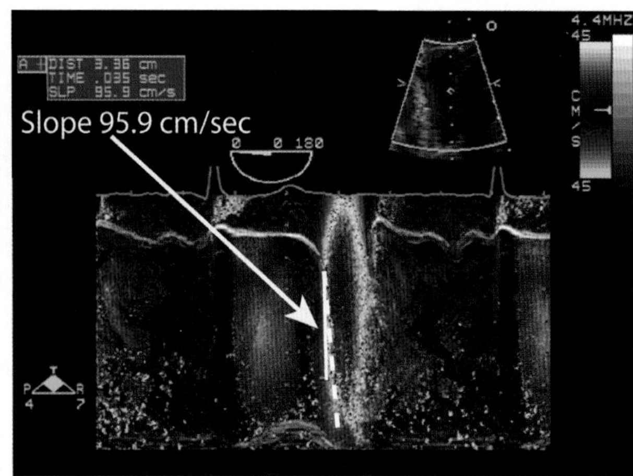

Figure 79.1.

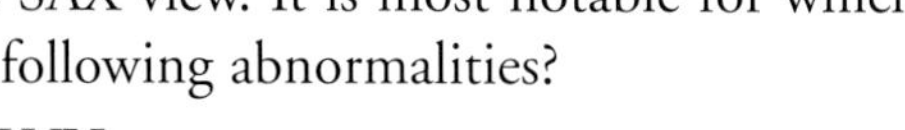

QUESTION 79.1. Part A: Video 79.1 shows a ME SAX view. It is most notable for which of the following abnormalities?

A. LVH
B. Septal bounce
C. Diastolic dysfunction
D. "Swinging heart sign"
E. RV diastolic collapse.

Part B: This abnormality is suggestive of:

A. HCM (hypertrophic cardiomyopathy) or HOCM use whichever is used elsewhere in the text
B. Large pericardial effusion
C. Tamponade physiology
D. Constrictive pericarditis
E. Restrictive cardiomyopathy

QUESTION 79.2. Figure 79.1 represents a still image from the same patient and is most supportive of the following diagnosis:

A. Cardiomyopathy secondary to cardiac amyloidosis
B. Severe mitral stenosis
C. Severe mitral insufficiency
D. Normal LV flow propagation in a patient with constrictive pericarditis
E. Normal LV flow propagation in a patient with a restrictive cardiomyopathy

QUESTION 79.3. What is the most sensitive and specific diastolic modality to make the diagnosis of constrictive pericarditis versus restrictive cardiomyopathy with TEE?

A. Transmitral pulse wave Doppler flow profile analysis
B. LV color M-mode (flow propagation [Vp])
C. Tissue Doppler imaging
D. Isovolemic relaxation time of the LV
E. Pulse wave Doppler assessment of the pulmonary vein flow profiles

ANSWERS AND DISCUSSION

QUESTION 79.1 A AND B: Correct answers are C: Diastolic dysfunction (severe) and D: Constrictive pericarditis: Septal bounce indicating diastolic dysfunction suggestive of constrictive pericarditis. The patient presented in the clinical vignette has symptoms of potentially both left (fatigue) and right (pedal edema) heart failure. TEE can provide an answer as to whether his symptoms may be related to either systolic dysfunction, diastolic dysfunction, or a combination of both. TEE is also beneficial in this clinical scenario to evaluate for endocarditis. Video 79.1 presents a TEE TG mid SAX cine loop of the LV and a portion of the RV. Most notable in the clip is an apparent septal bounce that is diagnostic of diastolic dysfunction and supportive of, but not totally specific for, the diagnosis of constrictive pericarditis. (A) In this case, the septal bounce is related to the LV inability to fill normally during diastole because of a markedly thickened pericardium (i.e., constrictive pericarditis). The "bouncing" occurs in two phases during diastole coincident with early ventricular filling and then the atrial kick. The septum appears to bounce because the normal heart muscle cannot expand to accept the diastolic flow from the LA. Careful inspection of the image will reveal a thickened segment of pericardium in the region of the anterior LV wall (indicated by the arrows in Fig. 79.2). More accurate estimation of pericardial thickness can be obtained using M-mode imaging (as demonstrated in Fig. 79.3). Normally, the pericardium is only 2 to 3 mm in thickness, whereas this pericardium is at least 10 mm thick in this image.

Patients with hypertrophic cardiomyopathy most commonly present with hypertrophied ventricular muscle tissue (e.g., ventricular wall thickness greater than 14 mm) that is not apparent in this cine loop. Patients with a dilated cardiomyopathy and restrictive diastolic dysfunction have a characteristically large (e.g., short-axis end-diastolic diameter greater than 55 mm) and thin-walled ventricle in contrast to the one presented in Video 79.1. There is no evidence of a pericardial effusion and a "swinging heart" sign in Video 79.1. Video 79.2 presents an example of the "swinging heart" sign in a patient with a significant pericardial effusion. Tamponade is incorrect since there is no evidence of either pericardial effusion or tamponade physiology. RV wall diastolic collapse is indicative of the early to middle stages of pericardial tamponade and can also be appreciated in Video 79.2.

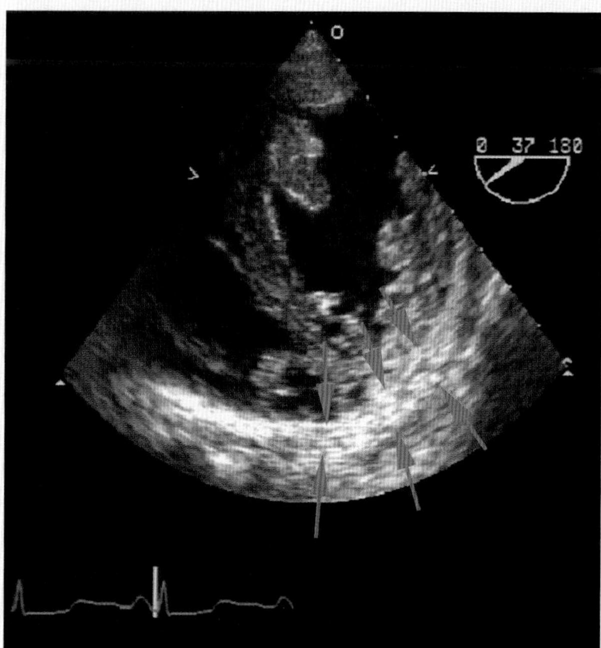

Figure 79.2.

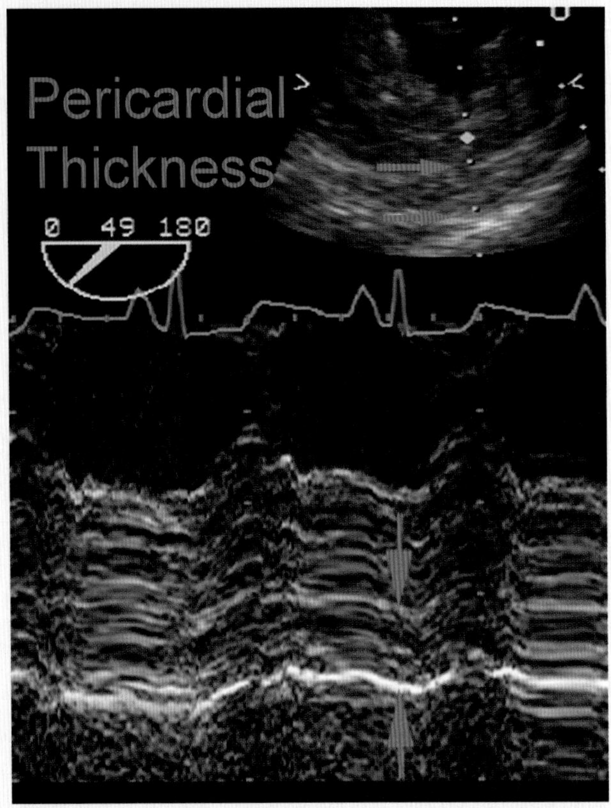

Figure 79.3.

QUESTION 79.2: The correct answer is D: Normal LV flow propagation in a patient with constrictive pericarditis. The image presented in Figure 79.1 is a color M-mode, or flow propagation (Vp), assessment of the LV in a patient with constrictive pericarditis. These patients generally have normal ventricular muscle, and thus the slope of their LV flow propagation profile is normal (greater than 100 cm/s) or nearly normal (greater than 45 cm/s), indicating appropriate relaxation of the muscle tissue. This patient presents with the normal Vp value of 95.9 cm/s. Despite the diastolic dysfunction that accompanies constrictive pericarditis, the majority of these patients will have similar flow propagation values. Performing a flow propagation assessment in an intubated patient will provide more consistent results if mechanical ventilation is interrupted during the measurement.

Cardiac amyloidosis is incorrect since it is similar to a hypertrophic cardiomyopathy. Both hypertrophic cardiomyopathy and cardiac amyloidosis are problems that are inherent to the muscle, which is noncompliant, and therefore will not demonstrate normal diastolic function; flow propagation values tend to be below 35 cm/s in these patients. Answer B is incorrect because patients with severe mitral stenosis will not have accurate flow propagation values related to the TMF acceleration that occurs as a result of the stenotic valve orifice. Mitral stenosis is a known pitfall to obtaining accurate flow propagation measurements. There is also a lack of evidence of mitral insufficiency in Figure 79.1, so answer C is incorrect. If there were any significant mitral insufficiency, a color Doppler signal would be seen above the echogenicity representing the mitral leaflet during systole. Unlike *constrictive* disease, individuals with a *restrictive* cardiomyopathy will have grossly abnormal flow propagation profiles. Color M-mode is one method used to differentiate the two conditions.

QUESTION 79.3: The correct answer is C: Tissue Doppler imaging.

Patients with a restrictive cardiomyopathy typically demonstrate a lateral mitral annular E_m velocity of greater than 8 cm/s (provided that the patient does not have a regional wall abnormality in this segment of muscle). Constrictive pericarditis is not a problem that is commonly associated with ventricular muscle abnormalities, thus the tissue Doppler imaging values will commonly be normal in these patients. Figure 79.4 presents a tissue Doppler image of a patient with constrictive pericarditis. Note that E_m is greater than 8 cm/s. In contrast, a patient with a restrictive cardiomyopathy will have a grossly abnormal tissue Doppler imaging value (i.e., E_m less than 8 cm/s).

Transmitral pulse wave Doppler assessment can be very useful to identify constrictive pericarditis, but it is considerably less sensitive (84%) and specific (91%) than tissue Doppler imaging to distinguish between constrictive and restrictive disease. In spontaneously breathing patients, there will be a *greater than 10% increase* (i.e., an increase of approximately 10% of the peak E-wave velocity is normal) in the transmitral peak E-wave velocity at *end expiration* and thus exaggerated respirophasic variation is observed. In constrictive pericarditis, patients who are being treated with

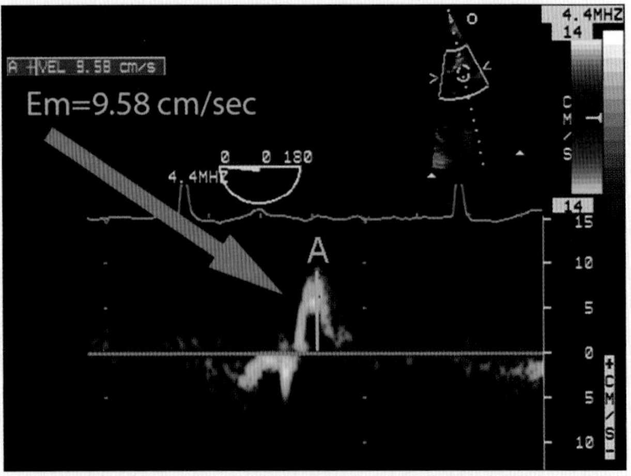

Figure 79.4.

positive pressure ventilation, there is commonly an exaggerated respirophasic variation that is opposite in direction to that observed in spontaneously breathing patients (i.e., there is a greater than 30% *decrease* in the peak E-wave velocity that is normally observed in intubated patients at *end expiration*). Figure 79.5 presents a transmitral Doppler profile of a patient with constrictive pericarditis that is being mechanically ventilated (note the 62% decrease in expiratory peak E-wave velocity). Such degrees of respirophasic variation are not observed in patients with restrictive cardiomyopathy.

Other methods such as color M-mode and isovolemic relaxation time are less sensitive and specific for distinguishing constrictive pericarditis from restrictive cardiomyopathy. Although pulse wave Doppler assessment of the pulmonary vein profiles has been noted to be useful in discerning constrictive pericarditis from restrictive cardiomyopathy, it is not as specific as tissue Doppler imaging. One transesophageal study demonstrated that there was an exaggerated respirophasic variation (i.e., greater than 18% increase during inspiration) of the peak pulmonic D-wave velocity in patients with constrictive pericarditis that has not been observed in patients with restrictive cardiomyopathy.

Figure 79.6 presents the pulmonary vein tracings from a patient with constrictive pericarditis that demonstrate the characteristic increased exaggerated respirophasic variation (i.e., 38% increase) observed in the peak D-wave velocity during inspiration.

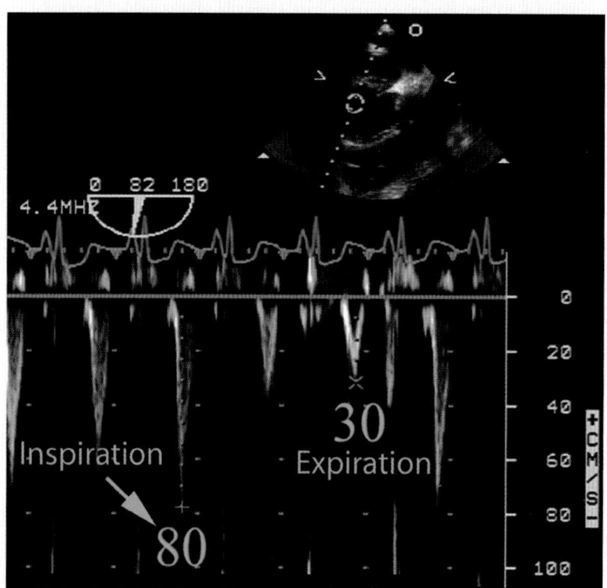

Figure 79.5.

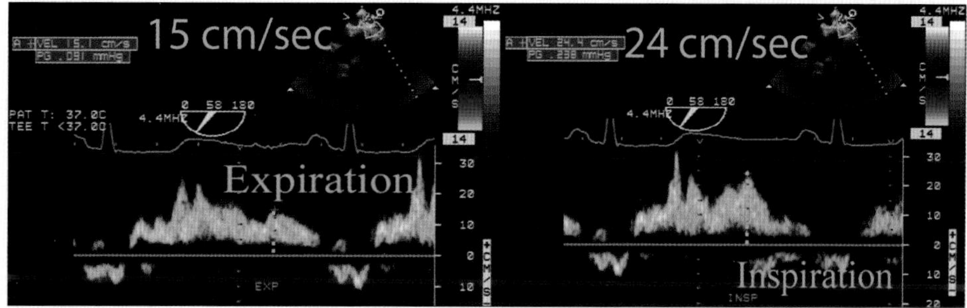

Figure 79.6.

TAKE-HOME LESSON:

Constrictive pericarditis and restrictive cardiomyopathy both result in diastolic dysfunction. Tissue Doppler imaging is the most sensitive and specific way to differentiate a filling problem due to constrictive disease or due to intrinsic myocardial dysfunction.

SUGGESTED READING

Klein AL, Cohen GI, Pietrolungo JF, et al. Differentiation of constrictive pericarditis from restrictive cardiomyopathy by Doppler transesophageal echocardiographic measurements of respiratory variations in pulmonary vein flow. *J Am Coll Cardiol.* 1993;22:1935–1943.

Lange RM, Bierig M, Devereux RB, et al. Recommendations for chamber quantification: a report from the American Society of Echocardiography's Guidelines and Standards Committee and the Chamber Quantification Writing Group, developed in conjunction with the European Association of Echocardiography, a branch of the European Society of Cardiology. *J Am Soc Echocardiogr.* 2005;18:1440–1463.

Otto C. Pericardial disease. In: Otto C, ed. *Textbook of Clinical Echocardiography.* 3rd ed. Philadelphia: Elsevier Saunders; 2004:259–275.

Rajagopalan N, Garcia MJ, Rodriguez L, et al. Comparison of new Doppler echocardiographic methods to differentiate constrictive pericardial heart disease and restrictive cardiomyopathy. *Am J Cardiol.* 2001;87:86–94.

Shernan S. Echocardiographic evaluation of pericardial disease. In: Konstadt SN, Shernan S, Oka Y, eds. *Clinical Transesophageal Echocardiography.* Philadelphia: Lippincott Williams & Wilkins; 2003:203–213.

Advanced

CASE 80

The patient was diagnosed with a congenital heart lesion at the age of 9. She remained uncorrected until the age of 36, at which time she developed increasing shortness of breath, fatigue, and chronic AFib. She is currently in your OR undergoing her repair.

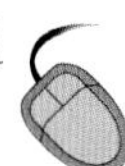

QUESTION 80.1. Based on Figure 80.1 and Video 80.1, her most likely diagnosis is:

A. Tetralogy of Fallot

B. AV canal defect

C. Ebstein anomaly

D. Transposition of the great arteries

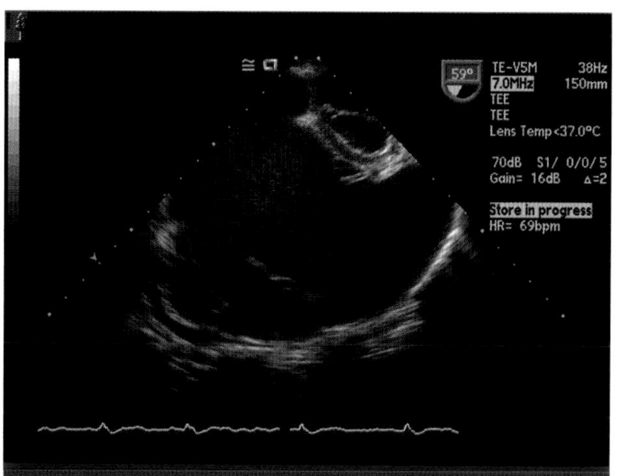

Figure 80.1.

She underwent a right and LA Maze procedure, a TV replacement, and dual-chamber pacemaker placement. The TEE of the prosthetic TV and RV shown in Videos 80.2 and 80.3 were obtained in the OR, following termination of CPB.

QUESTION 80.2. What would you ask the surgeon to do?

A. De-air the RV

B. Check the leaflets of the prosthetic valve

C. Assess the RCA

D. No intervention needed, proceed with chest closure

ANSWERS AND DISCUSSION

QUESTION 80.1: The correct answer is C: Ebstein anomaly.

Figure 80.1 and Video 80.1 show a ME RV inflow–outflow view of the enlarged RA, atrialized portion of the RV, and inferior displacement of the septal leaflet of the TV. Note also the abnormal attachment of the septal leaflet of the TV, the right atrial enlargement, and the extension of the RA into the RV, so-called atrialization of the RV. Figure 80.2 is a still image shown to illustrate the usual TV annulus and inferior displacement of the septal leaflet attachments.

QUESTION 80.2: The correct answer is C: Assess the RCA. Normally, the RCA travels from the right-facing sinus of the AV and courses posteriorly and laterally, adjacent to the TV annulus, then forms the predominant posterior descending branch. In many patients with Ebstein anomaly its course changes; it is deviated rightward or leftward and the posterior descending branch is not in its usual location in the interventricular groove. In addition, during plication procedures, risk to the RCA includes direct injury, stenosis, or kinking. The surgeon must be aware of the exact location of the RCA to prevent unintentional injury, the cause of RV dysfunction in this patient. Since the function of the RV is an important prognostic indicator in patients with Ebstein anomaly, any intraoperative compromise of the RCA should be immediately addressed. It is essential to note the baseline RV systolic function prior to operation.

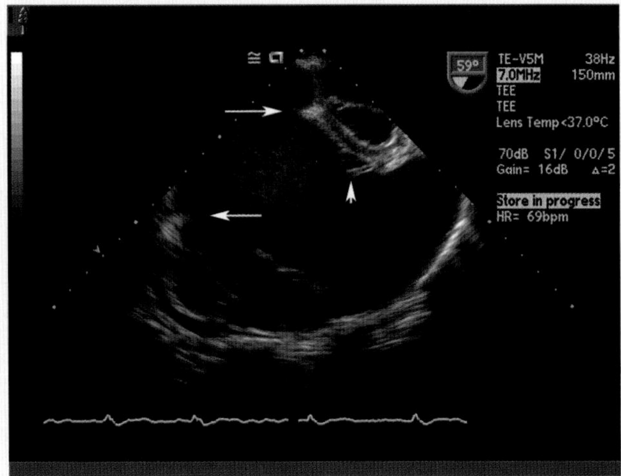

Figure 80.2. Still image of the TEE, ME RV inflow–outflow view. The long arrows mark the location of the TV annulus, the arrowhead marks the inferior attachment of the TV septal leaflet. These are the classic echo manifestations of a patient with Ebstein anomaly.

TAKE-HOME LESSON:

In many patients with Ebstein anomaly the RCA is aberrant. Injury, stenosis or kinking of the artery can occur and potentially lead to RV dysfunction.

SUGGESTED READING

Adachi I, Ho SY, McCarthy KP, et al. Coronary blood supply of the inferior wall of the right ventricle in hearts with Ebstein malformation: relevance to vertical plication. *J Thorac Cardiovasc Surg.* 2008;136(6): 1437–1441.

Brown ML, Dearani JA, Danielson GK, et al. Functional status after operation for Ebstein anomaly: the Mayo Clinic experience. *J Am Coll Cardiol.* 2008;52(6):460–466.

Chu D, Bakaeen FG. Reply to the Editor. *J Thorac Cardiovasc Surg.* 2009;138:513–514.

CASE 81

A 39-year-old male presents for elective AV surgery. As part of your preoperative TEE, you obtain the images shown in Figures 81.1 to 81.3.

QUESTION 81.1. The AV abnormality demonstrated on this echocardiogram is best described as:

A. Unicuspid acommissural AV
B. Unicuspid unicommissural AV
C. Bicuspid AV
D. Tricuspid AV

QUESTION 81.2. What is the etiology of the AV disease?

A. Congenital
B. Postinflammatory
C. Postinfectious
D. Degenerative ("calcific" or "senile")

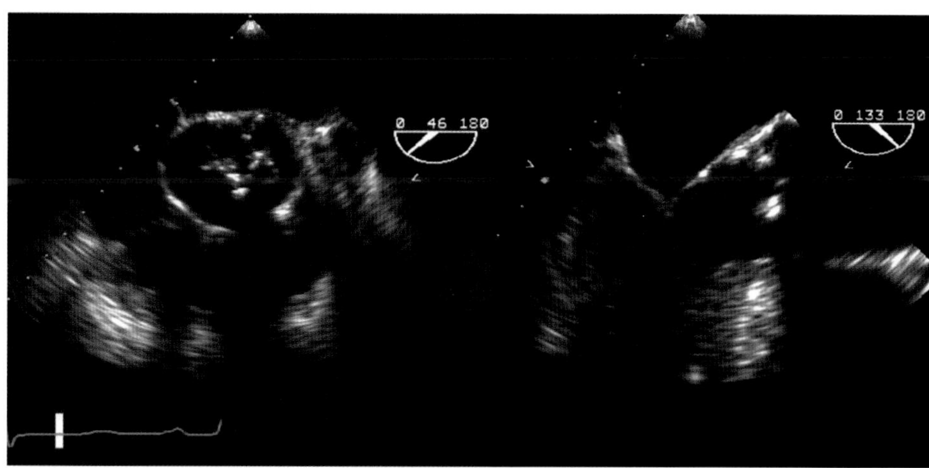

Figure 81.1. ME short- (on left) and long-axis (on right) views of the AV. See also Videos 81.1 to 81.4.

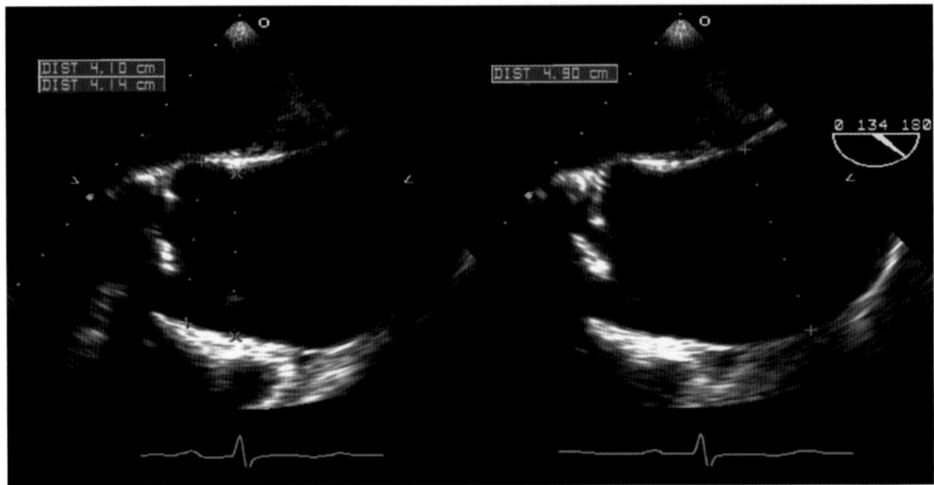

Figure 81.2. Upper esophageal LAX of the ascending aorta, demonstrating the measurements of the aortic root (on left) and ascending thoracic aorta (on right).

QUESTION 81.3. How significant is the valve stenosis?

A. Mild
B. Moderate
C. Severe
D. There is no abnormality

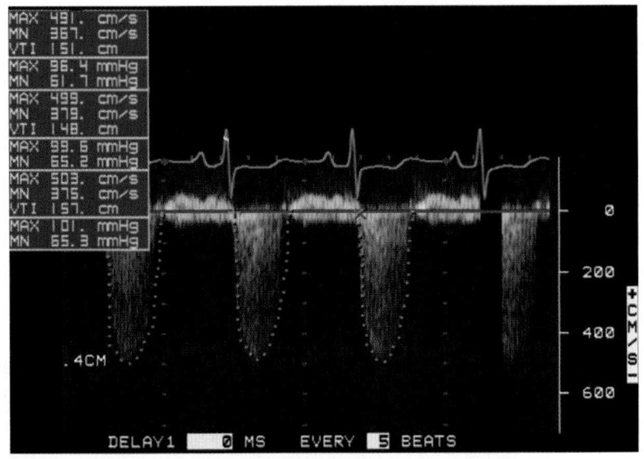

Figure 81.3. CW Doppler measurement across the AV, obtained from the deep TG view of the LV.

QUESTION 81.4. Which of the following statements best describes this abnormality?

A. It is an isolated AV disease
B. It is often associated with an aortopathy
C. It is only diagnosed in the pediatric age group
D. It is the leading cause of AS requiring AVR

QUESTION 81.5. In this case the surgical procedure you would recommend is:

A. An AVR
B. An AVR and an ascending aortic replacement
C. An AVR and an aortic root replacement
D. An AV repair

ANSWERS AND DISCUSSION

QUESTION 81.1: The correct answer is B: Unicuspid unicommissural AV. Only one commissure can be seen at the 12 o'clock position (posteriorly) on the AV. The AV can have anywhere from one to four cusps. In the unicuspid form, two subtypes are possible: *unicuspid acommissural*, in which there is no commissure but a central, often triangular, orifice, and *unicuspid unicommissural*, in which there is always a single commissure *posteriorly* directed. A raphe may be present that can be confused with a fused commissure. The acommissural subtype is more commonly found in pediatric populations, but adult cases have also been described. Although the overall incidence of unicuspid AV in the general adult population is low (0.02%), it is not that uncommon in the subgroup of patients who have AV disease. In a large series of surgically explanted AV in adult patients with *isolated AV disease*, unicuspid AV were present in 5% of patients (of which the vast majority were unicommissural). Moreover, in patients between the ages of 21 and 60, 19% of the valves were unicuspid. Patients with unicuspid valves were more likely to be male, more likely to have heavily calcified valves, and more likely to present at a younger age for surgery. One reason unicuspid AV is so rarely diagnosed formally at the time of surgery is that heavy calcifications may mask the unicuspid nature of the valve. Without careful pathologic examination, many of these valves may be called "functional bicuspid."

QUESTION 81.2: The correct answer is A: Congenital. Although the ultimate diagnosis can only be made with absolute certainty by pathologic examination, the appearance of the valve and the age of the patient strongly suggest a congenital origin. The valve appears to be a calcified and stenotic, with aliasing CFD in systole. The abnormal anatomy creates excessive structural stresses on the valve, resulting in calcification and stenosis. This is not a postrheumatic process (answer B), nor is it an infectious process (answer C), although unicuspid valves, like other valvulopathies, are at increased risk of developing endocarditis. Finally, degenerative AS is more prevalent in the geriatric population with normal TV, and it is unlikely to affect a 39-year-old patient. Figure 81.4 shows the pathologic specimen from this patient. Note that without careful pathologic examination, it may be difficult to differentiate between a bicuspid valve with a fused bottom commissure and a true unicuspid valve. Finally, Figure 81.5 and Video 81.5 present a nonstenosed unicommissural unicuspid AV for comparison.

QUESTION 81.3: The correct answer is C: Severe. The transvalvular velocities are very high with a peak velocity of over 5 m/s, suggesting severe AS. The calculated peak gradient is 100 mm Hg and the mean gradient is 65 mm Hg.

QUESTION 81.4: The correct answer is B: It is often associated with an aortopathy. In a series of 21 patients with a unicuspid AV, 48% had ascending *aortic dilation*.[1] Hence it is more than just an isolated aortic valve disease (thus, answer A is false). Like bicuspid AV, unicuspid valves are associated with an increased risk of *aortic*

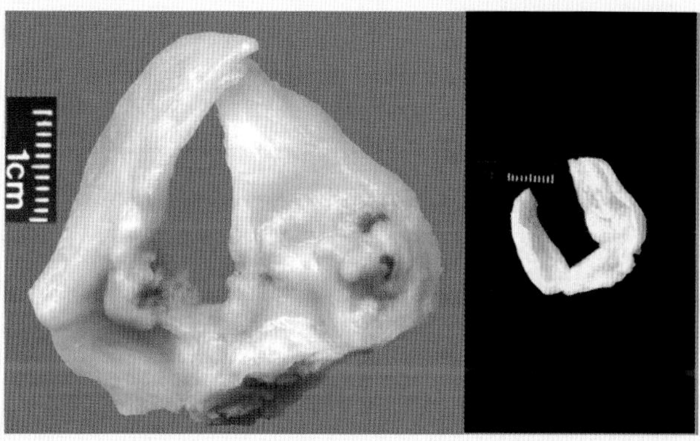

Figure 81.4. Pathologic specimens of this patient's valve (on left), and an example of a noncalcified, nonstenotic unicuspid unicommissural AV.

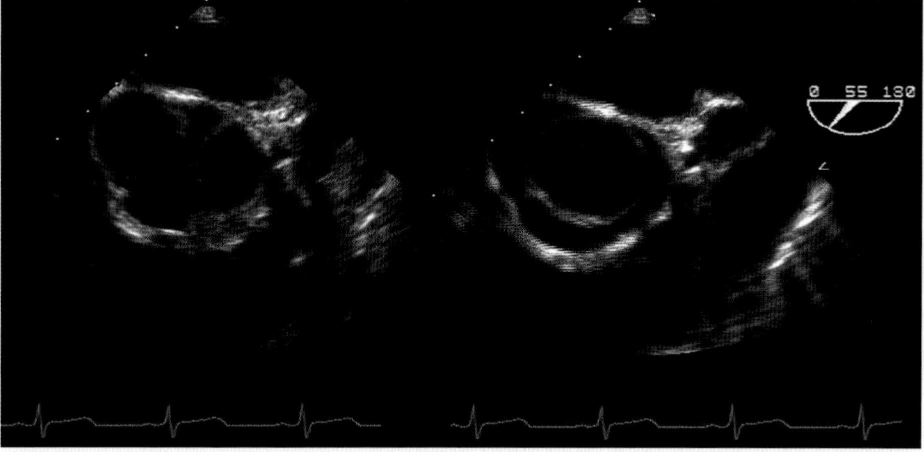

Figure 81.5. ME aortic short-axis view of a noncalcified, nonstenosed unicuspid AV in diastole (on left) and systole (on right).

dissection. In a large autopsy study, the incidence of *aortic dissection* in patients with unicuspid valves was 18 times higher than that found in patients with a tricuspid AV, and double that of patients with a bicuspid AV. It can be seen in young adults, but it is less frequent than bicuspid valve disease. Hence answers C and D are incorrect.

QUESTION 81.5: The correct answer is B: An AVR and an ascending aortic replacement. This patient has severe AS and requires an AVR. However, this patient also has significant dilation of the ascending aorta and milder dilation of the aortic root (Fig. 81.2). Although there are no specific recommendations dealing with aortopathy and unicuspid AV, the current guidelines for elective surgical repair of a dilated ascending aorta with a bicuspid AV suggest intervention when:

Aortic diameter >5.0 cm
Aortic diameter >4.5 cm with any of the following:

a. Expansion rate > 0.5 cm/year in an adult
b. Aortic coarctation
c. First-degree relative with ascending aortic dissection or rupture
d. Long smoking history especially with COPD
e. Small adult body size

Aortic diameter >4.0 cm with concomitant indication for elective AVR

Since the risk of aortic dissection is higher in unicuspid AV than in bicuspid valves it is appropriate to intervene. In addition to an AVR the ascending aorta should be replaced. The aortic root and the sinotubular junction both are also dilated, although not as severely as the ascending aorta. The necessity of replacing the root is less clear as it would entail a more complicated operation with re-implantation of the coronary arteries. Although dilation of the aortic root after ascending aortic and AVR in patients with AV disease and dilation of the ascending aorta have been described, the long-term results of replacement only of the AV and ascending aorta in patients who do not have Marfan syndrome and have no or only minimal dilation of the aortic root (like this patient) are very good. Depending on local surgical preference and expertise, answer C could also be acceptable. Answer D is incorrect: this valve is heavily calcified and thus is not amenable to repair.

TAKE-HOME LESSON:

In the unicuspid form, two subtypes are possible: acommissural and unicommissural. Acommissural, in which there is no commissure but a central, often triangular, orifice, and *unicuspid unicommissural*, in which there is always a single commissure *posteriorly* directed. A raphe may be present that can be confused with a fused commissure. Like bicuspid AV, unicuspid valves are associated with an increased risk of *aortic dissection*.

REFERENCE

1. Larson EW, Edwards WD. Risk factors for aortic dissection: a necropsy study of 161 cases. *Am J Cardiol.* 1984;53:849–855.

SUGGESTED READING

Houel R, Soustelle C, Kirsch M, et al. Long-term results of the Bentall operation versus replacement of the ascending aorta and aortic valve. *J Heart Valve Dis.* 2002;11(4):485–491.

Novaro GM, Mishra M, Griffin BP. Incidence and echocardiographic features of congenital unicuspid aortic valve in an adult population. *J Heart Valve Dis.* 2003;12:674–678.

Roberts WC, Ko JM. Clinical and morphological features of the congenitally unicuspid acommissural stenotic and regurgitant aortic valve. *Cardiology.* 2007;108:79–81.

Roberts WC, Ko JM. Frequency by decades of unicuspid, bicuspid, and tricuspid aortic valves in adults having isolated aortic valve replacement for aortic stenosis, with or without associated aortic regurgitation. *Circulation.* 2005;111:920–925.

Roberts WC, Ko JM. Weights of operatively excised stenotic unicuspid, bicuspid, and tricuspid aortic valves and their relation to age, sex, body mass index, and presence or absence of coronary artery bypass grafting. *Am J Cardiol.* 2003;92:1057–1065.

Sioris T, David TE, Ivanov J, et al. Clinical outcomes after separate and composite replacement of the aortic valve and ascending aorta. *J Thorac Cardiovasc Surg.* 2004;128:260–265.

Tadros TM, Klein MD, Shapira OM. Ascending aortic dilatation associated with bicuspid aortic valve: pathophysiology, molecular biology and clinical implications. *Circulation.* 2009;119:880–890.

Advanced

CASE 82

A 62-year-old man presents with a history of CHF. He is scheduled for AVR and CABG. His systolic blood pressure is 85 to 90 mm Hg and he cannot lie flat. Upon insertion of the TEE probe you observe the images shown in Figure 82.1 and Video 82.1.

QUESTION 82.1. What is the tentative diagnosis based on review of Figure 82.1 and video 82.1?

A. AS and insufficiency
B. Mitral insufficiency
C. Aortic and MV endocarditis
D. A and B

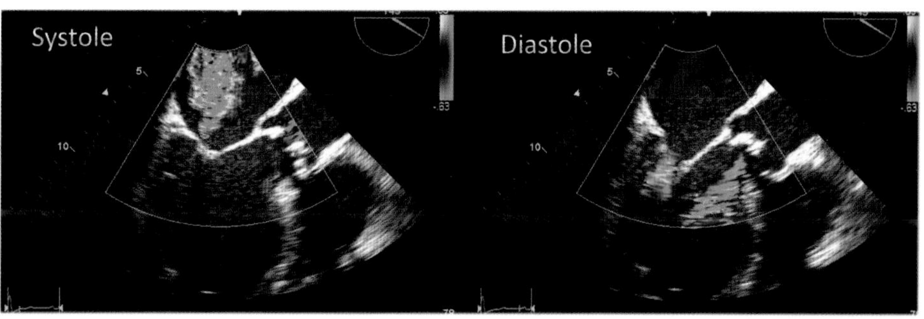

Figure 82.1. ME long axis with CFD in systole and diastole.

QUESTION 82.2. In order to assess the degree of stenosis, you perform a CW Doppler of the AV. Based on the mean and peak pressure gradients (Fig. 82.2) and an assessment of Figure 82.3 and Video 82.2, what is your conclusion?

A. Severe AS
B. Mild AS
C. Subvalvular AS
D. Unable to accurately assess degree of AS based on present information

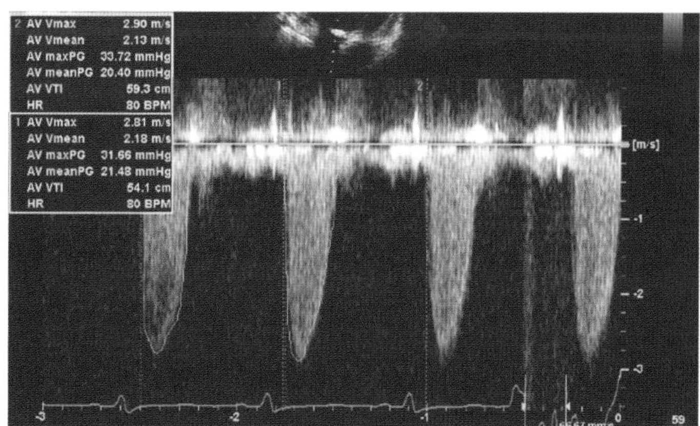

Figure 82.2. CW Doppler of the AV.

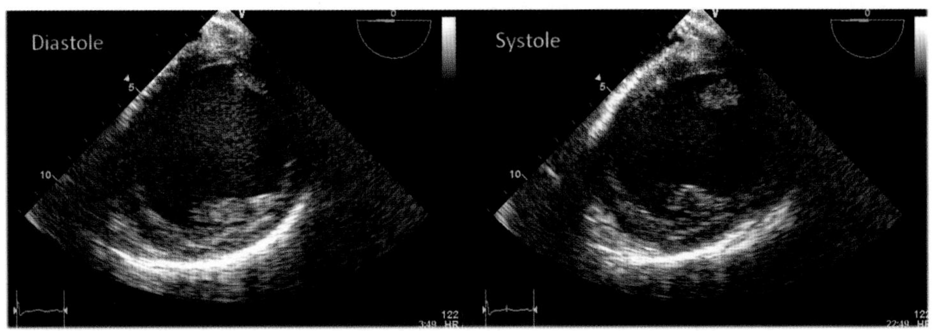

Figure 82.3. TG SAX view in systole and diastole. See also Video 82.2.

QUESTION 82.3. You measure the LVOT diameter to be 2.3 cm. With the information in Figures 82.2 and 82.4 and in light of Videos 82.1 and 82.2, which of the following statements is true?

A. Severity of AS may be overestimated due to poor LV function

B. Moderate-to-severe AS with AVA of 0.98 cm^2

C. AS severity cannot be accurately determined in the presence of aortic regurgitation

D. The severity of AS will be overestimated due to severe MR

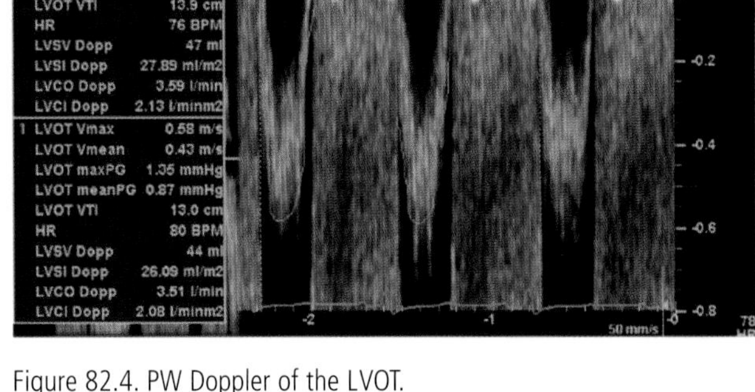

Figure 82.4. PW Doppler of the LVOT.

QUESTION 82.4. The accuracy of the LVOT measurement is uncertain due to suboptimal imaging. What alternative technique could be used to help determine the severity of AS?

A. PHT

B. Flow reversal in descending aorta

C. Pulse contour analysis

D. Dimensionless index

ANSWERS AND DISCUSSION

QUESTION 82.1: The correct answer is D: AS with insufficiency and mitral insufficiency.

The AV appears heavily calcified with limited mobility suggesting AS (Fig. 82.1, Video 82.1). There is also aortic and mitral insufficiency on CFD. Answer A is correct but incomplete. Answer B is correct but incomplete. Answer C is incorrect; no vegetations are detected on the valves. Of note, from Video 82.1 we can see that the LV is clearly dilated with poor function. The LV dilatation has contributed to bileaflet mitral leaflet restriction that is responsible for the MR.

QUESTION 82.2: The correct answer is D: Unable to conclude accurately with present information.

Having identified the calcified AV, the next goal should be to determine the transvalvular gradient. Using TEE, the best way to do this is to acquire a TG image (either 90-degree TG LAX or deep TG image) and obtain a CW Doppler tracing through the AV (Fig. 82.2). The mean pressure gradient measures ~21 mm Hg with an instantaneous peak pressure gradient of ~32 mm Hg. The mean pressure gradient indicates only mild AS (<30 mm Hg), where moderate stenosis: 30 to 50 mm Hg, severe > 50 mm Hg. However, the LV function in this patient is very poor (Videos 82.1 and 82.2). The depressed ventricular function may create a lower than expected mean and peak gradient (PG). In these cases a dobutamine challenge may be beneficial. In mild or moderate disease, the increase in flow through the valve following dobutamine administration may cause a greater opening of the valve leaflets (relative flexibility) for mild and moderate disease. However, in severe AS an increase in flow through the valve would not alter its orifice size and the pressure gradient would rise. Therefore with poor LV function, low flow rates may result in an overestimation of AS severity based on 2D appearance, while resulting in an underestimation based on velocity gradients.

Answer C is incorrect; in this patient, no subvalvular stenosis was noted in TEE views. This diagnosis can be confirmed by using PW doppler in the LVOT from the deep transgastric view if the 2D images are not conclusive.

QUESTION 82.3: The correct answer is A.

Measurement of the AVA by continuity requires a separate measurement of the LVOT VTI (velocity time integral) and diameter to determine the cross-sectional area (CSA). The diameter is best measured in the 120-degree ME LAX. It is extremely important to precisely measure the LVOT diameter as the calculation requires the squaring of the radius (πr^2) and therefore a squaring of the error. A PW Doppler measurement is made at the LVOT in the TG LAX or a deep TG view. These measurements can then be entered into the continuity equation and the AVA can be calculated using:

$$AVA = LVOT_{CSA} \times \frac{LVOT_{VTI}}{AV_{VTI}}$$

Using the above equation, the diagnosis of mild (valve area 1.5 to 2.0 cm^2), moderate (valve area 1.0 to 1.5 cm^2), or severe (valve area <1.0 cm^2) AS can be made. In the case presented, the calculated valve area was 0.98 cm^2 or moderate-to-severe AS based on the continuity equation using LVOT and AV VTI. In the presence of poor LV function, however, the AV may not open to its fullest due to poor SV. The calculated AVA will be small but may increase in the presence of improved SV. Administration of dobutamine (not routine in the OR) would result in an increase in flow at both the LVOT and the AV but the leaflets may open more in milder disease resulting in a smaller increase in velocity at the valve when compared to the LVOT. In severe disease, the increase in flow would not result in a change in AV opening. The increase in velocities at both the LVOT and the AV would be proportionate.

Answer B is not completely correct. The AVA of 0.98 cm^2 is correct using the continuity equation but the AVA may increase if the SV were higher. Dobutamine studies may help in determining the true grade of AS. Answer C is incorrect. The continuity equation would not be affected by AI. Even though the volume through the valve is increased due to the RV, this should not affect the continuity equation. Answer D is incorrect. The presence of MR would not affect the pressure gradient through the AV. The MR velocity contour, however, can be similar to that of the aortic velocity contour and has been mistaken for the interrogation of the AV. Great care must be taken in measuring the velocity profile.

QUESTION 82.4: The correct answer is D: Dimensionless index.

Calculation of a dimensionless index for AS involves measuring the ratio of the VTI of the LVOT and the AV's narrowest point ($LVOT_{VTI}/AS_{VTI}$). This approach is a variation of the continuity equation with the advantages of being less sensitive to hemodynamics. It does not require the measurement of the LVOT diameter as it is calculated as the ratio of LVOT flow to transvalvular flow. A ratio less than 0.25 indicates severe AS. Answer A, PHT is useful in mitral stenosis not AS. Answer B, flow reversal in descending aorta is used to determine the severity of aortic regurgitation. Answer C, pulse contour analysis has not been successfully applied to the assessment of AS.

TAKE-HOME LESSON:

Pressure gradients and AVA determinations for AS in the presence of poor LV function can lead to erroneous conclusions regarding severity of AS.

SUGGESTED READING

Cohen IS. Aortic stenosis. In: Perrino AC Jr, Reeves ST, eds. *A Practical Approach to Transesophageal Echocardiography*. 2nd ed. Philadelphia, PA: Lippincott Williams & Wilkins; 2008.

CASE 83

An 8-month-old child with Down syndrome presents to the hospital for surgical repair of a congenital heart lesion. The TEE images are shown in Videos 83.1 and 83.2 and in Figures 83.1 and 83.2.

QUESTION 83.1. What is the diagnosis?

A. ASD
B. VSD
C. AV canal
D. Tetralogy of Fallot

QUESTION 83.2. An AV canal is composed of which of the following?

A. Inlet VSD
B. Primum ASD
C. Abnormal AV valves
D. A and B only
E. A and C only
F. A, B, and C

QUESTION 83.3. The left-sided AV valve (Video 83.2, Fig. 83.2) would best be classified as

A. Rastelli A
B. Rastelli B
C. Rastelli C
D. Rastelli D

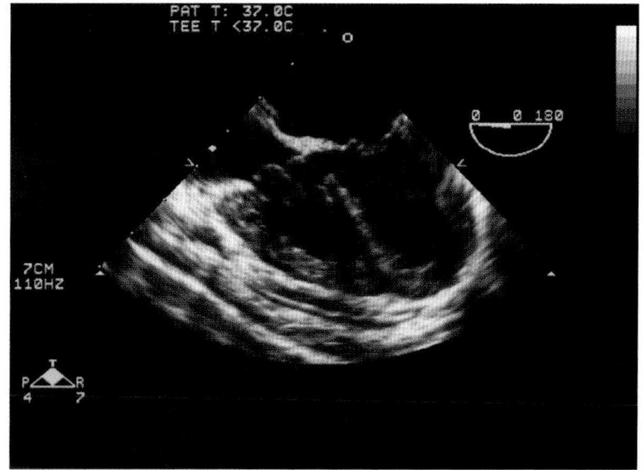

Figure 83.1.

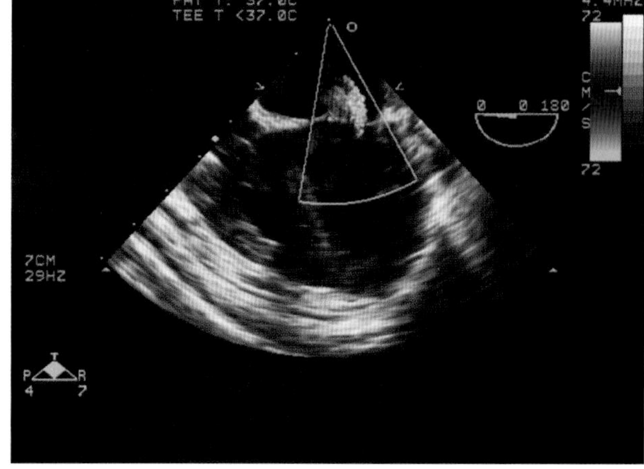

Figure 83.2.

ANSWERS AND DISCUSSION

QUESTION 83.1: The correct answer is C: AV canal. This condition is now commonly called AV canal defect. It results from the failure of the endocardial cushions to fuse during the fifth week of fetal development. It is associated in up to 20% of patients with Down, 15% of patients with Noonan, and 50% of patients with Ellis-van Creveld syndromes.

QUESTION 83.2: The correct answer is F: A, B, and C. A common atrioventricular canal (CAVC) defect is composed of a primum ASD, inlet ASD, and AV valve abnormalities. There are three types of CAVCs: partial, transitional, and complete.

QUESTION 83.3: The correct answer is C: Rastelli C. In a complete AV canal defect there is typically a large common single AV valve. The left AV segment of the valve usually contains a cleft that is insufficient. The Rastelli classification system is based on the chordal attachments of the anterior bridging leaflet of the common AV valve. In all Rastelli subtypes the LVOT is narrowed and elongated.

RASTELLI CLASSIFICATION

A: The anterior leaflet is attached to the crest of the ventricular septum by thin chordae tendinae.

B: The anterior leaflet is attached via chordae tendinae to a papillary muscle in the RV near the septum.

C: The anterior leaflet lacks any ventricular septal attachments and is perceived almost 'floating' above the septum. This is the most common type associated with trisomy 21.

D: Does not exist.

TAKE-HOME LESSON:

Due to the presence of typically a large common single atrioventricular valve, these patients frequently have residual or progressive MR post repair that may necessitate surgery later in life.

SUGGESTED READING

Andropoulos DB, Stayer SA, Russell IA, eds. *Anesthesia for Congenital Heart Disease*. Blackwell Futura; 2005.

CASE 84

A 76-year-old female with coronary artery disease, hyperlipidemia, and history of a previous stroke presents to your OR for an on-pump CABG.

QUESTION 84.1. The arrows in Figures 84.1 and 84.2 are pointing toward:

A. Type B aortic dissection
B. Descending thoracic aortic atheroma
C. Pleural effusion
D. Foreign body in aorta

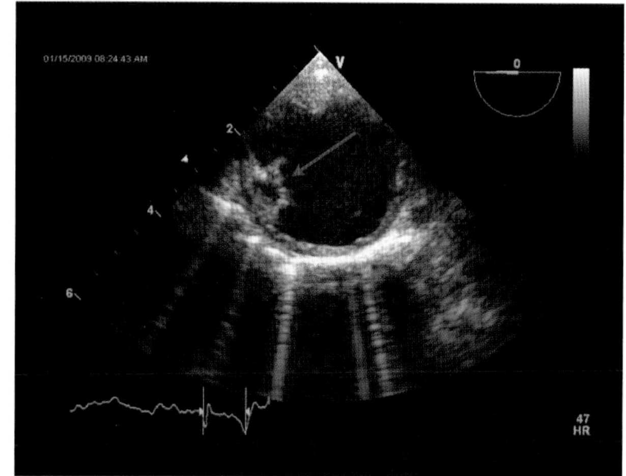

Figure 84.1. Short-axis view of descending thoracic aorta.

QUESTION 84.2. If the identified echo-dense object is an atheroma that moves within the aortic lumen, how would it be graded?

A. Grade I
B. Grade II
C. Grade III
D. Grade IV
E. Grade V

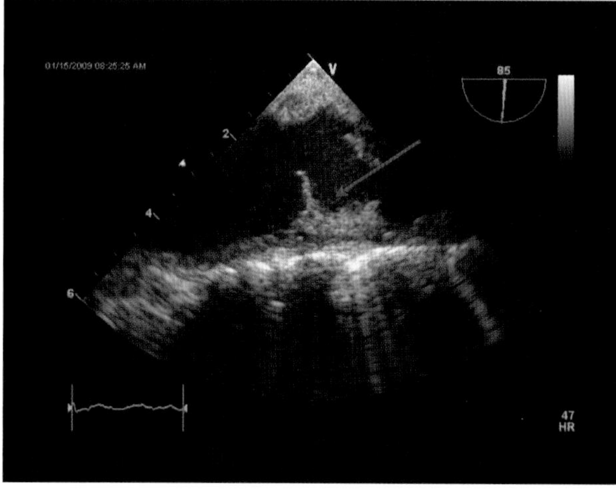

Figure 84.2. Long axis of descending thoracic aorta.

QUESTION 84.3. Risk factors for aortic plaque include:

A. Advanced age
B. Hypertension
C. COPD
D. Cerebrovascular disease
E. Renal insufficiency
F. All of the above

QUESTION 84.4. All of the following are indications for an epiaortic ultrasound exam of the ascending aorta except:

A. History of stroke
B. Grade III or greater descending aortic plaque
C. Evidence of calcified aorta by other imaging modality such as MRI, CT scan, or chest x-ray.
D. Palpation by surgeon reveals no plaque
E. TEE exam reveals no ascending aortic plaque

QUESTION 84.5. Identify the following structures in Figure 84.3:

Standoff ____
Anterior aortic wall ____
Posterior aortic wall ____
Lateral aortic wall ____
SVC ____
Right PA ____

QUESTION 84.6. The arrow in Figure 84.4 is pointing to a(n)

A. Aortic dissection
B. Mobile plaque
C. IABP
D. Artifact

QUESTION 84.7. Epiaortic echocardiography reveals an ascending aortic plaque, such as the one shown in Figure 84.5. As the echocardiographer, you suggest to the surgeon:

A. Alter cannulation site, cross clamp or cardioplegia location
B. Convert to off-pump CABG
C. Perform aortic endarterectomy
D. Some combination of the above that reduces aortic manipulation

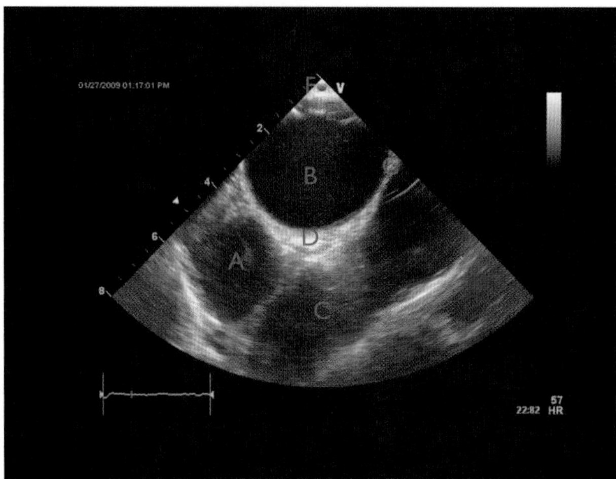

Figure 84.3. Short axis of aorta via epiaortic ultrasonography.

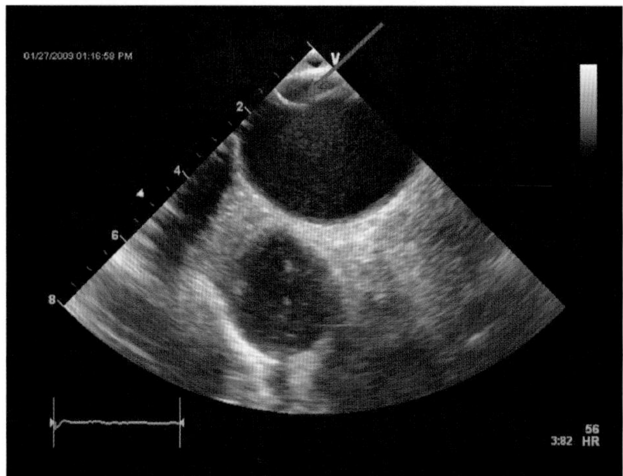

Figure 84.4. Short-axis epiaortic image.

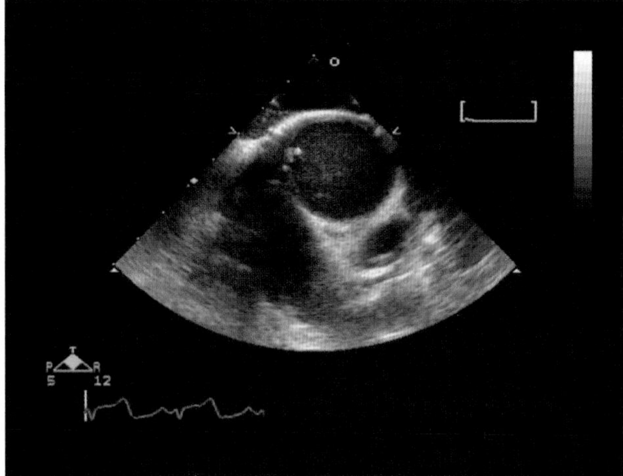

Figure 84.5. Short-axis epiaortic ultrasound. See Video 84.1 for mobile component of plaque. (Courtesy of Emory University.)

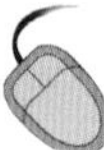

ANSWERS AND DISCUSSION

QUESTION 84.1: The correct answer is B. Figures 84.1 and 84.2 are TEE images of the descending thoracic aorta in short axis demonstrating a significant atheromatous burden. The arrow is pointing directly at a large atheroma. A Type B dissection would appear as a linear echo-dense object in the middle of the aortic lumen. A pleural effusion would not appear as an echo-dense object; rather, most often, it will appear as a semilunar-shaped echo-lucency outside of the aorta. This image is not consistent with a foreign body such as an IABP.

QUESTION 84.2: The correct answer is E. In 1992 Katz introduced a grading scale for aortic plaques that was recommended in 2008 as a standard scale by the American Society of Echocardiography (Table 84.1).

Table 84.1 Aortic Atherosclerosis Grading Scale

Grade I	Normal-to-mild intimal thickening
Grade II	Severe intimal thickening without protrusion
Grade III	Atheroma protruding <5 mm
Grade IV	Atheroma protruding ≥ 5 mm
Grade V	Any thickness with a mobile component

QUESTION 84.3: The correct answer is F. Advanced age, hypertension, COPD, renal insufficiency and cerebrovascular disease are all associated with an increased risk of aortic atherosclerosis.

QUESTION 84.4: The correct answer is D. Current indications for performing an epiaortic ultrasound exam include increased risk factors for stroke (age, female sex, history of cerebral vascular disease, diabetes, HTN and renal insufficiency) and evidence of aortic pathology (atherosclerosis or calcification) on other imaging modalities, including TEE. Additionally, surgical palpation has been proven to miss 50% of significant ascending aortic plaque when compared to epiaortic ultrasound. Given the favorable risk-benefit ratio of epiaortic ultrasonography it should be used for every patient who will have any degree of aortic manipulation.

QUESTION 84.5:

Standoff	F
Anterior aortic wall	E
Posterior aortic wall	D
Later aortic wall	G
SVC	A
Right PA	C

Epiaortic ultrasonography is accomplished by placing a TTE probe in a sterile sleeve in the surgical field. The probe is then placed directly on the aorta by the operator, most commonly by the surgeon. (The images in this case were obtained with a phased-array probe. A linear array probe can also be used. It does not require a standoff.) A standoff is created to allow a medium through which the ultrasound waves can pass from the probe to the aorta. Sterile ultrasound jelly or saline is used as a transducer medium within the sheath. Without the standoff, the anterior surface of the aorta is difficult to image. Because the probe is placed directly on the aorta, the structures located in the near field, or the top of the image, are anterior.

QUESTION 84.6: The correct answer is D. The echocardiographer must always be cognizant of artifacts introduced by the microbubbles in the standoff. If a dissection is suspected, always interrogate the aorta from multiple imaging angles and with another modality such as TEE. The artifact will disappear in more than one imaging plane while a true disease process will persist.

QUESTION 84.7: The correct answer is D. What the echocardiographer and the surgeon choose to do with the information varies greatly by institution and with practitioner preference. Some studies have shown that simply by decreasing aortic manipulation, stroke rates can be decreased by as much as 50%. The largest series investigating the influence of epiaortic ultrasound on outcomes retrospectively reviewed approximately 6000 cases and showed a significant decrease in stroke rate when epiaortic ultrasound was used. Off-pump CABG might be the best management strategy, but asking a surgeon to perform an off-pump CABG when they are not comfortable with the operation may increase morbidity and decrease graft patency rates. A rational combination of maneuvers such as altering cannulation, cardioplegia, or clamp sites or using no touch aortic techniques can be utilized when off-pump CABG is not feasible.

TAKE-HOME LESSON:

Current indications for performing an epiaortic exam include increased risk for stroke (age, female sex, history of cerebral vascular disease, diabetes, hypertension, and renal insufficiency) and evidence of aortic atherosclerosis or calcification by other imaging modality such as CT scan, chest x-ray, or TEE.

SUGGESTED READING

Glas KE, Swaminathan M, Reeves ST, et al. Guidelines for the performance of a comprehensive intraoperative epiaortic ultrasonographic examination: recommendations of the American Society of Echocardiography and the Society of Cardiovascular Anesthesiologists; Endorsed by the Society of Thoracic Surgeons. *Anesth Analg*. 2008;106(5):1376–1384.

Perino AC Jr, Reeves ST. *A Practical Approach to Transesophageal Echocardiography*. Philadelphia: Lippincott Williams & Wilkins; 2008.

Whitley WS, Glas KE. An argument for routine ultrasound screening of the thoracic aorta in the cardiac surgery population. *Semin Cardiothorac Vasc Anesth*. 2008;12(4):290–297.

Advanced

CASE 85

A 76-year-old patient with history of arterial hypertension and severe AS underwent AVR. During the prebypass period, PW Doppler examination of the mitral inflow (with a sample volume placed between the tips of mitral leaflets—ME 4CH view) showed the pattern in Figure 85.1. Arterial blood pressure was 135/87 mm Hg.

QUESTION 85.1. What is the diastolic function? What is the proper intervention?

A. Normal; do nothing
B. Abnormal; do nothing
C. Abnormal; decrease afterload
D. Indeterminate; further investigation needed

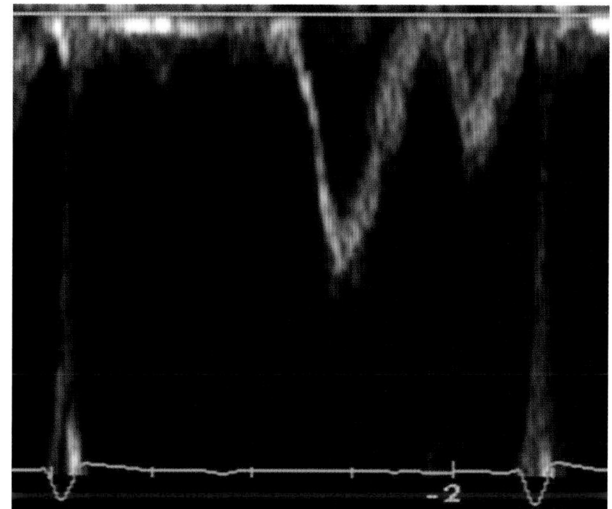

Figure 85.1.

QUESTION 85.2. Later on, during autologous blood withdrawal, you notice that the mitral inflow pattern has changed to the one shown in Figure 85.2. Does this patient have diastolic dysfunction?

A. No, the pattern is normal
B. Yes, the patient has impaired relaxation
C. Yes, the patient has a pseudonormal pattern
D. Yes, the patient has a restricted filling pattern

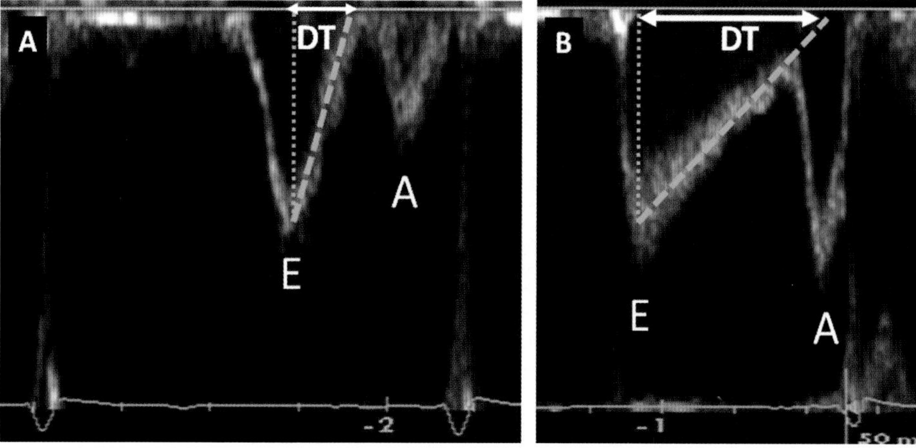

Figure 85.2.

QUESTION 85.3. Prior to autologous blood removal, would the pulmonary vein tracing shown in Figure 85.3 be consistent with this patient's diastolic function?

A. No, the s:d ratio would be reversed

B. No, there should not be an A wave

C. Yes, the s:d ratio would be expected

D. Yes, but only if the patient also had severe MR

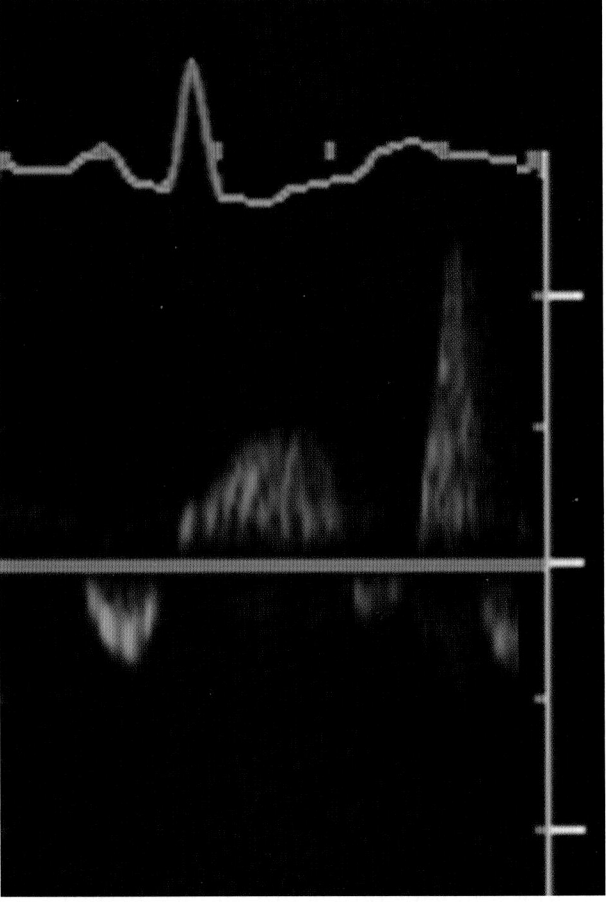

Figure 85.3.

ANSWERS AND DISCUSSION

QUESTION 85.1: The answer is D: Indeterminate; further investigation needed.

Diastole is composed of four separate stages: (1) isovolumetric relaxation, (2) early filling, (3) diastasis, and (4) atrial contraction. The blood flow into the LV can be measured during early filling and atrial contraction using PW Doppler. The "E" and "A" waves correspond to these two periods, and the influences on their shape are shown in Figure 85.4.

An early (E) to late (A) velocity ratio between 1 and 2 is considered to represent normal diastolic function in people younger than 50 to 60 years of age. However, load dependency of mitral inflow velocities can result in an E:A ratio between 1 and 2 even when diastolic function is impaired. This pattern is known as "pseudonormal." It is the result of higher LA pressures, producing a greater increase in the LA–LV pressure gradient, thus increasing the height of the E wave despite significant diastolic dysfunction. A pseudonormal pattern should be suspected if a "normal" E:A ratio is found in patients with known LV hypertrophy, high LVEDPs, or patients greater than 60 years old. Distinguishing between a normal and pseudonormal pattern requires either interrogating the pulmonary veins, decreasing preload (by using a Valsalva maneuver), or the use of tissue Doppler imaging.

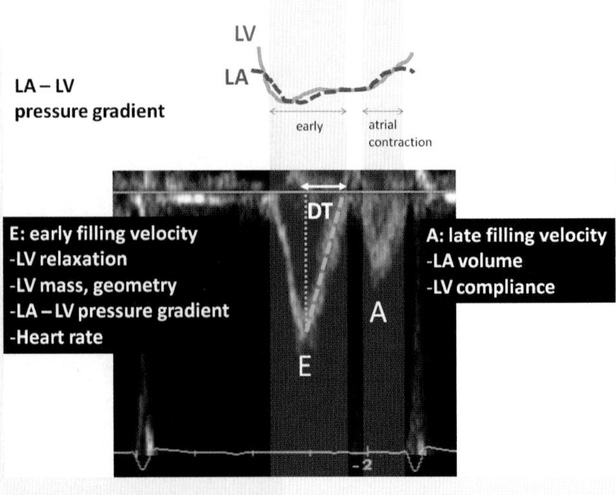

Figure 85.4.

QUESTION 85.2: The correct answer is C: Yes, the patient has diastolic dysfunction, as evidenced by a pseudonormal filling pattern. In this case, the initial filling pattern (Fig. 85.1) had an E:A ratio between 1 and 2. This pattern is found with normal diastolic function or when an increased LA pressure compensates for impaired relaxation (pseudonormal filling pattern). When the preload was decreased by removing the autologous blood, the E wave decreased in height and the deceleration time became prolonged (Fig. 85.2). If the patient had normal diastolic function, both the E and A waves would have decreased in amplitude. A restricted filling pattern is seen with extreme diastolic dysfunction and is the result of high LA pressures in addition to poor LV chamber compliance. The E:A ratio is >2 and usually much higher, while the E-wave deceleration time is very short. This pattern is shown in Figure 85.5.

QUESTION 85.3: The correct answer is C: Yes, the s:d ratio seen in Figure 85.3 would be expected.

This pulmonary vein tracing, produced using pulse wave Doppler located in the LUPV, shows the "s" (systolic) wave to be significantly reduced compared to the "d" (diastolic) wave. Normally, the "s" wave is larger or at least equal to the "d" wave, as shown in Figure 85.6. However, just like higher LA pressures will increase the "E" wave on mitral inflow, high LA pressures will also cause an increase in the "d" wave in the pulmonary veins. This produces an s:d ratio <1 and is one way to help distinguish normal mitral inflow from pseudonormal mitral inflow. Another marker for pseudonormalization is a pulmonary vein "a" wave greater than 35 cm/s. This "enlarged a wave" is caused by higher LA pressures exaggerating the reversal of flow during atrial contraction. Severe MR causes systolic reversal of the "s" wave.

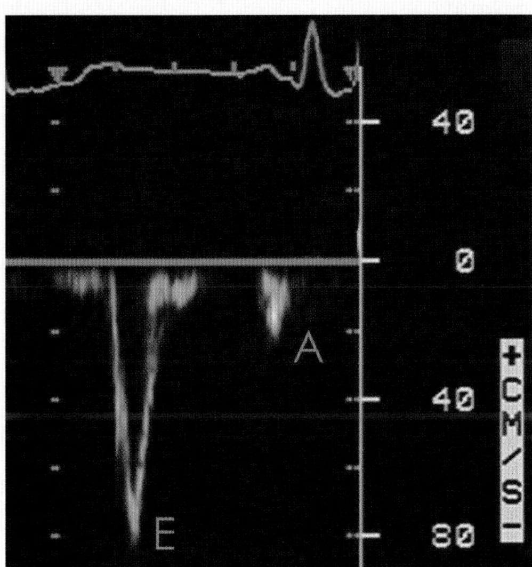

Figure 85.5.

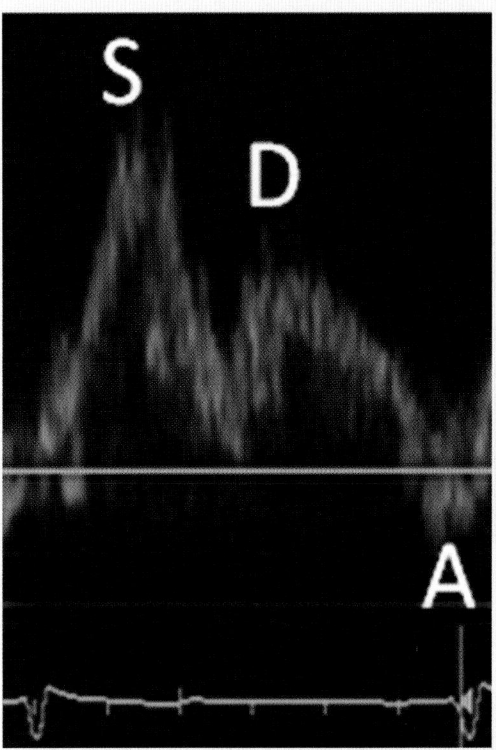

Figure 85.6.

TAKE-HOME LESSON:

An early (E) to late (A) velocity ratio between 1 and 2 is considered to represent normal diastolic function in people younger than 50 to 60 years of age. However, load dependency of mitral inflow velocities can result in an E:A ratio between 1 and 2 even when diastolic function is impaired. This pattern is known as "pseudonormal."

SUGGESTED READING

Maurer MS, Spevack D, Burkhoff D, et al. Diastolic dysfunction. Can it be diagnosed by Doppler echocardiography? *J Am Coll Cardiol.* 2004;44: 1543–1549.

Nagueh SF, Appleton CP, Gillebert TC, et al. Recommendations for the evaluation of left ventricular diastolic function by echocardiography. *J Am Soc Echocardiogr.* 2009;22:107–133.

CASE 86

A 26-year-old woman is evaluated for worsening dyspnea on exertion and syncope. Her past medical history is notable for repair of a membranous VSD at the age of 10 years. Exam reveals a loud systolic murmur. TEE is obtained for further work-up (Fig. 86.1).

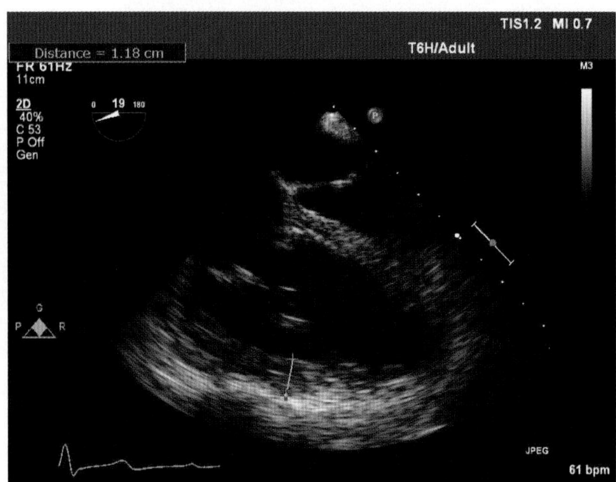

Figure 86.1. ME 4CH view of the heart. See also Video 86.1.

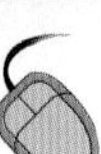

QUESTION 86.1. This patient has a RV free wall diameter and an interventricular septal wall diameter greater than 1 cm. What is the minimum definition of RV hypertrophy?

A. End-systolic RV free wall diameter of 0.5 cm thickness
B. End-diastolic RV free wall diameter of 0.7 cm thickness
C. Interventricular septal thickness of 1 cm
D. End-diastolic RV free wall diameter of 0.5 cm thickness

QUESTION 86.2. Examining the ME 4CH views (Figs. 86.1 and 86.2), what is the most likely cause of the right heart dilatation?

A. TR
B. Residual VSD
C. RV outflow obstruction
D. Unable to discern from the information available

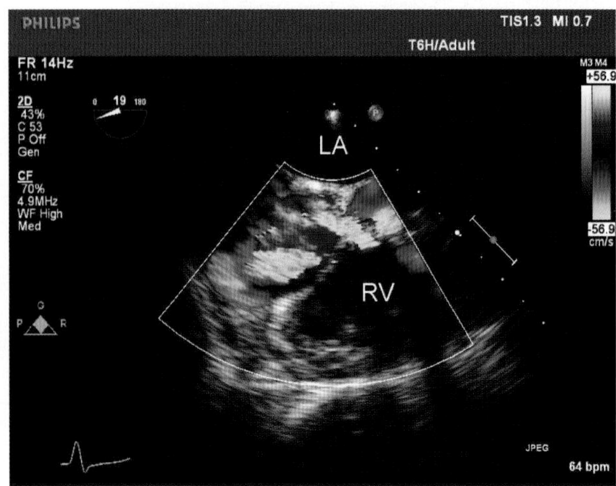

Figure 86.2. ME 4CH view with CFD. See also Video 86.2.

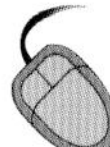

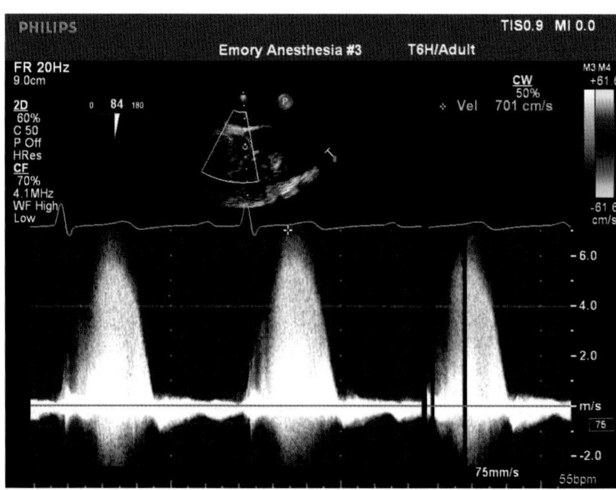

Figure 86.3. CW Doppler of the TR velocity.

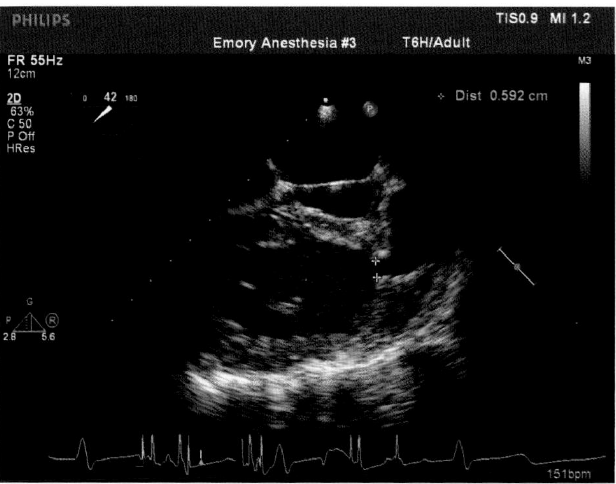

Figure 86.4. RV inflow–outflow view of the RV. See also Video 86.3.

QUESTION 86.3. CW Doppler of the TR revealed a peak, instantaneous velocity of the regurgitant jet of 7 m/s (Figure 86.3). What is the most likely cause of the TR?

A. Ebstein anomaly of the TV
B. Residual VSD
C. RV outflow obstruction
D. Pulmonic valve (PV) insufficiency

QUESTION 86.4. The pathology demonstrated in Figure 86.4 and Video 86.3 is most consistent with the diagnosis of which disease?

A. Tricuspid atresia
B. Carcinoid heart disease
C. Double-chamber RV
D. Residual VSD

ANSWERS AND DISCUSSION

QUESTION 86.1: The correct Answer is D: End-diastolic diameter of 0.5 cm thickness.

The normal RV free wall thickness is less than half of the LV and measures less than 5 mm at end diastole. RV hypertrophy is associated with pressure overload of the RV from RV outflow tract obstruction, pulmonary stenosis, or significant PA hypertension.

ANSWER A: Answer A—*End-systolic RV free wall diameter of 0.5 cm thickness*—is incorrect because end-systolic measurements will vary more with RV contractile function than end-diastolic diameters.

ANSWER B: Answer B—*End-diastolic RV free wall diameter of 0.7 cm thickness*—is incorrect. Severe RV hypertrophy is defined as 0.7 cm or greater.

ANSWER C: Answer C—*Interventricular septal thickness of 1 cm*—is incorrect as well. The interventricular septal diameter is more indicative of the LV thickness than the RV thickness.

QUESTION 86.2: The correct answer is D: Unable to discern from the information available. RV dilatation and RV hypertrophy are associated with multiple pathophysiological states. It is difficult to ascertain the root etiology without further examination. TR and residual VSD are both primarily diseases of RV volume overload and dilatation. Some secondary RV hypertrophy is possible with late stage pulmonary hypertension. RV outflow obstruction is strongly associated with dilatation secondary to pressure overload.

ANSWER C: Answer C is incorrect. *RV outflow obstruction* is strongly associated with dilatation of the RV secondary to chronic pressure overload. Long-standing pressure overload will frequently induce RV dilatation.

QUESTION 86.3: The correct answer is C: RV outflow obstruction.

The key to understanding this question is appreciating that the peak tricuspid regurgitant velocity is 7 m/s. The simplified Bernoulli equation states the peak pressure gradient is four times the square of peak instantaneous velocity. Solving for the pressure gives us: $4 \times (7 \text{ m/s})^2 =$ 196 mm Hg. The peak systolic pressure of the RV is 196 mm Hg greater than the central venous pressure (CVP)!

ANSWER A: Answer A is incorrect. Ebstein anomaly of the TV is associated with severe TR and volume overload of the RV. The TEE does not demonstrate an apically displaced TV and "atrialization" of the RV tissue.

ANSWERS B and D: Answers B and D are incorrect. *Residual VSD* and *pulmonic valve insufficiency* are both associated with volume overload of the RV and associated RV dilatation can cause severe TR.

Such high pressures could only be caused by a chronically progressive obstruction with compensatory RV hypertrophy. The obstruction in the distal RV or PV would shield the PA and lungs from such critically high pressures. Chronic volume overload of the RV can induce high RV pressures, but nowhere the magnitude of 200 mm Hg. The secondary PA hypertension would not be viable with life.

QUESTION 86.4: The correct answer is C: Double-chamber RV.

Double-chamber RV is an unusual congenital anomaly that is most commonly associated with VSDs. In this patient, it is likely that no significant obstruction was present at the time of surgical intervention for the VSD. The pathology is due to anomalous, hypertrophied muscle bundles that obstruct the RV outflow from the tricuspid to the pulmonary valve. Chronic pressure overload induces further hypertrophy and progression of the outflow obstruction until a murmur or symptoms are noted. The echocardiographic exam typically demonstrates an aberrant muscle bundle crossing the RV or an abnormal, band-like thickening of the RV outflow tract.

In effect, the RV is divided into a proximal high-pressure chamber and distal low-pressure chamber. The lungs are shielded from the high pressures and the symptoms can be dynamic, similar to HOCM.

ANSWER A: Answer A is incorrect. *Tricuspid atresia* is associated with total obstruction of the right heart outflow and an underdeveloped or absent RV. No gradient is established and the patient has single ventricle physiology.

ANSWER B: Answer B is incorrect. *Carcinoid heart disease* is associated with pulmonary stenosis and TR, but not the RV outflow obstruction demonstrated in Figure 86.4 and Video 86.3. The classic signs of severe, TV thickening are also not present in the previous figures.

ANSWER D: Answer D is incorrect. *Residual VSD* is not demonstrated by any figures or videos presented. The flow acceleration is in the RV just prior to the pulmonic valve and PA (Fig. 86.5).

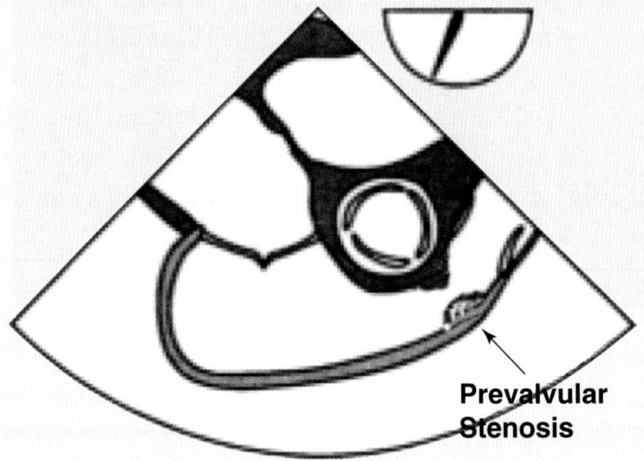

Figure 86.5. RV inflow–outflow view with prevalvular stenosis.

SUGGESTED READING

Galiuto L, O'Leary PW, Seward JB. Double-chambered right ventricle: echocardiographic features. *J Am Soc Echocardiogr.* 1996;9:300–305.

Restivo A, Cameron AH, Anderson RH, et al. Divided right ventricle: a review of its anatomical varieties. *Pediatr Cardiol.* 1984;5:197–204.

Schroeder RA, Sreeram GM, Mark J. Right ventricle, right atrium, tricuspid valve, and pulmonic valve. In: Perrino AC, Reeves ST, eds. *A Practical Approach to Transesophageal Echocardiography.* 2nd ed. Philadelphia: Lippincott Williams & Wilkins; 2007:281–295.

CASE 87

A 47-year-old male presents with a history of a cough, unresponsive to antibiotic therapy. In the last week, he has noted swelling in his legs and abdomen, which he believes is a drug reaction. On examination, a right-sided systolic murmur is appreciated. Following investigations, he is found to have severe TV regurgitation and a decision is made to take the patient to the OR. You perform a TEE before CPB (Figs. 87.1 and 87.2).

QUESTION 87.1. The echocardiogram is most consistent with which of the following?

A. Ebstein anomaly

B. Carcinoid disease of the TV

C. TV endocarditis

D. Myxomatous TV with a flail posterior leaflet

QUESTION 87.2. Based on the location of the lesion and the particular cross section presented, which structure is the most likely to be affected?

A. Eustachian valve

B. Anterior TV leaflet

C. Posterior TV leaflet

D. Septal TV leaflet

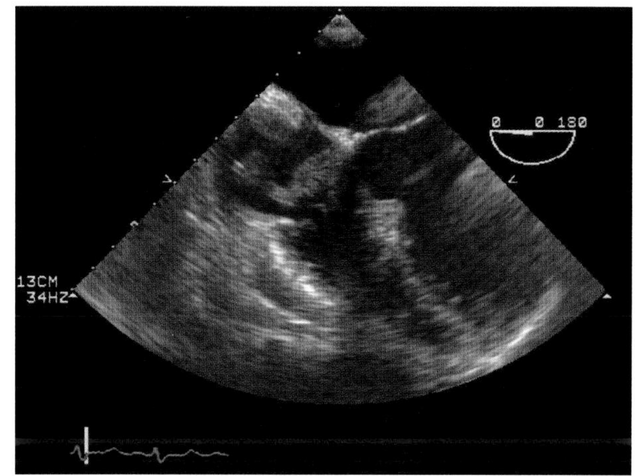

Figure 87.1. ME 4CH view, 2D. See also Video 87.1.

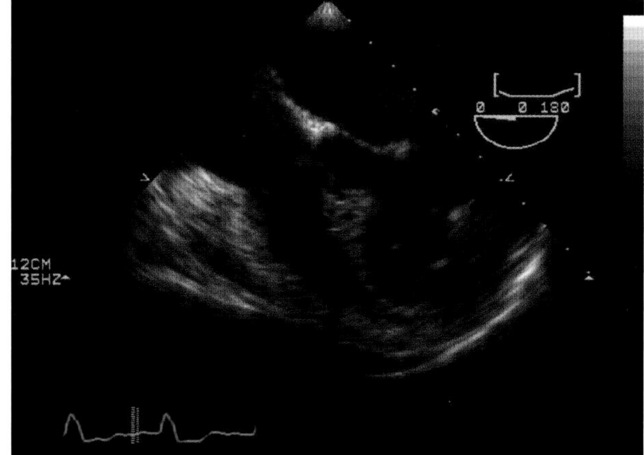

Figure 87.2. ME 4CH view with anteflexion, 2D. See also Videos 87.2 and 87.3.

QUESTION 87.3. The patient is noted to have a new *RBBB*. What other finding, demonstrated in Figure 87.2 and Videos 87.2 and 87.3, could be the cause of this electrocardiographic finding?

A. The presence of a PA catheter
B. Severe RV ischemia
C. Septal wall abscess
D. Small perimembranous VSD

The surgeon confirms the diagnosis of TV endocarditis firmly attached to the septal leaflet. Further inspection also demonstrates the presence of a septal abscess. The surgeon proceeds to patch the abscess and repair the TV. Upon separation from CPB, you obtain the TEE images shown in Figure 87.3.

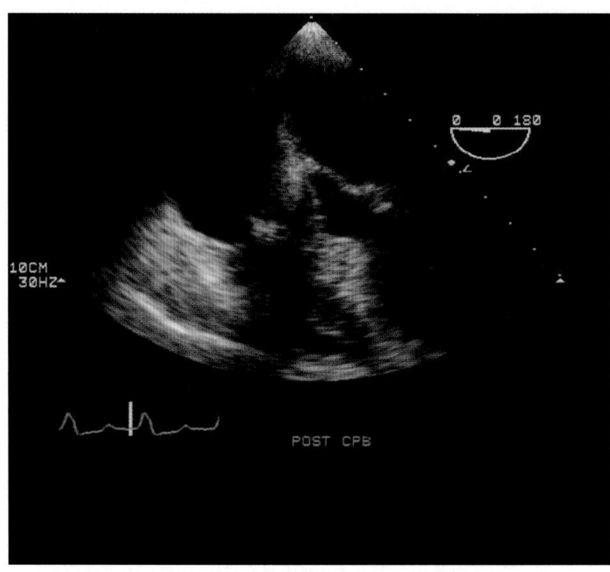

Figure 87.3. ME 4CH view, 2D, after repair of the TV. See also Video 87.4.

QUESTION 87.4. The echocardiographic appearance of Figure 87.3 (and Video 87.4) is most consistent with what type of repair?

A. Modified Alfieri repair of the TV
B. De Vega annuloplasty
C. Tricuspid replacement with a bioprosthesis
D. Excision of the entire TV without replacement

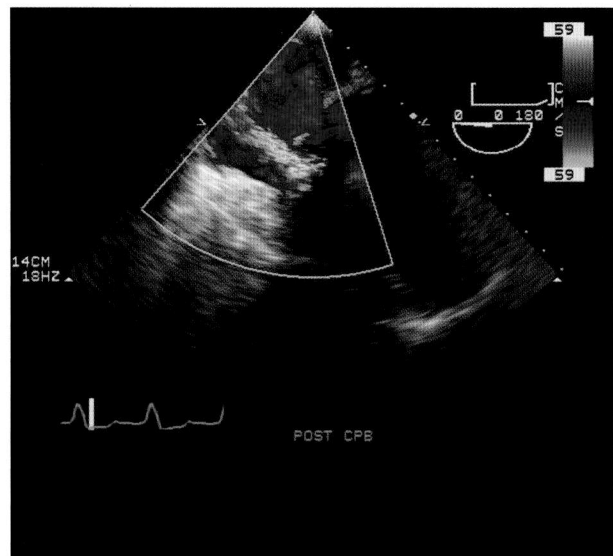

Figure 87.4. ME 4CH view, CFD; post TV procedure.

QUESTION 87.5. Based on the CFD information provided in Figure 87.4 and Video 87.5, what would you advise the surgeon to do?

A. Further surgical intervention is needed for tricuspid stenosis.
B. The valve repair should be revised due to moderate TR.
C. The valve should be replaced due to moderate TR.
D. Moderate TR is present, no further intervention is needed.

ANSWERS AND DISCUSSION

QUESTION 87.1: The correct answer is C: TV endocarditis. There is a large, mobile, echo-dense mass located on the right atrial aspect of the septal leaflet. Color Doppler demonstrates severe, eccentric TR. The differential diagnosis, here, includes other types of masses affecting the TV, such as thrombus or a tumor, myxoma being the most common one. Answer A is incorrect: Ebstein anomaly is often described as the *atrialization* of part of the RV. This occurs as the malformed tricuspid leaflets are displaced apically into the RV cavity. In many cases of Ebstein anomaly, the septal and posterior leaflets may be rudimentary or absent. This is clearly not the case in this patient. Answer B is incorrect: typical carcinoid changes include thickening and fibrosis of the whole valve. Leaflet mobility is usually restricted. In our case, the valve motion is not restricted. Answer D is incorrect: Although myxomatous changes can occur in the TV, the size, shape, and thickness of the leaflet/vegetation are not consistent with this diagnosis.

QUESTION 87.2: The correct answer is D: Septal TV leaflet. In the four-chamber view, the septal leaflet is the easiest to recognize, as it is the closest to the interventricular septum. The opposing leaflet is *usually* the anterior leaflet, but it can also be the posterior leaflet depending on the degree of retroflexion of the probe. In the ME RV inflow–outflow view, the posterior leaflet is usually displayed on the *left* and the other leaflet is either the septal or the anterior leaflet. Remember that the junctions between the leaflets of the TV are usually vague indentations, rather than frank commissures as seen on the MV. Answer A is incorrect: In Figure 87.1, the mass is seen near the interventricular septum, firmly attached to the septal leaflet. While much less common, Eustachian valve vegetations have been reported in 5 out of 152 patients in one series of right-sided endocarditis.[1] Of note, Eustachian valve endocarditis is *clinically indistinguishable* from tricuspid endocarditis and it is often missed by TTE.[2] Thankfully, TEE has successfully identified the Eustachian valve vegetations in all patients in which it was performed, thus highlighting the importance of diagnostic TEE in cases in which right-sided endocarditis is suspected.[3]

QUESTION 87.3: The correct answer is C: Septal wall abscess. On close inspection of the septal wall, one sees an area of irregular thickening in the basal interventricular septum (marked by the arrows in Fig. 87.5). Within that area of thickening, there is an echo-lucent center with a tract leading up the septal wall toward the septal leaflet. This appearance is consistent with an abscess. Now, given that the right bundle branch of the conduction system of the heart runs down the RV side of the interventricular septum, it is possible that an abscess in that location would affect electrical conduction. Answer A is incorrect: there is no pulmonary catheter visible in these images. However, PA catheters are known to cause an right bundle branch block (RBBB) in 3% to 12% of cases in which they are used. Answer B is incorrect: there is no RV dysfunction or regional wall motion abnormality suggestive of severe ischemia (can only be appreciated on the video). Finally, answer D is incorrect, as the color Doppler signal in Video 87.3 shows no evidence of a VSD.

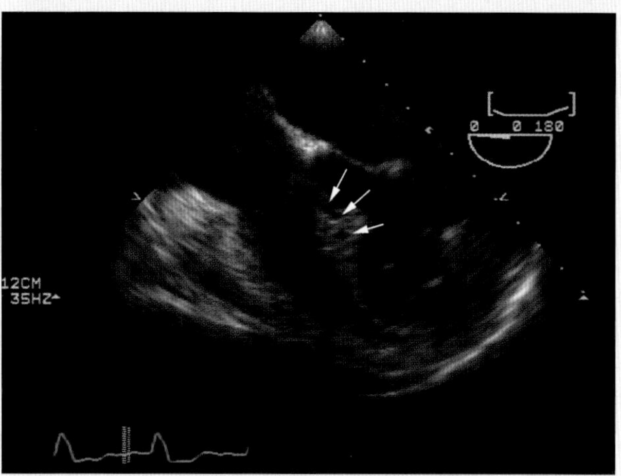

Figure 87.5. ME 4CH view demonstrating septal abscess *(arrows).*

QUESTION 87.4: The correct answer is A: Modified Alfieri repair. In Figure 87.3 and Video 87.4 there is obvious thickening in the center and the subvalvular area of the TV. This thickening is the result of suturing of the leaflet edges together, a technique analogous to a mitral Alfieri stitch (in fact, this patient underwent a complex repair, involving unroofing and patching of the abscess, resection of the septal leaflet, bicuspidization of the TV, and finally, an Alfieri-type suture between the remaining two leaflets of the TV). Answer B is incorrect: a De Vega annuloplasty is a circumferential suture around the TV annulus, to reduce the annular size. It is often used to treat functional TR. It is essentially *invisible* on echo and does not result in subvalvular thickening. Answer C is also incorrect: a bioprosthesis has a characteristic sewing ring and struts that are easily recognized on echo. Finally, answer D is incorrect, since TV tissue can clearly be seen. Although complete excision of the valve without replacement has been used in some centers, this was not the case here.

QUESTION 87.5: This question is open to differences of opinion and is somewhat surgeon dependent. The arguments presented here are intended to stimulate reflection by the reader. The *best* answer here is B: There is moderate residual TR and, *if feasible*, it should *ideally* be revised. A good repair is always the best solution.

There is good evidence in the literature that, in the context of MV disease (ischemic or rheumatic), functional TR is a prognostic marker of poor outcome. Patients with moderate-to-severe (3 to 4+) TR at the time of MV surgery have a greatly increased likelihood to have class III to IV heart failure in the future.[4,5] These patients tend to have a much better long-term prognosis if the TR is treated than if it is left alone, mostly due to the RV dysfunction that develops over time in untreated patients.[6,7] Moreover, moderate-to-severe functional TR is unlikely to resolve in most patients, following correction of mitral disease alone, making the choice to repair the tricuspid obvious.

Organic TV disease is rare, and the surgical repair is more complex than for functional disease. Tricuspid replacement is often the only alternative. Despite an increased *early mortality* with TV replacement, the long-term outcome appears to be similar in TV repair and TV replacement.[8,9]

Much more controversial is the choice between accepting a suboptimal repair and replacing the valve. Because the short-term prognosis is worse after replacement, some surgeons tend to reserve TV replacement for cases of unfixable severe tricuspid disease. If one belongs to that school of thought, answer D would be acceptable. The counterargument to this line of thought is that long-term observation of case series of TV repair has much *higher rates of recurrence* of severe, late TR than TV replacement.[8,10] Thus, if one believes that TV replacement is a short-term risk for a long-term gain, then answer C would be acceptable. Finally, one must not forget that this is a case of acute endocarditis and any form of foreign material (TV prosthesis) could be considered undesirable, leading one to accept more residual TR after repair than usual.

Answer A is incorrect as there is no significant aliasing of diastolic flow (the color is mostly dark blue), making tricuspid stenosis unlikely.

TAKE-HOME LESSON:

TV anatomy is more difficult to delineate as compared to the MV. In the ME 4CH view, the TV septal leaflet is the easiest to recognize, as it is the closest to the interventricular septum. The opposing leaflet is usually the anterior leaflet, but it can also be the posterior leaflet of the TV depending on the degree of retroflexion of the probe. In the ME RV inflow–outflow view, the TV posterior leaflet is usually displayed on the left and the other leaflet is either the septal or the anterior leaflet. Remember that the junctions between the leaflets of the TV are usually vague indentations, rather than frank commissures as seen on the MV.

REFERENCES

1. San Roman JA, Vilacosta I, Sarriá C, et al. Eustachian valve endocarditis: is it worth searching for? *Am Heart J.* 2001;142:1037–1040.
2. Bowers J, Krimsky W, Gradon JD. The pitfalls of transthoracic echocardiography. A case of Eustachian valve endocarditis. *Tex Heart Inst J.* 2001;28:57–59.
3. Sawhney N, Vachaspathi P, Raisinghani A, et al. Eustachian valve endocarditis: a case series and analysis of the literature. *J Am Soc Echocardiogr.* 2001;14:1139–1142.
4. Boyaci A, Gokce V, Topaloglu S, et al. Outcome of significant functional tricuspid regurgitation late after mitral valve replacement for predominantly rheumatic mitral stenosis. *Angiology.* 2007;58:336–342.
5. Ruel M, Rubens FD, Masters RG, et al. Late incidence and predictors of persistent or recurrent heart failure in patients with mitral prosthetic valves. *J Thorac Cardiovasc Surg.* 2004;128:278–283.
6. Calafiore AM, Gallina S, Iacò AL, et al. Mitral valve surgery for functional mitral regurgitation: should moderate-or-more tricuspid regurgitation be treated? a propensity score analysis. *Ann Thorac Surg.* 2009;87(3):698–703.

7. Shiran A, Sagie A. Tricuspid regurgitation in mitral valve disease incidence, prognostic implications, mechanism, and management. *J Am Coll Cardiol.* 2009;53(5):401–408.
8. Singh SK, Tang GH, Maganti MD, et al. Midterm outcomes of tricuspid valve repair versus replacement for organic tricuspid disease. *Ann Thorac Surg.* 2006;82:1735–1741.
9. Moraca RJ, Moon MR. Outcomes of tricuspid valve repair and replacement: a propensity analysis. *Ann Thorac Surg.* 2009;87(1):83–87.
10. Bajzer CT, Stewart WJ, Cosgrove DM, et al. Tricuspid valve surgery and intraoperative echocardiography: factors affecting survival, clinical outcomes, and echocardiographic success. *J Am Coll Cardiol.* 1998;32:1023–1031.

Advanced

CASE 88

A 62-year-old male presents with unstable angina and moderate-to-severe MR. Cardiac catheterization demonstrates three-vessel coronary artery disease and an LVEF of 30%.

The following values are obtained:

LV end-diastolic diameter: 60 mm
MV annulus (anteroposterior): 42 mm
MV annulus (bicommissural): 38 mm
Mitral tethering distance: 11 mm

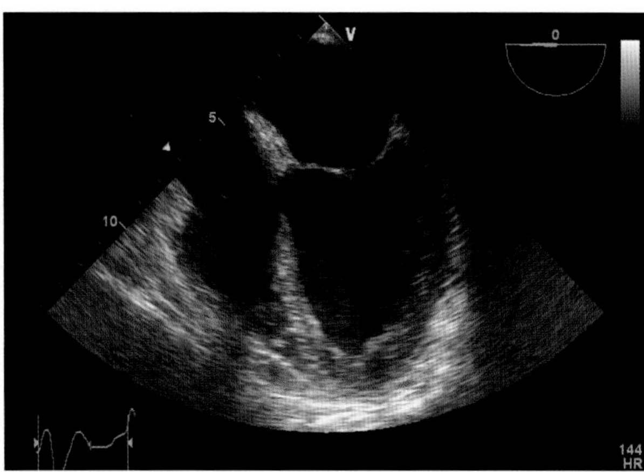

Figure 88.1. ME 4CH view, 2D. See also Video 88.1.

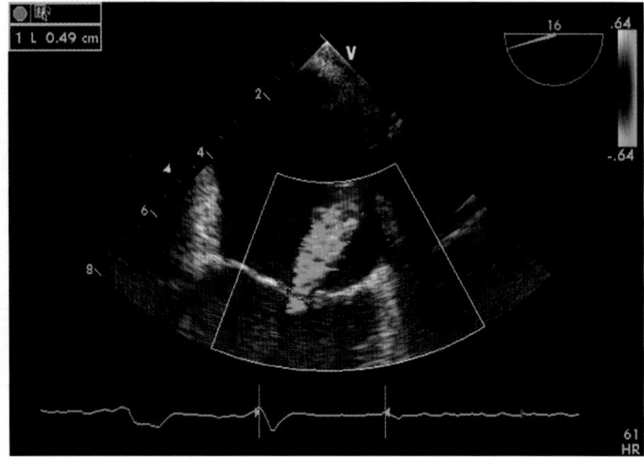

Figure 88.2. ME 4CH view with color Doppler and measurement of vena contracta.

QUESTION 88.1. Using Figures 88.1 and 88.2 and Video 88.1, as well as the measurements listed above, what is the mechanism of this patient's MR?

A. P2 prolapse (type 2)
B. Mitral annular dilation (type 1)
C. Leaflet restriction (type 3)
D. Perforated A2 segment (type 2)

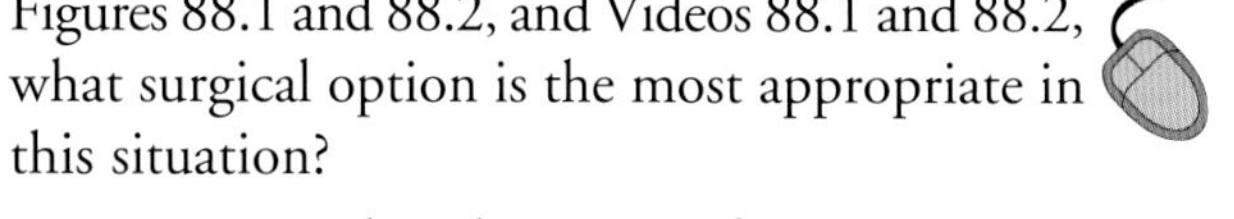

QUESTION 88.2. After reviewing the images from Figures 88.1 and 88.2, and Videos 88.1 and 88.2, what surgical option is the most appropriate in this situation?

A. P2 repair, plus placement of an annuloplasty ring
B. Coronary revascularization alone. No need to address the MV
C. Placement of an annuloplasty ring alone
D. MV replacement

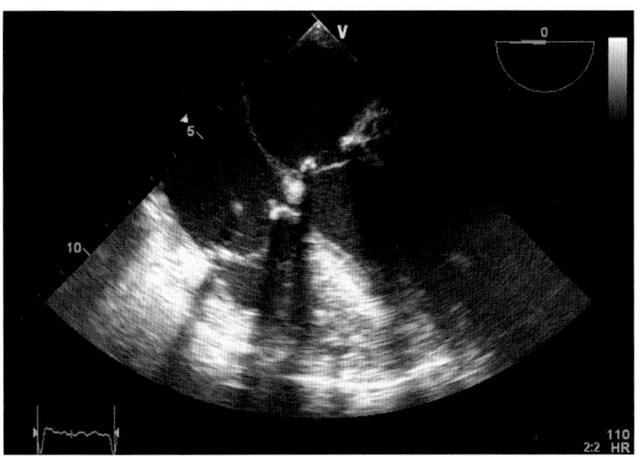

Figure 88.3. ME 4CH view, 2D.

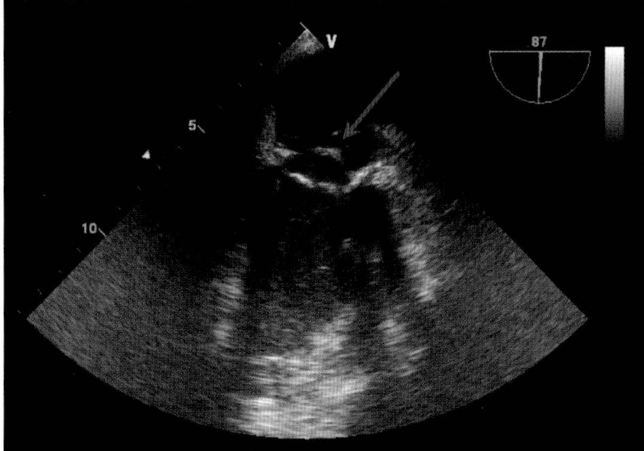

Figure 88.4. ME commissural view, 2D.

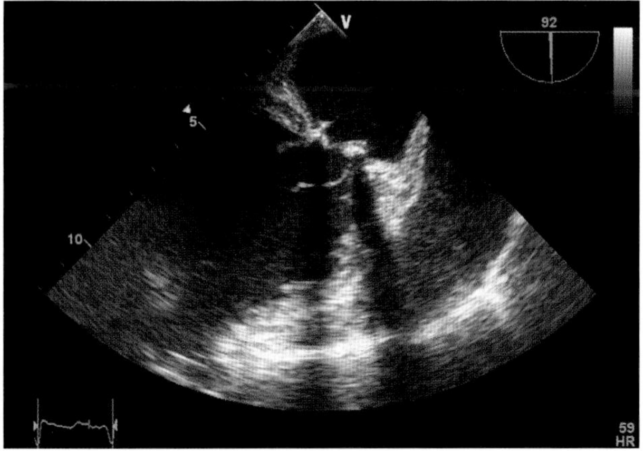

Figure 88.5. ME 2CH view, 2D.

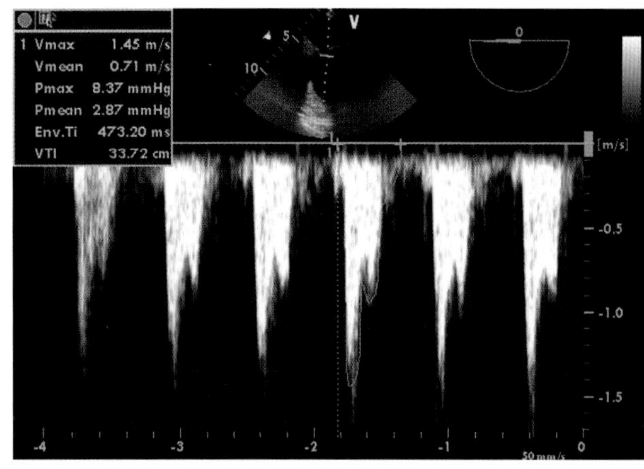

Figure 88.6. CW Doppler through the MV annulus.

QUESTION 88.3. Figures 88.3, 88.4, and 88.5 and Videos 88.2, 88.3, and 88.4 were obtained after separation from CPB. Paying special attention to the arrow in Figure 88.4, the echocardiographic images are most consistent with which type of surgical repair?

A. Placement of a Geoform ring
B. MV replacement
C. Placement of a Carpentier–Edwards ring
D. Placement of an ACORN device around the LV

QUESTION 88.4. Post-CPB echocardiographic examination of the valve using CW Doppler reveals a mean gradient of 2.87 mm Hg (Figure 88.6). What is considered the highest acceptable mean gradient with this type of device?

A. 2 mm Hg
B. 4 mm Hg
C. 8 mm Hg
D. 10 mm Hg

QUESTION 88.5. What is the *least* accurate way to assess the MV area following an annuloplasty repair?

A. CW Doppler
B. PISA
C. Continuity equation
D. PHT measurement

ANSWERS AND DISCUSSION

QUESTION 88.1: The correct answer is C: Leaflet restriction (type 3).

In the Carpentier classification of MR (see Figure 88.7), type 3b refers to cases where the mitral leaflets are *structurally normal*, but there is restriction of the leaflets in systole, due to *tethering* of the mitral leaflets. In chronic ischemic heart disease or dilated cardiomyopathy, the LV dilates, resulting in *posterior* and *apical* papillary muscle displacement and tethering of the mitral leaflets in systole. The subsequent failure of coaptation causes MR. In such cases, the jet is usually *central* or *slightly posteriorly* directed. Note that there is almost always annular dilatation associated with type 3b MR (as is the case here). The difference between type 1 and type 3b is the tethering of the leaflets. In some views, the chordae tendinae are tense and won't let the mitral leaflets come up to the level of the annulus. In Figure 88.1, one can see that the leaflets are not touching and are held below the mitral annulus. As the patient's LV dilated, it pulled on the leaflets and does not allow proper coaptation. Answers A (*P2 prolapse*) and D (*A2 perforation*) are incorrect: there is no evidence of prolapse of any segment of this MV, and the regurgitant jet originates *between* the leaflet tips, not *through* A2, as would be expected in a perforation. Finally, answer B (*annular dilatation, type 1*) is also incorrect: while a dilated mitral annulus of 38 mm × 42 mm can occur with *any type* of chronic MR, a *tethering distance of 11 mm* is strongly suggestive of type 3b MR.

QUESTION 88.2: The correct answer is C: Placement of an annuloplasty ring.

The surgical approach to the management of functional MR is controversial: Functional MR is a marker of the severity of a patient's LV dysfunction, and the most commonly used solution to this problem has been to address the MR directly by inserting an *undersized annuloplasty ring*. Various types of rings have been used. Because the MV is structurally normal and the etiology of functional MR is *ventricular disease*, some experts suggest that the treatment should rather be targeted at the ventricular dilatation, using various ventricular remodeling techniques as a way to improve the LV dysfunction and MR. Finally, others advocate coronary revascularization alone, unless the MR is severe and the patient has severe symptoms of heart failure.

The Alfieri stitch (Case 36) has been shown to reduce immediate postoperative MR; however, results from a Cleveland Clinic study judged its long-term success as unsatisfactory. It remains favored by some surgeons and, more recently, shows promise as a successful method for percutaneous MV repair. In addition, it does nothing to help reshape the LV. Valve repair is always superior to valve replacement.

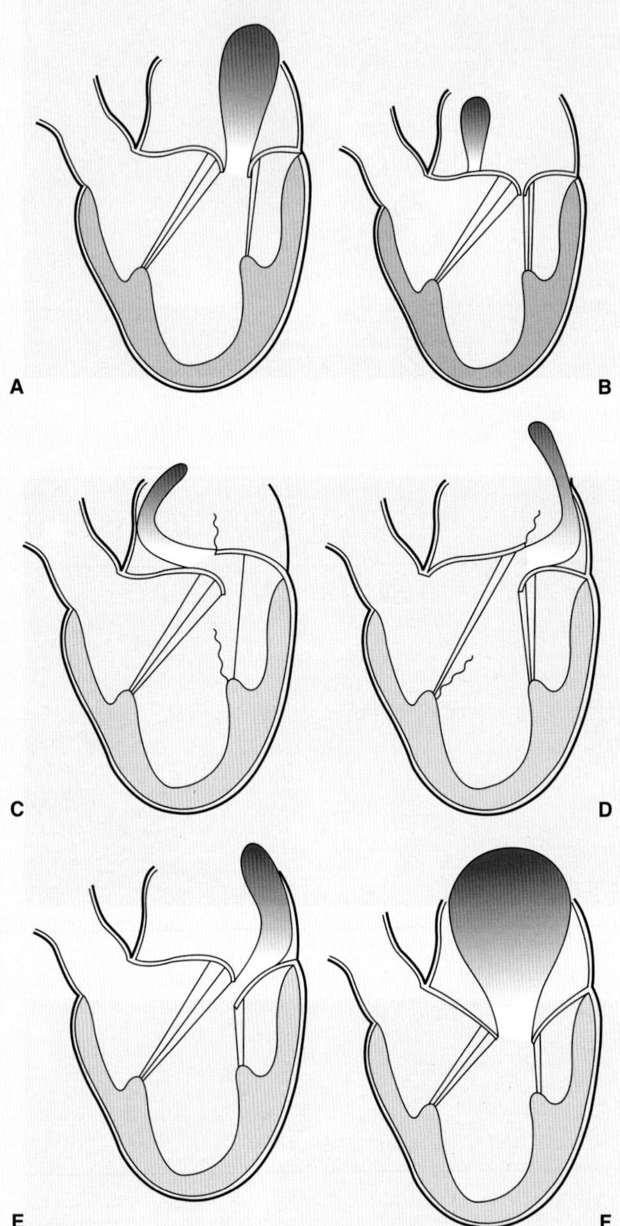

Figure 88.7. Carpentier's classification of MR based on leaflet motion. In type 1 **(A)**, the leaflet motion is normal and the MR jet tends to be central. In type 2 **(C,D)**, there is excessive leaflet motion and the MR jet is typically directed away from the diseased leaflet. In type 3 lesion, the leaflet motion is restricted leaflet motion and is further subdivided into type 3a (structural, E) and 3b (functional, F). In type 3 lesions, the regurgitant jet maybe directed away from the diseased leaflet if only one leaflet is affected, or it may be central if both mitral leaflets are equally affected. Adapted from Perrino AC, Reeves ST eds. *A Practical Approach to Transesophageal Echocardiography*. 2nd ed. Philadelphia: Lippincott Williams & Wilkins; 2008, Chapter 8, with permission.

QUESTION 88.3: The correct answer is A: Placement of a Geoform ring. Figures 88.3, 88.4, and 88.5 illustrate the postoperative appearance of a properly placed Geoform ring. The arrow highlights the echocardiographic appearance of the posterior elevation of the ring around the area of P2. It is important to recognize this as a *normal echocardiographic image* and not an improperly placed ring. Although no trial to date has demonstrated its superiority, many surgeons favor the Geoform ring for patients with ischemic MR. Shown in Figure 88.8, the Geoform ring is a dog bone–shaped ring with a unique elevation along the posterior aspect. The reduction of the anterior–posterior diameter of the mitral annulus brings the leaflets into close proximity and allows them to coapt. The posterior elevation is thought to help remodel a dilated ventricle. A standard, flat Carpentier–Edwards annuloplasty ring would neither significantly reduce the anterior–posterior dimension nor help reshape and remodel the LV. Answer B (*MV replacement*) is incorrect: this valve shows none of the hallmarks of either a mechanical or a bioprosthetic MV. Answer C (*Carpentier–Edwards ring*) is incorrect: As stated above, the various images in this patient demonstrate the posterior elevation of the ring, whereas the Carpentier–Edwards ring is flat. Finally, answer D is incorrect: the ACORN device is a circumferential mesh that is surgically applied to the heart to reduce its diameter. It does not involve a ring on the MV.

QUESTION 88.4: The correct answer is C: 8 mm Hg. Mitral stenosis can inadvertently be caused by using too small a ring with a small anterior–posterior diameter. CW Doppler should be used as a part of any postrepair echocardiographic examination of the valve. Mean gradients of between 4 and 6 mm Hg and sometimes up to 8 mm Hg are acceptable. A mean gradient higher than 8 mm Hg should be corrected prior to leaving the OR.

QUESTION 88.5: The correct answer is D: PHT measurement. Postvalvuloplasty, the measurement of PHT is *not a reliable estimate* of MV area. Frequent changes in LV compliance following CPB lead to inaccuracies in the formula 220/$PT_{1/2}$ and, therefore, it should not be used. Doppler measurements, estimations of the valve area by PISA, the continuity equation, and the Gorlin formula can all be used reliably.

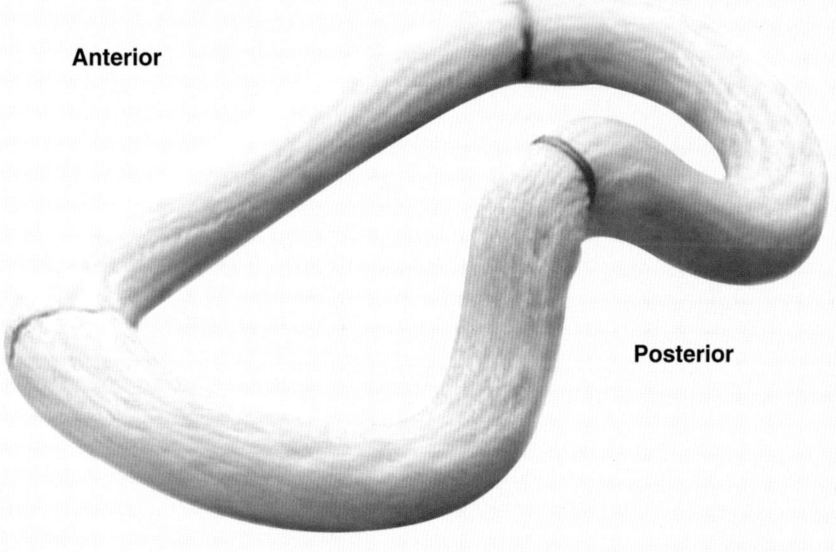

Figure 88.8. The Geoform ring.

TAKE-HOME LESSON:

In type 3b MR, the leaflet restriction is "functional" and proper coaptation is prevented by systolic tethering of the mitral leaflets as a result of a dilated LV and/or displaced papillary muscles. This lesion is most commonly associated with coronary artery disease (in which case it is referred to as *ischemic* MR), but can also result from other types of dilated cardiomyopathies. The Geoform ring was specifically designed in an attempt to correct the leaflet tethering encountered due to a dilated LV in ischemic MR.

SUGGESTED READING

Armen TA, Vandse R, Crestanello JA, et al. Mechanisms of valve competency after mitral valve annuloplasty for ischemic mitral regurgitation using the Geoform ring: insights from three-dimensional echocardiography. *Eur J Echocardiogr*. 2009;10:74–81.

Bhudia SK, McCarthy PM, Smedira NG, et al. Edge-to-edge (Alfieri) mitral repair: results in diverse clinical settings. *Ann Thorac Surg*. 2004;77:1598–1606.

Feldman T, Kar S, Rinaldi M, et al. EVEREST Investigators. Percutaneous mitral repair with the MitraClip system safety and midterm durability in the initial EVEREST (Endovascular Valve Edge-to-Edge REpair Study) Cohort. *J Am Coll Cardiol*. 2009;54:686–694.

Perrino AC, Reeves ST, eds. *A Practical Approach to Transesophageal Echocardiography*. 2nd ed. Philadelphia: Lippincott Williams & Wilkins; 2008:172–175.

Votta E, Maisano F, Bolling SF, et al. The Geoform disease-specific annuloplasty system: a finite element study. *Ann Thorac Surg*. 2007;84:92–101.

CASE 89

A small 76-year-old woman (5'0", 50 kg with a BSA of 1.4 m^2) presented to the OR for an AVR. Her baseline TEE examination confirmed severe AS with a valve area of 0.5 cm^2 and only a trace amount of aortic regurgitation. Her EF was >55% and there were no other significant findings.

QUESTION 89.1. In order to minimize the risk of patient prosthesis mismatch (PPM) in this patient, what is the minimum EOA the inserted valve should have?

A. 0.85 cm^2

B. 1.00 cm^2

C. 1.20 cm^2

D. PPM cannot be predicted

The operation proceeded uneventfully and she was successfully weaned from CPB on milrinone and norepinephrine. Her postprocedure TEE is shown in Video 89.1.

QUESTION 89.2. What type of AV prosthesis was inserted?

A. A stentless bioprosthetic valve

B. A stented bioprosthetic valve

C. A homograft

D. A bileaflet mechanical valve

Spectral Doppler tracings through the AV and LVOT are shown in Figure 89.1.

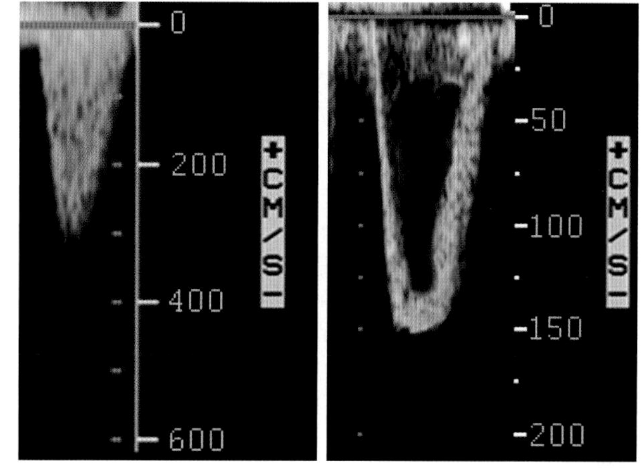

Figure 89.1.

QUESTION 89.3. What is the approximate peak gradient through the prosthesis?

A. 36 mm Hg

B. 30 mm Hg

C. 27 mm Hg

D. 20 mm Hg

QUESTION 89.4. What is the patient's dimensionless velocity index (DVI) and is it within normal limits?

A. The DVI is 0.5, which indicates valve dysfunction

B. The DVI is 0.5, which is normal

C. The DVI is 2, which indicates valve dysfunction

D. The DVI is 2, which is normal

QUESTION 89.5. Assuming the implanted valve gave the patient an indexed EOA of 0.86 cm^2 and taking into account the information provided in Questions 89.1 to 89.4, what is your recommendation to the surgical team?

A. Close the chest

B. There is likely some subvalvular stenosis that needs to be addressed

C. Measure the "true" gradient by placing a catheter in the LVOT and the aortic root

D. The valve is too small so a root enlargement procedure should be performed

ANSWERS AND DISCUSSION

QUESTION 89.1: The correct answer is C: 1.20 cm^2. Indexed EOA_i is the valve's EOA divided by the patient's BSA. Studies have shown that an $EOA_i > 0.85$ minimizes the risk of PPM. An EOA_i of 0.65 or less confers a significant risk of creating PPM. In this particular patient, with a BSA of 1.4 m^2, implanting a valve with an EOA of 1.2 cm^2 would give an EOA_i of 0.86 (1.2 divided by 1.4), which would minimize the risks of PPM. Implanting a smaller-sized valve than this would create the potential for PPM.

Currently, the best predictor of PPM is the EOA_i. The valve's EOA is usually determined in vitro and can be found in the valve's packaging. Many manufacturers also provide a table specific to each valve model such as the one shown in Figure 89.2. This allows the surgeon to easily see the risk of PPM with the planned implanted valve size. If the risk of PPM is high, a valve with a larger EOA is recommended. This may mean changing from a stented bioprosthetic to a mechanical valve, which would generally have a greater EOA for any given size. Placing a larger-sized bioprosthetic valve may also be an option. However, this often complicates the surgical procedure by necessitating a root enlargement procedure that can add to operative morbidity and mortality.

QUESTION 89.2: The correct answer is B: A stented bioprosthetic valve. The tissue leaflets can easily be seen in the ME AV LAX, as pointed out by the red arrow in Figure 89.3A. The valve can be differentiated from a stentless bioprosthetic valve by the struts of the valve seen best in the ME long AV short-axis view and pointed out by the blue arrows in Figure 89.3B. It is important to know what type of valve has been implanted when assessing prosthetic valves using Doppler. In general, stented bioprosthetic valves have the highest postoperative mean gradients for any given size. Mechanical valves come in second, with stentless bioprosthetics and homografts having the lowest mean gradients.

	EOA_i by Prosthesis size (mm)					
Prosthesis size (mm)	**19**	**21**	**23**	**25**	**27**	**29**
Average EOA (cm^2)	1.1	1.3	1.5	1.8	2.3	2.7
BSA (m^2)						
0.6	1.83	2.17	2.50	3.00	3.83	4.50
0.7	1.57	1.86	2.14	2.57	3.29	3.86
0.8	1.38	1.63	1.88	2.25	2.88	3.38
0.9	1.22	1.44	1.67	2.00	2.56	3.00
1	1.10	1.30	1.50	1.80	2.30	2.70
1.1	1.00	1.18	1.36	1.64	2.09	2.45
1.2	0.92	1.08	1.25	1.50	1.92	2.25
1.3	0.85	1.00	1.15	1.38	1.77	2.08
1.4	0.79	0.93	1.07	1.29	1.64	1.93
1.5	0.73	0.87	1.00	1.20	1.53	1.80
1.6	0.49	0.88	0.88	0.88	0.88	1.69
1.7	0.65	0.76	0.88	1.06	1.35	1.59
1.8	0.61	0.72	0.83	1.00	1.28	1.50
1.9	0.58	0.68	0.79	0.95	1.21	1.42
2	0.55	0.65	0.75	0.90	1.15	1.35
2.1	0.52	0.62	0.71	0.86	1.10	1.29
2.2	0.50	0.59	0.68	0.82	1.05	1.23
2.3	0.48	0.57	0.65	0.78	1.00	1.17
2.4	0.46	0.54	0.63	0.75	0.96	1.13
2.5	0.44	0.52	0.60	0.72	0.92	1.08

Figure 89.2.

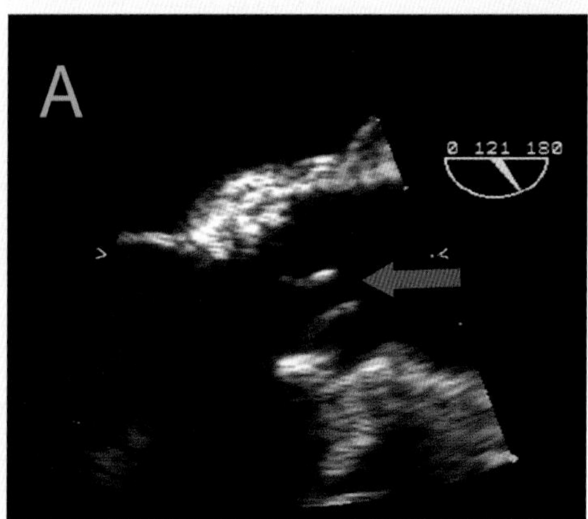

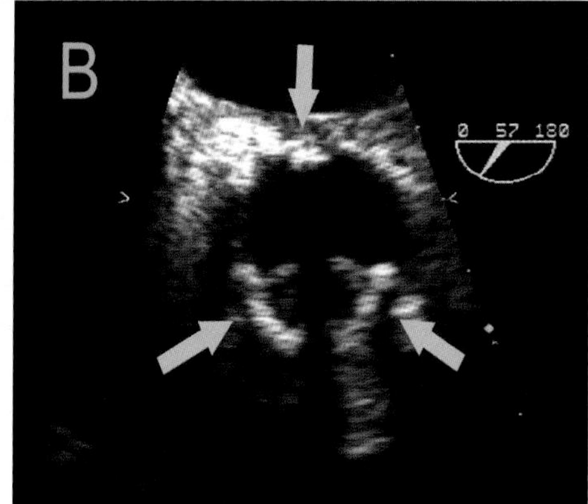

Figure 89.3.

QUESTION 89.3: The correct answer is C: 27 mm Hg. When using the simplified Bernoulli equation ($\Delta P = 4V^2$), it is important to remember that the equation is valid only when the velocity proximal to the obstruction (or valve in this case) is negligible. In situations of high flow, particularly in the case of a small LVOT in a patient on inotropes, ignoring the proximal velocity can result in an error of up to 30%. In these circumstances, the entire modified Bernoulli equation should be used: $\Delta P = 4(V_2^2 - V_1^2)$.

QUESTION 89.4: The correct answer is B: The DVI is 0.5, which is normal. The DVI is the ratio of the LVOT peak velocity to the peak velocity through the AV. This patient's DVI would therefore be 1.5:3, or 0.5. Typical DVIs immediately following CPB are in the 0.4 to 0.6 range. For long-term follow-up of prosthetic valves, DVIs $\geq$0.3 are considered normal. If valve leaflet dysfunction were present, the DVI would be significantly decreased as blood flow acceleration through the narrowed opening would increase the peak AV velocity. A DVI of $<$0.25 is consistent with significant valve obstruction. In contrast to peak Doppler gradients, DVI is not affected by high flow conditions. For this reason, it is a good screening method in the immediate post-CPB period.

QUESTION 89.5: The correct answer is A: Close the chest. The 2D examination of the valve, seen in Video 89.1, demonstrates a good opening of the valve leaflets and a stable annulus. No significant valvular regurgitation is shown when CFD is applied. Since the EOA_i is acceptable and the DVI is within expected limits, the valve is functioning properly and no further action is needed. An LVOT peak velocity of 1.5 m/s would not be uncommon in a small patient on inotropes and does not suggest subvalvular stenosis. The EOA_i is acceptable and trying to place a larger-size valve by enlarging the aortic root would provide little benefit to the patient.

There is often confusion between Doppler-derived gradients and catheter-derived gradients, with the former always higher than the later. One reason for this is the pressure recovery phenomenon, which can be significant in prosthetic valves. The total mechanical energy in blood flowing past a narrowing consists of kinetic energy (*K*) and pressure energy (*P*). As shown in Figure 89.4, as the blood enters the narrowed orifice (i.e., the prosthetic valve) it accelerates, increasing the kinetic energy while decreasing the pressure component. This is the point where Doppler gradients are sampled—the kinetic component at its highest and the pressure component at its lowest. As the blood moves beyond the narrowing, it slows and some of the kinetic energy is converted back to pressure energy. This is where catheter gradients are measured and since some pressure is "recovered," the ΔP (aka gradient) is smaller.

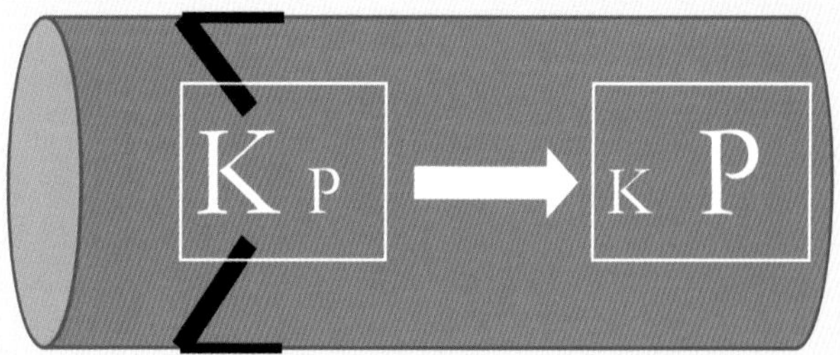

Figure 89.4.

TAKE-HOME LESSON:

Peak gradients through prosthetic valves following separation from CPB are frequently high, usually as a result of not using the entire modified Bernoulli equation: $\Delta P = 4(V_2^2 - V_1^2)$. The DVI, which is less flow dependent, is a better tool to screen for valve obstruction in this setting.

SUGGESTED READING

Pibarot P, Dumesnil JG. Prosthesis-patient mismatch: definition, clinical impact, and prevention. *Heart.* 2006;92:1022–1029.

Vandervoot PM, Greenberg NL, Pu M, et al. Pressure recovery in bileaflet heart valve prosthesis. *Circulation.* 1996;92:3464–3472.

Zoghbi WA, Chambers JB, Dumesnil JG, et al. Recommendations for evaluation of prosthetic valves with echocardiography and Doppler ultrasound. *J Am Soc Echocardiogr.* 2009;22:975–1014.

CASE 90

A 52-year-old male presents with severe CHF, NYHA IV, which is refractory to maximal medical therapy. Investigations confirm end-stage ischemic cardiomyopathy not amenable to revascularization. He is scheduled for insertion of a LVAD as a bridge to heart transplantation. You are the echocardiographer performing the CPB TEE.

QUESTION 90.1. Which of the following potential prebypass TEE findings would be *least likely* to affect his intraoperative management?

A. Moderate to severe (3+) mitral stenosis
B. Moderate (2+) AI
C. Moderate to severe (3+) MR
D. Small (2 mm), secundum ASD

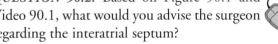

QUESTION 90.2. Based on Figure 90.1 and Video 90.1, what would you advise the surgeon regarding the interatrial septum?

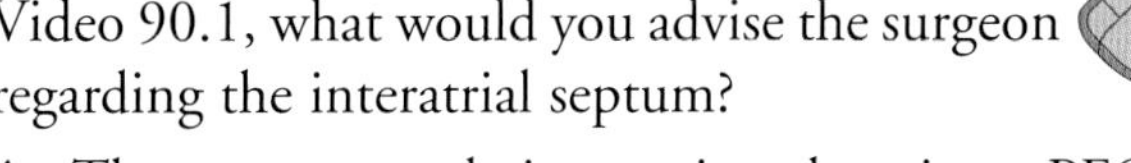

A. The contrast study is negative; there is no PFO
B. The contrast study is positive; there is a PFO
C. The contrast study is technically poor; surgical exploration of the interatrial septum is required
D. The contrast study is negative, but a PFO cannot be excluded

Post LVAD implantation, you confirm proper alignment of the inflow cannula in the ME 2CH and ME 4CH views. You continue to wean off CPB while increasing the LVAD support. You obtain the ME LAX and colour flow Doppler shown in Figure 90.2.

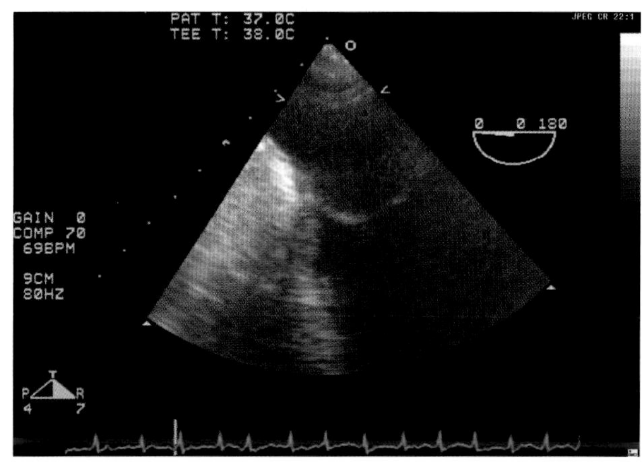

Figure 90.1. Agitated saline contrast study, ME 4CH view, focusing on interatrial and upper interventricular septum. See also Video 90.1.

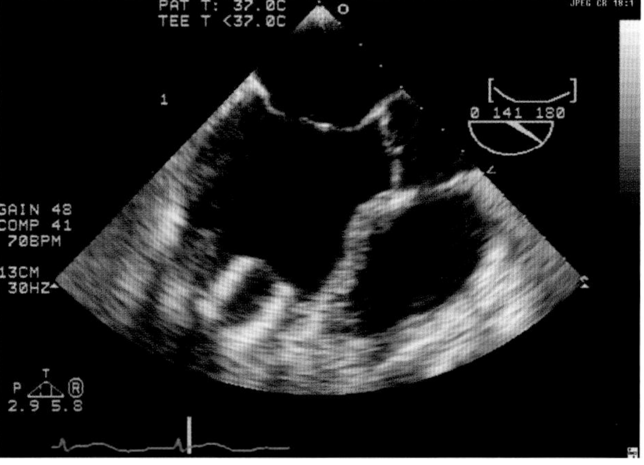

Figure 90.2. ME LAX of the LV, post LVAD insertion. See also Videos 90.2 and 90.3.

QUESTION 90.3. What can you conclude regarding the LVAD and cardiac function based on Figure 90.2 and Videos 90.2 and 90.3?

A. The echocardiographic findings are consistent with full LVAD support
B. The diastolic flow pattern is consistent with obstruction of the inflow cannula
C. There is inadequate LVAD support as there is no intermittent opening of the AV
D. There is an iatrogenic VSD located near the base of the anteroseptal wall

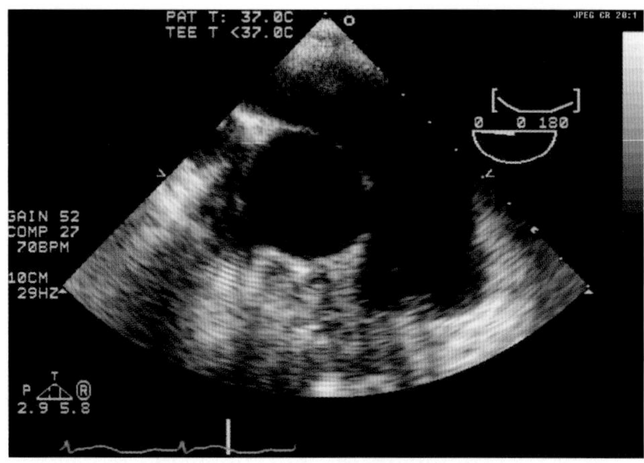

Figure 90.3. Short-axis view of the ascending aorta. See Video 90.4.

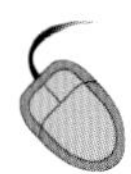

QUESTION 90.4. Based on Figures 90.3 and 90.4, as well as Video 90.4, which of the following statements is correct.

A. The patient has a pulsatile LVAD with normal flow velocity
B. The patient has a pulsatile LVAD with mild outflow valve regurgitation
C. The patient has a continuous flow LVAD with normal flow velocity
D. The patient has a continuous flow LVAD with kinking of the outflow cannula in systole resulting in elevated velocities

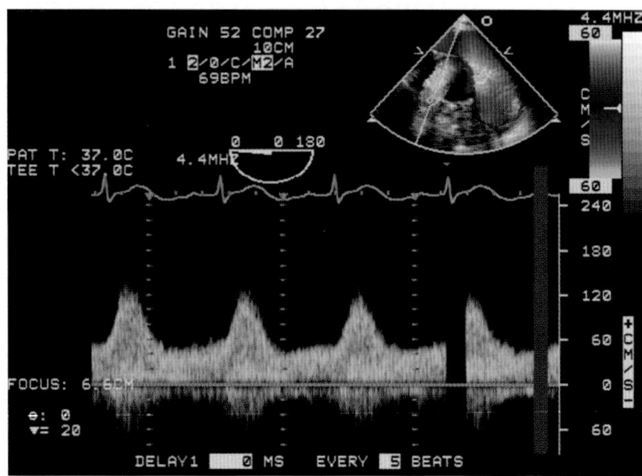

Figure 90.4. CW Doppler of the outflow cannula from the short-axis view of the ascending aorta.

Postoperatively, the patient does well, with small dose inotropic support and minimal bleeding. One day after surgery, you are called urgently to assess the patient as there is very low device flow despite several fluid boluses totaling 1.5 L. You perform a limited, focused TEE exam and the first image obtained (Fig. 90.5) is provided.

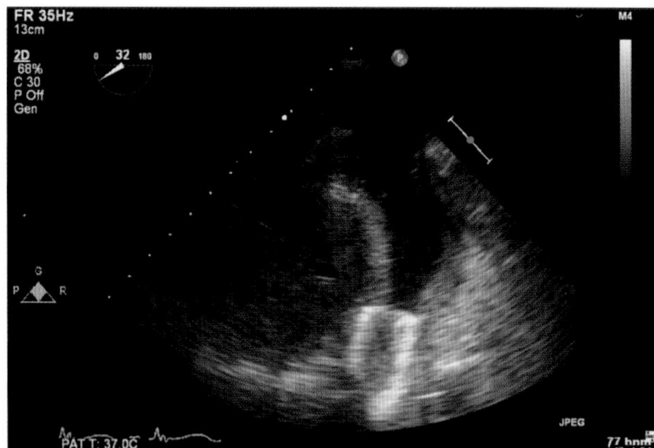

Figure 90.5. ME 4CH view, one day post-op in ICU. See also Video 90.5.

QUESTION 90.5. Based on Figure 90.5 and Video 90.5, what would you advise to immediately remedy the situation?

A. Administer another fluid bolus as the LV is severely underfilled
B. Administer more inotropes to stabilize RV function and improve LVAD filling
C. Increase the speed of the LVAD to improve cardiac output and pressure
D. Reduce the speed of the LVAD

ANSWERS AND DISCUSSION

QUESTION 90.1: The correct answer is C: Moderate to severe (3+) MR. Functional magnetic resonance (MR) of at least moderate severity is common in end-stage systolic heart failure, occurring in almost 40% of patients. Because ventricular contraction and device pulsation are dissociated, some concern has been expressed about the potential for MR when the LV contracts against a closed AV. Usually, there is a reduction in MR after LVAD insertion and once the LV is properly unloaded, this is rarely a problem. As such, MR pre-VAD rarely requires intervention for a successful surgery.

Answer A is incorrect. As mitral stenosis will impair filling of the LVAD inflow cannula at the ventricular apex, any significant mitral stenosis must be surgically corrected with either mitral commissurotomy or valve replacement.

Answer B is incorrect. It is recommended that all cases of severe and most cases of moderate AI be repaired prior to LVAD. What must also be appreciated is that the severity of aortic regurgitation in systolic heart failure may be significantly underestimated. This occurs because of the decreased transvalvular gradient that results from chronically elevated ventricular end diastolic pressures. It is recommended that the degree of AI pre-VAD be assessed *during CPB* as the transvalvular pressure gradient will more closely reflect the post-VAD state.

Answer D is incorrect. The presence of an ASD requires surgical closure, as it may cause a right-to-left shunt and systemic desaturation once the LV is unloaded.

QUESTION 90.2: The answer is D: The contrast study is negative, but a PFO cannot be excluded.

A contrast study is used to determine whether an atrial shunt, usually a PFO, is present or absent. Agitated bacteriostatic saline is injected as a contrast agent, and it crosses the atrial septum in the presence of a right-to-left shunt. A positive saline contrast study is defined by the presence of three or more contrast bubbles within the LA, occurring *within three beats* of the contrast medium entering the RA. In order to increase the right atrial pressure and the sensitivity of the test, a Valsalva maneuver can be performed. As there are no bubbles transmitted to the LA within three heartbeats, this study is negative. From a technical perspective, the study provided in the clips is technically sound, making *answers B and C incorrect*. However, it is important to remember that echocardiography can only detect the presence of an intracardiac shunt *if there is flow across it*. Due to the chronically elevated LA pressures encountered in end-stage systolic heart failure, it is possible that a saline contrast study will be negative pre-VAD, only to discover a widely PFO upon activation of the device. In a reported case series, 3 of 14 VAD patients had a PFO found at surgical inspection, despite negative bubble studies. Thus *answer A is incorrect*, as one cannot definitively rule out the possibility of a PFO based on a bubble study. For this reason, many surgeons routinely inspect the atrial septum during the insertion of an LVAD. If this is not performed, it is imperative to assess the septum for a PFO or other right-to-left shunt as soon as possible after weaning from CPB.

QUESTION 90.3: The answer is A: The echocardiographic findings are consistent with full LVAD support.

As previously stated, you had already confirmed proper alignment of the cannula in the two- and four-chamber views. Video 90.3 confirms that diastolic flow into the LVAD apical cannula is laminar, with no evidence of aliased flow. Although not included, one would confirm proper filling by CW Doppler measurement of the peak-filling velocity. The acceptable peak-filling velocities are below 2.3 m/s for pulsatile devices, and between 1 and 2 m/s for axial flow devices. Figure 90.2 and Video 90.2 are consistent with what is expected of full LVAD support. The RV is seen contracting in systole, the MV opens in diastole and closes in systole, often with a markedly decreased degree of MR, and the AV remains closed throughout the cardiac cycle, as all flow out of the ventricle occurs through the LVAD. If the LVAD was not properly unloading the ventricle, there would be an increase in LV pressure and flow would be directed either forward through the AV or backward through the MV.

Answer B is *incorrect* because there is no aliased diastolic flow to suggest cannula obstruction. Answer C is *incorrect*. The AV should not open intermittently with LVAD support unless one is attempting to wean the LVAD. This could occur if the VAD was placed as a bridge to recovery. Answer D is *incorrect*. There is no evidence of a VSD.

QUESTION 90.4: The correct answer is C: The patient has an axial flow (continuous flow) LVAD with normal flow velocity. Figure 90.3 demonstrates the outflow cannula entering the ascending aorta along the right anterolateral aspect with good orientation. This can further be confirmed on a LAX of the ascending aorta. The CW trace in Figure 90.4 demonstrates continuous, unidirectional, and slightly pulsatile flow, which is normal for this type of device. Continuous flow devices are often assumed to be constant flow devices; however, variations in flow and some pulsatility are the rule rather than the exception. Because the power and rotation speed of a continuous flow device are not subject to great variation, the main determinant of flow through the device becomes the gradient between the inflow and the outflow pressures. In Figure 90.4, peak velocity and flow occurs in systole, when the ventricular pressure is the greatest, and thus, the gradient between inflow (ventricular) pressure and outflow (aortic) pressure is the lowest.

Answer A is *incorrect* because a pulsatile device would generate a pulsatile CW trace; however, there would be no forward flow during device filling and, as such, measured velocities would return to zero prior to another cycle, which is not the case in Figure 90.4. Furthermore, the peak velocities measured would be higher, usually about 2.1 m/s in a well-functioning pulsatile device. Answer B is *incorrect*. There are no regurgitant velocities demonstrated in Figure 90.4. Regurgitant velocities occur during device filling and would indicate malfunction of the one way valve in the outflow component.

ANSWER D: Answer D is *incorrect*. As specified earlier, pulsatility will occur with variations in inflow and outflow pressures. Although, in theory, a partial obstruction of the outflow cannula would cause an increase in outflow velocity, this increase would be greater than that recorded in Figure 90.4, and, likely, greater than the accepted flow velocities of 1 to 2 m/s for continuous flow devices.

QUESTION 90.5: The correct answer is D: Reduce the speed of the LVAD.
Figure 90.5 and Video 90.5 provide an example of a suction event with partial occlusion of the inflow cannula. When the pump flow, controlled by pump speed, is progressively increased, the ventricle is unloaded to a greater extent. If, however, the speed is increased excessively, there will be the creation of suction forces, which can cause partial or complete collapse of the surrounding ventricular walls and partially or completely obstruct the inflow cannula. The septum is seen bulging into the LV cavity and partially occluding the inflow cannula. Turning down the device speed will immediately remedy the suction event, while permitting the echocardiographer to complete a thorough examination of all chambers, valves, and pericardial structures to determine the inciting cause of the suction event. Some possible causes include hypovolemia, intracardiac thrombus, misalignment of the inflow cannula, severe RV failure with septal bowing, and cardiac tamponade. Although not provided, the CW Doppler trace demonstrated elevated peak inflow velocities.

Answer A is incorrect. Although hypovolemia is often a cause of suction events, administration of fluid alone may not be enough to fix a suction event. The pump flows must be decreased to allow for equilibration of the pressure gradient before the ventricle fills properly. Answer C is incorrect. Further increasing the speed of the LVAD will exacerbate the degree of obstruction, further decreasing device flow and the resulting cardiac output.

Answer B is incorrect. Inotropes could potentially have two, frankly opposite effects. If severe RV failure is the cause of the suction event, this maneuver may improve LV filling by improving interventricular dependence. However, increasing the contractility of an already severely underfilled LV may further obstruct the inflow cannula, exacerbating the suction event. In either scenario, inotropes would not be the first-line therapy, but may be used in concert with other maneuvres to improve filling of the LV.

TAKE-HOME LESSON:

A comprehensive TEE examination is essential prior to LVAD insertion to determine potential contraindications or the need for additional procedures. Intracardiac shunts, apical thrombus, mitral stenosis, and AI may necessitate changes in management. TEE evaluation after insertion includes confirmation of correct cannula placement and function.

SUGGESTED READINGS

Bryant AS, Holman WL, Nanda NC, et al. Native aortic insufficiency in patients with left ventricular assist devices. *Ann Thor Surg*. 2006;81:E6–E8.

Chumnanvej S, Wood ML, MacGillivray TE, et al. Perioperative echocardiographic examination for ventricular assist device implantation. *Anesth Analg*. 2007;105:583–601.

Holman WL, Bourge RC, Fan P, et al. Influence of left ventricular assist on valvular regurgitation. *Circulation*. 1993;88:309–318.

Horton SC, Khodaverdian R, Chatelain P, et al. Left ventricular assist device malfunction: an approach to diagnosis by echocardiography. *J Am Coll Cardiol*. 2005;45:1435–1440.

Liao KK, Miller L, Toher C, et al. Timing of transesophageal echocardiography in diagnosing patent foramen ovale in patients supported with left ventricular assist device. *Ann Thorac Surg.* 2003;75:1624–1626.

Noon GP, Morley DL, Irwin S, et al. Clinical experience with the MicroMed DeBakey ventricular assist device. *Ann Thorac Surg.* 2001;71:133–138.

Rao V, Slater JP, Edwards NM, et al. Surgical management of valvular disease in patients requiring left ventricular assist device support. *Ann Thorac Surg.* 2001;71:1448–1453.

Scalia GM, McCarthy PM, Savage RM, et al. Clinical utility of echocardiography in the management of ventricular assist devices. *J Am Soc Echocardiogr.* 2000;13:754–763.

Advanced

CASE 91

A 38-year-old female with history of a previously repaired VSD presents with severe CHF after recovery from a recent upper respiratory infection. A presumptive diagnosis of viral myocarditis is made and a Tandem Heart percutaneous left ventricular assist device (pVAD) is placed emergently to manage this patient's deteriorating clinical status.

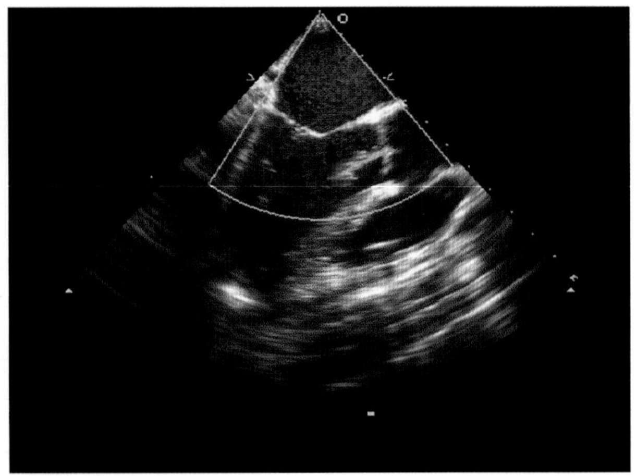

Figure 91.1. ME LAX.

QUESTION 91.1. Two weeks after initial placement of the pVAD, a little improvement is noted in the patient's cardiac function. The pVAD is being replaced with a more permanent HeartMate II LVAD as a bridge to transplantation. Prior to placement of the LVAD, the TEE image shown in Figure 91.1 and Video 91.1 is obtained. What is the most appropriate management?

A. Recommend surgical closure of the AV
B. Recommend replacement of the AV
C. Increase flow through the pVAD to 5.8 L/min
D. Decrease flow through the pVAD to 3.0 L/min

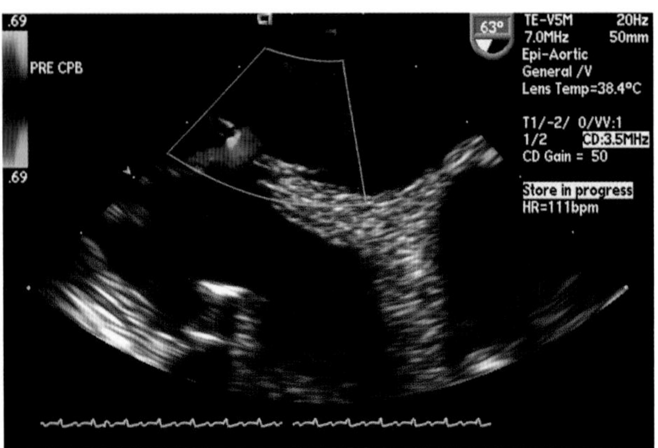

Figure 91.2. Zoom view of ME RV inflow-outflow.

QUESTION 91.2. The pVAD has been replaced with a HeartMate II LVAD. What is the most likely reason for the TEE finding (Fig. 91.2 and Video 91.2)?

A. Ostium secundum ASD
B. PFO
C. Traumatic ASD
D. Ostium primum ASD

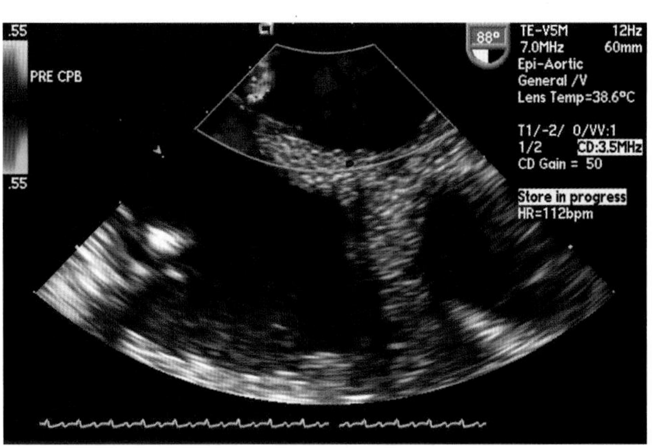

Figure 91.3. Modified ME bicaval view.

QUESTION 91.3. After weaning from bypass, the patient is persistently hypoxemic. LVAD flow is noted to be 5.6 L/min. Repeat TEE images are obtained (Fig. 91.3 and Video 91.3). What would be the most effective next step in the management of this patient?

A. Increase the FiO_2 from 0.8 to 1.0
B. Increase flow through the LVAD to 6.2 L/min
C. Decrease flow through the LVAD to 5.0 L/min
D. Perform a contrast study

QUESTION 91.4. Despite your best efforts, the patient continues to have refractory hypoxemia. What do you advise the surgeon to do now?

A. Close the chest and bring the patient to the ICU
B. Go back on bypass and surgically close the ASD
C. Close the chest and schedule occlusion of the ASD percutaneously
D. Decrease flow through the LVAD to 3.3 L/min

ANSWERS AND DISCUSSION

QUESTION 91.1: The correct answer is A: Recommend surgical closure of the AV. Severe AI can lead to decreased forward perfusion from the LVAD outflow cannula. Often the degree of AI in a patient with severe CHF can be difficult to determine as values can be underestimated secondary to high LV and low aortic diastolic pressures. Once an LVAD is placed, the AV experiences higher than normal pressures from the outflow cannula, exposing underlying AI. This patient's LVAD is being placed as a bridge to transplantation and there is no expectation for cardiac recovery. In this case, it would be most appropriate to simply close the AV with sutures or oversew the valve with a pericardial patch.

Answer B is incorrect. In a patient who is receiving an LVAD as a bridge to recovery, repair, or replacement of the AV would be most appropriate. Answer C is incorrect. Increasing flow through the outflow cannula will worsen the AI. Answer D is incorrect. Although decreasing flow through the outflow cannula may help, it is not a long-term solution.

QUESTION 91.2: The correct answer is C: Traumatic ASD. The Tandem Heart pVAD inflow cannula is placed through the femoral vein. The cannula is then advanced into the RA and across the atrial septum, providing inflow from the LA. Puncture of the atrial septum with a large inflow cannula can leave an atrial defect when removed. The Tandem Heart outflow cannula is placed through the femoral artery and it provides retrograde flow through the aorta. The major advantage of a pVAD versus a more permanent LVAD is the speed at which mechanical support can be established. Unfortunately, the device is only designed to provide support for up to 14 days and will need to be replaced with a more permanent LVAD if continued support is necessary.

Answer A is incorrect. Although the patient does have a history of a congenital cardiac defect and ostium secundum defects account for 70% of all ASDs, the clinical scenario is more likely to be associated with the direct trauma from placement of the pVAD. Answer B is incorrect. The perpendicular flow pattern to the atrial septum and location of the lesion are inconsistent with a PFO. The flow pattern for PFO tends to run parallel to the atrial septum under the flap between the septum primum and the septum secundum. Answer D is incorrect. Ostium primum defects occur near the AV junction and are more rare than secundum defects, accounting for only 20% of all ASD lesions.

QUESTION 91.3: The correct answer is C: Decrease flow through the LVAD to 5.0 L/min. Figure 91.2 shows the same traumatic ASD but CFD now suggests the blood flow is traveling from the RA to the LA (red color denotes flow toward the TEE transducer in this view). With a right-to-left shunt, the patient may have significant hypoxemia and will be at higher risk for embolic events. Often, decompression of the LV and atrium after placement of an LVAD can lead to right atrial pressure exceeding LA pressure and subsequent right-to-left shunt in patients with ASDs or PFO that have not been closed. By decreasing the LVAD flow slowly, LA pressure will rise and right-to-left shunt will decrease.

Answer A is incorrect. The patient has a pure right-to-left shunt, which will be refractory to an increased FiO_2. Answer B is incorrect. Increasing the LVAD flow will only worsen the situation by further decreasing the LA pressure. Answer D is incorrect. Although performing a bubble study might be helpful in further diagnosing the lesion, it is clear from the TEE and clinical scenario that an ASD exists. Treatment of the hypoxemia would be most appropriate.

QUESTION 91.4: The correct answer is B: Go back on bypass and surgically close the ASD. A patient with refractory hypoxemia is unstable and an immediate repair is needed. Attempting to transport a patient to an ICU or interventional cardiology procedure room with no pulmonary reserve could be disastrous. The best option would be to have the surgeons address the issue as soon as possible.

Answer A is incorrect. The patient's persistent hypoxemia necessitates correction of the lesion. Answer C is incorrect. Percutaneous closure of the ASD would be an option in a stable patient. Answer D is incorrect. Although decreasing LVAD flow further would increase LA pressure and potentially decrease the right-to-LA shunt, at only 3.3 L/min hypoperfusion to major organ beds is a risk.

TAKE-HOME LESSON:

The surveillance TEE exam prior to VAD placement is integral to its successful function. Prior procedures such as the placement of a percutaneous VAD can further complicate the successful conversion to a centrally cannulated VAD. Repeat TEE examination after VAD placement must confirm proper VAD function and rule out unexpected cardiac shunting of blood flow. In this patient, correction of the AI and the traumatic ASD was necessary for proper VAD function and perfusion of the patient.

SUGGESTED READING

Chumnanvej S, Wood MJ, MacGillivray TE, et al. Perioperative echocardiographic examination for ventricular assist device implantation. *Anesth Analg.* 2007;105:583–601.

CASE 92

A 51 year old male previously underwent placement of a mechanical MV due to infective endocarditis. The patient now presents with dyspnea. TEE was performed and it revealed the image shown in Figure 92.1.

QUESTION 92.1. The CFD jet in the LA represents what phenomenon (Video 92.1 and Figure 92.1)?

A. Severe mitral paravalvular leak
B. Stuck mechanical leaflet with wide open MR
C. Right superior pulmonary vein inflow
D. Large ASD with left-to-right shunting

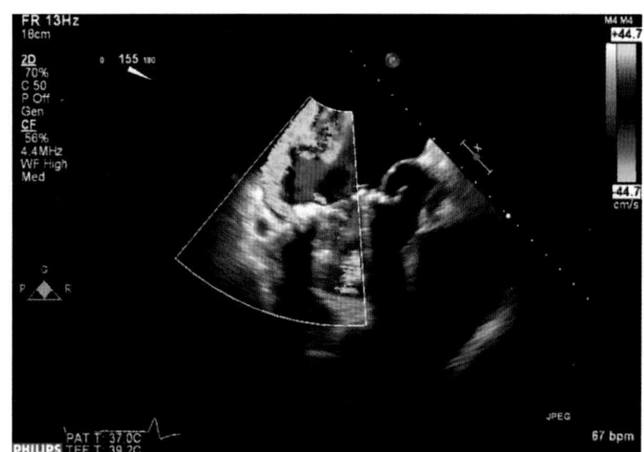

Figure 92.1. ME LAX with CFD (see Video 92.1).

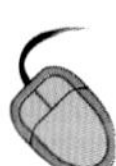

QUESTION 92.2. Which of the following is NOT a true statement with respect to paravalvular leaks?

A. It occurs more frequently with *bioprosthetic* implants
B. Patients are frequently anemic
C. Annular calcification is a risk factor
D. Oversizing the prosthesis with respect to the annulus is a risk factor

The patient was referred to an interventional cardiologist for percutaneous closure of the severe mitral paravalvular defect using an Amplatzer occlusion device. The image in Figure 92.2 was obtained before deployment of the Amplatzer device:

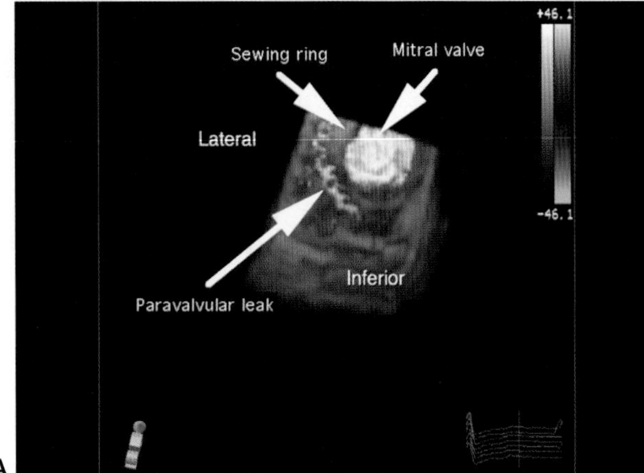

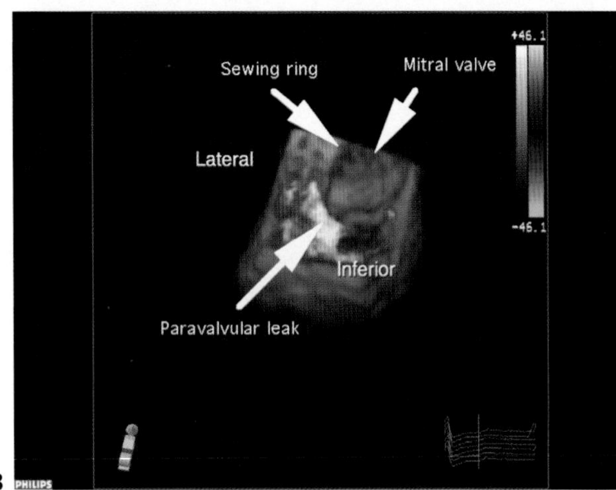

Figure 92.2. **A:** 3D reconstruction of the MV from the LA (early diastole) (see Video 92.2). **B:** 3D reconstruction of the MV from the LA (systole) (see also Video 92.2).

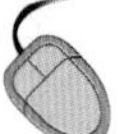

QUESTION 92.3. Which of the following complications might occur as a result of Amplatzer deployment for closure of paravalvular defects?

A. Stroke
B. Worsening MR
C. Mitral stenosis
D. ASD
E. All of the above

The paravalvular leak was unsuccessfully abolished after two attempted closures with successively larger Amplatzer occluders. Ultimately, the patient was referred for surgical intervention resulting in primary closure of the paravalvular defect. The images shown in Figures 92.3 to 92.5 and Videos 92.3 to 92.5 were captured immediately after attempted closure with the second Amplatzer device.

QUESTION 92.4. Why does this patient have persistent severe MR despite attempted closure of the paravalvular leak with an Amplatzer device?

A. The Amplatzer device was deployed in a second smaller paravalvular defect of clinical insignificance leaving the larger defect unaffected
B. The Amplatzer device is a pediatric septal occluder unsuitable for closure of adult paravalvular defects
C. The Amplatzer device did not deploy successfully
D. The Amplatzer device is geometrically mismatched to the defect

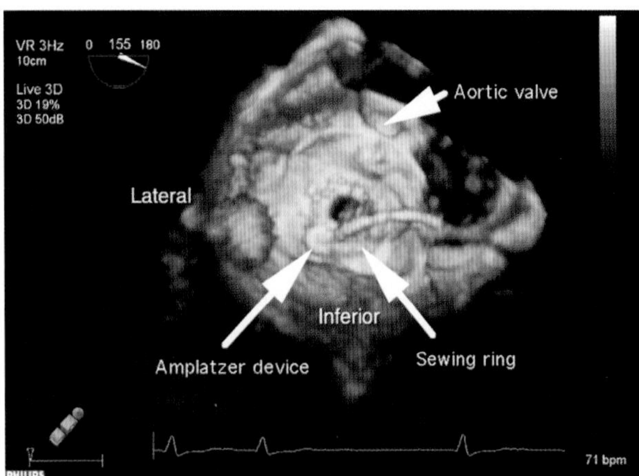

Figure 92.3. 3D view of MV with deployed Amplatzer occluder (see also Video 92.3).

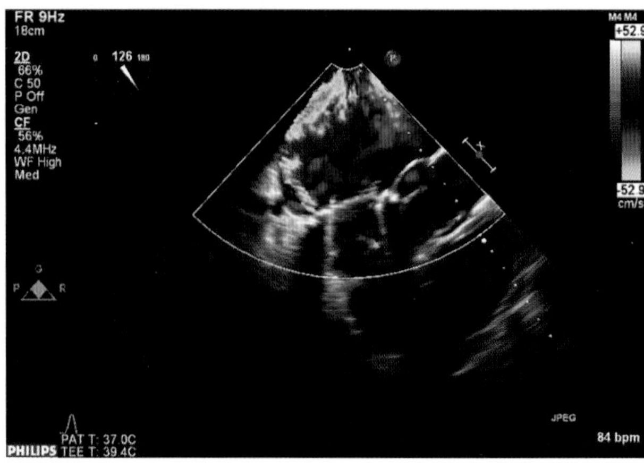

Figure 92.4. ME LAX view with CFD (see also Video 92.4).

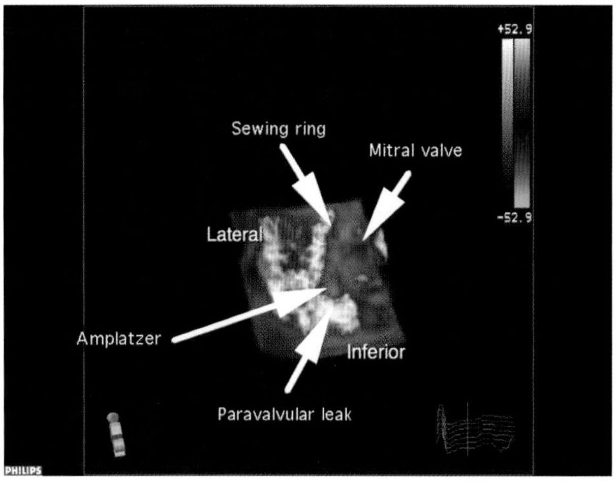

Figure 92.5. 3D reconstruction of the MV from the LA (systole) (see also Video 92.5).

ANSWERS AND DISCUSSION

QUESTION 92.1: The correct answer is A: Severe mitral paravalvular leak.

The color Doppler jet originates at the level of the mitral annulus outside of the sewing ring. This defines a paravalvular leak. The Nyquist limit is set at 45 cm/s, suggesting that the Doppler jet may be an overestimation of actual severity of the paravalvular leak. However, the Doppler jet adheres to the concave surface of the LA as it exits around the inferolateral aspect of the mitral annulus. This phenomenon is termed the Coanda effect and tends to minimize the jet area with respect to LA size—often leading to underestimation of the severity of eccentric jets. Therefore, the severity of the leak should be graded as severe.

The mechanical leaflets are not stuck and there is no significant regurgitation through the mechanical valve itself. Thrombus or pannus formation may be a source of malfunctioning prosthetic valve leaflets. Leaflets stuck in the open position would lead to significant MR whereas leaflets stuck in the closed position may lead to some degree of mitral stenosis. In this case, the regurgitant jet is outside of the sewing ring. The CFD jet has been described as a paravalvular leak. In addition, the jet is on the inferolateral wall of the LA. The right superior pulmonary vein is a medial structure. The CFD jet is hugging the inferolateral wall. The interatrial septum is not seen in the ME LAX view.

QUESTION 92.2: The correct answer is A: It occurs more frequently with *bioprosthetic* implants.

Paravalvular leaks occur more frequently with mechanical prosthetic valves. A large prospective trial of 575 patients randomized to receive either mechanical or bioprosthetic valve replacements at Veterans Affairs Hospitals published 15-year follow-up data in 2000. The incidence of mitral paravalvular leak was significantly higher with mechanical valve replacement compared with their bioprosthetic counterparts (17% vs. 7%, $p = 0.05$). For AV replacements, there was a trend toward an increased incidence of paravalvular leak with mechanical implants (8% vs. 2%, $p = 0.09$).

Paravalvular defects create high velocity jets. Shear stress on red blood cells may cause hemolysis. Patients who present with fatigue and shortness of breath are often found to be anemic on laboratory evaluation. Annular calcification is a risk factor for paravalvular leak. Leaks are created when the seal between the sewing ring and the annulus is incomplete. Debridement of MAC may create an uneven annular surface leading to paravalvular defects. Similarly, infected or friable tissue may prevent a tight seal from forming with the sewing ring. Fitting an oversized prosthetic valve into a smaller annulus places torque on the valve. This can prevent an adequate seal with the annulus or weaken valve sutures. This can ultimately lead to paravalvular leak.

QUESTION 92.3: The correct answer is E: All of the above.

ANSWER A: Deployment of Amplatzer devices for the closure of paravalvular defects may lead to a number of complications. Amplatzer occluders seal anatomic holes on both sides of a defect by seating their rim around a lip of tissue. Accidental misfiring of the device without seating the rims on both sides of the defect can predispose to distal embolization. Even an initially properly seated device can later become dislodged. Embolization to the arterial tree and cerebral vasculature is a dreaded complication.

ANSWER B: Deployment of an Amplatzer occluder for a paravalvular leak may increase the severity of the leak. Oversizing the Amplatzer device with respect to the defect may cause dehiscence of the sewing ring from the mitral annulus—exacerbating the paravalvular leak. Alternatively, paravalvular leaks often have a crescentic shape, whereas Amplatzer occluders are circular. The geometric mismatch between a circular device and crescentic defect may have the same effect as oversizing the device—fracture of the annulus from the sewing ring. In this case, Figure 92.3 demonstrates the crescentic nature of the paravalvular defect as the convex sewing ring separates from the concave annulus.

ANSWER C: An oversized Amplatzer device may also lead to mitral stenosis. Despite successful deployment, extension of the Amplatzer rim may impinge on the prosthetic orifice and obstruct inflow. Trapping of mechanical MV leaflets in the closed position has also been documented.

ANSWER D: Iatrogenic ASD is a common result of percutaneous closure of mitral paravalvular defects. Access to the LA is usually achieved via cannulation of the femoral vein. Once the RA is entered, trans-septal puncture allows for passage of the guide wire and catheters to the LA.

QUESTION 92.4: The correct answer is D: The Amplatzer device is geometrically mismatched to the defect. The defect in this case is cresentic in shape. An appropriately defect in this case was crescentic in nature. An appropriately sized circular Amplatzer occluder will fail to abolish a leak in the setting of a geometric mismatch. On the contrary, deployment of circular occluders in oblong crescentic defects may actually predispose to further separation of the sewing ring from the annulus, worsening the leak. The need for oblong-shaped occluders has been recognized and their development is currently underway. Three-dimensional echocardiography may be useful in identifying potential device-defect geometric mismatch and aid in the appropriate deployment of novel oblong devices.

Persistent severe MR is not secondary to a misplaced Amplatzer device. Figure 92.3 clearly shows the location of the deployed device around the inferolateral portion of the sewing ring. This is the location of the original paravalvular leak identified on both 2D imaging and 3D color full-volume reconstructions (Figs. 92.1 and 92.2). The device was placed in the appropriate defect and not in a smaller clinically insignificant one.

Pediatric Amplatzer septal occluders are commonly used for closure of adult paravalvular defects. Adult paravalvular defects are smaller than Amplatzer occluders used to close atrial septal defects in adults. In this case, the defect was sized and closure was attempted with successively larger pediatric septal occluders. An adult-sized septal occluder was not an appropriate size match and would not have led to resolution of this patient's leak.

Figure 92.3 clearly shows successful deployment of the Amplatzer device.

TAKE-HOME LESSON:

Paravalvular leaks of a mechanical prosthetic valve are multifactorial and not uncommon. Appropriate diagnosis of valve malfunction versus paravalvular leak requires a careful exam of the valve. A sewing ring dehiscence can often be crescent shaped and not conducive to repair with a catheter-based closure device such as an Amplatzer occluder.

SUGGESTED READING

Bhindi R, Bull S, Schrale RG, et al. Surgery insight: percutaneous treatment of prosthetic paravalvular leaks. *Nat Clin Pract Cardiovasc Med.* 2008;5:140–147.

Hammermeister K, Sethi GK, Henderson WG, et al. Outcomes 15 years after valve replacement with a mechanical versus a bioprosthetic valve: final report of the Veterans Affairs randomized trial. *J Am Coll Cardiol.* 2000;36:1152–1158.

CASE 93

A 58-year-old woman presents to the OR for MV surgery and MAZE procedure. She has New York Heart Association (NYHA) class III symptoms of CHF and gives a history of rheumatic fever. She also has a history of chronic AFib and two previous strokes. Preoperative coronary angiogram revealed normal coronary arteries. After induction of anesthesia, you obtain the TEE images shown in Figures 93.1 and 93.2.

QUESTION 93.1. Which of the following best describes the MV leaflet motion in this patient according to the Carpentier classification?

A. Type I
B. Type II
C. Type IIIa
D. Type IIIb

QUESTION 93.2. Based on Figure 93.3 and Video 93.3, how much TR does this patient have?

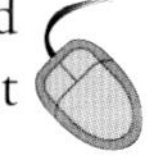

A. None
B. Mild
C. Moderate
D. Severe

The surgeon would like to know if the tricuspid annulus is dilated and if there is significant tethering of the leaflets.

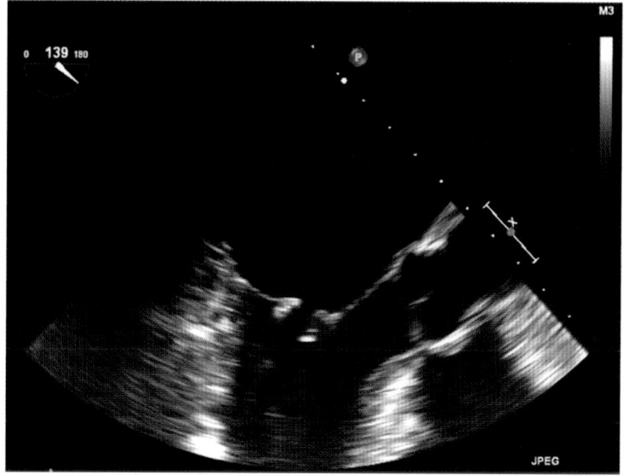

Figure 93.1. ME LAX of the MV, 2D, in systole. See also Video 93.1.

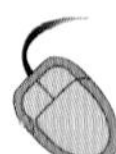

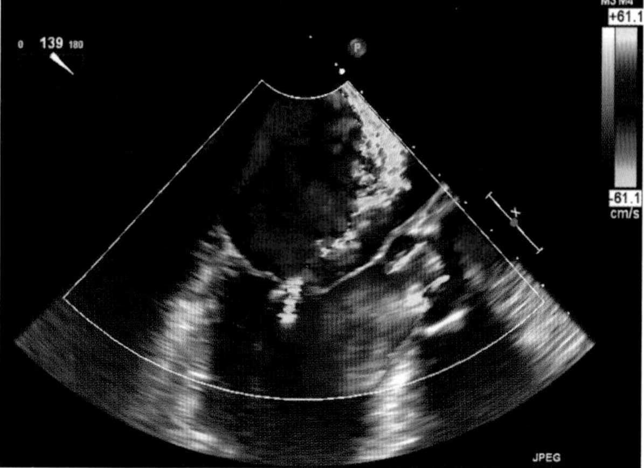

Figure 93.2. ME LAX, 2D, in systole, with CFD. See also Video 93.2.

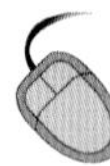

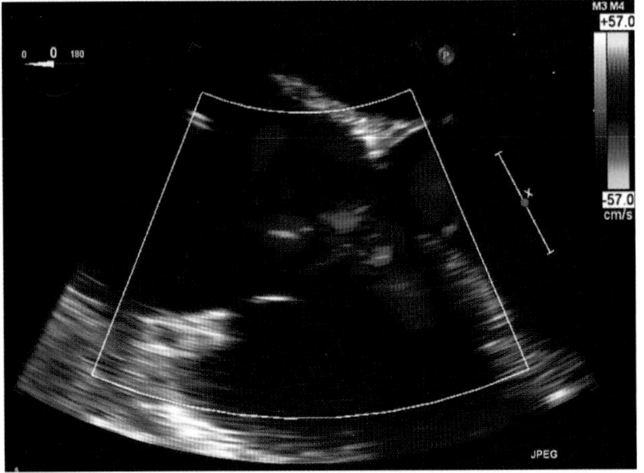

Figure 93.3. ME 4CH view, rotated to the right to demonstrate the TV with CFD in systole. See also Video 93.3.

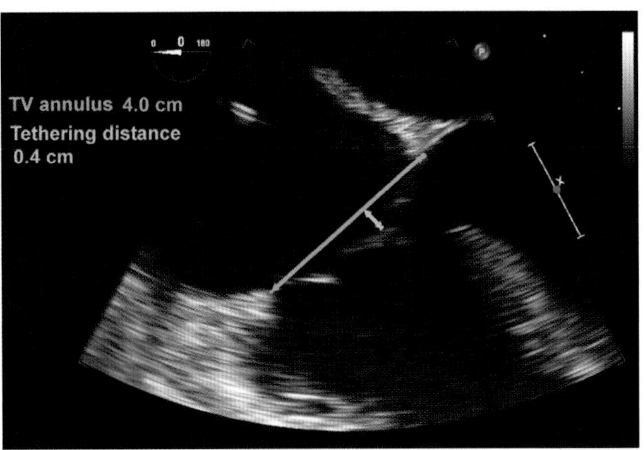

Figure 93.4. TV annular dimensions.

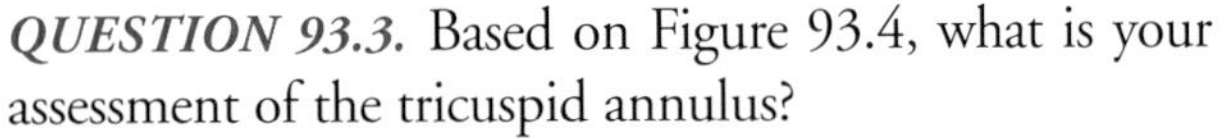

QUESTION 93.3. Based on Figure 93.4, what is your assessment of the tricuspid annulus?

A. Normal TV annular dimension, no significant tethering
B. Dilated TV annular dimension, significant tethering
C. Dilated TV annular dimension, no significant tethering
D. Normal TV annular dimension, significant tethering

QUESTION 93.4. Given the complete echo assessment of both tricuspid and MV, what are the surgical options on how to manage the TV?

A. There is no TR; leave it alone
B. There is no TR; but you should still repair the valve to prevent the late development of TR
C. This patient has rheumatic valve disease; you should replace the TV to prevent the late development of tricuspid stenosis
D. None of the above

QUESTION 93.5. In addition to replacing the MV and performing a MAZE procedure, the surgeon repairs the TV using a modified De Vega technique (Gore-Tex pledgeted annuloplasty suture) to reduce the annular diameter (see Fig. 93.5). What is the rationale for repairing the TV?

A. To prevent late TR
B. To improve the patient's functional status
C. To improve the patient's survival
D. All of the above

QUESTION 93.6. The tricuspid annulus after repair measures 2.8 cm in the four-chamber view. The mean diastolic pressure gradient is 1 mm Hg. What mean pressure gradient is acceptable after TV repair?

A. Less than 1 mm Hg
B. Less than 5 mm Hg
C. Less than 10 mm Hg
D. You cannot rely on the gradient following tricuspid repair

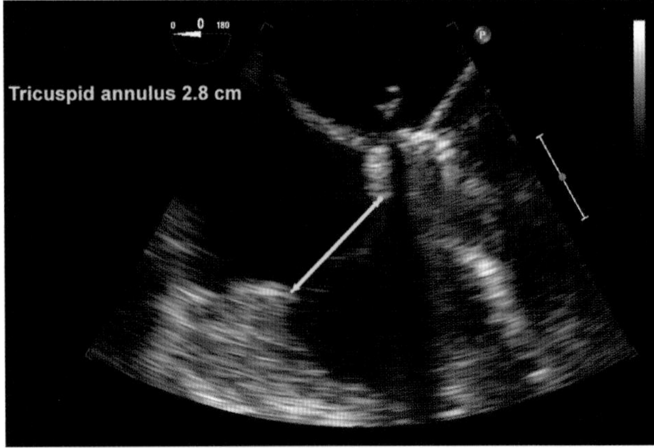

Figure 93.5. ME 4CH view of TV, post repair with a modified De Vega suture. See also Video 93.4.

ANSWERS AND DISCUSSION

QUESTION 93.1: The correct answer is C: Type IIIa. The functional classification of Carpentier describes MV leaflet motion relative to the mitral annular plane. Type I pathology involves *normal* leaflet motion as seen with leaflet perforation or cleft, or with pure annular dilatation. Type II pathology involves *excessive* leaflet motion as seen with leaflet prolapse or flail. Type III pathology involves *restricted* leaflet motion. Type IIIa refers to restricted leaflet motion during diastole and systole (as seen with rheumatic mitral valvular disease), whereas Type IIIb refers to restricted leaflet motion during systole (typically seen in functional MV regurgitation associated with ischemic heart disease). This patient has rheumatic valve disease and the TEE exam demonstrates a mix of mitral stenosis and regurgitation. On Figures 93.1 and 93.2 and Videos 93.1 and 93.2, both leaflets (especially the posterior) are severely restricted, both in systole and diastole.

QUESTION 93.2: The correct answer is A: None. Although one should always look at multiple views of a valve before deciding on the amount of regurgitation, based on this view alone, using CFD and with an adequate Nyquist limit, there appears to be no TR.

QUESTION 93.3: The correct answer is B: Dilated TV annular dimension, no significant tethering. The normal tricuspid annular (TA) dimension (as measured in the ME 4CH view) is 2.8 cm ± 0.5 cm. This patient's TA dimension is 4.0 cm. It is recommended to report the greatest dimension during the cardiac cycle (generally end-diastole). A tricuspid tethering height of greater than 0.5 cm is considered significant. This patient falls just short of that value. The significance of the tethering height is that some surgeons alter their repair technique when annular dilatation and tethering are both present, in the hope of improving the durability of their repair. For example, a simple ring or suture annuloplasty may be used in a case of isolated annular dilatation, while an edge-to-edge repair plus a ring may be chosen when both pathologies are present.

QUESTION 93.4: In the author's view, the most correct answer is B: There is no TR, but you should still repair the valve to prevent the late development of TR. The ACC/AHA and European Society of Cardiology (ESC) give a class I recommendation to TV repair only in patients with *severe* TR undergoing MV surgery. The ACC/AHA give a class IIb recommendation to TV repair in patients with less than severe TR undergoing MV surgery, whereas the ESC gives a class IIa recommendation to TV repair with a TA diameter >40 mm or moderate TR undergoing MV surgery.[1,2] However, recent studies support a more aggressive approach to TV repair in the setting of MV surgery than recommended by current guidelines. In a recent review, Shiran and Sagie[3] recommend TV annuloplasty with a ring at the time of MV surgery, to *correct or prevent* TR, if the TA diameter is ≥3.5 cm *regardless of the severity of the regurgitation.*[4] The goal is threefold: to prevent late TR, to improve functional capacity, and to offer a late survival benefit. The discussion of Question 93.6 expands on this topic. If one strictly adheres to the current ACC/AHA guidelines, answer A (*do nothing*) is also correct: a repair is reasonable, but not mandatory. Answer C (*TV replacement to prevent TS*) is incorrect: if the patient has no sign of tricuspid rheumatic involvement at this stage, she is unlikely to develop it later in life. She is at much higher risk of developing TR.

QUESTION 93.5: The correct answer is D: *All of the above.* As stated in the discussion of Question 93.4, a recent review recommends a more aggressive approach to dilated TVs in the context of MV surgery, even in the absence of significant TR.[4] The goal is to *prevent late TR*, to *improve functional capacity,* and to offer a *late survival* benefit. One of the studies supporting this recommendation was published by Dreyfus et al.[5] The TA diameter was measured on bypass (from the anteroseptal commissure to the anteroposterior commissure—the long axis of the valve) and the valve was electively repaired if the annular diameter was ≥7 cm (this is *equivalent to about 4 cm by ME 4CH view*), *regardless of the severity* of the regurgitation. At 10-year follow-up, patient whose TV was repaired tended to have *better survival* (90.3% vs. 85.5%), had significantly *less TR* (0.7% vs. 34% grade 3 or 4 TR), and significantly *better functional capacity* (0% vs. 14% functional class III or IV.

QUESTION 93.6: The correct answer is B: Less than 5 mm Hg. The echocardiographic evaluation of tricuspid stenosis is difficult in the best of circumstances and even more so following TV repair. Most techniques and associated normal values used in TEE evaluation of tricuspid stenosis are extrapolated from the evaluation of mitral stenosis, some of which may or may not be applicable to the TV. Moreover, the echocardiographic parameters of RV loading and diastolic function are less well understood than on the left side, making the evaluation of tricuspid inflow uncertain. As a result, a gradation of severity of tricuspid stenosis is difficult to establish, and many authorities suggest that a "cut-off" level of *hemodynamically significant stenosis* is probably more clinically relevant. Within that context, the recently published EAE/ASE guidelines on the echocardiographic assessment of valve stenosis[6] describe a *mean* pressure gradient of *5 mm Hg* as a generally accepted threshold of hemodynamically significant tricuspid stenosis. Normal tricuspid inflow velocity is rarely more than 0.7 m/s, and a value ≥1.0 m/s should prompt a careful evaluation of the valve. Finally, a PHT ≥190 msec and a valve area (calculated by continuity equation) ≤1.0 cm^2 are described as suggestive of significant tricuspid stenosis, but more scientific validation is required.

TAKE-HOME LESSON:

Tricuspid valve pathology accompanies mitral pathology on a regular basis. Intervention for dilated annulus with no regurgitation is advocated by some centers.

REFERENCES

1. Anwar AM, Soliman OI, Nemes A, et al. Value of assessment of tricuspid annulus: real-time three-dimensional echocardiography and magnetic resonance imaging. *Int J Cardiovasc Imaging.* 2007;23:701–705.
2. Baumgartner H, Hung J, Bermejo J, et al. Echocardiographic assessment of valve stenosis. *Eur J Echocardiogr.* 2009;10(1):1–25.
3. Shiran A, Sagie A. Tricuspid regurgitation in mitral valve disease. *J Am Coll Cardiol.* 2009;53:401–408.
4. Bonow RO, Carabello BA, Chatterjee K, et al. ACC/AHA 2006 guidelines for the management of patients with valvular heart disease: a report of the American College of Cardiology/American Heart Association Task Force on Practice Guidelines. *J Am Coll Cardiol.* 2006;48:e1–e148.
5. Dreyfus GD, Corbi PJ, Chan KM, et al. Secondary tricuspid regurgitation or dilatation: which should be the criteria for surgical repair? *Ann Thorac Surg.* 2005;79:127–132.
6. Vahanian A, Baumgartner H, Bax J, et al. Guidelines on the management of valvular heart disease: the Task Force on the Management of Valvular Heart Disease of the European Society of Cardiology. *Eur Heart J.* 2007;28:230–268.

CASE 94

A 62-year-old woman is undergoing open-heart surgery for AS. Intraoperative TEE shows that she has a bicuspid AV with moderate to severe AS and mild to moderate AI. During examination of the aorta you notice the abnormality as shown in Figures 94.1 and 94.2, and Videos 94.1 and 94.2 in the upper esophageal LAX.

QUESTION 94.1. Which is the most likely diagnosis in this patient?

A. PDA
B. Abnormal origin of left coronary artery (White–Bland–Garland syndrome)
C. Surgically created shunts
D. Aortopulmonary window

QUESTION 94.2. What important hemodynamic information cannot be calculated from Figure 94.3, a CW Doppler of the anomaly?

A. Shunt timing
B. Shunt direction
C. Peak pressure gradient
D. Shunt fraction

QUESTION 94.3. From Figure 94.3 and the information provided, calculate the PA systolic pressure. BP: 95/60 RAP: 10

A. 32 mm Hg
B. 46 mm Hg
C. 62 mm Hg
D. Cannot be calculated

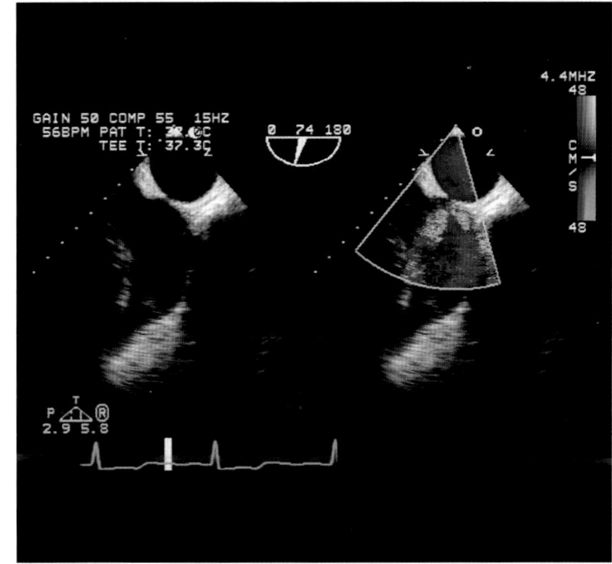

Figure 94.1.

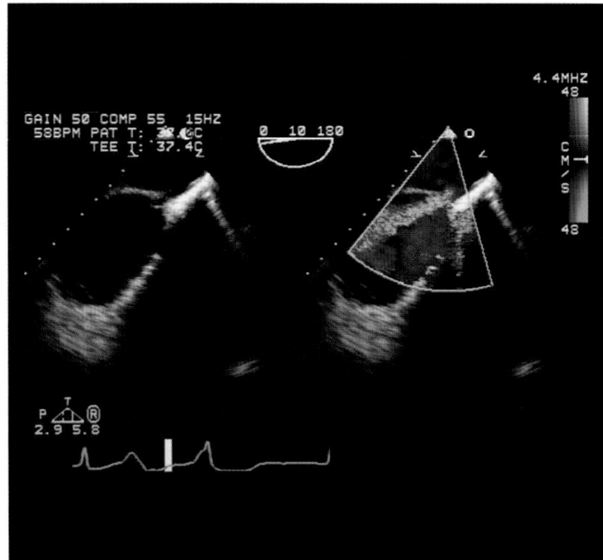

Figure 94.2.

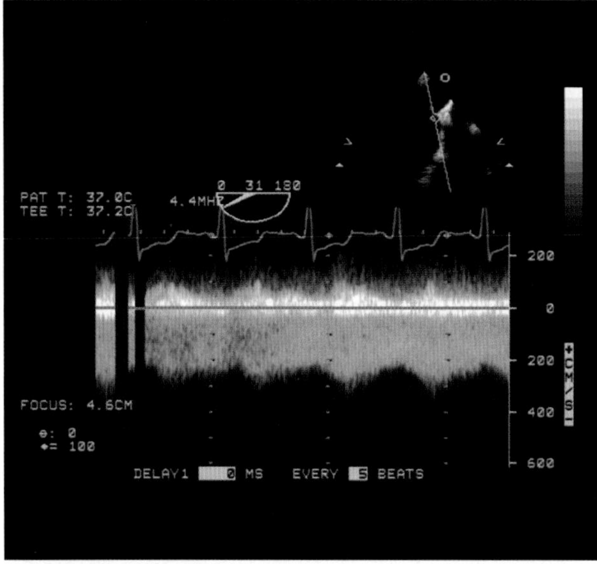

Figure 94.3.

QUESTION 94.4. The recommended management of this patient will be

A. Leave without intervention

B. Perform AVR and PDA closure surgically via sternotomy

C. Perform AVR and refer patient for intervention in cath lab after surgery

D. Turn patient on the side and manage it surgically via lateral thoracotomy

QUESTION 94.5. The surgical management of this type of lesion is recommended in a

A. Calcified lesion

B. Aneurysmal lesion

C. Small narrow lesion

D. Lesion coexisting with fixed pulmonary hypertension

ANSWERS AND DISCUSSION

QUESTION 94.1: The correct answer is A: PDA.

The ductus arteriosus is an essential part of the fetal circulation and usually closes after birth. A PDA is defined as a persistent communication between the descending aorta (near the origin of left subclavian artery) and the main or proximal left PA. In cases not complicated by pulmonary hypertension, pressure in the aorta is higher than the PA and creates a left-to-right shunt through the PDA. A PDA can be an isolated lesion or occurs in association with other congenital heart lesions, such as VSD and ASD. In this case, the PDA is associated with a bicuspid AV. Adequate visualization of PDA can be difficult as it travels anterior to the trachea. Figure and video 94.1 includes a LAX of the PA, showing the characteristic high-velocity jet arising from the ductus during diastole. In Figure and video 94.2, rotation of the probe shows the origin of the abnormal flow from the aorta to the PA. This jet creates the reversed (antegrade) flow toward the pulmonic valve. Figure 94.3 shows the presence of continuous flow between the aorta and the PA with the CW Doppler cursor aligned along the ductus.

Any condition creating abnormal diastolic flow in the PA could be confused with PDA flow. Answer D is incorrect as an aortopulmonary window is a rare congenital condition that involves an abnormal connection between the ascending aorta and the PA. In an aortopulmonary window, there is a flow disturbance in the aorta at the site of the variably sized fenestration. The flow is usually perpendicular to the long axis of the PA and expands rapidly. Answer B is incorrect as an anomalous origin of a coronary artery from the PA usually arises in one of the sinuses of pulmonic valve and there is retrograde flow from the anomalous vessel within the PA. The other normally connected coronary artery is usually dilated. Answer C is incorrect as surgically created shunts may have flow patterns similar to the PDA; the site of the shunt is usually remote from the site of the ductus.

QUESTION 94.2: The correct answer is D: Shunt fraction.

To calculate the shunt fraction would require information about both systemic (Qs) and pulmonary flow (Qp). The ductal shunt flow can be calculated as below:

$$\text{Ductal shunt flow} = \text{pulmonary blood flow} - \text{systemic blood flow}$$

Pulmonary flow in these cases equals systemic flow plus PDA shunt flow. It must be noted that the shunt flow in PDA occurs downstream from the pulmonic valve; as a result, flow through the pulmonic valve is equal to systemic flow (not pulmonary flow) and flow through the AV is a measure of pulmonary flow. Alternatively, flows through the TV or MV can be used to calculate shunt fraction with flow through TV representing systemic flow and flow through MV representing pulmonary blood flow.

Doppler techniques are used to further confirm the diagnosis of a PDA, assess the direction and timing of the flow, measure the pressure gradient between the aorta and the PA. The UE Aortic Arch SAX view at 90 degrees provides excellent alignment for Doppler technique (Fig. 94.2). Doppler can also quantify the volume of shunt flow. The ME Asc Ao SAX view obtained by pulling back the probe from a four-chamber view at 0 degree discloses a dilated main, right, and left PA.

Color Doppler in the distal main PA reveals mosaic flow. A PW Doppler sample volume positioned at the mouth of the ductus reveals high velocity flow present during both systole and diastole. Positioning the sample volume within the ductus offers additional help in detecting the shunt direction. The peak systolic gradient between the aorta and the PA can be calculated from the peak velocity of shunt flow using the simplified Bernoulli equation with a CW Doppler trace. Color M-mode along the ductal flow can further confirm the continuous flow. The mosaic reverse flow in the PA may decrease in the presence of severe pulmonary hypertension; CW Doppler usually shows bidirectional flow across the duct in these cases.

QUESTION 94.3: The correct answer is B: 46 mm Hg.

PA systolic pressure can be calculated by applying the Bernoulli equation. The measured gradient across the PDA is the difference in pressure between the aorta and the PA during systole, as follows:

$$4(V_{PDA})^2 = \text{Systolic BP} - \text{PASP}$$
$$\text{PASP} = \text{Systolic BP} - 4(V_{PDA})^2$$
$$\text{PASP} = 95 - 4 \times (3.5) \times (3.5) = 46 \text{ mm Hg}$$

QUESTION 94.4: The correct answer is B: Perform AVR and PDA closure surgically via sternotomy.

The PDA was closed on CPB, which was required for the AVR. Answer A is incorrect as leaving the PDA unrepaired during this case can cause excessive bleeding in the surgical field and LV distension from increased venous return through the pulmonary circulation.

In adults, the management of a PDA depends on the magnitude and direction of the shunt flow and PA pressure. When a PDA occurs in isolation, device closure is the treatment of choice. When a PDA is associated with other intracardiac lesions, it may be closed at the time of cardiac surgery. However, preoperative device closure of the PDA should be considered, given the potential anatomic difficulties often encountered with the PDA in the adult population and also the presence of comorbidities that could adversely affect the surgical risk.

It is reasonable to proceed with device closure in an adult with a small asymptomatic PDA. Closure of the PDA is not indicated in an adult patient with pulmonary hypertension and right-to-left shunting.

In the adult, PDA is associated with the presence of calcification and general tissue friability in the area of the aortic isthmus and PA; as a result, surgical manipulation is more hazardous in the adult than in the child. Fortunately, the need for surgical closure of a PDA in the adult is uncommon.

QUESTION 94.5: The correct answer is B: Aneurysmal lesion.

The currently preferred method of PDA closure is with the use of a device in the cardiac catheterization lab. Surgical closure is less commonly performed and is only reserved for most difficult cases, for example a PDA that is large, aneurysmal, distorted, or previously infected (endarteritis). A congenital cardiac surgeon should preferably perform the operative management. The primary surgical approach may be via thoracotomy (VATS or open) or sternotomy, with or without CPB. Ligation and division of the PDA or patch closure from inside the main PA or inside the aorta are possible surgical techniques. Recanalization is rare.

Answer A is incorrect as a calcified lesion increases the risk of surgical repair, which can be complicated by aortic/PA perforation. It is a strong indication for device closure. If surgical repair is pursued, it is recommended to be performed with the use of CPB. Answer C is incorrect as an asymptomatic tiny PDA without an audible murmur probably should be left alone and closely followed up or considered for device closure. Answer D is incorrect as the presence of fixed pulmonary hypertension is a well-established contradiction for any intervention in PDA.

TAKE-HOME LESSON:

The presence of abnormal flow in the PA should prompt a thorough examination for a PDA.

SUGGESTED READING

Rouine-Rapp K, Miller-Hance WC. Transesophageal echocardiography for congenital heart disease in the adult. In: Perrino A, Reeves ST, eds. *A Practical Approach to Transesophageal Echocardiography.* 2nd ed. Philadelphia: Lippincott Williams & Wilkins; 2008:380–381.

CASE 95

A 69-year-old man comes to the OR for a MV replacement. He has a history of a long-standing murmur and had rheumatic fever as a child. After inserting the TEE probe, you obtain the images shown in Figure 95.1A,B and Video 95.1.

QUESTION 95.1. Based on the echocardiogram, the most likely mechanism of MR in this patient is:

A. Type 1
B. Type 2
C. Type 3a
D. Type 3b

After inspecting the MV, the surgeon decides that it cannot be repaired and opts for MV replacement. Figure 95.2 and Video 95.2 are obtained after separation from CPB.

QUESTION 95.2. Figure 95.2 was obtained after CPB. What type of prosthesis did the surgeon insert in the mitral position?

A. Mechanical single tilting disc prosthesis
B. Mechanical bileaflet prosthesis
C. Bovine pericardial bioprosthesis
D. Mitral homograft

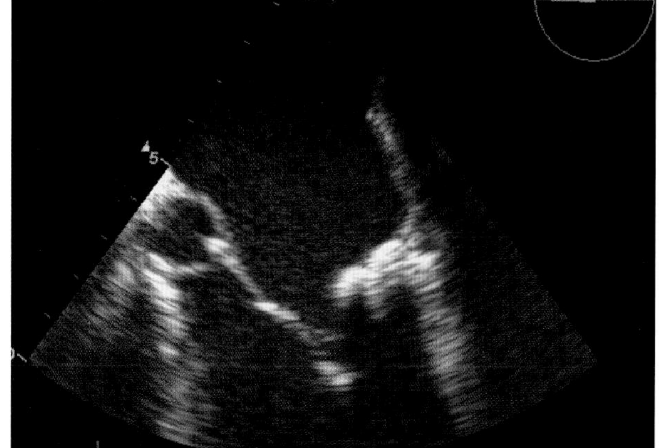

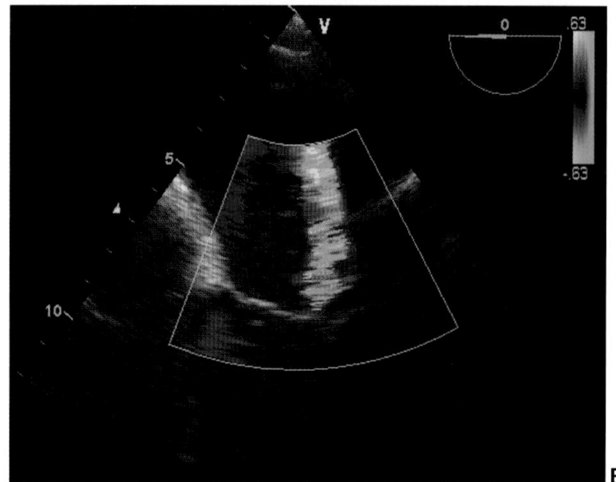

Figure 95.1. **A,B:** ME 4CH view, zooming in on the MV (see also Video 95.1).

QUESTION 95.3. The CFD image of the MV prosthesis (Fig. 95.3) is most consistent with which of the following:

A. Normal "washout" regurgitant jets
B. Excessive intravalvular leaking due to a stuck leaflet
C. Aliasing diastolic flow consistent with stenotic restricted diastolic flow
D. A paravalvular leak

QUESTION 95.4. Based on these same images, what is the location of the paravalvular leak?

A. Posterolaterally, in the area of the native P2 scallop
B. Anteromedially, adjacent to the AV
C. Straight anterior, in the area of the native A1 segment
D. Straight posterior, near the native posteromedial commissure

QUESTION 95.5. Based on the above echo, the most appropriate course of action would be:

A. Give protamine, since this is a completely normal prosthesis
B. Immediately return to bypass to repair this stuck prosthetic valve
C. Return to bypass and replace the valve with a larger one
D. Give protamine; this is a very small paravalvular leak

After discussing with your surgeon, the decision is made to give protamine and to close the chest. At the time of sternal closure, you take another look at the mitral prosthesis and you obtain the image shown in Figure 95.4 and Video 95.4.

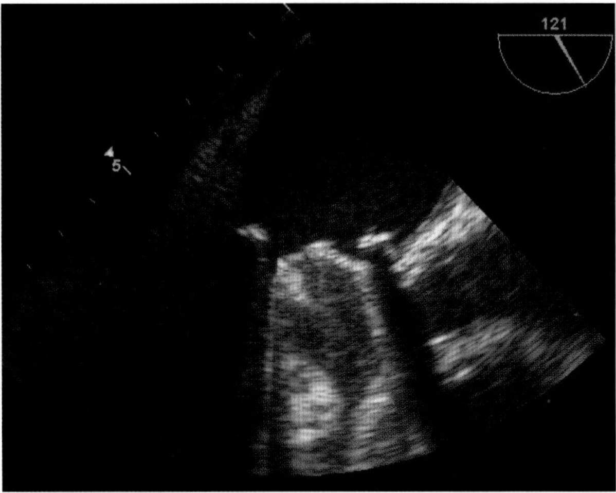

Figure 95.2. 2D ME LAX of the MV (see also Video 95.2).

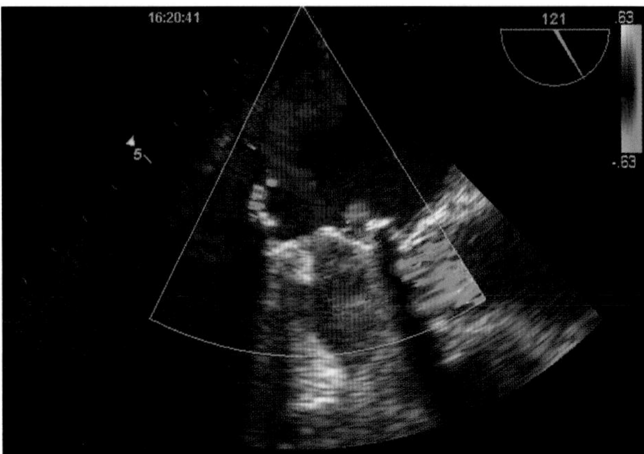

Figure 95.3. CFD ME LAX of the MV (see also Video 95.3).

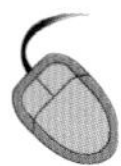

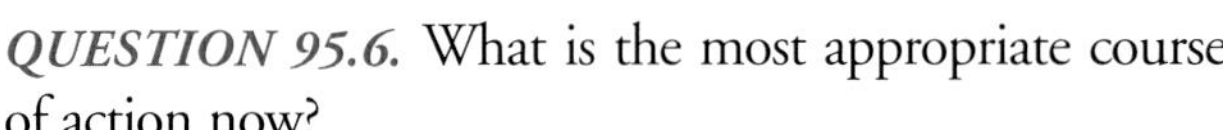

QUESTION 95.6. What is the most appropriate course of action now?

A. Holy cow! A suture must have let go. We need to reopen the chest and fix this
B. Continue closing the chest; nothing has changed
C. Continue closing the chest, as paravalvular leaks often get worse after sternal closure
D. None of the above

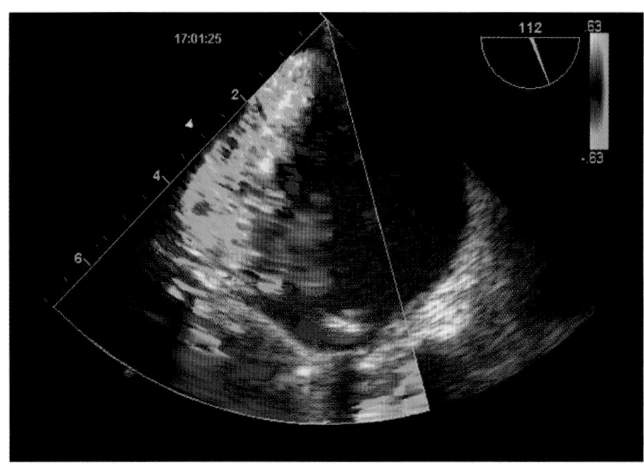

Figure 95.4. CFD ME LAX of the MV (see also Video 95.4).

ANSWERS AND DISCUSSION

QUESTION 95.1: The correct answer is C: Type 3a.

The widely used Carpentier classification of MR is based on leaflet motion: Type 1 involves normal leaflet motion and is often the result of pure annular dilatation or leaflet perforation. Type 2 represents excessive leaflet motion, like leaflet prolapse or flail. Finally, Type 3 refers to MR caused by restricted leaflet motion. In Type 3a, the restriction is structural and most often the result of rheumatic disease. In Type 3b, the restriction is functional, meaning that the leaflets themselves are normal but they are tethered, as a result of apical and posterior displacement of the papillary muscles. In this example, the image shows a posterior mitral leaflet that is thick, calcified, and very restricted. In this case, the video shows a posterior mitral leaflet that is thick, calcified and restricted (Video 95.1). The color Doppler image also shows a posteriorly directed jet, consistent with a posterior leaflet restriction.

QUESTION 95.2: The correct answer is B: Mechanical bileaflet prosthesis.

The image is oriented such that both leaflets can clearly be seen head on. In order to obtain this image, the valve is placed in the center of the sector scan and the angle of rotation is advanced until both leaflets can be visualized. A single disc mechanical valve, as its name implies, has only one visible leaflet that covers the entire orifice. A bioprosthesis, be it porcine or bovine pericardial, has characteristic thin leaflets and three struts that extend into the LV. Finally, a mitral homograft can be indistinguishable from a native MV on TEE.

QUESTION 95.3: The correct answer is D: A paravalvular leak. All mechanical prosthetic valves are designed to have normal regurgitant jets to decrease the risk of thrombosis. They typically appear as small, relatively low velocity jets, arising *inside* the sewing ring of the valve. Bileaflet mechanical prostheses typically have as many as three such small regurgitant "washout" jets and one of these can be seen on the right-hand side of the image. The small jet on the left of the image clearly arises *outside* of the sewing ring and represents a *paravalvular* leak. A leaflet stuck in the open position would cause a large *intravalvular* leak, similar to the MR jet that was present at the beginning of the case (Fig. 95.1B). Diastolic flow restriction would result in *diastolic* aliasing, but there is no such jet on this echo. Moreover, the 2D image clearly shows both leaflets of the prosthesis opening widely.

QUESTION 95.4: The correct answer is A: Posterolaterally, in the area of the native P2 scallop.

A preferred method to identify the location of a mitral paravalvular leak with the probe in the ME position is to image the valve in the center of the sector scan, activate CFD, and slowly rotate the imaging array from 0 to 180 degrees, until the leak is visible. *If the valve is centered*, the degree of rotation provides a guide to the location of the leak. Figure 95.5 is a drawing of the MV seen from the perspective of the LA, with the various scanning planes from 0 to 150 degrees. It is useful in each patient to "calibrate" the scanning planes to neighboring structures (i.e., at what scanning plane is the AV transected 135 or 150 degrees) to more precisely guide the surgeon to the location of the specific

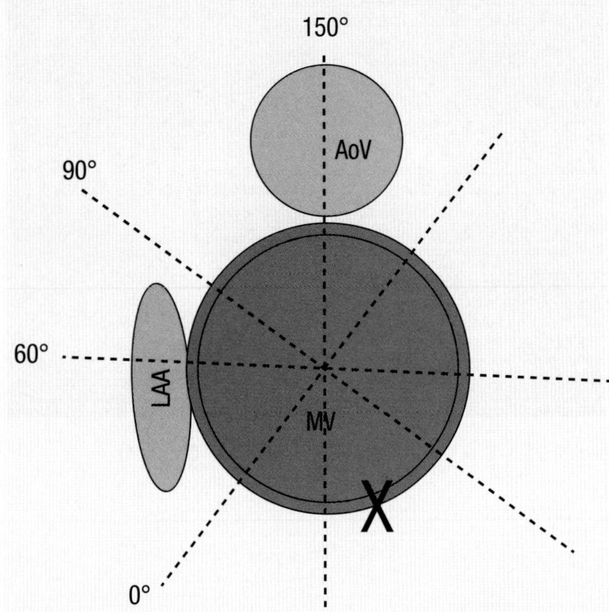

Figure 95.5. Drawing of the MV.

leak. The "X" marks the location of the paravalvular leak in this patient, posteriorly (on the left of the image) at 125 degrees of transducer rotation. This roughly corresponds to the area of the P2 scallop on the native MV.

QUESTION 95.5: The correct answer is D: Give protamine; this is a very small paravalvular leak. This is indeed a small paravalvular leak and it is appropriate to not intervene. While one would ideally want *no* paravalvular leak, minor leaks (1+) are unlikely to cause significant hemodynamic or hemolytic complications, and should be ignored given the known risks of intervention. Also, if the annulus is particularly calcified (as is often the case in rheumatic valves), a picture-perfect result may not be achievable. Answer B, a stuck leaflet, whether it is open or closed, mandates immediate return to bypass. Finally, answer A is incorrect since there is a paravalvular leak, this is not a completely normal prosthesis.

QUESTION 95.6: The correct answer is A: We need to reopen the chest and fix this. Over the course of about 40 minutes (note the times on images 3 and 4), the paravalvular leak has increased from mild to severe. This is most likely the result of a suture suddenly breaking or tearing through the tissues. Closure of the sternum in itself wouldn't cause such a major change. This is a serious problem that requires returning to bypass for repair. Heparin was given, the patient was recannulated, and the valve was re-inspected. The diagnosis of broken suture was confirmed, additional sutures were placed to reinforce the implant, and the patient came off bypass with no apparent paravalvular leak.

TAKE-HOME LESSON:

Mitral paravalvular leaks can be insignificant or they can cause hemodynamic compromise. They are usually readily visible by TEE examination. A systematic postbypass examination of the valve will reveal their presence and may indicate the need for surgical correction.

SUGGESTED READING

Cheung A. Prosthetic valves. In: Perrino AC Jr, Reeves ST, eds. *A Practical Approach to Transesophageal Echocardiography.* 2nd ed. Philadelphia: Lippincott Williams & Wilkins; 2008:257–278.

Savage R, et al. Assessment in mitral valve surgery. In: Savage R, Aronson S, et al., eds. *Comprehensive Textbook of Intraoperative Transesophageal Echocardiography.* Philadelphia: Lippincott Williams & Wilkins; 2005:443–533.

CASE 96

A 20-year-old woman was first diagnosed with a systolic heart murmur at 10 days of age. She was previously treated with medical therapy and now presents with symptoms of palpitations, fatigue, and dyspnea. An exercise test showed inducible ventricular tachycardia.

QUESTION 96.1. After reviewing Figures 96.1 (ME 4Ch) and 96.2 (ME 4Ch with CFD) and Video 96.1 (four chambers) and Video 96.2 (TG basal short axis), what is your diagnosis?

A. Acute myocarditis

B. Myxomatous MV

C. Congenitally corrected transposition of the great arteries (cc-TGA)

D. D-Transposition of the great arteries (D-TGA)

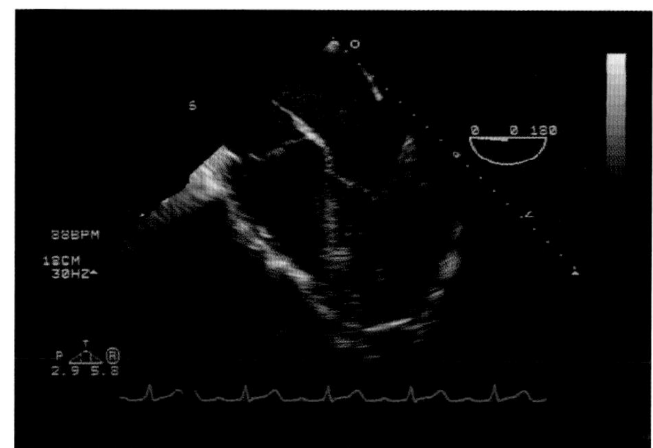

Figure 96.1.

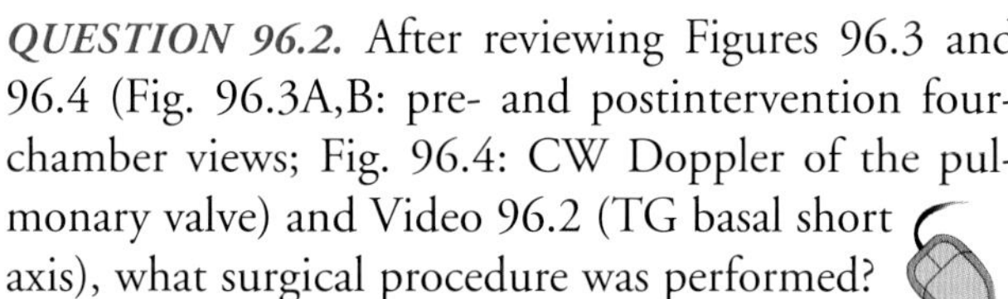

QUESTION 96.2. After reviewing Figures 96.3 and 96.4 (Fig. 96.3A,B: pre- and postintervention four-chamber views; Fig. 96.4: CW Doppler of the pulmonary valve) and Video 96.2 (TG basal short axis), what surgical procedure was performed?

A. MV replacement

B. Pulmonary artery banding (PAB)

C. MV repair

D. TV replacement

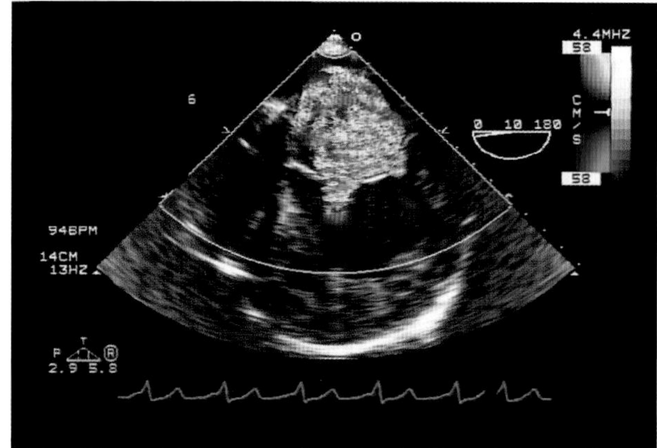

Figure 96.2.

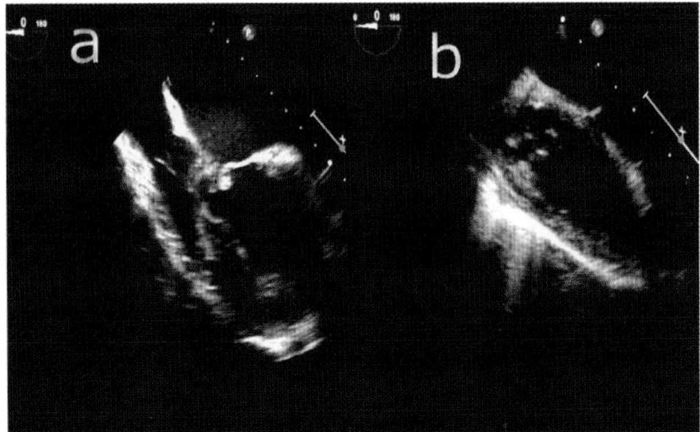

Figure 96.3.

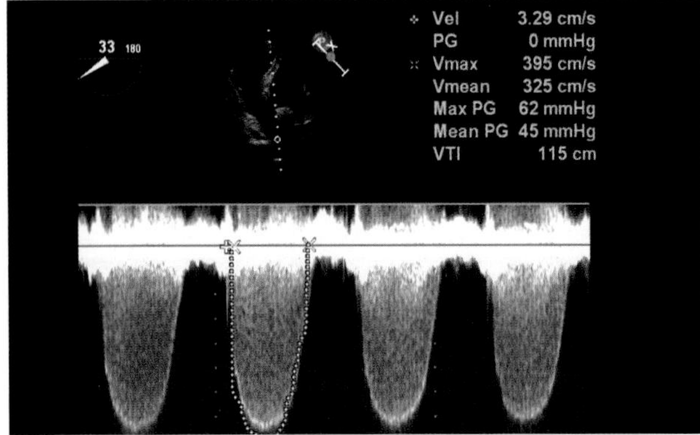

Figure 96.4.

QUESTION 96.3. Comparing presurgical (Fig. 96.3A) and postsurgical (Fig. 96.3B) procedure, what do these views represent?

A. Unloading of the morphological LV
B. Decrease in MR
C. Septal shift
D. Increase in TR

QUESTION 96.4. Following the surgical procedure a CW Doppler trace (Fig. 96.4) through an outflow tract shows a peak gradient of 62 mm Hg. The systemic blood pressure is 90 mm Hg. What possible outcomes exist for this patient?

A. Complete repair at a later date
B. Tighten the PA band
C. No further intervention
D. Loosen the PA band

QUESTION 96.5. What additional structural anomaly is least likely to be found in this patient?

A. TV abnormalities
B. MV abnormalities
C. VSD
D. Pulmonic stenosis

ANSWERS AND DISCUSSION

QUESTION 96.1: The correct answer is C: cc-TGA.

Patients with cc-TGA are born with atrioventricular (AV) discordance as well as ventricular-arterial (VA) discordance. The RA connects to the morphological LV, which gives rise to the PA, and the LA connects to the morphological RV, which gives rise to the aorta. The term "corrected" refers to the physiologically normal direction of blood flow caused by this "double discordance." The morphological RV therefore functions as the systemic ventricle, whereas the morphological LV functions as the pulmonary ventricle.

The atrio-ventricular valves best determine ventricular morphology, as a TV always enters a morphological RV. In Figures 96.1 and 96.2, four-chamber views at 0 degree, the TV appears to the right of the display and is inferior, closer to the cardiac apex (Video 96.1). In addition, it can be differentiated from the MV by chordal attachments to the inlet septum and the absence of distinct papillary muscle attachments. In the basal short-axis view instead of the bileaflet MV, the trileaflet TV is seen (Video 96.2). The abnormal great artery relationship is also pathognomonic of TGA: the aorta (and AV) lies anterior and to the left of the PA (and pulmonic valve) so both valves are coplanar (Fig. 96.5 and Video 96.3).

Answer A is incorrect because one would expect both ventricles to be dilated and hypofunctioning in the presence of acute myocarditis. Answer B is incorrect because in this patient, the MV is the valve for the pulmonary circulation and appears normal on the left of the display. Answer D is incorrect as D-TGA is characterized by AV concordance and VA discordance.

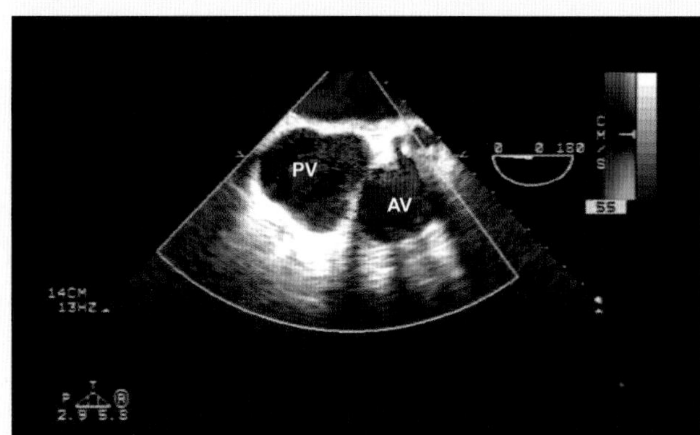

Figure 96.5.

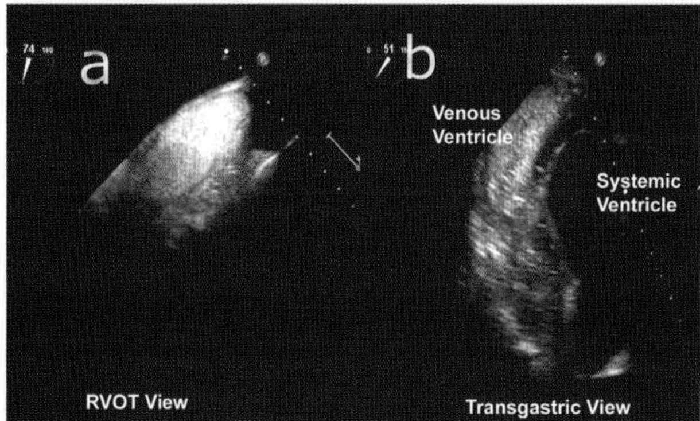

Figure 96.6.

The systemic and pulmonary circulations run in parallel with some form of communication between the two circulations.

TIP: Injection of agitated saline can aid the examiner in the determination of the venous atria, venous ventricle, and PA as shown in Figures 96.6A and B respectively.

QUESTION 96.2: The correct answer is B: PAB.

PAB is more commonly performed to reduce pulmonary blood flow in the case of a VSD, thus preventing permanent damage to the lung vasculature and irreversible PA hypertension. The rationale behind PAB procedure in patients with cc-TGA (Fig. 96.7, Video 96.4 [pulmonary ban, arrow]) is to train the morphological LV to manage the increased afterload of the systemic circulation, allowing for future possible double-switch procedure, thus restoring normal anatomy and preventing further impairment of the RV.

Consideration of PAB in patients with cc-TGA is indicated when CHF secondary to a failing RV is present. The exact mechanism of systemic ventricular failure is unknown but may relate to microscopic structural features and fiber orientation of the RV myocardium. Other possibilities include coronary perfusion mismatch, because the cardiac hypertrophy

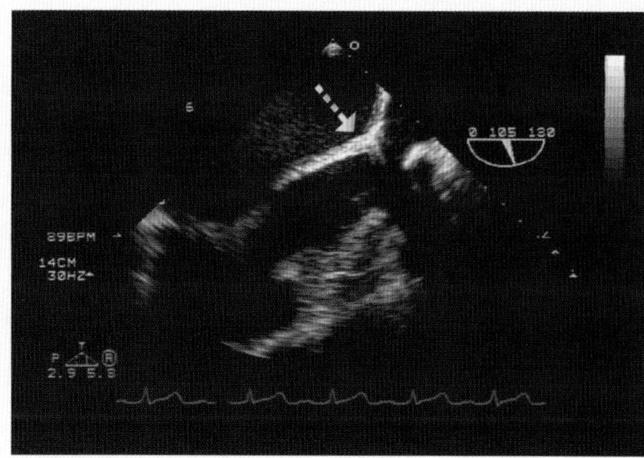

Figure 96.7.

caused by the added pressure load on the morphological RV may outstrip the coronary artery oxygen supply, which comes mainly from the RCA.

QUESTION 96.3: The correct answer is C: Septal shift. In Figure 96.3A, the abnormal ventricular septum displacement from the high-pressure RV toward the low-pressure LV (leftward shift) contributes to "pulling" the septal leaflet away from adequate TV coaptation resulting in worsening TR in these patients. Following PAB (Fig. 96.3b) the morphologic LV is more distended from the increased afterload displacing the septum to a more neutral position thus reducing the amount of TR. Answers A and B are incorrect because the morphologic LV is being loaded by the PAB and may develop worsening MR.

QUESTION 96.4: The correct answer is C: No further intervention.

The LV function must be assessed during the PAB. This is usually obtained in the OR by a catheter placed in the morphological LV to assess pressure volume loops as the PA band is tightened. The banding is thus calibrated to an afterload associated with the junction between the linear and the nonlinear portions of the systolic pressure–volume relationship, in the subpulmonary morphologic LV.

The PAB is generally tightened to a point where the morphologic LV pressure is 80% of the systemic ventricular pressure, with acceptance of only mild systolic dilatation of the LV. In our example, there is a significant dilatation of the morphologic LV and displacement of the septum into the morphologic RV in the systemic position. The subsequent echo evaluations should show normal LV mass and ventricular wall thickness, indexed for weight and age.

When these criteria are not met, PAB can be repeated. Patients would be ultimately listed for transplantation if morphologic LV dysfunction is observed, and/or PAB is not tolerated. Candidates to transplant would be those with end-stage heart failure, deteriorating functional class, or with a limited life expectancy. PAB as a sole treatment modality can improve morphological RV function and reduce TR, thus acting as a destination therapy or as a bridge to transplant.

The post-PAB echo evaluation of this patient shows an inadequate LV/RV pressure ratio (below 0.8). It also showed moderate MR and the subsequent lack of increase in the LV muscle mass, thus not favoring a double-switch procedure, but destination therapy. A double-switch procedure would involve anatomic correction meaning an atrial switch (Mustard or Senning procedure) and an arterial switch (Jatene procedure).

Answers B and D are incorrect, because further tightening of the PA band could lead to LV failure, while loosening the PA band brings TR toward the initial levels.

QUESTION 96.5: The correct answer is B: MV abnormalities.

In this patient the systemic atrio-ventricular valve (SAVV) is not the MV, which appears normal, but the TV that is regurgitant.

Abnormality of the TV or the SAVV occurs in 90% of patients. Most commonly, the valve is displaced inferiorly toward the cardiac apex. With time, there is an increasing regurgitation, and this is often concordant with worsening degrees of RV function.

A VSD occurs in 70% of patients and is usually perimembranous and may extend into the inlet septum. Pulmonic stenosis (PS) occurs in 40% of patients and is often subvalvular. Abnormalities of the pulmonic valve often coexist with obstruction in the subpulmonary region: either an aneurysm of the membranous septum, a fibrous membrane, or mobile subpulmonary tissue "tags," which also contribute to obstruction.

TAKE-HOME LESSON:

Identification of the systemic and venous ventricles is essential in diagnosing and managing congenitally corrected transposition of the great arteries.

SUGGESTED READING

Rouine-Rapp K, Miller-Hance WC. Transesophageal echocardiography for congenital heart disease in the adult. In: Perrino AC Jr, Reeves ST, eds. *A Practical Approach to Transesophageal Echocardiography.* 2nd ed. Philadelphia: Lippincott Williams & Wilkins; 2008:389–393.

CASE 97

A 68-year-old man is undergoing urgent surgical revascularization for triple-vessel disease and unstable angina. Flotation of the Swan–Ganz catheter intraoperatively revealed unexpected moderate-to-severe pulmonary hypertension.

An intraoperative TEE examination is performed and some of the findings are shown in Figures 97.1, 97.2, and 97.3 and Video 97.1. 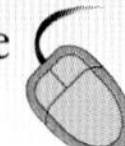

QUESTION 97.1. What could be the cause of RV dilation in this patient?

A. Intracardiac shunt
B. Severe MR
C. Grade III diastolic dysfunction
D. Severe LV systolic dysfunction
E. Pulmonary embolism
F. All of the above

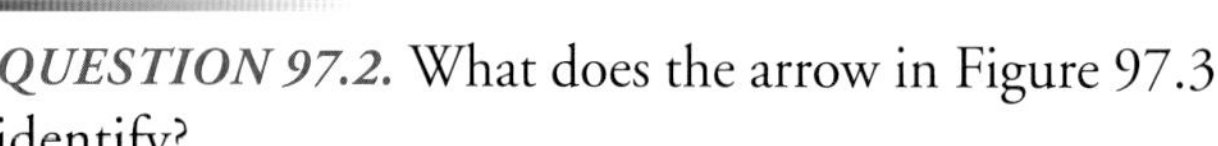

QUESTION 97.2. What does the arrow in Figure 97.3 identify?

A. Artifact
B. Protruding atheroma in the ascending aorta
C. Protruding mass in the right PA
D. Protruding mass in the left PA

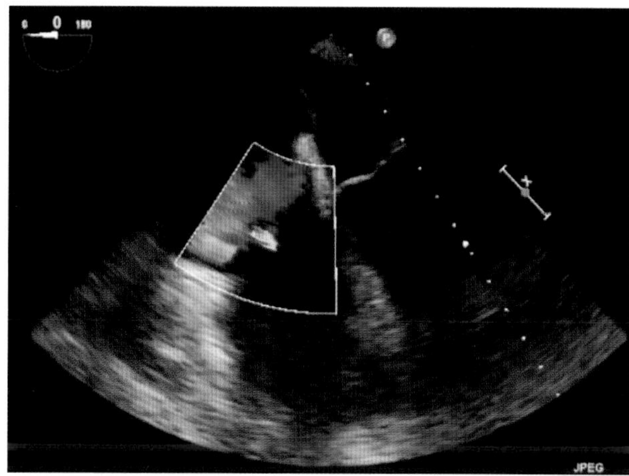

Figure 97.1. ME 4CH view.

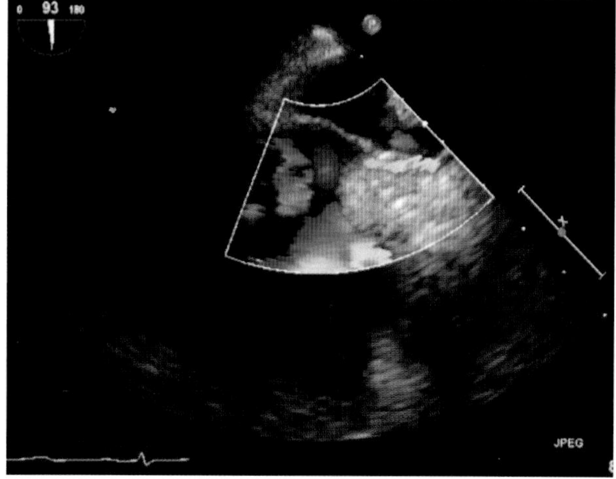

Figure 97.2. ME bicaval view; a PFO is visualized by CFD.

QUESTION 97.3. How would you advise the surgeon?

A. The patient should undergo off-pump surgical revascularization
B. The case should be cancelled
C. The patient should undergo pulmonary embolectomy
D. The initial surgical plan should not be altered

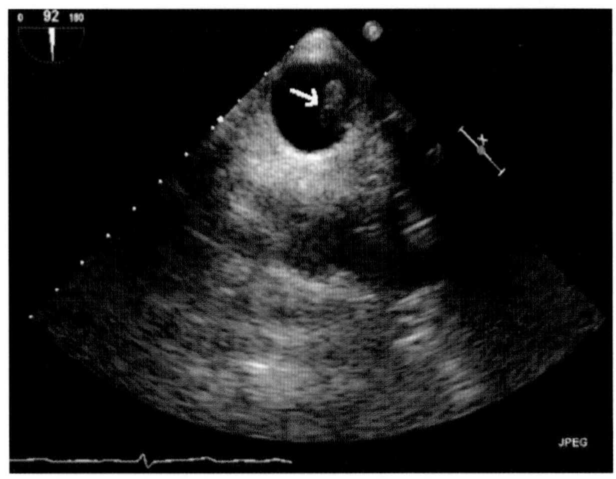

Figure 97.3. ME LAX.

ANSWERS AND DISCUSSION

QUESTION 97.1: The correct answer is F. Figure 97.1 shows flattening of the interventricular septum and RV dilation. Generally, the differential diagnosis for RV dilation could include intracardiac shunt (as shown in Fig. 97.2), severe MR, grade III diastolic dysfunction, severe LV systolic dysfunction, pulmonary embolism, primary pulmonary hypertension, or secondary pulmonary hypertension due to obstructive sleep apnea or lung disease. Performance of a comprehensive intraoperative TEE examination is needed to determine an etiology for the unexpected pulmonary hypertension.

QUESTION 97.2: The correct answer is C.

Examination of the great vessels in the ME short-axis and LAX of the ascending aorta revealed a mass in the right PA (Fig. 97.3 and Video 97.1). The ascending aorta is not seen at 90 degrees, eliminating aortic atheroma as a choice. The possibility of an artifact has been excluded by examination in various views, by injection of agitated saline (Fig. 97.4), and ultimately by epivascular examination (Fig. 97.5). The left PA is rarely seen on TEE due to interposition of the airways.

QUESTION 97.3: In light of the intraoperative TEE findings, the diagnosis of acute pulmonary embolism can be made. The patient should undergo pulmonary arteriotomy and embolectomy in addition to closure of the PFO and surgical revascularization.

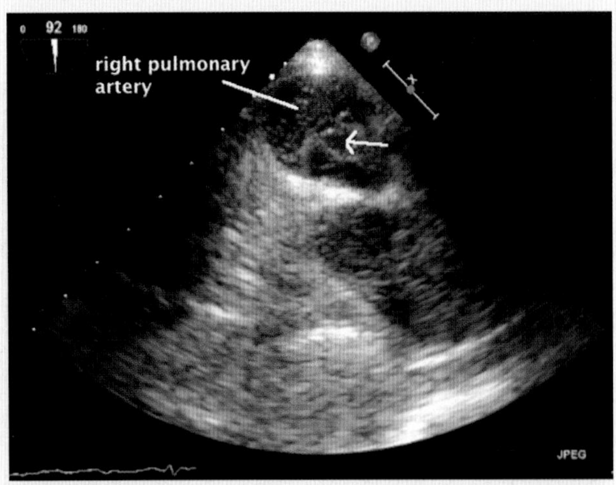

Figure 97.4. ME LAX of the ascending aorta after injection of agitated saline. The arrow identifies the filling defect caused by the protruding mass in the right PA.

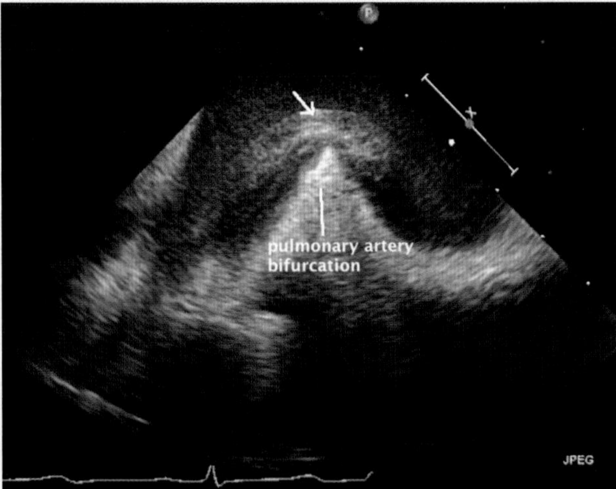

Figure 97.5. Epivascular view of the PA bifurcation. The arrow identifies the saddle thrombus.

TAKE-HOME LESSON:

TEE is beneficial in the diagnosis of unexpected pulmonary hypertension.

Evidence of pulmonary embolism includes mass(es) in the RA, RV, and PA, with RV dysfunction being common. Examination of the atrial septum to rule out shunts and paradoxical embolus is warranted.

Patients with pulmonary embolus need urgent intervention. Whether that intervention occurs in the OR or interventional radiology suite is dependent on the extent of disease and availability of equipment and personnel.

SUGGESTED READING

Allyn JW, Lennon PF, Siegle JH, et al. The use of epicardial echocardiography as an adjunct to transesophageal echocardiography for the detection of pulmonary embolism. *Anesth Analg*. 2006;102(3):729–730.

Rosenberger P, Shernan SK, Body SC, et al. Utility of intraoperative transesophageal echocardiography for diagnosis of pulmonary embolism. *Anesth Analg*. 2004;99(1):12–16.

Stein PD, Sostman HD, Bounameaux H, et al. Challenges in the diagnosis of acute pulmonary embolism. *Am J Med*. 2008;121(7):565–571.

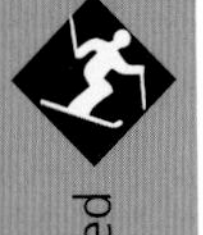

Advanced

CASE 98

A 62-year-old man with a history of smoking and COPD presented to the OR for AVR. Preoperative cardiac catheterization revealed no coronary artery disease, but moderately elevated PA pressures. Initial TEE examination in the OR showed severe AS, but no other valvular abnormalities.

QUESTION 98.1. Prior to initiation of CPB, a ME 4CH view and corresponding M-mode image (shown in Fig. 98.1) were obtained. What significant finding is shown?

A. Ebstein anomaly

B. A VSD

C. An ASD

D. RV hypertrophy

E. Tricuspid stenosis

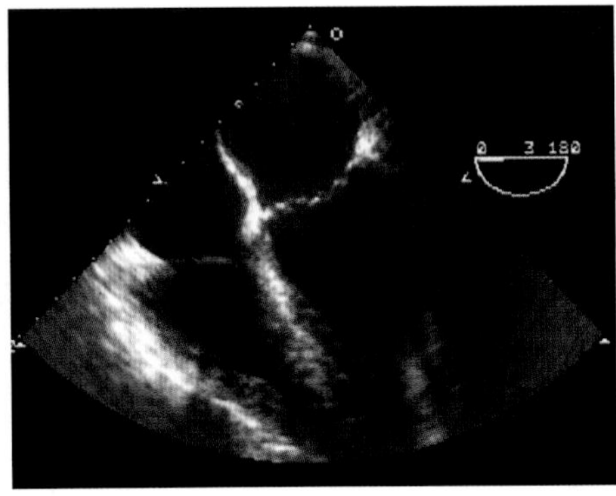

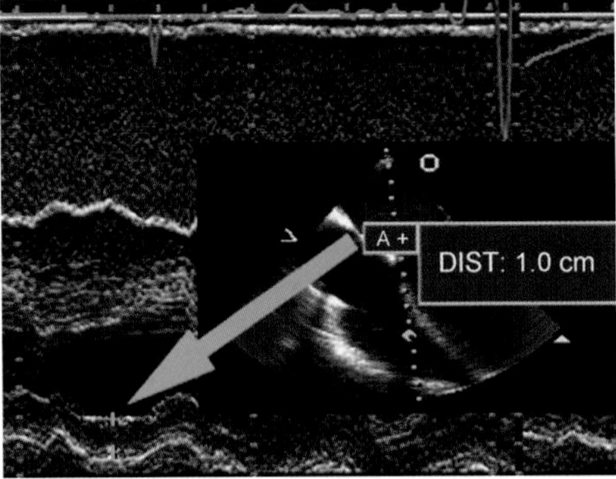

Figure 98.1.

QUESTION 98.2. Despite initially separating from CPB without inotropes, hypotension becomes a problem prior to closing the patient's chest. Interrogation of the new AV with TEE is unremarkable. However, a comprehensive examination shows the images seen in Video 98.1. What is the most likely cause of ongoing hemodynamic instability?

A. A newly created VSD
B. Emboli down the left main coronary artery
C. RV failure
D. Pericardial effusion
E. Massive MR

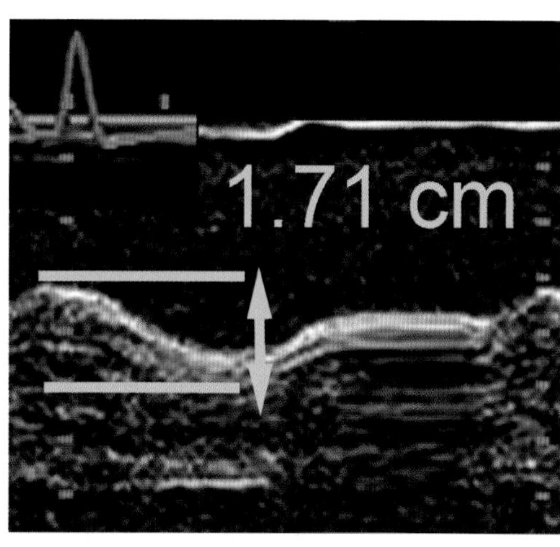

Figure 98.2.

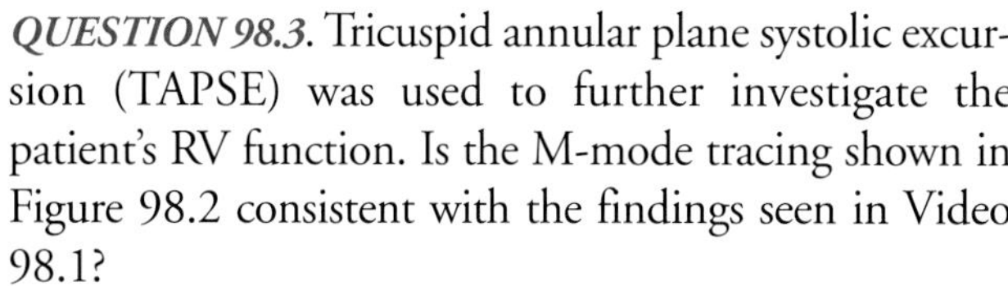

QUESTION 98.3. Tricuspid annular plane systolic excursion (TAPSE) was used to further investigate the patient's RV function. Is the M-mode tracing shown in Figure 98.2 consistent with the findings seen in Video 98.1?

A. Yes, a TAPSE less than 20 mm is consistent with RV dysfunction
B. Yes, a TAPSE less than 20 mm is consistent with moderate TR
C. No, the TAPSE would be expected to be greater than 20 mm
D. No, the M-mode cursor should be placed through the septal part of the TV annulus
E. TAPSE is not a valid measure of RV function

QUESTION 98.4. According to the information provided by TEE, what would be the most appropriate treatment for the patient's hemodynamic instability?

A. Administer crystalloid for volume expansion
B. Start an inotrope infusion such as epinephrine
C. Return to CPB and perform a CABG to the patient's LAD
D. Return to CPB for repair of the new VSD
E. None of the above

ANSWERS AND DISCUSSION

QUESTION 98.1: The correct answer is D. Figure 98.1 shows *RV hypertrophy.*

A good rule of thumb is that the RV wall thickness should be less than half of the LV wall thickness. However, in this particular patient with a hypertrophied LV, it can be harder to notice a hypertrophied RV. So, another guideline is that normal RV wall thickness at end diastole should be less than 5 mm. No tricuspid pathology is seen in Figure 98.1, nor are any ASDs or VSDs apparent.

QUESTION 98.2: The correct answer is C. The patient has *RV failure.*

The first part of Video 98.1 shows a dilated RA (note the bowing of the interatrial septum toward the left) in the ME 4CH view with a significant amount of new TR. The RV is also significantly dilated compared to the size of the LV. The second half of the video is the RV inflow–outflow view, also with a significant amount of TR. Also, note that the free wall of the RV has decreased movement. There is no evidence of a VSD or pericardial effusion. Emboli down the left main coronary artery would be expected to result in LV dysfunction. Massive MR would likely result in high LA pressure, causing the interatrial septum bow toward the RA, not the left.

QUESTION 98.3: The correct answer is A. TAPSE is a useful method to evaluate the RV, and a *TAPSE less than 20 mm is consistent with RV dysfunction.* During systole, the long axis of the RV shortens, bringing the tricuspid annulus downward to the apex. Figure 98.3

demonstrates this, showing the RV at the beginning (A) and end (B) of systole. Normally, the lateral aspect of the tricuspid annulus descends about 25 mm, but anything less than 20 mm is indicative of significant systolic impairment. In Question 98.3, the figure demonstrates an M-mode tracing that has been placed through the tricuspid annulus along the free wall of the RV (not the septal wall). The distance from the highest point of the annulus to the lowest point of the annulus is indicated to be less than 20 mm, which is consistent with the patient's RV failure. TAPSE has been validated as having a good correlation with RV systolic function as assessed by radionucleotide angiography. TAPSE is not used to assess TR.

QUESTION 98.4: The correct answer is B. The most logical treatment for this patient would be to *start an inotrope such as epinephrine* in order to increase systolic function of the RV. Volume expansion would be less helpful since the TEE already demonstrates an overloaded RV with decreased function. A coronary graft to the LAD would not likely be helpful since the LAD does not supply the RV. No new VSD is shown in any of the figures or the video.

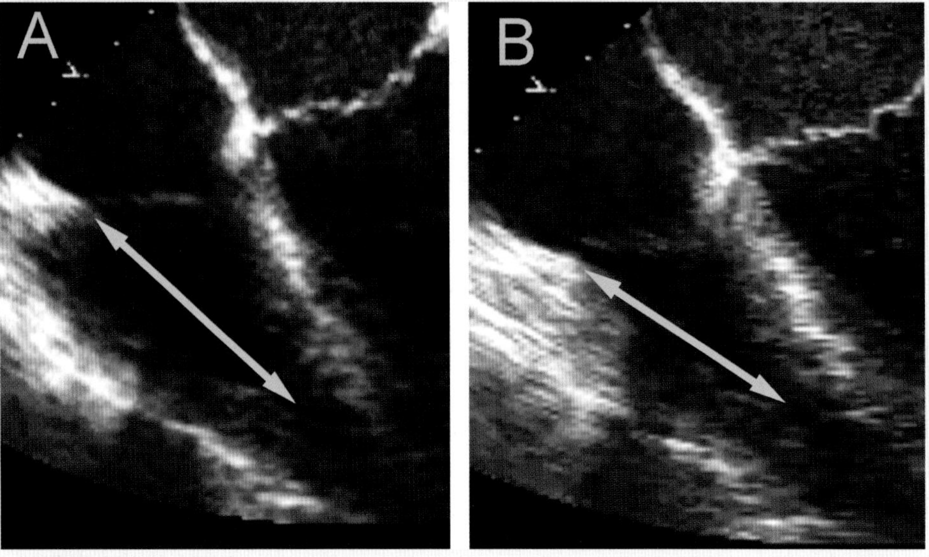

Figure 98.3.

TAKE-HOME LESSON:

TAPSE is a useful method to evaluate the RV, and TAPSE less than 20 mm is consistent with RV dysfunction.

SUGGESTED READING

Haddad F, Hunt SA, Rosenthal DN, et al. Right ventricular function in cardiovascular disease, part I: Anatomy, physiology, aging, and functional assessment of the right ventricle. *Circulation*. 2008;117:1436–1448.

Miller D, Farah DG, Liner A, et al. The relation between quantitative right ventricular ejection fraction and indices of tricuspid annular motion and myocardial performance. *J Am Soc Echocardiogr*. 2004;17:443–447.

CASE 99

A 21-year-old woman presented with increasing fatigue and shortness of breath. Physical examination demonstrated a RV heave, a prominent systolic flow murmur across the pulmonary outflow tract, and fixed splitting of the second heart sound. The TTE examination was not diagnostic and a TEE was performed.

QUESTION 99.1. Representative TEE images (bicaval view) in this patient, as shown in Figure 99.1A, B (Video 99.1A,B), demonstrate the following:

A. A VSD

B. A secundum ASD

C. False drop-out in the region of the atrial septum

D. A sinus venosus defect

E. A PFO

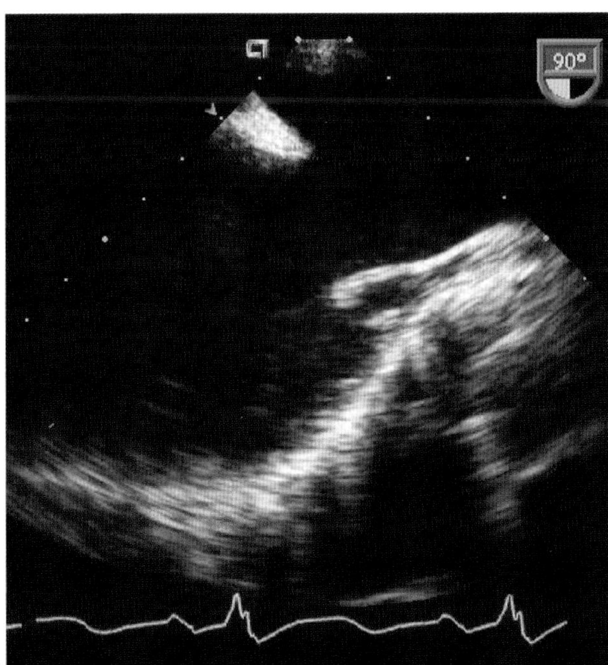

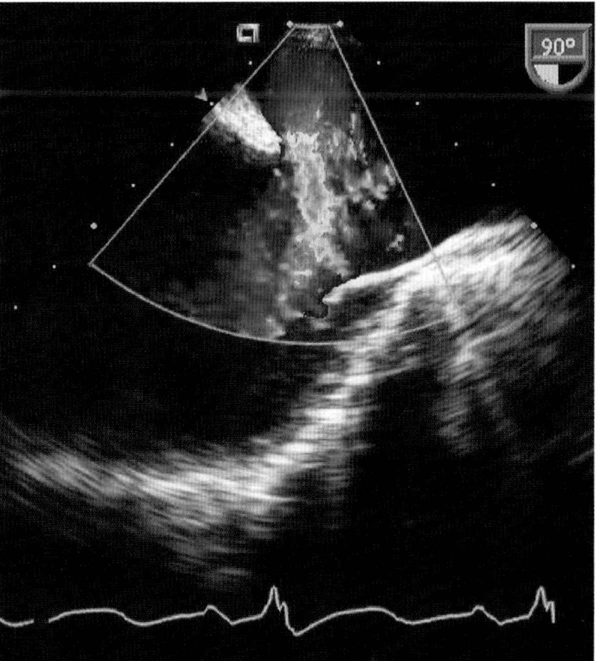

Figure 99.1.

QUESTION 99.2. In association with this particular type of congenital heart defect, you might expect to see any or all of the following *except*:

A. Anomalous attachment of the pulmonary veins
B. Proximity to the SVC to the interatrial communication
C. A trifoliate morphology of the left AV valve
D. Evidence of right-sided volume overload
E. A left-to-right atrial level shunt

QUESTION 99.3. The definitive approach in patients with this malformation consists of:

A. Surgical intervention
B. Medical management of heart failure
C. Transcatheter closure of the defect by device occlusion
D. Observation and close follow-up
E. Aspirin prophylaxis to prevent the risk of paradoxical embolization

ANSWERS AND DISCUSSION

QUESTION 99.1: The correct answer is D: A sinus venosus defect. The TEE images in Figure 99.1A,B (Video 99.1A,B) display the characteristic features of a sinus venosus defect as shown in a longitudinal scan of the atrial septum (bicaval view). 2D imaging demonstrates what appears to be a deficiency of tissue at the superior aspect of the interatrial septum, resulting in a large defect. There is immediate proximity of the mouth of the SVC to the interatrial communication, also described as a biatrial or overriding connection. This location is typical of sinus venosus defects of the superior type. The presence of shunting across this region is confirmed by color Doppler interrogation. Although typically included among the spectrum of interatrial communications, some consider that anatomically this congenital lesion does not represent a true ASD since the deficiency is due to the absence of the anterior wall of the right upper pulmonary vein and the posterolateral wall of the cardiac end of the SVC.

Atrial septal defects can be found anywhere within the interatrial septum, can be of any size, and may be single or multiple. The most frequent defect resulting in atrial shunting is the secundum defect. This is generally centrally located within the fossa ovalis (Fig. 99.2A, Video 99.2A). In contrast, sinus venosus defects are found outside the confines of the fossa ovalis. Primum atrial septal defects represent a form of VSD or endocardial cushion defect. The region of shunting is at the inferior aspect of the interatrial septum (Fig. 99.2B, Video 99.2B). A PFO, an essential interatrial communication in fetal life, is considered to be present in approximately 25% of the general population (Fig. 99.2C, Video 99.2C). Although false or artificial echocardiographic drop-out may mimic the appearance of septal defects, this is unlikely to occur when the imaging plane is perpendicular to the anatomic structures being interrogated.

QUESTION 99.2: The correct answer is C. All the choices listed are true regarding sinus venosus defects except for their association with a left common AV valve of trifoliate morphology. The left AV valve in patients with sinus venosus defects is of the typical mitral morphology. This is in contrast to the characteristic trifoliate appearance of the left AV valve in VSD related to the presence of a cleft, frequently associated with various degrees of valvular regurgitation (Fig. 99.3A,B and Video 99.3A,B).

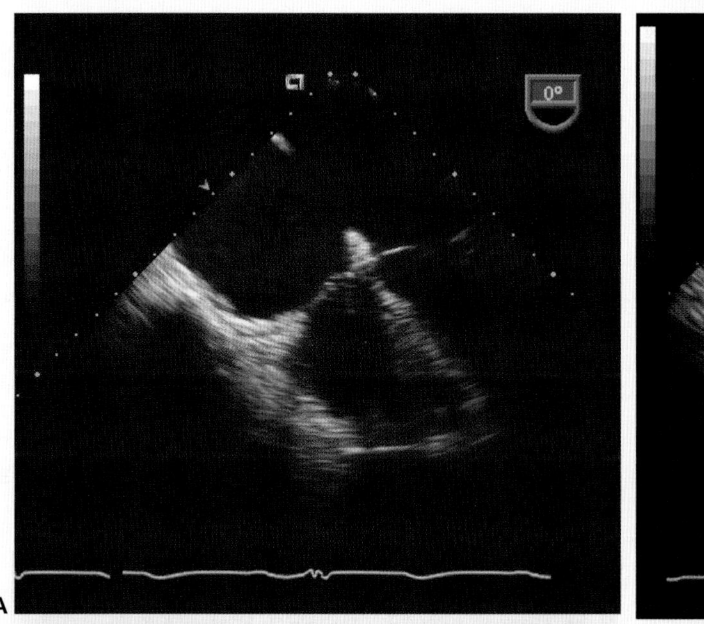

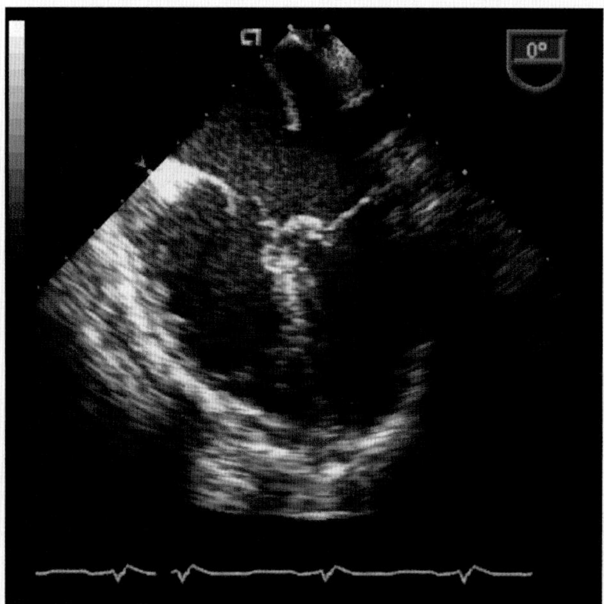

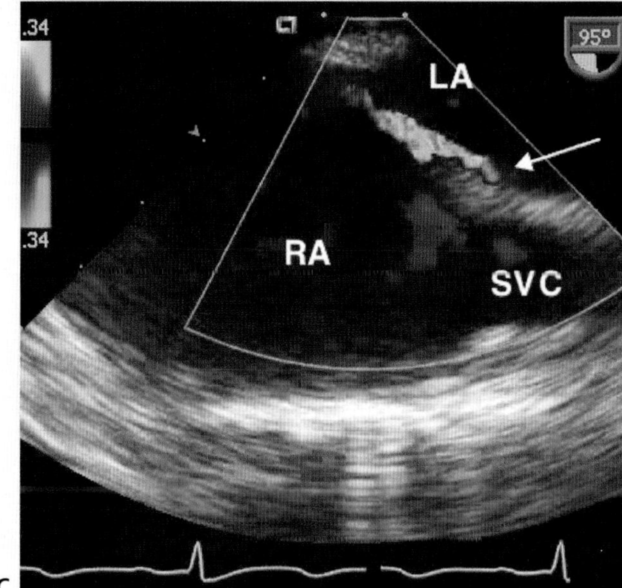

Figure 99.2. **A:** ME 4CH view displaying a large secundum ASD. Note the centrally located interatrial communication with rims of atrial tissue surrounding the defect. See also Video 99.1C. **B:** ME 4CH view demonstrating primum ASD. Note inferior location of the defect just above the level of the AV valves. See also Video 99.1D. **C:** CFD interrogation of the atrial septum in the bicaval view demonstrating flow across a PFO. See also Video 99.1E.

A defect located at the superior aspect of the interatrial septum (superior sinus venosus defect), at the junction of the SVC and the RA, is more common than the IVC type of defect (located posteriorly at the junction of IVC and the RA). In the majority of patients these defects are associated with anomalous pulmonary venous connection(s) (80% to 90% of cases) from the right lung. In the superior type of defect, the partially anomalous venous connection is from the right upper pulmonary vein into the SVC (Fig. 99.3C and Video 99.3C). Moderate- to large-size defects lead to chronic volume overload, manifested by right atrial and RV dilation (Fig. 99.3D and Video 99.3D). TEE has been recommended for any patient with unexplained dilatation of the right side of the heart.

QUESTION 99.3: The correct answer is A: Surgical intervention. Cumulative experience has documented essentially no operative mortality and minimal morbidity on long-term surgical follow-up. In view of the location of the defect with respect to the SVC or IVC and anomalous pulmonary venous drainage, care must be taken to avoid obstruction to systemic venous flow into the RA and pulmonary venous drainage into the LA, while at the same time obliterating the interatrial communication (Fig. 99.4A–C and Video 99.4). This should be the focus of the postoperative TEE examination. The excellent surgical results have favored this approach over observation and medical management. In contrast to catheter-based approaches for

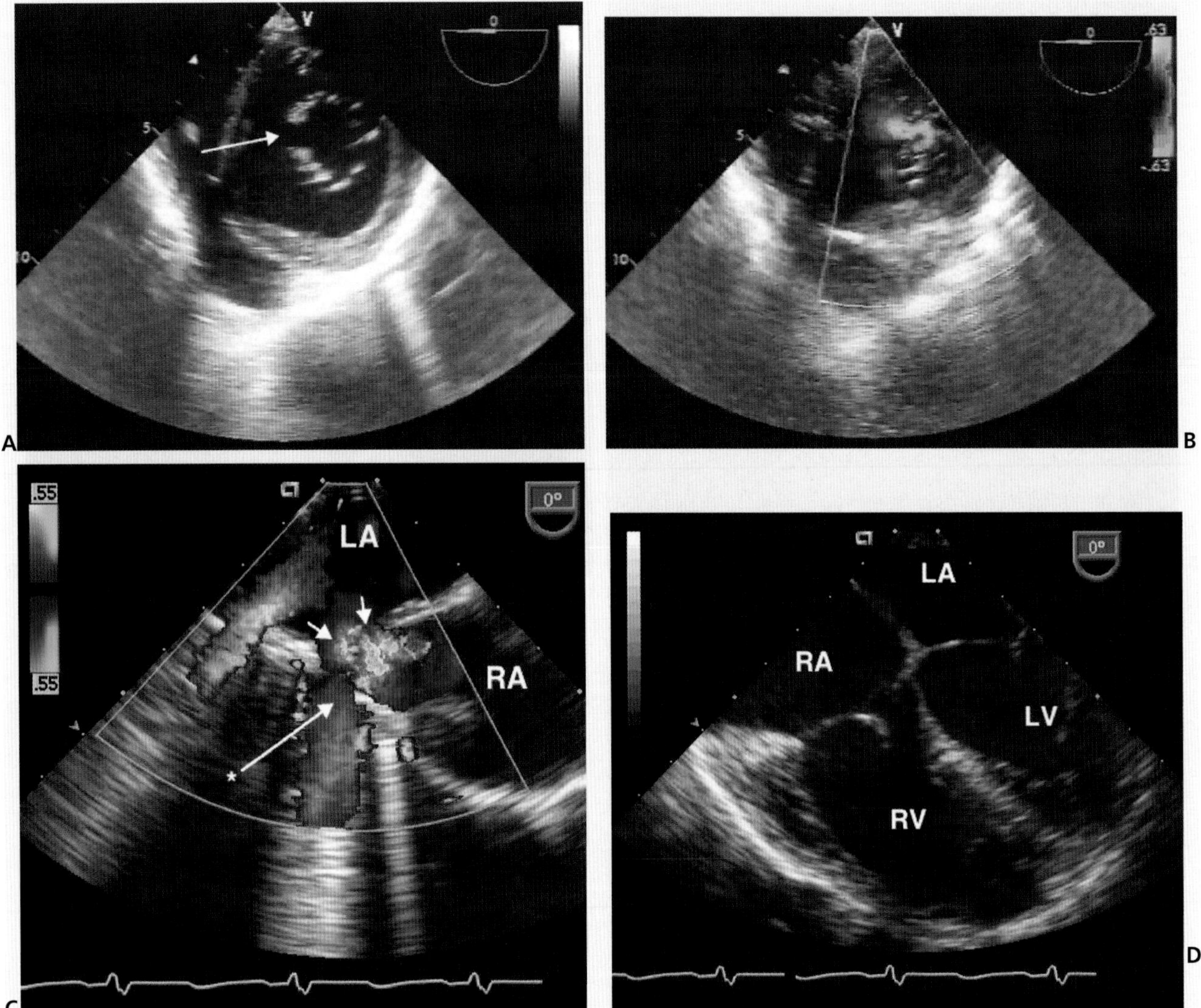

Figure 99.3. **A:** TG basal short-axis view in patient with primum ASD. The arrow indicates cleft in the left AV MV. See also Video 99.2A. **B:** CFD imaging demonstrating regurgitation across MV cleft. See also Video 99.2B. **C:** TEE with CFD obtained from the midesophagus by rotating the imaging plane to the right from the four-chamber view demonstrates anomalous attachment of the right upper pulmonary vein *(large arrow with asterisk)* into the roof of the RA in association with an interatrial communication *(small arrows)*. A separate pulmonary vein is also seen draining into the LA. See also Video 99.2C. **D:** ME 4CH view displaying dilated right-sided cardiac chambers. See also Video 99.2D.

secundum atrial septal defects, these procedures are not applicable to sinus venosus defects due to the immediate proximity of venous structures to the defect and lack of anchoring septal tissue precluding safe deployment of such devices. Although the potential risk of paradoxical embolization is present in patients with intracardiac communications, no prophylactic therapy has been advocated to reduce this risk.

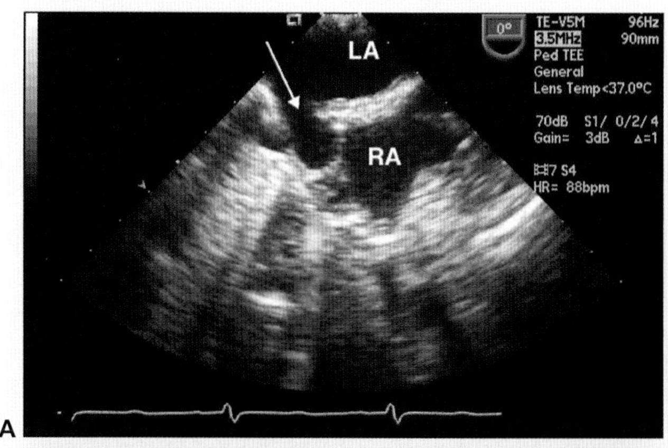

A

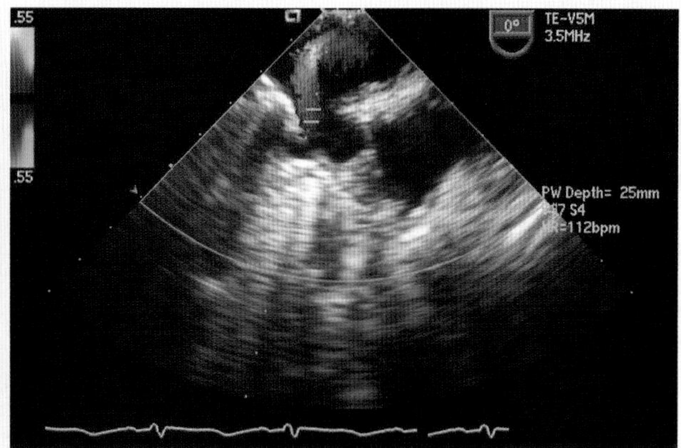

B

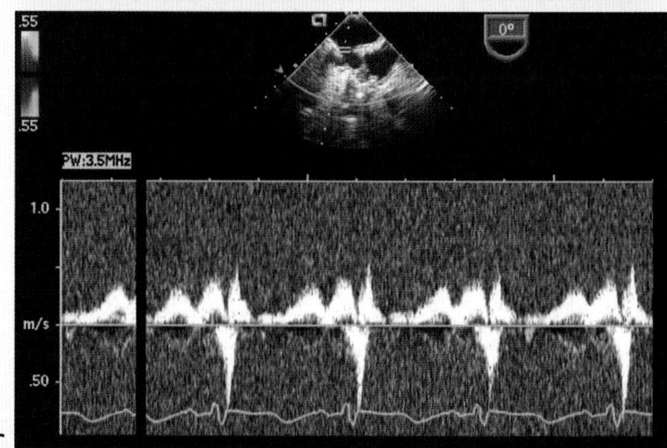

C

Figure 99.4. Postoperative TEE images from a modified ME view obtained after clockwise transducer rotation of a four-chamber view demonstrating the pericardial baffle that allows for drainage of the anomalous pulmonary veins into the LA (*arrow*, **A**). In this patient the SVC was transected and directly anastomosed to the right atrial appendage (Warden procedure). CFD and spectral Doppler interrogation demonstrate no evidence of obstruction to drainage from the anomalous veins through the baffle into the LA **(B,C)**. See also Video 99.3.

TAKE-HOME LESSON:

A sinus venosus defect is due to the absence of the anterior wall of a pulmonary vein and the posterolateral wall of the SVC or IVC. Hence one needs to look for this defect adjacent to the entrance of the SVC or IVC into the RA.

SUGGESTED READING

Agrawal SK, Khanna SK, Tampe D. Sinus venosus atrial septal defects: surgical follow-up. *Eur J Cardiothorac Surg*. 1997;11:455–457.

al Zaghal AM, Li J, Anderson RH, et al. Anatomical criteria for the diagnosis of sinus venosus defects. *Heart*. 1997;78:298–304.

Ammash NM, Seward JB, Warnes CA, et al. Partial anomalous pulmonary venous connection: diagnosis by transesophageal echocardiography. *J Am Coll Cardiol*. 1997;29:1351–1358.

Crystal MA, Al Najashi K, Williams WG, et al. Inferior sinus venosus defect: echocardiographic diagnosis and surgical approach. *J Thorac Cardiovasc Surg*. 2009;137:1349–1355.

Kharouf R, Luxenberg DM, Khalid O, et al. Atrial septal defect: spectrum of care. *Pediatr Cardiol*. 2008;29:271–280.

Kronzon I, Tunick PA, Freedberg RS, et al. Transesophageal echocardiography is superior to transthoracic echocardiography in the diagnosis of sinus venosus atrial septal defect. *J Am Coll Cardiol*. 1991;17:537–542.

Maxted W, Finch A, Nanda NC, et al. Multiplane transesophageal echocardiographic detection of sinus venosus atrial septal defect. *Echocardiography*. 1995;12:139–143.

Pascoe RD, Oh JK, Warnes CA, et al. Diagnosis of sinus venosus atrial septal defect with transesophageal echocardiography. *Circulation*. 1996;94:1049–1055.

Watanabe F, Takenaka K, Suzuki J, et al. Visualization of sinus venosus-type atrial septal defect by biplane transesophageal echocardiography. *J Am Soc Echocardiogr*. 1994;7:179–181.

Advanced

CASE 100

A 53-year-old female with a history of hypertension presented with worsening chest pain and shortness of breath. On review of systems, she admitted to several pre-syncopal episodes prior to admission. TTE revealed a normal EF with moderate LVH and asymmetric septal hypertrophy (septal wall thickness of 2.3 cm). The instantaneous gradient across the AV estimated with CW Doppler was 120 mm Hg. Left heart catheterization revealed normal coronary anatomy and confirmed normal ventricular function. The patient was referred for ventricular septal myomectomy.

Intraoperative TEE revealed the images shown in Figures 100.1 to 100.4.

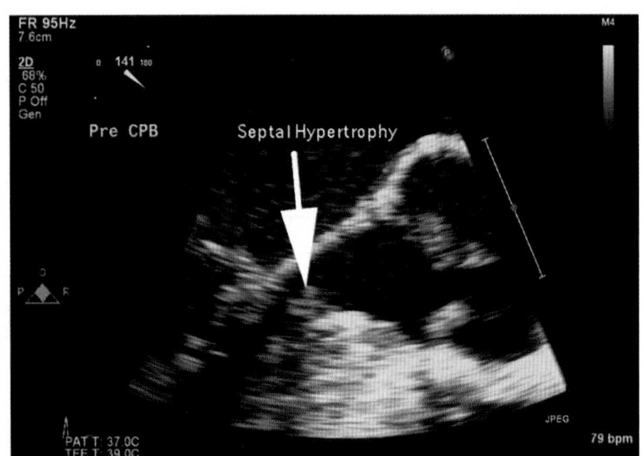

Figure 100.1.

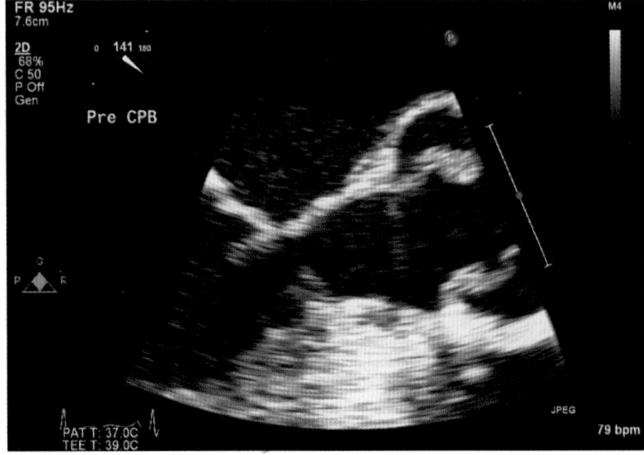

Figure 100.2.

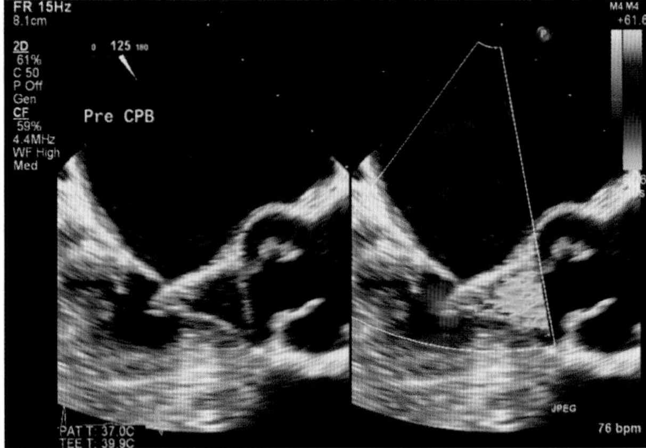

Figure 100.3.

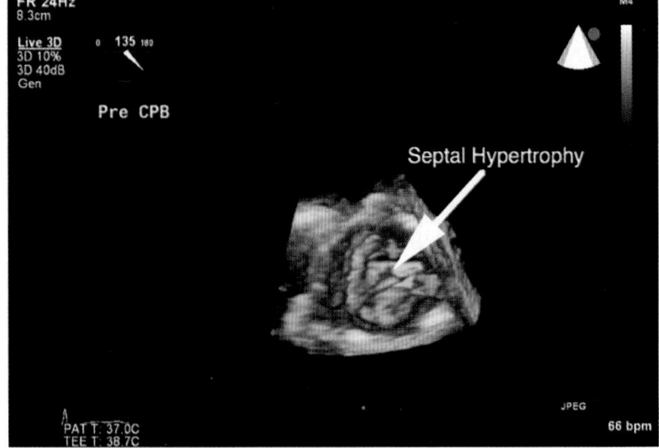

Figure 100.4.

QUESTION 100.1. Which of the following additional diagnoses should be called to the surgeon's attention?

A. VSD

B. Subaortic membrane

C. Cleft anterior leaflet of MV

D. Moderate-to-severe AI

QUESTION 100.2. Subaortic stenoses are known to be associated with all of the following congenital problems *except:*

A. Bicuspid AV

B. Aortic coarctation

C. Perimembranous VSD

D. Williams syndrome

QUESTION 100.3. Pathophysiologic effects of subaortic membranes include all of the following *except:*

A. AI

B. Asymmetric septal hypertrophy

C. *Late* systolic closure of the AV

D. Thickened anterior MV leaflet

QUESTION 100.4. Which of the following is NOT a cause for discrepancy between Doppler-derived pressure gradients and catheter-derived values in patients with subaortic stenosis?

A. The modified Bernoulli equation ($\Delta P = 4V^2$) fails to take into account proximal velocity

B. The pressure recovery phenomenon

C. The presence of an associated VSD

D. Measurement of peak instantaneous gradient as opposed to peak-to-peak values

QUESTION 100.5. Figure 100.5 was obtained after separation from CPB. Which of the following statements is TRUE?

A. The tracing is a PW Doppler

B. Further surgical intervention is warranted

C. Inotropic support should be initiated

D. The elevated gradient is indicative of increased stroke distance (volume) and further volume loading is inappropriate

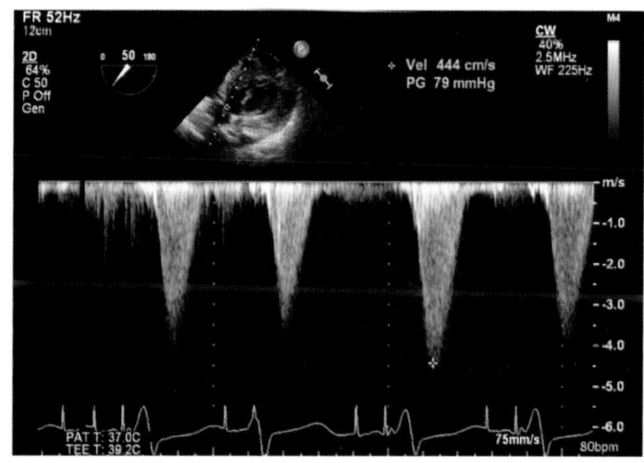

Figure 100.5. Doppler evaluation of LVOT gradient.

ANSWERS AND DISCUSSION

QUESTION 100.1: The correct answer is B.

Consistent with the preoperative TTE, the ME AV LAX of the TEE reveals evidence of significant LVOT obstruction. The ventricular septum in the LVOT is significantly hypertrophied with flow acceleration visible on CFD. Intraoperative CW Doppler interrogation also revealed a peak instantaneous gradient of 120 mm Hg.

However, closer inspection of the ME AV LAX and deep TG views reveals a thin linear band traversing the LVOT within close proximity to the AV. This finding is consistent with a discrete subaortic membrane.

Morphologically, subaortic stenoses are divided into three categories.

Type 1: A discrete fibrous membrane located immediately below the AV with an otherwise normal LVOT. It usually bows toward valve during systole and into the ventricle during diastole. The thin membrane is more easily visualized with TTE using apical four-chamber view or with TEE using a deep TG view. These planes place the membrane perpendicular to the path of the ultrasound beam—enhancing spatial resolution.

Type 2: A thick fibrous ring located 1 cm below the valve and extending 1 to 2 cm down the LVOT. It is often associated with muscular hypertrophy. Diffuse hypertrophy may ultimately encroach on the MV.

Type 3: A long fibromuscular tunnel several centimeters long in the LVOT. The subaortic stenosis seen in this patient is a combination of types 1 and 2. A discrete subaortic membrane is visualized distal to a narrowed and hypertrophied LVOT. This is not an uncommon scenario, as the increased pressure gradient secondary to a discrete membrane may ultimately lead to compensatory septal hypertrophy along the LVOT, compounding the stenosis. Alternatively, type 2 subaortic stenosis may cause abnormal flow patterns in the LVOT, leading to formation of a type 1 membrane more distally.

Type 1 subaortic stenoses are amenable to simple surgical resection, whereas types 2 and 3 require more extensive resection and remodeling of the LVOT.

Answers A, C, and D are incorrect. In this case, there is no evidence of VSD. The anterior mitral leaflet is thickened, but not cleft. Cleft anterior MV leaflets do not occur with this condition, rather they are associated with primum ASD. There is trace AI.

QUESTION 100.2: The correct answer is D. Williams syndrome is a genetic syndrome caused by deletion of the long arm of chromosome 7. One of the twenty-six missing genes in this syndrome codes for the protein elastin. A lack of elastin ultimately leads to connective tissue abnormalities and narrowing of large arteries. *Supravalvular* AS is seen as a manifestation of this narrowing, but subvalvular stenosis has not been linked to this condition.

Answers A and B are incorrect. Subaortic stenoses are known to be associated with abnormalities of the aorta, including bicuspid AV and aortic coarctation. Answer C is incorrect. Abnormalities of the ventricular septum can occur, including VSDs and RVOT obstruction.

QUESTION 100.3: The correct answer is C.

Early systolic closure of the AV may frequently be associated with subaortic stenosis. It is neither a sensitive nor a specific sign. Other conditions such as aortic root dilatation may also be associated with early systolic closure of the valve. Bicuspid aortic valves and thickened AV leaflets often fail to demonstrate this sign in the presence of subaortic stenosis. This sign is best documented with M-mode and the mechanism remains unclear.

With subaortic stenosis, abnormal flow eddies, and high velocity jets directed toward the AV leaflets may cause thickening of the AV leaflets resulting in malcoaptation. This may lead to varying degrees of AI. As seen in this case, a discrete subaortic membrane causing outflow tract obstruction may induce septal hypertrophy along the outflow tract, increasing the gradient further and worsening symptoms. Subaortic stenosis may involve part of the anterior mitral leaflet. The anterior mitral leaflet makes up the posterior boundary of the LVOT. Septal hypertrophy in conjunction with an anteriorly displaced mitral annulus may cause repetitive friction of the anterior mitral leaflet against the hypertrophied fibrous septum during both systole and diastole. In conjunction with abnormal accelerated flow patterns, this may lead to thickening of the anterior MV leaflet—as seen in this case.

QUESTION 100.4: The correct answer is C.

A concurrent perimembranous VSD proximal to the subaortic stenosis will serve as a "pop off" valve in the LVOT. Flow across the VSD will decrease forward systemic flow and the resultant gradient across the subaortic stenosis. This may lead the clinician to underestimate the severity of the stenosis, but will not affect the calculated gradient per se. Catheter-derived gradients in the presence of a VSD will also be lower than in the absence of a VSD.

The modified Bernoulli equation $\Delta P = 4V^2$, where ΔP is the change in pressure and V is the peak velocity, used to calculate peak instantaneous pressure gradient fails to take into account the velocity of blood flow proximal to any given stenosis. Under normal circumstances, where the proximal velocity is less than 1 m/s, its contribution to pressure is less than 4 mm Hg and can be ignored. When the proximal velocity is greater than 1.5 m/s, its contribution to the pressure gradient becomes greater than 10 mm Hg and should not be ignored. The equation $\Delta P = 4(V_2^2 - V_1^2)$, where V_2 = distal velocity and V_1 = proximal velocity, should be used in its place. Disregarding proximal velocity in circumstances where there is significant proximal flow acceleration leads to an overestimation of the actual pressure gradient across the distal narrowing. Therefore, using the first equation in rare clinical combinations of LVOT obstruction in the setting of AS and our case of LVOT obstruction in the setting of subaortic membrane will overestimate the actual gradient of the more distal obstruction. Catheter-derived measurements are more accurate and may easily calculate the gradient for each serial narrowing.

In a perfect Venturi system where a pressure drop occurs across a mechanical narrowing, very little kinetic energy is dissipated as heat and may be reconverted to pressure after the narrowing in a phenomenon called pressure recovery. Stenoses in vivo dissipate as much as 85% of kinetic energy as heat, leaving very little energy to contribute to post-stenotic pressure by the mechanism of pressure recovery. Therefore, instantaneous peak pressure gradients measured at the orifice may be extrapolated to the system as a whole. Longer tubular stenoses, as found in the subaortic LVOT, more closely approximate the flow characteristics of a Venturi system. Therefore, pressure recovery may result in a lower overall pressure drop in the system as kinetic energy is reconverted into pressure after the narrowing. TEE Doppler-derived instantaneous peak gradients measure only the pressure drop at the vena contracta before the recovery of pressure. Therefore, with subaortic stenosis, overestimation of the true pressure gradient when compared to catheter-derived values may occur.

TEE Doppler-derived peak instantaneous gradients are inherently larger than their catheter-derived counterparts. Doppler-derived gradients are more physiologic and may not occur at the maximal LV systolic pressure. They measure the maximal velocity during the cardiac cycle and convert that to the maximal pressure gradient between the LV and proximal aorta. Catheter-derived gradients measure the peak LV systolic pressure and subtract from it the peak aortic systolic pressure. Peak LV and aortic systolic pressures may occur at different points in the cardiac cycle and may not be a true physiologic measurement. For this reason, peak-to-peak catheter-derived measurements are usually slightly smaller. This holds true for all stenoses and is not just limited to those of the subaortic region.

The surgeon performed a resection of a 3-mm discrete subaortic membrane as well as a 1-cm ventricular septal myomectomy for severe asymmetric septal hypertrophy. Immediately after separation from CPB, the patient became hemodynamically unstable. Doppler interrogation from a deep TG window revealed the following (Fig. 100.5).

QUESTION 100.5: The correct answer is B.

The surgical result is unacceptable. Although the subaortic membrane was resected, significant LVOT obstruction remained despite the septal myomectomy. Since significant outflow tract obstruction and asymmetric septal hypertrophy were present before surgery, the persistent gradient most likely represents suboptimal surgical resection rather than new dynamic outflow tract obstruction resulting from SAM of the MV. Therefore, the treatment should be further surgical intervention rather than medical management.

The above Doppler tracing depicts a high velocity tracing with a full envelope characteristic of CW Doppler. There is no sampling volume and so the velocities measured may occur anywhere along the path of the ultrasound beam. In the setting of stenosis, the highest velocity is most likely to occur at the stenotic orifice. In this case, the myomectomy was incomplete and severe residual subaortic stenosis is evidenced by a pressure gradient of 80 mm Hg. Inotropic support is not first-line therapy. Management of residual LVOT obstruction in subaortic stenosis before return to CPB should be treated in the same manner as dynamic outflow tract obstruction. Therefore, volume loading with slower heart rates and lower inotropic states will attenuate hemodynamic compromise more than reduced preload states, tachycardia, and inotropic support. As stated above, the increased pressure gradient is due to residual subaortic stenosis. Volume restriction is contrary to hemodynamic goals.

The patient was returned to CPB. The aortotomy was reopened and a more extensive septal myomectomy was performed. Separation from CPB the second time was uneventful. The immediate postoperative gradient across the AV was 12 mm Hg. The patient was seen 1 month after surgery with complete resolution of her symptoms.

TAKE-HOME LESSON:

Morphologically, subaortic stenoses are divided into three types. Type 1 is a discrete fibrous membrane located immediately below the AV with an otherwise normal LVOT. Type 2 is a thick fibrous ring located 1 cm below the valve and extending 1 to 2 cm down the LVOT. Finally, type 3 is a long fibromuscular tunnel several centimeters long in the LVOT.

SUGGESTED READING

Reeves ST, Shanewise J, eds. *Fundamental Applications of Transesophageal Echocardiography*. SCA 2005 monograph on DVD. Philadelphia: Lippincott Williams & Wilkins; 2005.

CASE 101

A 63-year-old patient diagnosed with AS and pulmonic stenosis is scheduled for AVR and possible pulmonic valve repair. An intraoperative prebypass TEE examination is performed.

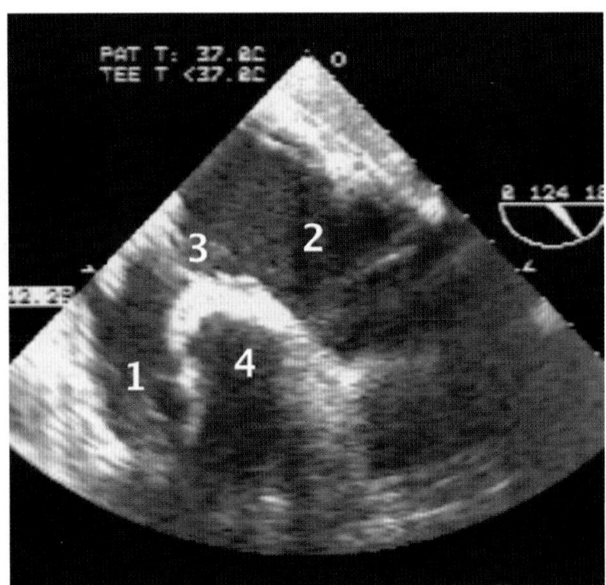

Figure 101.1. TG RV inflow–outflow view. See also Video 101.1.

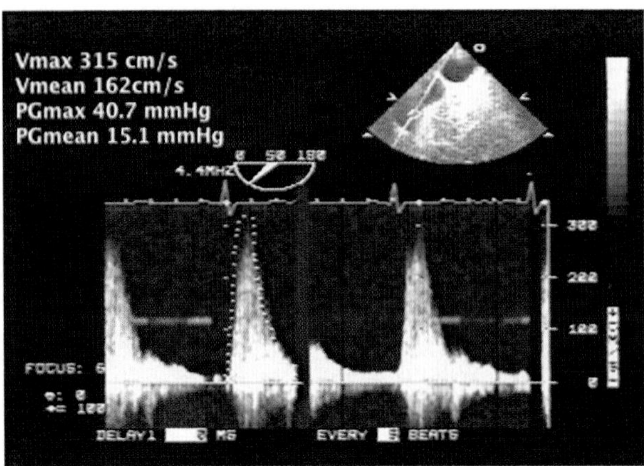

Figure 101.2. Upper esophageal aortic arch SAX with CW Doppler.

QUESTION 101.1. Regarding Figure 101.1 (see also Video 101.1), which of the following statements is true?

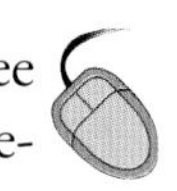

A. The structure identified by number 1 is the AV
B. The structure identified by number 2 is the LA
C. The structure identified by number 3 is the RVOT
D. The structure identified by number 4 is the PA

QUESTION 101.2. Figures 101.2 and 101.3 and Video 101.2 describe which of the following situations?

A. Normal pulmonic valve, normal pulmonic valve gradient
B. Abnormal pulmonic valve, abnormal pulmonic valve gradient
C. Normal pulmonic valve, abnormal pulmonic valve gradient
D. LVOT obstruction

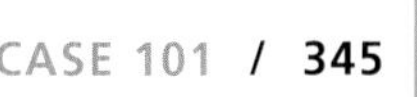

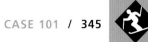

Advanced

QUESTION 101.3. Postbypass findings, as seen in Video 101.3 and Figures 101.4 and 101.5, suggest:

A. Adequate surgical repair; give protamine

B. Persistent pulmonic valve gradient; return to CPB

C. The Doppler spectra shown in the Figure 101.5 represent TMF

D. Figure 101.5 shows AV gradient

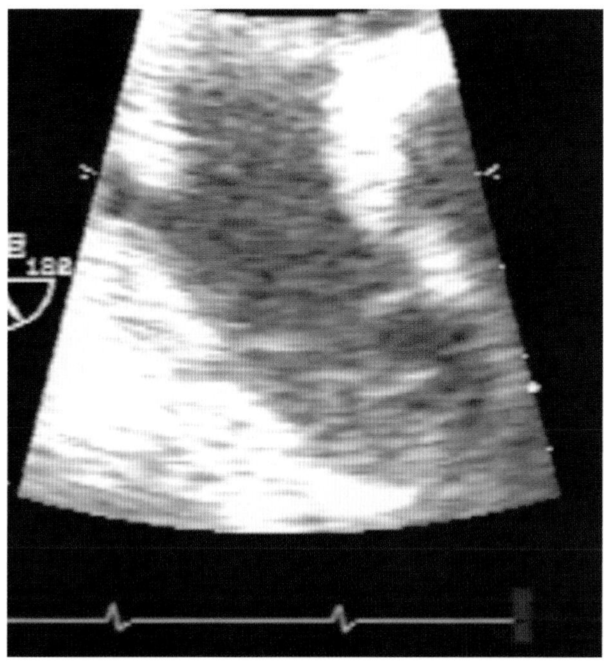

Figure 101.3. Zoom of pulmonic valve in TG RV inflow–outflow view. See also Video 101.2.

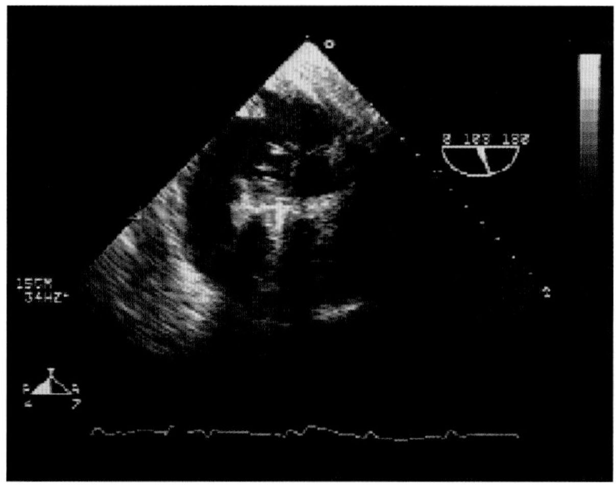

Figure 101.4. Postbypass TG RV inflow–outflow view. See also Video 101.3.

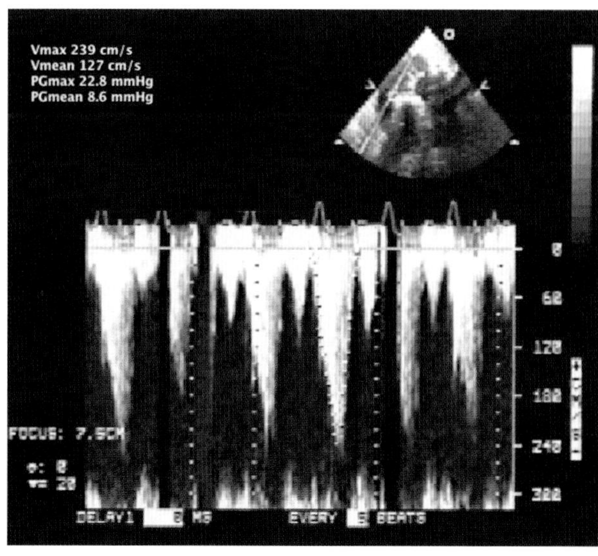

Figure 101.5. Postbypass CW Doppler of RVOT from TG RV inflow–outflow view.

ANSWERS AND DISCUSSION

QUESTION 101.1: The correct answer is C: The structure identified by number 3 is the RVOT. Figure 101.1 shows the TG RV inflow–outflow view (TG RV inflow–outflow), a modified view of the TG RV inflow recommended by the guidelines of the American Society of Echocardiography and the Society of Cardiovascular Anesthesia for performing a comprehensive intraoperative TEE examination. The TG RV inflow–outflow view is obtained by advancing the probe to the TG midpapillary level, turning the probe rightward, and rotating the multiplane angle to about 120 degrees. This view images the same structures that are seen in the ME RV inflow–outflow view, namely RA, TV, RV inflow, RVOT, pulmonic valve, and the main PA. The TG RV inflow–outflow, however, offers a better alignment of the blood flow with the Doppler beam through both the pulmonary valve and the RVOT, and is thus useful in the assessment of gradients across (both these structures) the pulmonic valve and RVOT. In the image shown, 1 is the RVOT, 2 is the TV and 4 is the proximal ascending aorta.

QUESTION 101.2: The correct answer is C: Normal pulmonic valve, abnormal pulmonic valve gradient. CW Doppler interrogation across the pulmonic valve (Fig. 101.2) revealed high velocities with a maximum velocity of 3.2 m/s and a peak pressure gradient of 40 mm Hg consistent with moderate pulmonic valve stenosis. In order to meet criteria for severe disease the peak velocity should exceed 4 m/s and the peak pressure gradient should exceed 64 mm Hg.[1] However, Figure 101.3 shows a normal appearing, pliable pulmonic valve. Inspection of the RVOT in the TG RV inflow–outflow (Video 101.4) shows a thickened infundibular septum bulging into the outflow tract. These findings, consistent with subpulmonic stenosis, altered the surgical plan. In lieu of a pulmonic valve repair/replacement the patient underwent pulmonary arteriotomy and infundibular myomectomy. The Doppler spectrum in Figure 101.2 has the same "dagger-shaped" envelope as the Doppler profile of the velocities usually seen across the LVOT in HOCM.

QUESTION 101.3: The correct answer is A: Adequate surgical repair. As shown in Figure 101.5 the velocities across the RVOT still demonstrate a dagger-like profile; however, the maximum velocity has decreased to 2.39 m/s corresponding to a peak pressure gradient of 22 mm Hg. As the velocity is less than 3 m/s and the peak pressure gradient is less than 36 mm Hg there is only mild grade of stenosis.[1] Interpretation of Doppler findings, including derived pressure gradients, in the immediate postbypass period should take into consideration that increased velocities may result from a number of factors, in particular inotropes. A thorough postbypass examination is paramount in patient's status post infundibular myomectomy. In addition to residual obstruction, complications include acquired VSD and damage to the pulmonic valve with new onset pulmonic insufficiency.

TAKE-HOME LESSON:

In addition to pulmonic stenosis, elevated right heart ejection velocities can also be caused by subvalvular or supravalvular stenoses. TEE provides several useful views to assess this region and identify the pathology at hand.

REFERENCE

1. Baumgartner H, Hung J, Bermejo J, et al. Echocardiographic assessment of valve stenosis: EAE/ASE recommendations for clinical practice. *J Am Soc Echocardiogr*. 2009;22(1):1–23; quiz 101-102.

CASE 102

A 20-year-old male who was diagnosed with AS 5 years ago was subsequently lost to follow-up. He then presented in acute heart failure and was urgently intubated and underwent an aortic valvuloplasty in the cardiac catheterization lab.

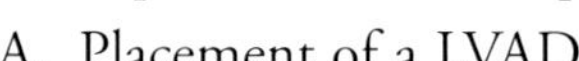

QUESTION 102.1. After reviewing Figure 102.1 (see also Video 102.1) and Figure 102.2, what other procedure has the patient undergone?

A. Placement of a LVAD

B. Placement of an IABP

C. Placement of a percutaneous left ventricular assist device (PLVAD)

D. Placement of a right ventricular assist device (RVAD)

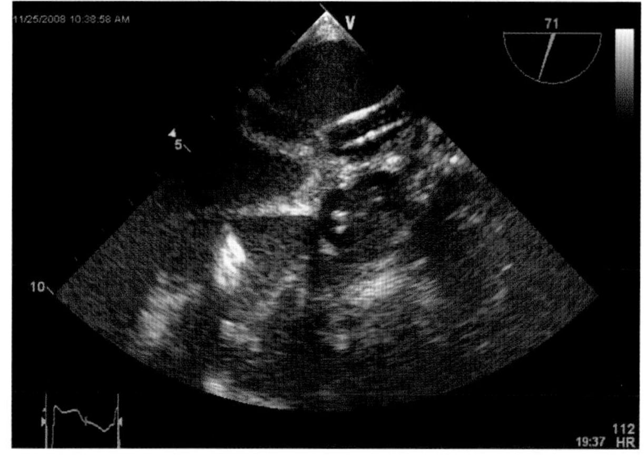

Figure 102.1.

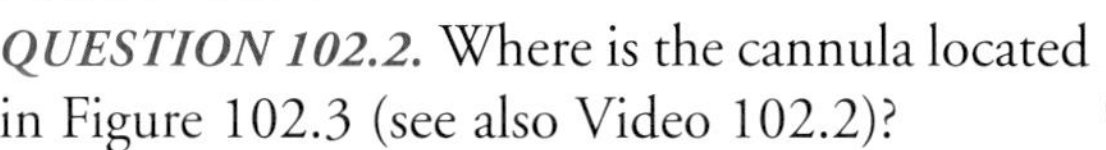

QUESTION 102.2. Where is the cannula located in Figure 102.3 (see also Video 102.2)?

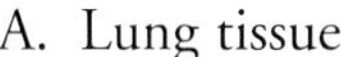

A. Lung tissue

B. IVC

C. Liver parenchyma

D. Hepatic vein

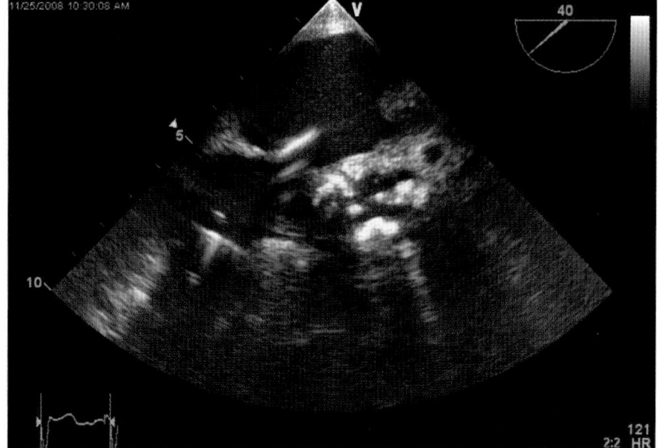

Figure 102.2.

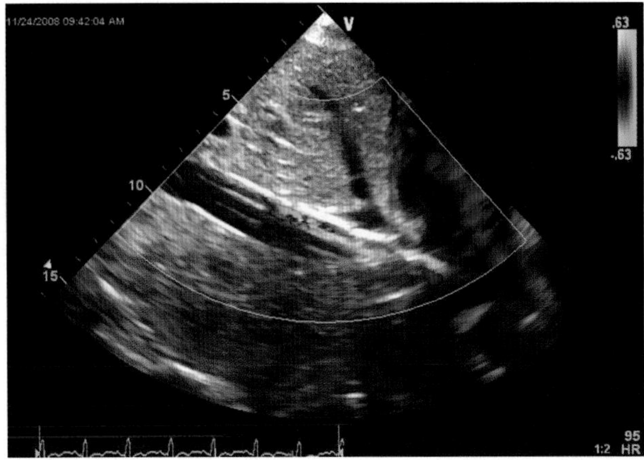

Figure 102.3.

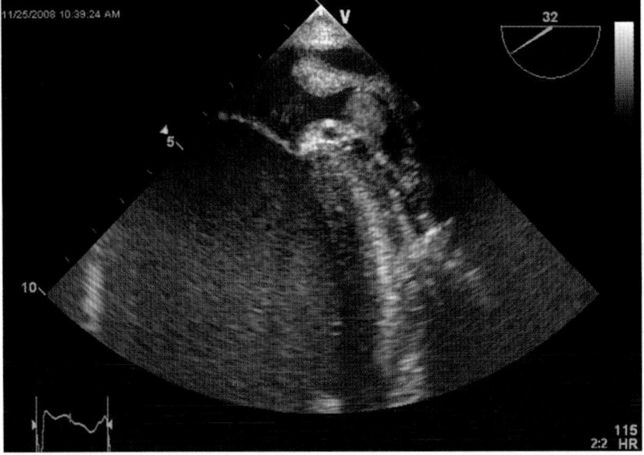
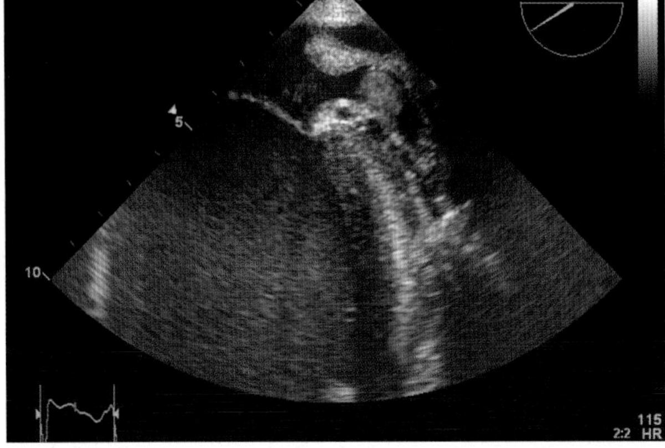

Figure 102.4.

QUESTION 102.3. Figure 102.4 (see also Video 102.3) is a potential complication of

A. LVAD
B. AFib
C. PLVAD
D. All of the above

ANSWERS AND DISCUSSION

QUESTION 102.1: The correct answer is C: Placement of a PLVAD (TandemHeart, CardiacAssist, Pittsburgh, PA). A PLVAD provides rapid and significant circulatory support within 30 minutes via LA to femoral artery bypass. Indications include high-risk percutaneous coronary intervention (PCI), cardiogenic shock in the setting of acute myocardial infarction, heart failure, as well as the perioperative period for cardiac surgery. The PLVAD can be utilized for a duration of up to 14 days. *Answer A is incorrect.* The placement of the LVAD inflow cannula (such as the TCI HeartMate VAD or Novacor VAD) would be into the LV apex. The placement of the LVAD inflow cannula (Abiomed VAD) would be to the LA (the most common LA placement is entry through the interatrial groove), right superior pulmonary vein, or the LV apex. In Figure 102.2 the cannula enters the LA from the RA across the interatrial septum and is a trans-septal cannula with one large end hole and multiple side holes for aspiration of oxygenated blood from the LA. *Answer B is incorrect.* An IABP is placed within the descending aorta. The TEE window shown is a modified ME RV inflow–outflow view, which doesn't visualize the descending aorta. In this window, however, you can visualize the AV in the short axis. *Answer D is incorrect.* The placement of the inflow cannula in an RVAD would be either the RA or the RV.

QUESTION 102.2: The correct answer is B: IVC. In this view, obtained by TTE, the inflow cannula of the PLVAD (TandemHeart) is visualized in the IVC entering the RA. *Answer A is incorrect*: This is liver, not lung; however, you can visualize lung tissue in the descending aortic SAX view obtained via TEE. *Answer C is incorrect*: This is liver parenchyma, yet the cannula is within the IVC not the parenchyma itself. The image was obtained via TTE with the probe in the subcostal position. *Answer D is incorrect*: Even though a hepatic vein is visualized in this subcostal four-chamber view obtained by TTE, the cannula is located in the IVC.

QUESTION 102.3: The correct answer is D: All of the above. Thrombus is located within the LAA and is a consequence of answers A, B, and C in which LA stasis occurs due to significantly depressed atrial mechanical function.

TAKE-HOME LESSON:

The use of TEE is becoming essential in the placement of the PLVAD. TEE assists in the trans-septal puncture and the correct placement of the trans-septal cannula from the RA into the LA. It is also useful in prevention, and/or to provide early detection, of the complications associated with the placement and use of a PLVAD. TEE is also used to identify the contraindications to the placement of a PLVAD.

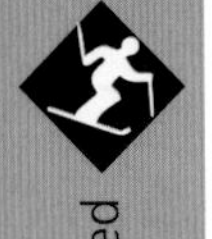

CASE 103

A 69-year-old woman is undergoing off-pump coronary artery revascularization. A TEE probe is inserted, and a comprehensive exam is performed. In the ME LAX view, a sample volume is positioned between the tips of the mitral leaflets in mid-diastole, and the spectral Doppler display of the mitral inflow velocities is shown in Figure 103.1A. Following that, the echocardiographer places the sample volume next to the mitral annulus, on the basal inferolateral LV segment. This spectral Doppler display is shown in Figure 103.1B.

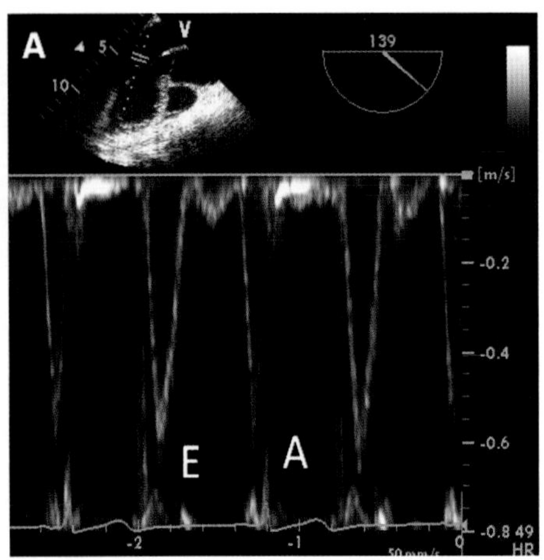

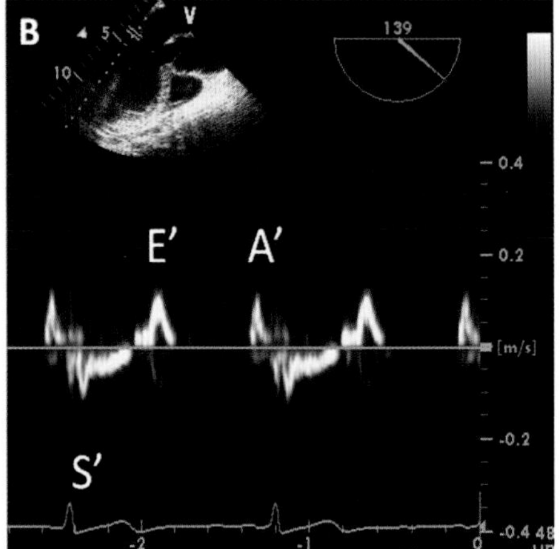

Figure 103.1.

QUESTION 103.1. Which of the following statements comparing the Figure 103.1 waveforms is true?

A. The tracing in Figure 103.1A has higher amplitude than the tracing in Figure 103.1B

B. The tracing in Figure 103.1B has higher velocities than the tracing in Figure 103.1A

C. The tracing in Figure 103.1B has lower velocities than the tracing in Figure 103.1A

D. The velocities and amplitudes are the same in both tracings

QUESTION 103.2. Each wave of the two tracings in Figure 103.1 is identified in Figure 103.2. Which of the following statements is true?

A. In a normal ventricle, E' precedes E

B. E' is independent of myocardial relaxation

C. In an ischemic ventricle, the ratio E'/A' is always larger than 1

D. S' and E' are generally preload independent

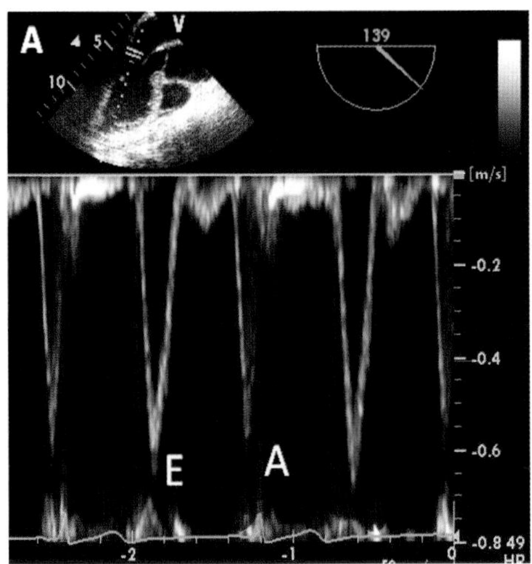

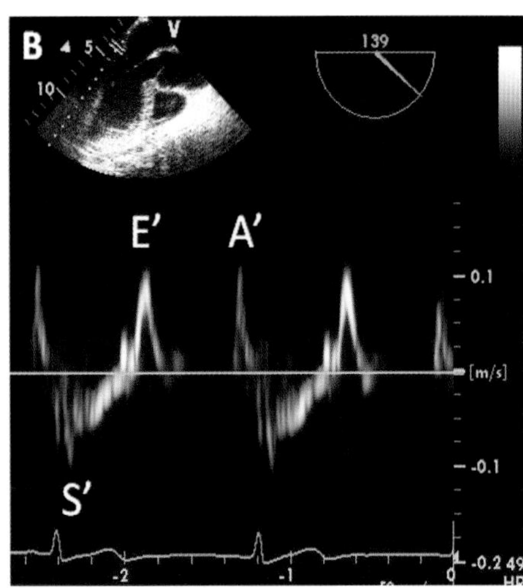

Figure 103.2.

QUESTION 103.3. The ratio E/E' reflects

A. Myocardial relaxation
B. LV filling pressure
C. Regional myocardial contractility
D. Intraventricular asynchrony

QUESTION 103.4. Using the information in Figure 103.2 and given that the average value of E' is 11 cm/s, what is the LV filling pressure?

A. Low: <8 mm Hg
B. Normal: between 8 and 15 mm Hg
C. Elevated: higher than 15 mm Hg
D. Not possible to tell

QUESTION 103.5. The average value of S' is 5 cm/s in the above patient. The LVEF is

A. Less than 35%
B. Between 35% and 45%
C. Between 45% and 55%
D. Higher than 55%

ANSWERS AND DISCUSSION

QUESTION 103.1: The correct answer is C. Doppler measures velocity of a moving target, based on the shift between the emitted and reflected frequencies. The default spectral Doppler settings on most TEE machines are adjusted so that the *high* velocity, *low* amplitude signal of blood flow is recorded and displayed. Myocardial motion also produces Doppler signals, which have *low* velocity but *higher* amplitude than blood. These myocardial Doppler signals are not visible on the classical spectral Doppler displays, because they are filtered out. Adjustments to the spectral Doppler setting can be made so that the moving myocardium can be recorded by focusing on the low velocity/high amplitude signals instead of filtering them out. Figure 103.1A displays the mitral inflow (conventional Doppler) and Figure 103.1B the myocardial motion (called tissue Doppler). Notice the lower velocity (usually less than 20 cm/s) and higher intensity (higher amplitude) of the myocardial signal. Myocardial velocity signals can be recorded by placing a sample volume (usually 5 mm) over the desired area, and activating the PW Doppler mode (compare Fig. 103.3A with Fig. 103.3B). Almost all of the current echocardiographic platforms are equipped with a default DTI mode, which, upon activation, displays a crisp spectral velocity envelope from the desired area (compare Fig. 103.3C with Fig. 103.3A and Fig. 103.3B). DTI "obeys" the Doppler rules: any deviation of more than 20 degrees between the plane of myocardial motion and Doppler beam results in underestimation of the recorded velocities. When using TEE, DTI velocities can be recorded in ME views from all basal segments, lateral to the mitral annulus. Mid- and apical segment DTI velocities are more difficult to record, because the curvature and direction of the wall segment deviate from a parallel incidence with the Doppler beam. Cardiac translation and the immobile sample volume make DTI recordings in the TG views unreliable.

QUESTION 103.2: The correct answer is A. DTI *E′* is related to myocardial relaxation, the first part of diastole, which is energy-dependent. Thus, answer B is incorrect. In a normal ventricle, myocardial relaxation precedes early blood flow, and DTI *E′* appears earlier than *E*. The longer the delay between *E* and *E′*, the worse the diastolic function of the ventricle. Myocardial motion is in the opposite direction of blood flow. That is why early (*E′*) and late (*A′*) diastolic myocardial velocities are oppositely directed from the

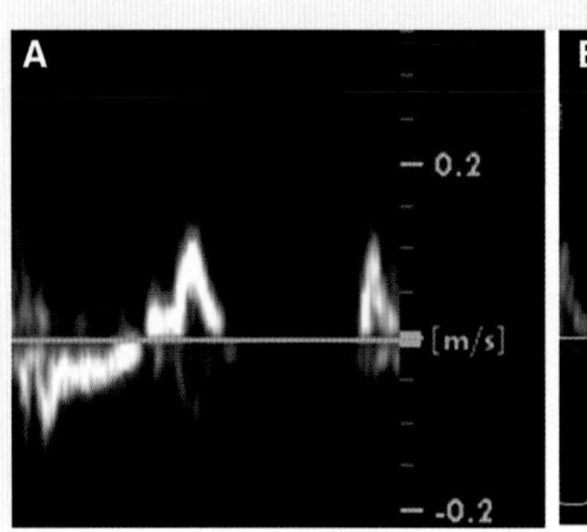

Conventional

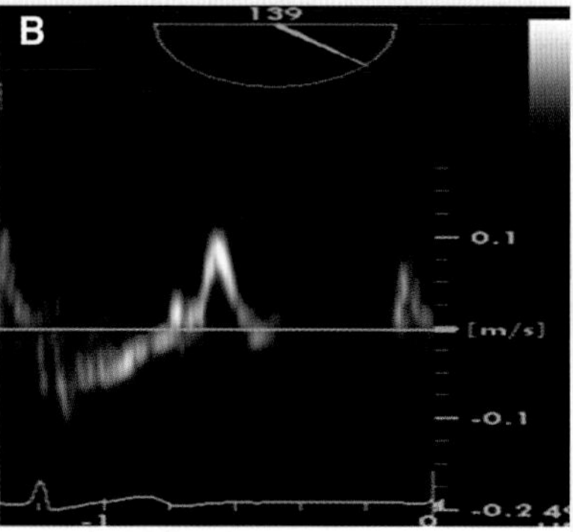

Low gain/amplitude

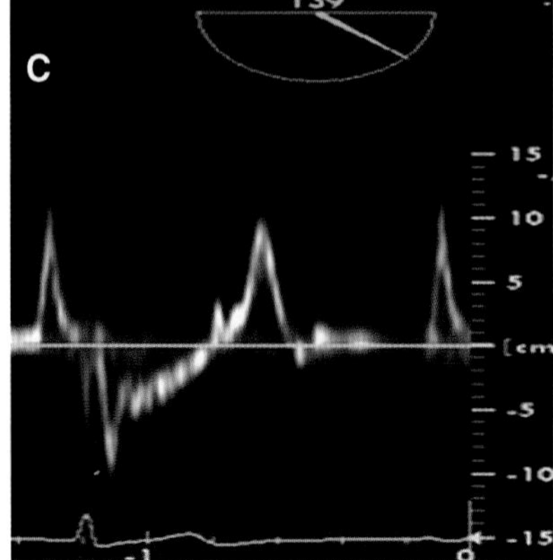

Doppler Tissue Imaging (DTI)

Figure 103.3.

mitral inflow early (E) and late (A) blood velocities (shown in Fig. 103.2).

In a normal ventricle, E' is preload dependent and the ratio E'/A' is greater than 1. Once there is diastolic impairment, the ratio E'/A' becomes lower than 1 and remains lower despite any pseudonormalization of the mitral inflow ratio E'/A' due to volume compensation. Another reason for E'/A' to become less than 1 is regional ischemia, which affects myocardial relaxation. Therefore an ischemic ventricle will always have E'/A' ratio <1, *not* >1, as stated in answer C. Although DTI velocities are angle dependent, their ratio is not. It is therefore quite useful to monitor the DTI signal from different myocardial segments for signs of ischemia. A baseline E'/A' ratio >1 that becomes <1 without obvious preload changes should immediately warn the physician that the patient's heart is ischemic.

Answer D—S' and E' are generally preload independent—is incorrect. In a *normal* ventricle, S' and E' velocities *are* preload dependent so long as cardiac function is intact. On the other hand, in a ventricle with decreased systolic function, E' becomes preload independent.

QUESTION 103.3: The correct answer is B. Mitral inflow E velocity is influenced by both myocardial relaxation and preload. DTI E' is relatively preload independent if cardiac function is impaired and expresses only myocardial relaxation. It has been proven, when compared to invasive LV hemodynamic measurements, that the ratio E/E' reflects the mean LA (and LV diastolic) pressure. The ratio E/E' is being extensively used by echocardiographers to estimate the mean LV pressure with the formula: mean LV diastolic pressure $= 2 + (1.3 \times E/E')$, with E' calculated as the average of as many basal LV segments as possible.

Answer A—Myocardial relaxation—is incorrect because it is E', not E/E' ratio that reflects myocardial relaxation. Answer C—Regional myocardial contractility—is incorrect because the systolic velocity S' reflects regional myocardial contractility. However, S', like E' and A', is recorded from an immobile sample volume placed over the moving myocardium. Tethering of the basal to the mid- and apical segments results in the basal S' velocity reflecting the systolic motion and contractility of the entire myocardial wall. That is, presence of motion cannot differentiate between active and passive motion of a segment. Answer D—Intraventricular asynchrony—is also incorrect. Presence of temporal delay in systolic contraction and diastolic relaxation can be estimated by calculating the difference between an ECG marker (usually the R wave) and the onset of S' wave among the various segments.

QUESTION 103.4: The correct answer is B. As described above, the LV pressure can be calculated using the formula:

$$\text{Mean LVEDP} = 2 + (1.3 \times E/E')$$

As is seen in Figure 103.1A, mitral inflow E velocity is 60 cm/s, therefore the mean LV pressure is 9 mm Hg. As a quick evaluation, if the ratio E/E' is >10, then the mean LV diastolic pressure is >15 mm Hg. This formula is valid for patients in AFib as well as those with atrial tachycardia.

QUESTION 103.5: The correct answer is B. S' is analogous to the concentration of β-adrenergic receptors. Using invasive hemodynamic measurements, the average of S' from two, diametrically opposite segments (or all six basal segments) is related to LVEF (%EF) with the equation:

$$\%EF = 8.2' S' + 3.$$

TAKE-HOME LESSON:

The Doppler principle can be used to record myocardial motion, which will produce waveforms with lower velocities and higher amplitude than blood flow. Tissue Doppler systolic and diastolic velocities can be used to detect ischemia, to estimate myocardial relaxation, and to calculate filling pressure and EF.

SUGGESTED READING

Skubas N. Intraoperative Doppler tissue imaging is a valuable addition to cardiac anesthesiologists' armamentarium: a core review. *Anesth Analg*. 2009;108: 48–66.

Advanced

CASE 104

A 68-year-old gentleman presents with progressive dyspnea on exertion secondary to MR and is scheduled for MV repair with CPB. Cardiac catheterization shows a right dominant coronary circulation and no evidence of significant coronary stenosis. Prebypass TEE is performed (see Figs. 104.1 to 104.4 and Videos 104.1 to 104.4).

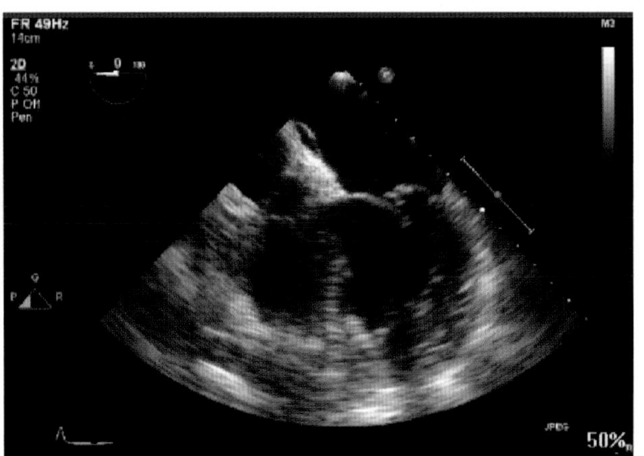

Figure 104.1. Prebypass ME 4CH systole.

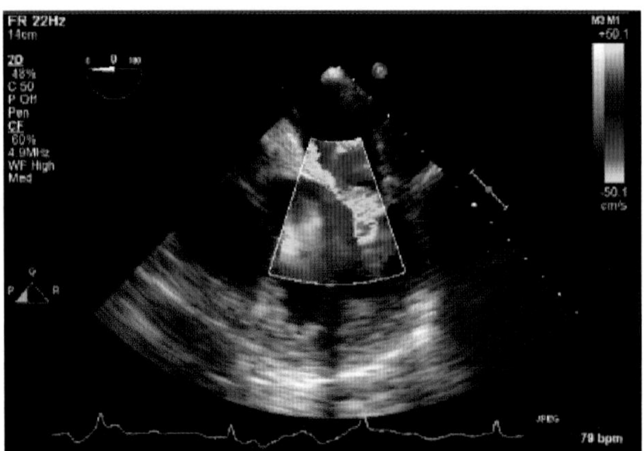

Figure 104.2. Prebypass ME 4CH with CFD.

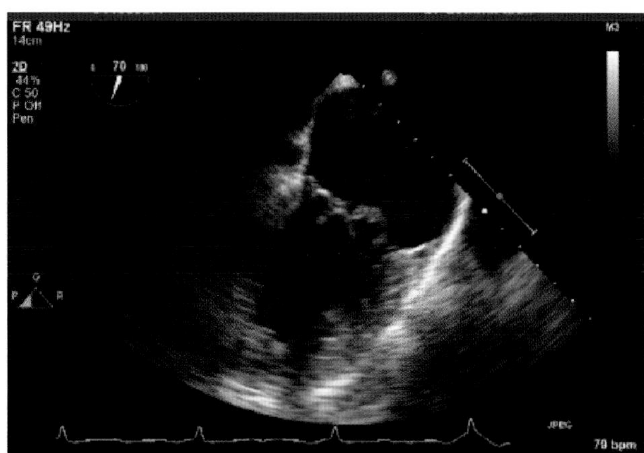

Figure 104.3. Prebypass ME 4CH commissural.

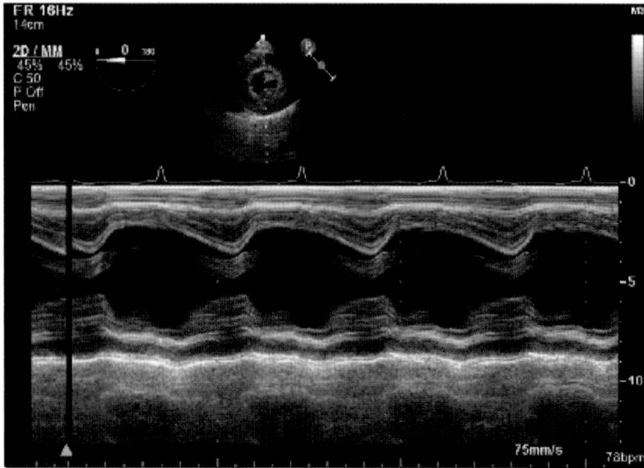

Figure 104.4. Prebypass TG SAX mid-papillary M-mode.

QUESTION 104.1. What Carpentier class best describes the MR in this patient?

A. Type I
B. Type II
C. Type IIIa
D. Type IIIb

QUESTION 104.2. What is the etiology of this patient's MV regurgitation?

A. Ischemic MR
B. Endocarditis with perforation of the anterior leaflet
C. Myxomatous degeneration with posterior MV prolapse
D. Rheumatic mitral insufficiency

The surgeon performs a complicated repair, including a quadrangular resection and sliding plasty of the posterior leaflet, insertion of an artificial Gortex neochord to repair a redundant anterior leaflet, and the insertion of an annuloplasty ring. The repair is completed within 127 minutes; an intraoperative saline injection leak test shows a competent repair, and the patient is weaned off of CPB with inotropic support. A postbypass echocardiographic examination is performed.

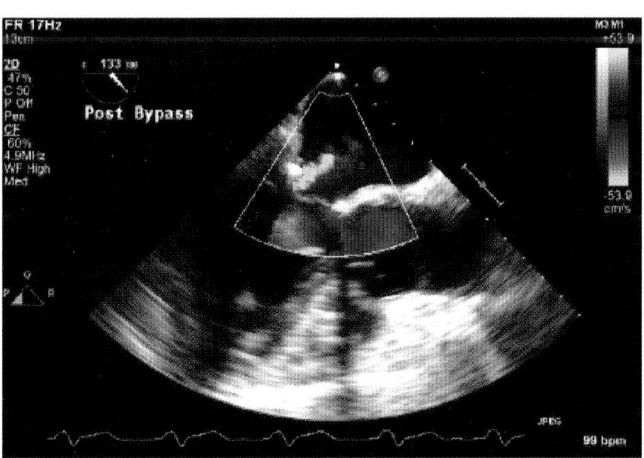

Figure 104.6. Postbypass ME LAX with CFD.

QUESTION 104.3. If chordal or papillary muscle damage was suspected from the repair, which of the following views provides the best imaging of the chordae tendinae?

A. ME 4CH view
B. ME LAX
C. TG two-chamber view
D. TG basal short-axis view

Evaluation of the chordae and papillary muscles is normal but as shown in the following postrepair images, there is persistent MR (see Figs. 104.5 to 104.7 and Videos 104.5 to 104.9).

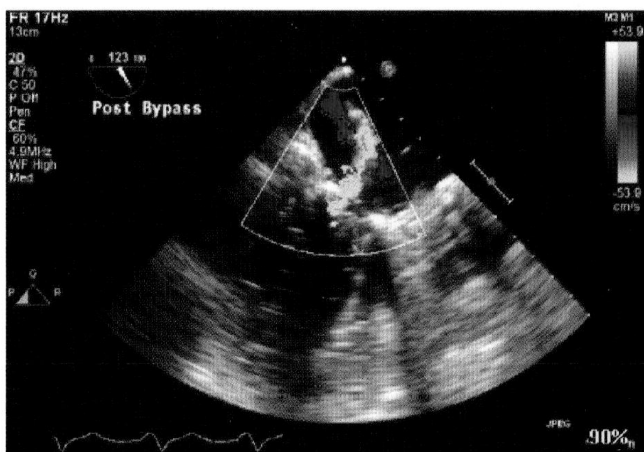

Figure 104.5. Postbypass ME LAX.

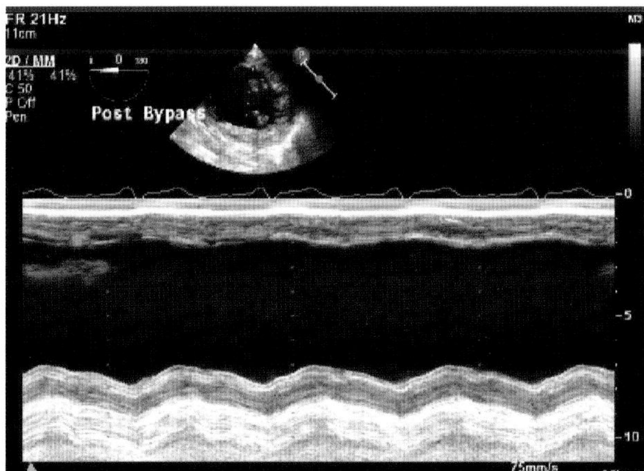

Figure 104.7. Postbypass TG SAX mid-papillary M-Mode.

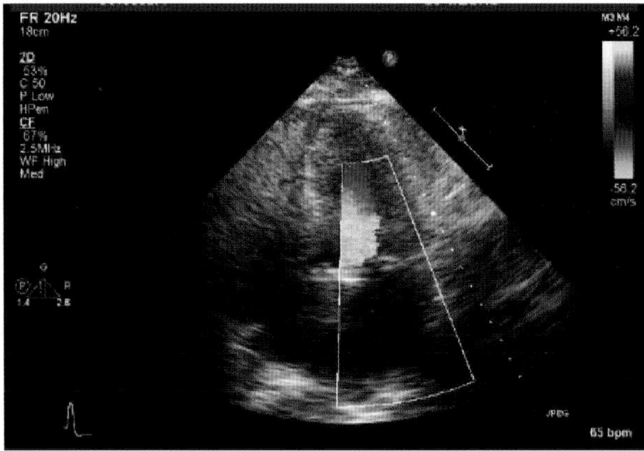

Figure 104.8. Postoperative transthoracic image with color Doppler.

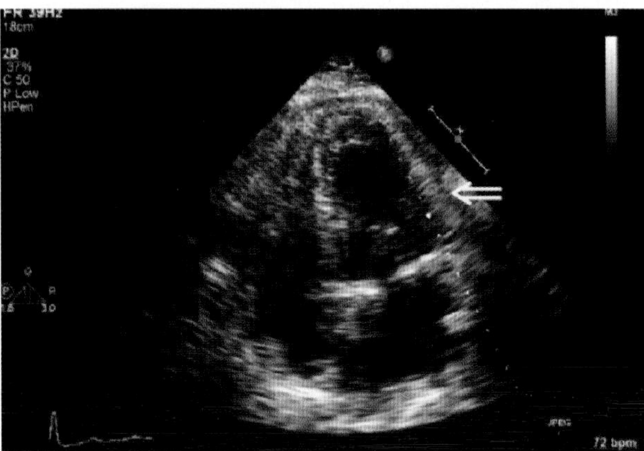

Figure 104.9. Postoperative transthoracic image.

QUESTION 104.4. The above mitral regurgitant jet vena contracta is measured to be 0.22 cm. Based on the provided images and data what recommendation would you offer to the surgeon?

A. Return to CPB for repair revision; this degree of MR indicates a failed repair
B. Give protamine; this amount of MR is acceptable
C. Instruct the perfusionist to give a volume bolus; this patient is experiencing SAM
D. Return to CPB for coronary revascularization of the circumflex artery

QUESTION 104.5. What would you inform the surgeon as to the responsible mechanism for the MR?

A. Ischemic MR
B. Posterior mitral leaflet prolapse
C. SAM of the anterior MV leaflet
D. Anterior leaflet perforation

QUESTION 104.6. MR due to ischemia is best described by what mechanism(s)?

A. Increased tethering of the mitral leaflets
B. Decreased ventricular ejection force
C. Both
D. Neither

The patient was continued on inotropic support without further intervention and transferred to the cardiothoracic ICU. On postoperative day 2, a transthoracic echo was performed (see Figs. 104.8 and 104.9, and Videos 104.10 and 104.11).

QUESTION 104.7. What view is seen in the above images?

A. Apical four-chamber view
B. Apical two-chamber view
C. Parasternal LAX
D. Subcostal view

QUESTION 104.8. Which wall is indicated by the arrow?

A. Lateral wall

B. Anterior wall

C. Septal wall

D. Inferior wall

QUESTION 104.9. What degree of MR is demonstrated by CFD in Figure 104.8?

A. None

B. Mild

C. Moderate

D. Severe

ANSWERS AND DISCUSSION

QUESTION 104.1: The correct answer is B: Type II.

Carpentier describes four classes of MR. Type I is due to annular dilation with failure of coaptation resulting in a central regurgitant jet. Type II is due to excessive motion of one or both of the leaflets overriding the plane of the annulus usually causing an eccentric jet away from the diseased leaflet. Type IIIa is due to restriction of the leaflets during both systole and diastole such as seen in rheumatic heart disease. Type IIIb is due to restriction of the leaflets during systole, commonly the result of ischemic cardiomyopathy.[1] From Figures 104.1 to 104.3 and Videos 104.1 to 104.3, one can see that the posterior leaflet is prolapsing above the annular plane causing an eccentric anteriorly directed jet, consistent with Carpentier classification II.

QUESTION 104.2: The correct answer is C: Myxomatous valvular disease.

Upon examination of Figures 104.1 to 104.3 and Videos 104.1 to 104.3, one can see the leaflets are thickened and redundant with some annular dilation. This is consistent with myxomatous degeneration of the MV.[2] Ischemic MR is unlikely given the MR jet is not central and no wall motion abnormality is seen in the provided images (Fig. 104.4 and Video 104.4). Endocarditis is unlikely due to the clinical presentation and no vegetations are visualized. Rheumatic disease of the MV is also unlikely as the leaflets lack the characteristic calcification and restriction associated with this disease.

QUESTION 104.3: The correct answer is C: TG two-chamber view.

The papillary muscles and chordal apparatus are commonly best imaged in the TG two-chamber view (Fig. 104.10 and Video 104.9). In this view, the cords and papillary muscles lie perpendicular to the ultrasound beam creating strong specular reflections and thereby superior image quality. This view is obtained by inserting the probe into the stomach and anteroflexing the probe to obtain the TG SAX) mid-papillary. Adjusting the multiplane transducer array to between 80 and 100 degrees images the TG two-chamber view. Other views, such as the ME LAX, can provide additional information and be useful in further evaluating the subvalvular apparatus and its attachment to the leaflets.

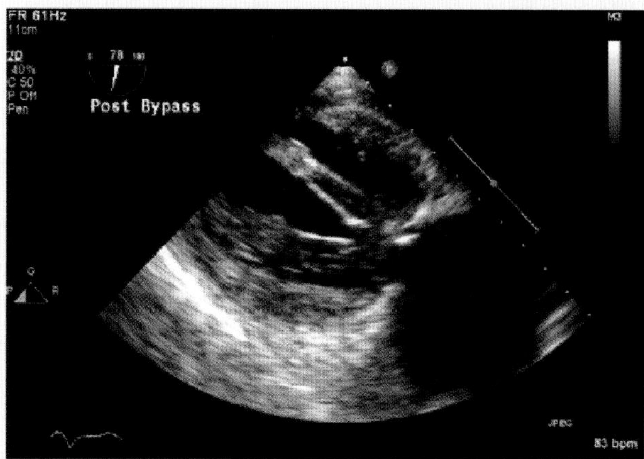

Figure 104.10. TG two-chamber view demonstrating the papillary muscles, chords and their attachments to the MV.

QUESTION 104.4: The correct answer is B: Give protamine; this is an acceptable amount of MR.

Despite conflicting reports in the literature, most cardiac centers consider mild MR after MV repair to be a successful intervention. There is evidence to suggest that there is no increase in long-term mortality in patients with persistent mild MR after repair.[3] In addition, any benefit of another repair must be weighed against the potential harm that a second bypass run could have on the heart and that a second attempt at repair may make the regurgitation worse, necessitating additional interventions such as MV replacement and increased bypass time. Answer C is incorrect. SAM of the anterior mitral leaflet is not visualized. Answer D, grafting of the circumflex artery is an important consideration following MV repair when there is high suspicion that the circumflex artery was ligated with a suture from the annuloplasty ring insertion. This complication is of most concern in patients with left or codominant coronary circulations as the circumflex artery lies significantly closer to the annulus in this group.[4] It usually presents as new onset lateral wall ischemia. This patient does have new RWMA, but the ischemia is inferior not lateral. This patient has a RCA dominant circulation that suggests the inferior wall ischemia is more likely due to problem with the RCA rather than occlusion of the circumflex.

QUESTION 104.5: The correct answer is A: Ischemic MR.

The echocardiographic exam supports the diagnosis of acute ischemic MR. This diagnosis is supported by the findings of a central MR jet in conjunction with new onset dilation of the LV and inferior wall motion abnormalities. In this patient without coronary artery disease, the possible etiologies for the regional wall abnormalities include poor myocardial protection with a long CPB run and/or intracoronary air emboli. Intracardiac air bubbles can be seen in Figure 104.5 and Video 104.5 and these emboli most commonly migrate (i.e., float) into the RCA as it its orifice is the most anterior of the coronary vessels. Unlike CABG procedures, this valve procedure required the surgeon to open the heart to access the MV. Access to the MV is done either through the RA and interatrial septum or the LA directly. Despite a thorough echocardiographic examination for intracardiac air collections and deairing maneuvers prior to discontinuation of CPB, air emboli are a frequent problem during intracardiac surgical procedures. One way to limit the impact of this complication is to continuously flood the field with carbon dioxide gas, as CO_2 emboli are absorbed much more quickly in the circulation. Another technique is to maintain the patient on 100% oxygen during ventilation in an attempt to denitrogenate the patient that facilitates the absorption of air emboli. Once the patient is weaned from bypass, increasing the blood pressure and thus the coronary artery driving pressure facilitates clearing gas embolic occlusions in the coronary circulation. Answer B, posterior mitral leaflet prolapse, is incorrect. There are no abnormalities in the valve leaflets that would lead to further intervention. There is no prolapse of the posterior leaflet and the anterior leaflet is coapting with the posterior leaflet without any evidence of SAM obstruction of the LVOT; therefore answer C is also incorrect (Fig. 104.6 and Videos 104.5 and 104.6). Answer D, anterior leaflet perforation, is not visualized in the images.

QUESTION 104.6: The correct answer is C: Both increased tethering and decreased ventricular contractile force.

Ischemic MR is a dynamic process. Tethering of the mitral leaflets preventing complete closure of the valve is the unifying principle. The exact mechanism of ischemic MR is debatable. Some believe direct stiffening of the papillary muscles is responsible, whereas others feel ventricular wall ischemia with dilation of the ventricle pulling the entire papillary muscle away from the valve is the cause. Regardless, the endpoint is the same, the leaflets become tethered and complete closure is not attained. As the systolic ventricular function decreases, so does the closing force on the mitral leaflets, further exacerbating the inability of the valve to close, and increasing the severity of the MR.[5]

QUESTION 104.7: The correct answer is A: Apical four-chamber view.

Transthoracic imaging is performed from four main anatomical locations; these are the parasternal, apical, subcostal, and suprasternal areas. The apical area images are comparable to the ME images in that the four cardiac chambers are visualized allowing the echocardiographer to assess overall biventricular function and the function of the mitral and TV(see Fig. 104.11). The probe is placed at the point of maximal impulse on the chest wall with the patient in a left lateral decubitus position.

QUESTION 104.8: The correct answer is A: Lateral wall.

Similar to the ME 4CH view, the standard image orientation is right to left, resulting in the lateral wall appearing on the right side of the screen opposite the RV and septal wall. The anterior and inferior walls are not in plane and are best imaged in the apical two-chamber view.

QUESTION 104.9: The correct answer is A: None.

There is no CFD signal seen retrograde into the LA. The CFD signal that is seen in Figure 104.8 is due to flow acceleration toward the AV in the LVOT captured in this systolic frame. Video 104.10 also does not reveal a regurgitant jet with CFD. These findings support the diagnosis of acute intraoperative ischemic MR that resolved by postoperative day 2.

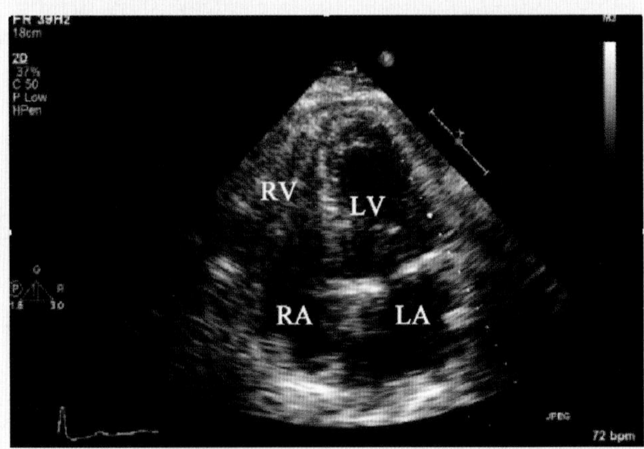

Figure 104.11. TTE apical four-chamber view labeled.

TAKE-HOME LESSON:

Examination of the MV leaflets, subvalvular apparatus, as well as ventricular function is essential to assess the etiology of MR.

REFERENCES

1. Lambert AS. Mitral regurgitation. In: Perrino AC, Reeves ST, eds. *Practical Approach to Transesophageal Echocardiography*. Philadelphia: Lippincott Williams & Wilkins; 2008:171–186.
2. Iglesias I. Intraoperative TEE assessment during mitral valve repair for degenerative and ischemic mitral valve regurgitation. *Semin Cardiothorac Vasc Anesth*. 2007;11:301–305.
3. Fix J, Isada L, Cosgrove D, et al. Do patients with less than "echo-perfect" results from mitral valve repair by intraoperative echocardiography have a different outcome? *Circulation*. 1993;88:II.39–II.48.
4. Virmani R, Chun PK, Parker J, et al. Suture obliteration of the circumflex coronary artery in three patients undergoing mitral valve operation. Role of left dominant coronary artery. *J Thorac Cardiovasc Surg*. 1982;84:773–778.
5. Levine RA, Schwammenthal E. Ischemic mitral regurgitation on the threshold of a solution from paradoxes to unifying concepts. *Circulation*. 2005;112:745–758.

CONTENTS

CONTENTS

AORTA

LEFT VENTRICLE

MITRAL VALVE REGURGITATION

MITRAL VALVE STENOSIS

AORTIC VALVE REGURGITATION

CATHETERS

MASSES

ARTIFACTS

IMAGE OPTIMIZATION

COMPLICATIONS

Index

Page numbers followed by *f* indicate figures

M

S

T